Smooth Muscle Excitation

Smooth Muscle Excitation

edited by

T. B. BOLTON

Department of Pharmacology and Clinical Pharmacology
St George's Hospital Medical School
London, UK

T. TOMITA

Department of Physiology
School of Health Sciences
Fujita Health University
Toyoake, Aichi, Japan

ACADEMIC PRESS

Harcourt Brace & Company, Publishers
London   San Diego   New York   Boston
Sydney   Tokyo   Toronto

ACADEMIC PRESS LIMITED
24/28 Oval Road
LONDON NW1 7DX

United States Edition published by
ACADEMIC PRESS INC.
San Diego CA 92101

A CIP record for this book is available from the British Library

ISBN 0–12–112360–X

This book is printed on acid-free paper

Every effort has been made to check the concentrations in this book.
However, as it is possible that errors may have been missed, the reader is
advised to consult other literature

Typeset by Mackreth Media Services, Hemel Hempstead
Printed and bound in Great Britain by Hartnolls Ltd, Bodmin, Cornwall

Contents

Contributors

P. I. Aaronson *Department of Pharmacology, United Medical & Dental Schools of Guy's & St Thomas's Hospitals, London SE1 7EH, UK*

I. Abe *Second Department of Internal Medicine, Faculty of Medicine, Kyushu University, Maidashi 3-1-1, Higashi-ku, Fukuoka 812, Japan*

C. Austin *Department of Physiology, University of Liverpool, Crown Street, PO Box 147, Liverpool, L69 3BX, UK*

D. J. Beech *Department of Pharmacology, University of Leeds, Leeds, LS2 9JT, UK*

T. B. Bolton *Department of Pharmacology & Clinical Pharmacology, St George's Hospital Medical School, Cranmer Terrace, London SW17 0RE, UK*

A. D. Bonev *Department of Pharmacology, University of Vermont, 55A South Park Drive, Colchester, Vermont, VT 05405, USA*

A. F. Brading *Department of Pharmacology, University of Oxford, Mansfield Road, Oxford, OX1 3QT, UK*

N. Bramich *Department of Pharmacology, University of Oxford, Mansfield Road, Oxford, OX1 3QT, UK*

J. E. Brayden *Department of Pharmacology, University of Vermont, 55A South Park Drive, Colchester, Vermont, VT 05405, USA*

C. van Breemen *Department of Pharmacology & Therapeutics, Faculty of Medicine, University of British Columbia, 2176 Health Sciences Mall, Vancouver, BC V6T 1Z3, Canada*

T. V. Burdyga *AV Palladine Institute of Biochemistry, 9 Leontovich Street, Kiev 30, Ukraine*

R. A. R. Bywater *Department of Physiology, Monash University, Clayton, Victoria 3168, Australia*

R. Casteels *Laboratorium voor Fysiologie, KUL Campus Gasthuisberg, B-3000 Leuven, Belgium*

H. A. Coleman *Department of Physiology, Monash University, Clayton, Victoria 3168, Australia*

H. M. Cousins *Department of Zoology, University of Melbourne, Parkville, Victoria 3052, Australia*

M. J. Crowe *Faculty of Medicine and Health Services, University of Newcastle, University Drive, Callaghan, Newcastle, NSW 2308, Australia*

S. Das   *Department of Biomedical Sciences and Intestinal Disease Research Programme, McMaster University, Hamilton, Ontario L8N 3Z5, Canada*

J. Eggermont   *Laboratorium voor Fysiologie, KUL Campus Gasthuisberg, B-3000 Leuven, Belgium*

L. Farraway   *Department of Biomedical Sciences and Intestinal Disease Research Programme, McMaster University, Hamilton, Ontario L8N 3ZS, Canada*

B. K. Fleischmann   *Department of Animal Biology, University of Pennsylvania, 3800 Spruce Street, Philadelphia, PA 19104-6046, USA*

K. Fujii   *Second Department of Internal Medicine, Faculty of Medicine, Kyushu University, Maidashi 3-1-1, Higashi-ku, Fukuoka 812, Japan*

M. Fujishima   *Second Department of Internal Medicine, Faculty of Medicine, Kyushu University, Maidashi 3-1-1, Higashi-ku, Fukuoka 812, Japan*

K. Furukawa   *Department of Physiology, Monash University, Clayton, Victoria 3168, Australia*

V. Ya. Ganitkevich   *Department of Physiology, University of Cologne, Robert Koch Str. 39, Köln 41, D-50931, Germany*

C. J. Garland   *Department of Pharmacology, University of Bristol, University Walk, Bristol, BS8 1TD, UK*

G. Grégoire   *Institut de Pharmacologie Moléculaire et Cellulaire, CNRS UPR 411, 660 route des Lucioles, 06560 Valbonne, France*

H. Hashitani   *Department of Physiology, Medical School, Nagoya City University, Mizuho-ku, Nagoya 467, Japan*

D. F. van Helden   *Faculty of Medicine & Health Sciences, University of Newcastle, University Drive, Callaghan, Newcastle, NSW 2308, Australia*

S. Henmi   *Department of Chemical Pharmacology, Faculty of Pharmaceutical Sciences, Nagoya City University, 3-1 Tanabedori, Mizuho-ku, Nagoya 467, Japan*

G. D. S. Hirst   *Department of Zoology, University of Melbourne, Parkville, Victoria 3052, Australia*

M. E. Holman   *Department of Physiology, Monash University, Clayton, Victoria 3168, Australia*

B. Horowitz   *Department of Physiology, University of Nevada School of Medicine, Reno, NV 89557, USA*

J. D. Huizinga   *Intestine Diseases Research Unit and Department of Biomedical Sciences, McMaster University, Hamilton, Ontario L8N 3Z5, Canada*

M. Iino   *Department of Pharmacology, Faculty of Medicine, University of Tokyo , Bunkyo-ku, Tokyo 113, Japan*

Y. Imaizumi   *Department of Chemical Pharmacology, Faculty of Pharmaceutical Sciences, Nagoya City University, 3-1 Tanabedori, Mizuho-ku, Nagoya 467, Japan*

R. Inoue   *Department of Pharmacology, Faculty of Medicine, Kyushu*

University, Fukuoka 812, Japan

S. Ito Laboratory of Pharmacology, Graduate School of Veterinary Medicine, Hokkaido University, North 18, West 9, Sapporo 060, Japan

Y. Ito Department of Pharmacology, Faculty of Medicine, Kyushu University, Fukuoka 812, Japan

T. Itoh Department of Pharmacology, Medical School, Nagoya City University, Mizuho-ku, Nagoya 467, Japan

M. Kamouchi Departments of Internal Medicine and Pharmacology, Faculty of Medicine, Kyushu University, Fukuoka 812-82, Japan

H. Karaki Department of Veterinary Pharmacology, Graduate School of Agriculture and Life Sciences, University of Tokyo, Bunkyo-ku, Tokyo 113, Japan

S. Kitajima Department of Veterinary Pharmacology, Graduate School of Agriculture and Life Sciences, University of Tokyo, Bunkyo-ku, Tokyo 113, Japan

K. Kitamura, Department of Dental Pharmacology, Fukuoka Dental College, 2-15-1 Tamura, , Sawara -ku , Fukuoka 814-01, Japan

U. Klöckner, Department of Physiology, University of Cologne, Robert Koch Str. 39, Köln 41, D-50931, Germany

S. Komori Laboratory of Pharmacology, Department of Veterinary Science, Faculty of Agriculture, Gifu University, 1-1 Yanagido, Gifu 501-11, Japan

M. I. Kotlikoff Department of Animal Biology, School of Veterinary Medicine, University of Pennsylvania, 3800 Spruce Street, Philadelphia, PA 19104-6046, USA

H. Kuriyama Departments of Internal Medicine and Pharmacology, Faculty of Medicine, Kyushu University, Fukuoka 812-82, Japan

R. J. Lang Department of Physiology, Monash University, Clayton, Victoria 3168, Australia

J. F. C. Lee Department of Biomedical Sciences and Intestinal Disease Research Programme, McMaster University, Hamilton, Ontario L8N 3Z5, Canada

L. Li Department of Pharmacology and Therapeutics, Faculty of Medicine, The University of British Columbia, 2176 Health Sciences Mall, Vancouver, BC V6T 1Z3, Canada

L. W. C. Liu Department of Biomedical Sciences and Intestinal Disease Research Programme, McMaster University, Hamilton, Ontario L8N 3Z5, Canada

G. Loirand Institut de Pharmacologie Moléculaire et Cellulaire, CNRS UPR 411, 660 route des Lucioles, 06560 Valbonne, France

J. Lorenz Department of Molecular & Cellular Physiology, University of Cincinnati, College of Medicine, 231 Bethesda Avenue, Cincinnati, OH 45267-0576, USA

D. J. K. Lyster Department of Physiology, Monash University, Clayton,

Victoria 3168, Australia

N. Macrez-Leprêtre   *Laboratoire de Physiologie Cellulaire et Pharmacologie Moléculaire, UFR Sciences Pharmaceutiques, 146 rue Léo Saignat, Université de Bordeaux II, 33076 Bordeaux, France*

J. Malysz   *Department of Biomedical Sciences and Intestinal Disease Research Programme, McMaster University, Hamilton, Ontario L8N 3Z5, Canada*

J. G. McCarron   *Department of Pharmacology, University of Vermont, 55A South Park Drive, Colchester, Vermont, VT 05405, USA*

D. McHugh   *Department of Pharmacology, University of Leeds, Leeds, LS2 9JT, UK*

C. Mironneau   *Laboratoire de Physiologie Cellulaire et Pharmacologie Moléculaire, UFR Sciences Pharmaceutiques, 146 rue Léo Saignat, Université de Bordeaux II, 33076 Bordeaux, France*

J. Mironneau   *Laboratoire de Physiologie Cellulaire et Pharmacologie Moléculaire, UFR Sciences Pharmaceutiques, 146 rue Léo Saignat, Université de Bordeaux II, 33076 Bordeaux Cedex, France*

L. Missiaen   *Laboratorium voor Fysiologie, KUL Campus Gasthuisberg, B-3000 Leuven, Belgium*

H. Miyoshi   *Department of Nutrition, School of Medicine, University of Tokushima, Kuramoto-cho, Tokushima 770, Japan*

J. Mostwin   *Department of Pharmacology, University of Oxford, Mansfield Road, Oxford, OX1 3QT, UK*

K. Muraki   *Department of Chemical Pharmacology, Faculty of Pharmaceutical Sciences, Nagoya City University, 3-1 Tanabedori, Mizuho-ku, Nagoya 467, Japan*

N. Nagano   *Department of Chemical Pharmacology, Faculty of Pharmaceutical Sciences, Nagoya City University, 3-1 Tanabedori, Mizuho-ku, Nagoya 467, Japan*

Y. Nakaya   *Department of Nutrition, School of Medicine, University of Tokushima, Kuramoto-cho, Tokushima 770, Japan*

S. Nakayama   *Department of Physiology, School of Medicine, Nagoya University, 65 Tsuruma-cho, Showa-ku, Nagoya 466, Japan*

Y. Nakazato   *Laboratory of Pharmacology, Graduate School of Veterinary Medicine, Hokkaido University, North 18, West 9, Sapporo 060, Japan*

M. T. Nelson   *Department of Pharmacology, University of Vermont, 55A South Park Drive, Colchester, Vermont, VT 05405, USA*

R. Ogata   *Departments of Internal Medicine and Pharmacology, Faculty of Medicine, Kyushu University, Fukuoka 812-82, Japan*

H. Ohashi   *Laboratory of Pharmacology, Department of Veterinary Science, Faculty of Agriculture, Gifu University, 1-1 Yanagido, Gifu 501-11, Japan*

T. Ohkubo   *Department of Dental Pharmacology, Fukuoka Dental College, 2-15-1 Tamura, Sawara-ku, Fukuoka 814-01, Japan*

T. Ohta *Laboratory of Pharmacology, Graduate School of Veterinary Medicine, Hokkaido University, North 18, West 9, Sapporo 060, Japan*

Y. Ohya *Second Department of Internal Medicine, Faculty of Medicine, Kyushu University, Maidashi 3-1-1, Higashi-ku, Fukuoka 812, Japan*

T. Osa *Department of Physiology, School of Medicine, Yamaguchi University, Ube 755, Japan*

H. Ozaki *Department of Veterinary Pharmacology, Graduate School of Agriculture and Life Sciences, University of Tokyo, Bunkyo-ku, Tokyo 113, Japan*

P. Pacaud *Institut de Pharmacologie Moléculaire et Cellulaire, CNRS UPR 411, 660 route des Lucioles, 06560 Valbonne, France*

Y-W. Pang *Department of Physiology, School of Medicine, Nagoya University, 65 Tsuruma-cho, Showa-ku, Nagoya 466, Japan*

H. C. Parkington *Department of Physiology, Monash University, Clayton , Victoria 3168, Australia*

J. B. Parys *Laboratorium voor Fysiologie, KUL Campus Gasthuisberg, B-3000 Leuven, Belgium*

R. J. Paul *Department of Molecular & Cellular Physiology, University of Cincinnati, College of Medicine, 231 Bethesda Avenue, Cincinnati OH 45267-0576, USA*

F. Plane *Department of Pharmacology, University of Bristol, University Walk, Bristol, BS8 1TD, UK*

J. M. Quayle *Department of Cell Physiology & Pharmacology, University of Leicester, School of Medicine, Medical Sciences Building, University Road, P.O. Box 138, Leicester, LE1 9HN, UK*

L. Raeymaekers *Laboratorium voor Fysiologie, KUL Campus Gasthuisberg, B-3000 Leuven, Belgium*

C. A. Rattray-Wood *Department of Physiology, Monash University, Clayton, Victoria 3168, Australia*

K. M. Sanders *Department of Physiology & Cell Biology, University of Nevada School of Medicine, Reno, NV 89557, USA*

M. Shibata *Department of Dental Pharmacology, Fukuoka Dental College, 2-15-1 Tamura, Sawara-ku, Fukuoka 814-01, Japan*

I. Sienaert *Laboratorium voor Fysiologie, KUL Campus Gasthuisberg, B-3000 Leuven, Belgium*

H. de Smedt *Laboratorium voor Fysiologie, KUL Campus Gasthuisberg, B-3000 Leuven, Belgium*

S. V. Smirnov *Department of Pharmacology, United Medical & Dental Schools of Guy's and St Thomas's Hospitals, London SE1 7EH, UK*

L. M. Smith *Department of Physiology, School of Medicine, Nagoya University, 65 Tsuruma-cho, Showa-ku, Nagoya 466, Japan*

H. Suzuki *Department of Physiology, Medical School, Nagoya City University, Mizuho-ku, Nagoya 467, Japan*

M. J. Taggart   *Department of Physiology, University of Liverpool, Crown Street, PO Box 147, Liverpool L69 3BX, UK*

A. Takai   *Department of Physiology, School of Medicine, Nagoya University, 65 Tsurumai-cho, Showa-ku, Nagoya 466, Japan*

G. S. Taylor   *Department of Physiology, Monash University, Clayton, Victoria 3168, Australia*

N. Teramoto   *Department of Pharmacology, University of Oxford, Mansfield Road, Oxford, OX1 3QT, UK*

T. Tomita   *Department of Physiology, School of Health Sciences, Fujita Health University, Toyoake, Aichi 470-11, Japan*

K. Tsuruda   *Department of Dental Pharmacology, Fukuoka Dental College, 2-15-1 Tamura, Sawara-ku, Fukuoka 814-01, Japan*

K. Tsutai   *Department of Physiology, School of Medicine, Sapporo Medical University, Sapporo 060, Japan*

H. Verboomen   *Laboratorium voor Fysiologie, KUL Campus Gasthuisberg, B-3000 Leuven, Belgium*

Y. Waniishi   *Department of Pharmacology, Faculty of Medicine, Kyushu University, Fukuoka 812, Japan*

S. M. Ward   *Department of Physiology and Cell Biology, University of Nevada School of Medicine, Reno, NV 89557, USA*

M. Watanabe   *Department of Chemical Pharmacology, Faculty of Pharmaceutical Sciences, Nagoya City University, 3-1 Tanabedori, Mizuho-ku, Nagoya 467, Japan*

Y. Watanabe   *Department of Pharmacology, Medical School, Nagoya City University, Mizuho-ku, Nagoya 467, Japan*

M. J. Watson   *Department of Physiology, Monash University, Clayton, Victoria 3168, Australia*

P-Y. von der Weid   *Faculty of Medicine and Health Sciences, University of Newcastle, University Drive, Callaghan, Newcastle, NSW 2308, Australia*

S. Wray   *Department of Physiology, University of Liverpool, Crown Street, P.O. Box 147, Liverpool L69 3BX, UK*

F. Wuytack   *Laboratorium voor Fysiologie, KUL Campus Gasthuisberg, B-3000 Leuven, Belgium*

H. Yabu   *Department of Physiology, School of Medicine, Sapporo Medical University, Sapporo 060, Japan*

Y. Yamamoto   *Department of Physiology, Medical School, Nagoya City University, Mizuho-ku, Nagoya 467, Japan*

M. Yoshino   *Department of Biology, Tokyo Gakugei University, Koganei 184, Tokyo, Japan*

H-L. Zhang   *Department of Pharmacology and Clinical Pharmacology, St George's Hospital Medical School, Cranmer Terrace, London SW17 0RE, UK*

A. V. Zholos   *Department of Pharmacology and Clinical Pharmacology, St George's Hospital Medical School, Cranmer Terrace, London SW17 0RE, UK*

Preface

Until recently the progress of electrophysiological research on smooth muscle has lagged far behind that of other excitable cells mainly because of the small fibre diameter and complex inter-fibre or inter-bundle interactions. The introduction of the patch-clamp method in the early 1980s gave a major breakthrough in the area of smooth muscle research which is now comparable to or even more active than those of nerve and cardiac muscle. Another field of rapid advances is the analysis of intracellular calcium and pH by the introduction of calcium- or pH-sensitive fluorescent dyes such as fura-2 and BCECF, respectively. With these methods the properties of calcium stores and control mechanisms of calcium release are being analysed in great detail. Now, we are facing difficulties in dealing with a flood of new information in these areas which appears in nearly every issue of physiological journals. Critical review articles are certainly needed to cope with this problem.

When the second joint meeting between the Physiological Societies of Japan and of Great Britain and Eire was held at Nagoya University in Japan on April 1st and 2nd, 1995, we organized a symposium on smooth muscle on an international scale, as one of the 12 selected subjects. This was followed by an extra meeting on smooth muscle at Izu near Mount Fuji on the 4th April to make the gathering more fruitful. We organizers considered that this was a good opportunity to ask the major participants at these meetings to write a review article on their own field. Nearly everybody we asked has accepted our idea and contributed to this book, for which we are very grateful. The title of the book is 'Smooth Muscle Excitation' but the articles actually cover rather wide topics such as ionic channels, receptor transduction, intracellular calcium release, rhythmic activity, neuromuscular transmission and endothelial interaction. We hope this is a useful book to obtain up-to-date information on the many active fields of smooth muscle research.

Looking to the future we should consider what outstanding problems need to be tackled. While some understanding has been gained of the general properties of smooth muscles, a deep understanding of their idiosyncrasies is far from being achieved; smooth muscles are each exquisitely adapted to perform particular functions. At present, the major thrusts of research are largely analytical and at some stage a more integrated understanding of tissue function will need to be reached. This applies to electrophysiology and to intracellular events. There are many unsolved problems, such as the origin and mechanism of slow electrical changes, as well as their interaction with as yet unsuspected intracellular events. When these and other problems are solved we will be some way towards a fuller understanding of how each smooth muscle contributes uniquely to organ function and so to the integrated function of the whole body.

T. Tomita   T. B. Bolton
Nagoya, Japan   London, UK

ACKNOWLEDGEMENT

We are grateful for generous financial support from Chugai Pharmaceutical Company and from The Wellcome Trust without which the Smooth Muscle Symposium in Nagoya/Izu and the publication of this book would not have been possible.

Introduction

M. E. HOLMAN

Department of Physiology, Monash University, Clayton, Victoria, Australia

In his introduction to the 1992 Symposium dedicated to our colleague Hirosi Kuriyama, Tadao Tomita wrote '*There is a mood of optimism today in biology stemming largely from insights rapidly being gained into biophysics, biochemistry, and molecular biology. Stubborn questions are beginning to yield to biochemical probing . . . This tendency is also true in the field of smooth muscle electrophysiology,*' (Tomita, 1992). Such a mood dominated the Symposium on Smooth Muscle held this year in honour of Tadao that began in Nagoya, as part of the joint meeting of the Physiological Societies of Great Britain, Japan and Eire and concluded in Ito City on the Izu Peninsula. The main theme of this Symposium is the regulation of intracellular calcium ion concentration, $[Ca^{2+}]_i$. It is appropriate that many of the presentations are concerned with electrophysiology since this approach to our understanding of smooth muscle function has been central to Tadao Tomita's work. Much of the present revolution in the interest of medical research in this field can be traced back to Edith Bülbring's laboratory in Oxford where Tadao worked during the 1960s. Those of us who used 'sharp' intracellular electrodes in order to investigate the physiology/pharmacology of smooth muscle at that time continue to be astonished and very pleased by the dramatic increase in the frequency of publication of papers on smooth muscle during the last few years. Many of these concern studies on the ionic membrane currents recorded with 'patch' electrodes from single smooth muscle cells that have been isolated from a variety of sources, both vascular and visceral. The suitability of smooth muscle cells for this technique, together with the evolution of fluorescent dyes that make possible the image analysis of localized concentrations of Ca^{2+}, have lead to the burgeoning of studies on smooth muscle physiology that continues today.

Forty years ago there seemed to be many problems in the use of sharp microelectrodes to record membrane potential of smooth muscles. It is interesting to speculate now as to why it was felt, initially, to be so difficult to successfully impale these cells. One partial explanation may be that we were influenced by our colleagues working on striated muscles who emphasized the need to use low resistance electrodes – mainly because of the lack of sophistication of the electronic equipment that was available to us at that time. In general, we were restricted to recording spontaneous activity with a 'stationary spot' on the cathode ray oscilloscope and moving film to record its deflections on the y axis. A huge amount of information was lost despite the long lengths of recording film that dangled down our stairwells while they were drying out. Responses to, for example, nerve stimulation could be recorded as a result of a 'triggered' single sweep on a fast time base by a cathode ray oscillograph, but in that mode spontaneous background activity (e.g. spontaneous miniature junction potentials) was lost. The introduction of computers for data acquisition and analysis has been a huge step forward. In those early days we were uncertain as to how to interpret our data. In other excitable cells action potentials were all-or-none events of similar magnitude. In well-stretched preparations of, for example, guinea-pig taenia coli (caeci), action potentials might vary from fast 'spikes' of 60 mV or more showing a reversal of membrane potential at their peak (overshoot) to small, apparently attenuated, spike-like potentials of 20 mV or less in amplitude. It is still not entirely clear today why these patterns of activity occur. But it is now certain that these records were not an artefact of our recording methods.

One of the first problems that confronted us was the ionic basis of the action potential. During the early 1960s it became apparent that there were many similarities between the action potentials of smooth muscle and crustacean skeletal muscle which had been studied by Fatt & Ginsborg (1955) in London and by Hagiwara and his school in Los Angeles (Hagiwara & Naka, 1964). The definitive proposal that the inward current causing the upstroke of the action potential was carried by Ca^{2+} ions was published in a paper by Brading et al. (1969). This was among the earliest of the many decisive contributions that Tadao has made to smooth muscle research.

The diversity of voltage-dependent Ca^{2+} channels in smooth muscle is now generally acknowledged. Dihydropyridine-sensitive Ca^{2+} channels of the L-type appear to predominate in visceral smooth muscle whereas various dihydropyridine-insensitive Ca channels may also occur in some vascular smooth muscles. Current studies are beginning to clarify the molecular structure of the smooth muscle L channel but little is known as yet about the molecular basis of its regulation. This is one of the questions that are addressed by this Symposium. L-channel activity is generally depressed by an increase in $[Ca]_i$ which also activates the ubiquitous voltage-dependent 'big' K^+ channels (BK). These large conductance channels (conductance of about 200 ps at 0 mV for symmetrical concentrations of high K^+) are expressed by most smooth muscles and probably contribute to the repolarization of action potentials of the spike form. It is now clear that smooth muscles can express a variety of other K^+ channels that can be distinguished according to their Ca^{2+}-sensitivity and/or voltage-sensitivity as well as their pharmacology. These include Ca^{2+}-sensitive SK channels with a smaller conductance that are blocked by apamin and may be important in determining the afterhyperpolarization associated with the action potentials of some smooth muscles. A delayed rectifier channel, K_V, is somewhat similar to those of other excitable cells and inactivates very slowly during maintained depolarization. In contrast, a transient K^+ current that is blocked by 4 aminopyridine, occurs when K_A channels are opened. Some smooth muscles also demonstrate inward rectification owing to the presence of K_{IR} channels which are important in determining the effect of relatively small changes in external K^+ concentration on the membrane potential. The regulation of many of these channels as a consequence of G-protein activation is under investigation and this aspect of smooth muscle was discussed by a number of contributors to this Symposium.

Some smooth muscle cells, especially those isolated from blood vessels, also have K^+ channels that are gated by a fall in intracellular ATP concentration. Similar channels were first observed in pancreatic β cells. When blood glucose rises these channels (K_{ATP}) close and the cells are depolarized leading to Ca^{2+} influx and exocytosis of insulin. These channels are blocked by glibenclamide and are opened by drugs such as cromakalim and pinacidil. Currently, there is a great deal of interest by the pharmaceutical industry in 'K-channel openers' in the light of their possible use in hypertension and certain types of cardiac arrhythmias. Several papers in the Symposium deal with the regulation of these channels by, for example, second messengers such as cAMP. A further type of K^+ channel that appears to be gated by ADP (and other nucleotide di-phosphates) in the presence of Mg^{2+} is also discussed.

A further problem that became apparent during the early days of smooth muscle electrophysiology and still awaits solution is that of the coupling between individual smooth muscle cells. Perhaps as a result of work with large extracellular stimulating electrodes Tadao Tomita decided to follow up earlier studies on the spread of electrotonus in smooth muscle by exploiting long thin preparations of taenia caeci that could be polarized with large extracellular electrodes. In providing a logical and elegant description of the passive electrical properties of smooth muscle he yet again demonstrated his capacity to come up with a beautiful hypothesis and the appropriate experimentation to test this hypothesis He argued that if current could flow from cell to cell through low resistance pathways, a suitable pair of polarizing electrodes could lead to the uniform polarization of the tissue in a radial direction. Longitudinally directed current would then flow through the smooth muscle strip, beyond the polarizing electrodes, in accordance with the cable equations of Hodgkin and Rushton (1946). This approach made it possible to estimate values for a number of parameters including R_M (membrane resistance, Ωcm^2), C_M (membrane capacitance, μFcm^{-2}), λ (length constant, cm) and τ (membrane time constant, s). At Monash we still use a 'Tomita bath' when we need to polarize a segment of smooth muscle. We have an original version in our archives that was given to us by Tadao.

It soon became clear that the value of R_M for smooth muscle was very much higher than that, for example, of mammalian skeletal muscle (100–200 KΩcm^2 compared with 1–2 KΩcm^2). The value for C_M eventually turned out to be about $1\mu F$ cm^{-2} – a value now known to be common to most excitable cells. The length constant λ was between 1 and 2 mm, very similar to that of striated muscles. Attempts to measure longitudinal tissue impedance in both smooth and cardiac muscle with alternating currents showed that this is frequency dependent, decreasing for frequencies of greater than 10 Hz. This suggests that the coupling between cells is shunted by a capacitative element and an adequate explanation for this observation is still unclear. Tomita first drew attention to this problem in 1969.

The estimates of R_M and C_M found from cable analysis can adequately account for the value of the input resistance and capacitance found when patch electrodes are used to record from single cells. The value for the input resistance of a single smooth muscle cell is of the order of 2–5 GΩ. If one attempts to measure the input resistance of the same cell, when it is coupled to its neighbours *in situ*, the value obtained is very low, of the order of KΩ. This is due to the syncytial structure of most, if not all, smooth muscles (Holman *et al.*, 1990). Recent work, especially on uterine smooth muscle suggests that smooth muscles can express connexon proteins that are similar to those of cardiac muscle. The conductance of a typical cardiac connexon pair is approximately one-quarter of the input resistance of a single smooth muscle cell. Hence, very few connexon pairs with open pores would be required to bring about effective cell coupling. Smooth muscle connexon channels are similar to other ion channels and they may be in the open or closed state. So far there is no known morphological method for determining their density or their state! Perhaps one of the simplest approaches to this problem is the intracellular injection of current into the tissue and the estimation of input resistance. A greater understanding of the molecular biology of the structures responsible for intercellular coupling and their regulation appears to be a topic that needs urgent attention.

It has long been recognized that some smooth muscles, especially those of the gastrointestinal tract of many species, show a unique type of spontaneous activity whose frequency appears to be remarkably stable. The origin of this form of electrical activity, known variously as slow waves, minute rhythms, pace-setter potentials, basic electrical rhythm etc., has intrigued many physiologists including Bozler *et al.*, Prosser, Ed Daniel and Grahame Taylor. Much of the early electrophysiological work on smooth muscle was devoted to this problem. Tadao summarized the 'state of the art' in the early 1980s in his chapter in the second Bülbring book (Tomita, 1982). This chapter is still an essential source of information for anyone working in this field and, from some points of view, it shows that we have made rather little progress during the last 15 years.

In late 1973, Tadao spent some time with us at Monash University. Prior to his visit, Grahame Taylor had made a number of interesting observations on the slow waves of rabbit small intestine. Working together they confirmed Grahame's finding that it was possible, on a few occasions, to record large slow waves from cells near the myenteric plexus, whose amplitude was twice that of the slow waves recorded throughout the bulk of the longitudinal layer. Professor Ed Daniel joined us in 1974 and he worked with Grahame using the 'Tomita bath' to study the nature of the electrical coupling between longitudinal and circular layers. Ed recalls

> 'we also occasionally found such cells as we pushed our electrodes through the myenteric plexus and into the circular muscle. We also found evidence that the two muscle layers were not well coupled electrically; i.e., the two layers had different membrane potentials by about 10 mV, IJPs (inhibitory junction potentials) in the circular did not spread into the longitudinal layer and electrotonic potentials in any given layer failed to spread into the other. This work, later elaborated and completed in my new laboratory at McMaster by Don Cheung, led us to suggest that the pacemaker driving slow waves to occur simultaneously in the two muscle layers was located between them. Of course, the possibility occurred to us that these strange cells with large slow waves and IJPs were either the pacemakers or smooth muscle cells closely coupled to them'
>
> (E.E. Daniel, 1995, personal communication).

Nowadays there is overwhelming evidence that the cells which drive the slow waves in the gastrointestinal tract are the interstitial cells of Cajal, a proposition first put forward by Lars Thuneberg (1982). For many years these cells were thought to be a thin layer of fibroblasts closely associated with the enteric plexuses. It has long been recognized that smooth muscles and fibroblasts are closely related. Some of the pictures of de-differentiating smooth muscle cells in Geoff Burnstock's article in the second Bülbring book look just like interstitial cells (Burnstock, 1982). Isolated preparations of ICCs have been studied with the patch-clamp technique and there is evidence that those obtained from canine colon express different types of inward current channels from those of neighbouring smooth muscle cells. In ICCs a 'hump' could be detected on the I-V curve that peaked at around -50 mV and this was blocked by low concentrations of nickel ions thus showing some similarities with the properties of T-type Ca^{2+} channels (Lee & Sanders, 1993). Recently, it has been possible to breed a strain of mice that lack or have only a minimal contingent of interstitial cells in their gastrointestinal tracts. These heterozygotes survive although their stomach and intestines lack slow waves. The abnormal electrical activity that characterizes their intestinal smooth muscle is discussed during the Symposium (see chapters in this volume by Sanders & Ward, and Huizinga et al.). That the onward movement of the contents of the gut can still proceed in the absence of slow waves clearly demonstrates the essential function of the enteric nervous system.

One novel approach to our understanding of the oscillator that drives the slow waves involves computer simulation. My colleagues Rick Lang and Colin Rattray-Wood have developed a model based on the known properties of the voltage-dependent Ca^{2+} and K^+ channels found in smooth muscle including their Ca^{2+}-dependence. Their model assumes that the Ca^{2+} concentration that regulates the ion channels is that of a submembrane compartment whose $[Ca^{2+}]$ varies with Ca^{2+} influx through L-channels and a variable but restricted rate of diffusion of Ca^{2+} out of this compartment into the bulk of the cytoplasm. While this model can reproduce electrical activity, including some wave forms that closely resemble slow wave activity, it has yet to mimic the stability of the frequency of the slow wave oscillator. Perhaps this involves the activity of a voltage-independent ion channel that we have yet to identify but one that has been postulated for many years.

The key to this simulation is the existence of a submembrane compartment whose $[Ca^{2+}]$ may be very different from that calculated for the average Ca^{2+} concentration of the cytoplasm. The nonuniform distribution of ions in smooth muscle cells is certainly one of the most important issues considered during the Symposium. Tools are now available to enable the direct measurement of the submembrane concentrations of Na^+ and Ca^{2+} and it is clear that local ion gradients across the cell membrane may be very different from those suggested by measurements on whole cells. These data will have very significant implications for the role of the Na^+,Ca^{2+}-exchanger and the membrane Na^+, K^+-ATPase in controlling submembrane Ca^{2+} concentration and hence the activity of a number of ion channels. Similarly, methods are now available for measuring the Ca^{2+} content of the sarcoplasmic reticulum (SR) and mitochondria. When these advances are considered along with the range of pharmacological tools which target different Ca^{2+} stores and which inhibit specific membrane transport processes one can predict the rapid development of a dynamic model for the handling of Ca^{2+} by smooth muscle cells.

Just as recent work has drawn attention to the localized concentrations of intracellular Ca^{2+} and Na^+, this Symposium also reminds us of Tadao Tomita's contributions to the continuing debate about the role of aerobic glycolysis in smooth muscle function and the possibility that the metabolism of smooth muscle cells is 'compartmentalized'. The suggestion that a cascade of the enzymes responsible for glycolysis might be associated with the cell membrane whereas the enzymes responsible for the production of ATP by oxidative phosphorylation may be more generally distributed came from the work of Rick Paul and his colleagues. Rick Paul has written

'Although the invoking of 'compartmentation' is often proportional to one's lack of information, several well-established lines of evidence support this hypothesis in smooth muscle'

(Paul, 1989).

Evidence is accumulating that supports the view that the ATP generated by glycolysis fuels membrane Na^+,K^+-ATPase and the membrane Ca^{2+} pumps whereas O_2-dependent respiration is more closely linked to actomyosin–ATPase and the development of tension and shortening.

The nature and regulation of intracellular Ca^{2+} stores has been a central aspect of smooth muscle research since various groups began to study the properties of the mitochondrial and microsomal fractions of subcellular preparations made from smooth muscle during the 1960s. Avril and Andrew Somlyo drew our attention to the involvement of non-mitochondrial intracellular stores in excitation-contraction coupling when they defined pharmaco–mechanical coupling in 1968 (Somlyo & Somlyo, 1994). We now know that the complexity and diversity of Ca^{2+} stores in different smooth muscles is just as diverse as the properties of different smooth muscles themselves.

It is generally agreed that most, if not all smooth muscles have a Ca^{2+} store that releases Ca^{2+} in response to the binding of inositol 1,4,5-trisphosphate (IP_3) to its receptor on the cytoplasmic surface of the sarcoplasmic reticulum. It is also agreed that the ability of IP_3 to release Ca^{2+} from this store depends on the $[Ca^{2+}]$ of the cytoplasm, being facilitated as cytoplasmic $[Ca^{2+}]$ rises from very low levels but inhibited at high levels of $[Ca^{2+}]$. The action of IP_3 also depends on the Ca^{2+} content of the stores which, *inter alia*, appears to be able to influence the entry of Ca^{2+} across the sarcolemma (capacitative Ca^{2+} entry). There is also evidence that there are Ca^{2+} stores in smooth muscle that release Ca^{2+} following activation of a ryanodine receptor by cytosolic Ca^{2+} (calcium induced calcium release CICR). Because CICR plays such an important role in the regulation of the contractions of cardiac muscle, it is not surprising that attention has been paid to this process in smooth muscle.

The model of Ca^{2+} processing by smooth muscle that is evolving at the present time, comes partly from comparisons with striated muscles but, perhaps more importantly, from work on typical eukaryotic nonmuscle cells. Molecular biologic techniques are playing an increasingly important role that eventually they will enable us to understand the structure and function of the proteins that are involved, together with their natural history. At present, it seems that nonmitochondrial calcium stores may be represented as independent 'sacs' of sarcoplasmic reticulum (SR) lying within the cytoplasm at various distances from the plasma membrane. In common with that of striated muscles, the lumen of smooth muscle SR contains Ca^{2+}-binding proteins which increase its storage capacity. Although studies on the ultrastructure of smooth muscle suggest that its SR is a continuous structure (Somlyo & Somlyo, 1994) it may be possible to model smooth muscle SR by a series of independent stores as a consequence of the distribution of its Ca^{2+}-binding proteins. In some regions the SR membrane comes into very close proximity with the plasma membrane and bridging structures have been reported to occur between them.

There is evidence from nonmuscle cells that the density and/or sensitivity of IP_3 receptors may vary for functionally different stores (Taylor, 1992). Much work is presently underway on the molecular biology of the IP_3 receptor and it is becoming clear that its molecular architecture has a number of features in common with the ryanodine receptor. The interplay between these two receptors and their differential distribution could lead to highly localized variations in cytosolic Ca^{2+} concentration and it is now possible to detect local Ca^{2+} levels as a function of time at the millisecond level of resolution.

The Ca^{2+}-ATPases of the SR exist in a number of isoforms and one of the many interesting observations discussed during this Symposium is the predominant expression of the 2b isoform in smooth muscle since this is characteristic of the endoplasmic reticulum of nonmuscle cells. The nonuniform distribution of 2a and 2b forms of SR Ca^{2+}-ATPase could lead to a diversity in the kinetics of the loading of Ca^{2+} by different stores. Uptake of Ca^{2+} into mitochondrial stores and the SR may be the most immediate consequence of an increase in cytosolic Ca^{2+} by Ca^{2+} influx across the cell membrane due to the activation of voltage-dependent Ca^{2+} channels or receptor-operated nonspecific cation channels. Membrane Ca^{2+}-ATPases and the Na^+,Ca^{2+}- transporter are implicated in the maintenance of the steady state calcium content of smooth muscle. The Na^{2+},Ca^{2+}- transporter may be involved in the fast clearance of submembrane Ca^{2+}, especially in smooth muscles with relatively sparse SR. Now that a specific inhibitor of this transporter is available ('XIP' – exchanger inhibiting peptide, see, for example, DiPolo & Beauge, 1994) it should be possible to define its role in regulating cytosolic Ca^{2+} very precisely. As a result of electronmicroscope studies with antibodies to the Na^+,Ca^{2+}- transporter and Na^+,K^+-ATPase it has been established that these membrane proteins are not uniformly distributed but are clustered in regions of the membrane that appear to be in close apposition to the superficial SR (Moore *et al.*, 1993).

Much progress has been made recently in our understanding of the events that occur following the binding of agonists to both muscarinic receptors and α-adrenoceptors in different smooth muscles. Families of these receptors have been cloned and their pharmacological properties are being defined. Different subtypes appear to act through different signal transduction pathways, emphasizing the fact that molecular biology is opening up new chapters in our approach to pharmacology and the more accurate targetting of the new drugs of the future. Several aspects of muscarinic receptor activation are discussed during the Symposium. In the gastrointestinal tract one prominent feature is the opening of a cation channel that is gated by an increase in G-protein α-subunit concentration. Muscarinic receptors are also linked to G_q whose activation leads to the release of IP_3 and diacylglycerol, a potent stimulator of protein kinase C. The increase in cytosolic Ca^{2+} due to the release of IP3 may then activate one or more Ca^{2+}-sensitive ion channels including the highly voltage-dependent BK channels mentioned above and Ca^{2+}-sensitive Cl^- channels. The actions of muscarinic receptors in the smooth muscles studied to date can be mimicked by GTP but we still need to know more about the consequences of an increase in cytosolic Ca^{2+} in different smooth muscles. Further work on the analysis of the Ca^{2+} oscillations that are observed in many cells in response to agonist–receptor interaction may provide insights onto this problem.

In her introduction to the first 'Bülbring book' in 1970 Edith Bülbring quoted G. L. Brown's comments –

> *'I am only too fully aware of the difficulties confronting the electrophysiologist when dealing with cells of the size and complexity of those surrounding hollow organs, but the paucity of even the most elementary information holds out the promise of rich rewards to the experimenter with a sufficient temerity to begin such an investigation'.*

This Symposium confirms that we have made some progress towards the fulfillment of Edith's *'guiding motive: to establish the electrophysiological basis for an investigation of the mode of action of drugs'* (Bülbring, 1970).

Smooth muscles *in vivo* are under the control of a variety of nervous influences. In many cases it now appears likely that target tissues may be exposed for a short time (milliseconds) to a high local concentration of neurotransmitter at sites where nerve terminal varicosities make close contacts (approximately 50 nm) with the opposing smooth muscle membrane. This is also true for cardiac muscle. Diffusion away from such a close contact will be rapid and the concentration of neurotransmitter reaching receptors several microns away may become comparable with those commonly used to activate receptors on isolated cells (see Hirst & Edwards, 1989). However, we still have a great deal to learn about the effects of highly localized high concentrations of neurotransmitters and whether or not close contacts are associated with specialized functional receptors.

One of the properties of smooth muscle that Edith Bülbring found especially interesting was the response of this tissue to stretch. It now appears that several membrane ion channels are sensitive to this stimulus. Much work still remains to be done before this fundamentally important property of smooth muscle is fully resolved. The long-term effects of even the smallest distension of the smooth muscle components of the hollow organs of the body, including blood vessels, are of great significance in our understanding of a variety of clinical conditions, including hypertension.

Optimism in the future of research into the functioning of smooth muscle that was epitomized by this Symposium was accentuated by the wonderful view of Mount Fuji that awaited us on our trip from Nagoya to Ito. We are privileged and proud to acknowledge our debt to Tadao Tomita who has been an outstanding role model and leader in this key field of medical research. He is greatly respected by us all for his uncompromising insistence on the need to establish the facts before indulging in fanciful theories and for his courage in tackling the most difficult problems presented by this ubiquitous but most essential tissue that we call 'smooth muscle'. We are very grateful to Tadao, to Tom Bolton and their many colleagues including Hirosi Kuriyama, Akira Takai, Shinsuke Nakayama and Lorraine Smith for organizing a most memorable and stimulating meeting in Japan during cherry-blossom time in 1995.

REFERENCES

Brading, A.F., Bülbring, E. & Tomita, T. (1969). The effect of sodium and calcium on the action potential of the smooth muscle of the guinea-pig taenia coli. *J. Physiol.* **200**, 621–635.

Bülbring, E. (1970). Introduction. In *Smooth Muscle* (Bülbring, E., Brading, A.F., Jones, A.W. & Tomita, T., eds) pp. xi–xix. Edward Arnold, London.

Burnstock, G. (1982). Development of smooth muscle and its innervation. In *Smooth Muscle: An Assessment of Current Knowledge* (Bülbring, E., Brading, A.F., Jones, A.W. and Tomita, T. (eds), pp. 431–457. Edward Arnold, London.

DiPolo, R. & Beauge, L. (1994). Cardiac sarcolemmal Na/Ca – inhibiting peptides XIP and FMRF-amide also inhibit Na/Ca exchange in squid axons. *Am. J. Physiol.* **267**, C307–311.

Fatt, P. & Ginsborg, B.L. (1955). The ionic requirement of the production of action potentials in crustacean muscle fibres. J. Physiol. **142**, 516–543.

Hagiwara, S. & Naka, K. (1964). The initiation of spike potential in barnacle muscle fibres under low intracellular Ca^{2+}. *J. Gen. Physiol.* **46**, 141–162.

Hirst, G.D.S. & Edwards, F.R. (1989). Sympathetic neuroeffector transmission in arteries and arterioles. *Physiol. Rev.* **69**, 546–604.

Hodgkin, A.L. and Rushton, W.A.H. (1946). The electrical constants of a crustacean nerve fibre. *Proc. Roy. Soc. B.* **133**, 444–479.

Holman, M.E., Nield, T.O. & Lang, R.J. (1990). On the passive properties of smooth muscle. In *Frontiers in Smooth Muscle Research* (Sperelakis, N. & Wood, J.D., eds), pp. 379–398. Alan R. Liss, New York.

Lee, H.K. & Sanders, K.M. (1993). Comparison of ionic currents from interstitial cells and smooth muscle cells of canine colon. *J. Physiol.* **460**, 135–152.

Moore, E.D.W., Etter, E.F., Phillipson, K.D., Carrington, W.A., Fogarty, K.E., Lifshitz, L.M. & Fay, F.S. (1993). Coupling of the Na^+/Ca^{2+} exchanger, Na^+/K^+ pump and sarcoplasmic reticulum in smooth muscle. *Nature* **365**, 657–660.

Paul, R.J. (1989). Introduction: energetics of smooth muscle. In *Muscle Energetics* (Paul R.J. Elzinga G. & Yamada K., eds), pp. 235–237. Alan R. Liss, New York.

Somlyo, A.P & Somlyo, A.V. (1994). Signal transduction and regulation in smooth muscle. *Nature* **372**, 231–236.

Taylor, G.S. (1992). Kinetics of Inositol 1,4,5-Trisphosphate stimulated Ca^{2+} mobilization. In *Advances in Second Messenger and Phosphoprotein Research* Vol. 26 (Putney, J.W.Jr, ed.), pp. 109–142. Raven Press, New York.

Thuneberg, L. (1982). Interstitial cells of Cajal: intestinal pacemaker cells? *Adv. Anat.*

Embryolog. Cell Biol. **71,** 1–130.

Tomita, T. (1982). Electrical activity (spikes and slow waves) in gastrointestinal smooth muscles. In *Smooth Muscle: An Assessment of Current Knowledge* (Bülbring, E., Brading, A.F., Jones, A.W. and Tomita, T., eds), pp. 127–156. Edward Arnold, London.

Tomita, T. (1992). Advances in smooth muscle electrophysiology. *Proc. Int. Symp. 'Smooth Muscle' Japanese J. of Pharmacol.* **58**(Supp II), 1P–6P.

1

Voltage-dependent L-type Calcium Channels in Smooth Muscle Cells

U. KLÖCKNER

Department of Physiology,
University of Cologne,
Cologne, Germany

Among six functional subclasses of voltage dependent calcium channels (VDCCs), so far described (T-, L-, N-, P-, Q-, and R-type VDCCs), two have been identified in smooth muscle cells: T- and L-type channels (but see Smirnov *et al.*, 1992). The T-type VDCC is a low voltage activated channel; it is activated, inactivated, and reaches maximum amplitude at more negative potentials than the L-type. In addition, the relative amplitude of T- versus L-type current is small (McDonald *et al.*, 1994). T-type VDCCs are not present in every smooth muscle tissue. Even in tissues where T-type channels were described, they were only found in a fraction of the cells examined.

In contrast to T-type, L-type VDCCs play an important role in the excitation–contraction coupling of smooth muscle cells. Located in the plasmalemma, they serve as a major pathway for calcium ions to enter the cytosol upon a depolarization of the cell membrane. L-VDCCs have been found in all smooth muscle cells examined to date. L-VDCC's were identified on the basis of sensitivity to 1,4-dihydropyridine type calcium antagonists and agonists (Triggle, 1991). L-type calcium channels activate at more positive membrane potentials and inactivate along a slower time course (for details see Bolton *et al.*, 1988; McDonald *et al.*, 1994). In addition to their well established role of mediating calcium entry via action potentials in excitable cells, L-type VDCCs may also be responsible for calcium entry over the physiological range of membrane potentials, providing smooth muscle cells with sufficient calcium to maintain a steady tone (Nelson *et al.*, 1990). In smooth muscle cells isolated from coronary artery of the guinea pig, single channel activity can be recorded at −50 mV, i.e. close to the resting potential of the cells (Ganitkevich and Isenberg, 1990).

Single channel activity in smooth muscle cells were recorded routinely

SMOOTH MUSCLE EXCITATION
ISBN 0-12-112360-X

using isotonic (110 mM) Ba^{2+} solutions to maximize the amplitude of the unitary current and to increase the signal to noise ratio, although it is known that the amplitude of the single channel current and the gating behaviour for the channel depend on the species and the concentration of the charge carrier. To facilitate stable recording conditions, single channel studies were mostly done at 22°C. At room temperature, with 110 mM Ba^{2+} as the charge carrier, the single channel conductance of L-type VDCCs is around 25 pS (McDonald et al., 1994). With physiological levels of divalent cation concentration in the recording pipette, elementary calcium currents appeared to be too small to be resolved. For example, nonstationary noise analysis in bovine chromaffin cells at a membrane potential of -12 mV yielded an expected elementary calcium channel amplitude of -0.027 pA in 1 mM $[Ca^{2+}]_o$ and -0.086 pA in 5 mM $[Ca^{2+}]_o$ (Fenwick et al., 1982). Despite these estimations, it has recently been shown that under adequate experimental conditions it is possible to record calcium channel activity in smooth muscle and cardiac myocytes with very low concentrations of a charge carrier, (Gollasch et al., 1992; Rose et al., 1992). However, these studies were performed at room temperature and extrapolation of the gating behaviour and the single channel amplitude to physiological conditions may be not appropriate.

In order to characterize the activity of single smooth muscle L-type VDCCs at 36°C, single channel recordings were performed on cells isolated from the urinary bladder of the guinea pig in the cell-attached configuration of the patch-clamp technique (see Klöckner and Isenberg, 1991). The analysis of the single channel current amplitude was favoured by the occurrence of long openings without the application of a calcium channel agonist.

Figure 1 demonstrates the difference between commonly used and 'physiological' recording conditions. The currents flow through L-type VDCC since the probability of the channel open state was sensitive to micromolar concentrations of 1,4-dihydropyridine type calcium channel agonists and antagonists. With 110 mM Ba^{2+} as the charge carrier the mean amplitude of the current through calcium channels is -2.4 pA recorded at a membrane potential of 0 mV (Figure 1, left). This amplitude is about twice as large as has been reported for the amplitude of L-type calcium channels (McDonald et al., 1994). However, this behaviour can be simply attributed to the higher experimental temperature (36°C), as it has been shown that the amplitude of single calcium channel currents, independently of the charge carrier, increase by a factor of about two when the temperature is elevated from 22°C to 36°C (Klöckner et al., 1990). At the same potential of 0 mV, with 1 mM Ca^{2+} as the charge carrier, the mean amplitude of the single channel amplitude amounts only to -0.32 pA (Figure 1, right). Although this value is about eight times lower than the single channel amplitude with

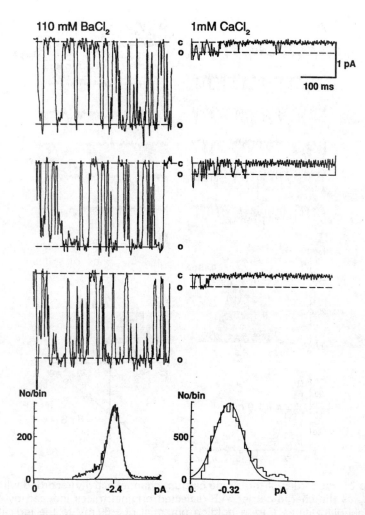

Figure 1 Dependence of single channel gating behaviour and amplitude on the charge carrier. The selected records were induced by 400-ms-long depolarizations of the patch membrane from −60 to 0 mV; 'c' indicates the closed, 'o' the open configuration of the channel. For the amplitude histograms the distribution of the closed state was subtracted. The cut-off filter frequency was 1 kHz. The membrane potential was zeroed by a high potassium solution.

isotonic barium solution, it is surprisingly high, suggesting that the apparent affinity constant for calcium ions is very low.

A more detailed analysis of the calcium channel activity recorded with a 'near- physiological' $[Ca^{2+}]_o$ is presented in Figure 2. In Figure 2A six original traces are shown induced by depolarizations from −60 to −10 mV. The

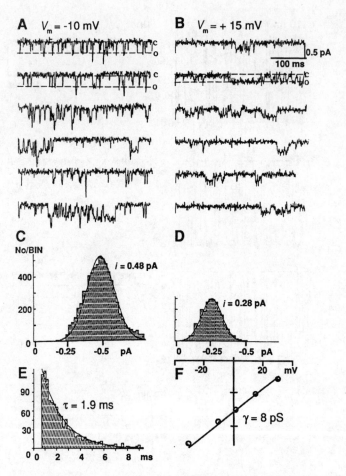

Figure 2 Properties of the single calcium channel activity recorded with 2 mM [Ca^{2+}]$_o$ as the charge carrier. A,B: selected original traces induced by 400-ms-long depolarizations from a holding potential of -60 mV to the indicated test potential; 'c' indicates the closed, 'o' the open configuration of the channel. C,D: amplitude histograms compiled at -10 and 15 mV. The distribution of the closed state is subtracted. E: open time histogram evaluated with a bin width of 0.2 ms and a threshold of 50% of the mean single channel amplitude, obtained from C. F: typical dependence of the mean amplitude of the single channel current on the test potential (current voltage relationship) with 2 mM [Ca^{2+}]$_o$ as the charge carrier. The slope of the straight line indicates a conductance of 8 pS.

superposition of two current amplitudes in all traces suggests that at least two channels were present in the patch. After substraction of the distribution of the closed channel, the amplitude histogram is fitted with a gaussian to a mean value of -0.48 pA at a test potential of -10 mV (Figure 2C). In Figure

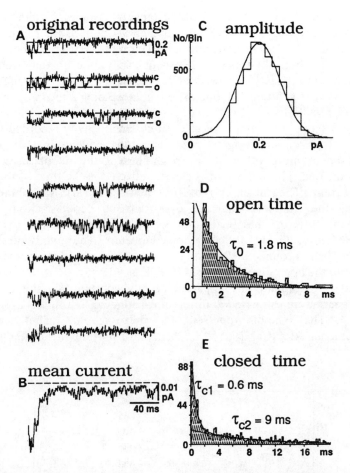

Figure 3 Properties of the single calcium channel activity recorded with 0.5 mM $[Ca^{2+}]_o$ as the charge carrier. A: selected original traces induced by 400-ms-long depolarizations from a holding potential of −60 mV to 0 mV. 'c' indicates the closed, 'o' the open configuration of the channel. The records were digitally filtered at 500 Hz. B: Mean current obtained by averaging the 200 traces of the experiment. C: amplitude histogram at 0 mV. The distribution of the closed state is subtracted. D: open time histogram evaluated with a threshold of 50% of the mean single channel amplitude, obtained from C. E: closed time histogram.

2B six original traces are displayed recorded at a test potential of +15 mV. At this potential the mean amplitude of the current through the open calcium channel amounted to −0.28 pA (Figure 2D). From similar amplitude distributions as shown in Figure 2C and D at a series of potentials between

−30 and 30 mV, a single channel conductance of 8 pS was obtained (Figure 2F). At 0 mV, recorded at 36°C and with 2 mM $[Ca^{2+}]_o$ as the charge carrier, the amplitude of the single calcium channel current is -0.4 ± 0.05 pA ($n = 7$). This value is about 15 times larger than has been estimated from noise analysis in 1 mM $[Ca^{2+}]_o$ (Fenwick et al., 1982). At −10 mV the life time of the open state was fitted with one exponential yielding a mean open time of 1.9 ms (Figure 2E).

Figure 3 shows an example of calcium channel activity recorded with 0.5 mM $[Ca^{2+}]_o$. From the original recordings it is evident, that the calcium channel opens more often at the beginning of the depolarization than towards the end. This behaviour is clearly reflected in the time course of the mean current. The mean current (ensemble average) was obtained by averaging the channel behaviour over the 200 depolarizations of this experiment. With 0.5 mM $[Ca^{2+}]_o$, at 36°C the mean current activates and inactivates very quickly, although not completely. The amplitude with 0.5 mM $[Ca^{2+}]_o$ is around -0.2 pA. The open time of 1.8 ms was not very different to the open time with 2 mM $[Ca^{2+}]_o$ at −10 mV.

In order to estimate the apparent affinity constant K_d, single channel conductances were estimated at different calcium concentrations as shown in Figure 4. The symbols represent the mean ± SEM of at least five measurements. At a $[Ca^{2+}]_o$ of 50, 15, 5, 2, and 1 mM the mean conductances

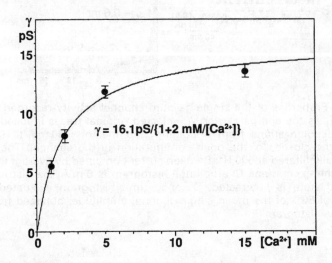

Figure 4 Dependence of the single channel conductance for L-type VDCCs on the concentration of Ca^{2+} in the patch pipette (mean ± SEM, data from 5–7 patches). The continuous line is a least-square fit according to the indicated equation.

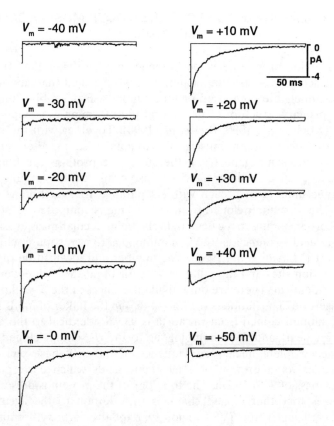

Figure 5 Mean currents obtained from a macropatch containing at least three channels. The currents were the average of 25 recordings. The holding potential was −60 mV. The filter cut-off frequency was 4 kHz.

were 16.0, 13.0, 11.5 8.0, and 5.5 pS, respectively. Fitting the data points with a Langmuir saturation curve yielded a saturating conductance of 16.1 pS and an apparent K_d value of 2 mM $[Ca^{2+}]_o$.

The activation and inactivation kinetics of the single channel current was studied with mean currents from macropatches containing more than three active channels (data filtered at 4 kHz and sampled at 20 kHz). The mean currents followed an activation–inactivation time course closely resembling the one of the whole-cell calcium currents (Klöckner & Isenberg, 1985). During steps to 0 mV, the mean current peaked within less than 1.5 ms. At 36°C, the activation time course was too fast to be adequately resolved. However, the inactivation followed a double-exponential time course (fast exponential 8 ms, slow exponential 40 ms time constant).

MOLECULAR STRUCTURE OF THE SMOOTH MUSCLE CALCIUM
CHANNEL

Recently, major progress has been made in identifying the structure of smooth muscle L-type calcium channels. It is suggested that smooth muscle calcium channels are composed of four subunits. From rabbit lung and rat aorta the primary structure of the central pore-forming α_1 subunit has been reported (Koch et al., 1990; Biel et al., 1990). Together with the cardiac α_1 subunit, the two smooth muscle α_1 subunits arise as alternative splice products of the same gene (α_{1C}), therefore, the proteins are homologous. Like their cardiac counterparts the isoforms contain four repeating hydrophobic units (I–IV), each with six putative transmembrane segments (S1–S6). The α_1 subunit cloned from rabbit lung is composed of 2166 amino residues corresponding to a calculated relative molecular mass of 242 516 Da. The amino acid sequence is 97.2% homologous to a α_1 subunit cloned from rabbit heart (Mikami et al., 1989). The number and localization of potential N-glycosylation sites and the putative sites for the cAMP-dependent protein kinase are identical. There are only small differences at the 5'-end, IS6, IVS3, and an insert of 75 nucleotides (nt 1391–1465) in the linker of motif I and II.

The α_1 subunit cloned from rat aorta is 93.9% identical to the α_1 subunit from rabbit heart and 98% homologous to the α_1 subunit cloned from rat brain. The complete nucleotide sequence of the 8305-base pair aortic α_1 subunit codes for a protein of 2169 amino acids which corresponds to a molecular mass of 243 615 Da. The topology of the protein is presumed to be the same as for other cloned channels. In addition to the occurrence of alterative splicing in the IVS3 region, part of the carboxyl-terminal tail is different in the aortic clone from the cardiac clones. However, the five phosphorylation sites found in the vascular α_1 subunit are also present in the cardiac isoform.

Injection of cRNA of the cardiac or the smooth muscle α_1 subunits into *Xenopus* oocytes leads to the expression of L-type VDCCs which are inhibited by calcium channel blockers (Mikami et al., 1989; Biel et al. 1990; Itagaki et al., 1992). Co-expression of the α_1 subunit with the α_2 and the β-subunit increased the current densities by a factor of 10 and accelerates the inactivation time constants. No major differences has been observed in the basic electrophysiological and pharmacological properties of the three isoforms including the amplitude of the whole cell and the single channel current, steady state activation and inactivation. Stable expression of the lung isoform in CHO cells also revealed no major differences (Welling et al., 1993b). The existence of two more splicing variants in the L-type α_1 subunit of rabbit intestinal smooth muscle has been reported using RT/PCR (Feron et al., 1994). The cDNA of the intestine α_1 subunit motif-IV clone, contains an open reading frame (314 aa) which is 99.8% and 93.6% identical to those of rabbit lung and rat aorta. No functional consequences associated with the splicing variants have been reported so far, with one exception: it has been shown that the 1,4-dihydropyridine nisoldipine inhibits the barium currents through the α_1 subunit at over 10-fold lower concentration compared with the current through cardiac α_1 subunit (Welling et al., 1993a). The authors speculate, that the different IVS3 sequences might contribute to the observed sensitivity toward dihydropyridines of smooth muscle and cardiac α_1 subunits. This finding was unexpected because the putative binding sites for DHP derivative (Tang et al., 1993) are identical in the two isoforms. Furthermore, the presumptive vascular smooth muscle calcium channel (Koch et al., 1990) does not contain the regions caused by splice variations in the lung.

The α_2/δ subunit (1080 aa) of the skeletal muscle calcium channel is a glycosylated membrane protein of 125 kDa. Apparently, the α_2/δ subunit is synthesized as a propeptide that is cleaved near the carboxy terminus to form the α_2 (1–934 aa) and the δ subunit (935–1080 aa). The transmembrane δ subunit anchors the α_2 protein by disulfide bridges at the extracellular site of the plasma membrane. Northern blot analysis has shown that identical α_2/δ subunits exist in heart, vascular and intestinal smooth muscle (see Hofmann et al. 1994). Co-expression of the α_1 subunit with a α_2/δ subunit results predominantly in an increase of the expressed currents by a factor of about two (Itagaki et al., 1992, but see Welling et al., 1993b).

Similar to the α_1 subunit there is evidence that different β subunits are present in different tissues. The β subunit isolated from skeletal muscle is a 55 kDa protein. Up to now transcripts of four different genes have been identified (β_1–β_4). In smooth muscle cells, β_2 and β_4 subunits have been detected. Transcripts of the β_2 gene exist in heart and to a lower degree in aorta, trachea and lung (Hofmann et al., 1994; Perez-Reyes and Schneider, 1994). Because transcripts of β_3 have been detected predominantly in aorta, trachea, lung, and colon, and only to a lesser degree in other tissue, it is speculated that this β subunit might be linked to the α_1 subunits expressed in smooth muscle cells (Hofmann et al., 1994). Remarkably, the β_3 protein does not contain consensus protein kinase A (PKA) phosphorylation sequences. Co-expression of the α_1 subunit with a β-subunit resulted in an increase of the current density by a factor of 5–10 and a shift of the steady-state activation and inactivation curves by 5–10 mV to more negative potentials (Bosse et al., 1992; Itagaki et al., 1992; Welling et al., 1993b).

The electrophysiological and biophysical properties of the native cardiac and smooth muscle L-type VDCCs are very similar (for references see McDonald et al., 1994). Despite these similarities the regulation of the activity of the channels in both tissues is quite different. Phosphorylation-mediated increase of the cardiac L-type calcium channel activity by a cAMP-dependent PKA is the major mechanism underlying the β-adrenergic stimulation of the heart beat. In contrast, in most smooth muscle cells studied to date there is no evidence for a PKA mediated phosphorylation of the calcium channel, i.e. there is no evidence for an increase in I_{Ca} dialysing the cells with cAMP or the catalytic subunit of PKA (for references see McDonald et al., 1994; but see Tewari & Simard, 1994). This discrepancy is astonishing, as the cloned cardiac and smooth muscle calcium α_1 subunits have identical phosphorylation sites.

In a study performed in *Xenopus* oocytes it was demonstrated that without co-expression of the β subunit the cardiac calcium channel current – induced by the expression of the α_1 subunit alone – cannot be modulated by a cAMP dependent phosphorylation (Klöckner et al., 1992). Only when co-expressed with the β subunit of the skeletal calcium channel the current can be increased by injection of cAMP. This finding was confirmed by a report showing that voltage-dependent facilitation of neuronal α_{1C} L-type calcium channels, which is thought to be caused by a PKA dependent phosphorylation reaction, required the co-expression of a calcium channel β subunit (Bourinet et al., 1994). The second important finding of this study was that smooth muscle calcium channel currents (induced by the expression of a smooth muscle α_1 subunit) can be 'transformed' into a cardiac type calcium channel current when co-expressed with the skeletal β subunit, i.e. cAMP causes an increase in the calcium channel current. Because the β_3 subunit has no PKA consensus sites it is tempting to speculate that it is the existence of different β-subunits in smooth muscle cells, compared with cardiac myocytes, which is responsible for the different regulation of the native calcium channels via PKA. Another possibility could be that the presence of a β subunit changes the conformation of the α_1 subunit in such a way that the protein is now accessible to protein kinase A. However, this work was criticized because the results do not exclude with the last condition the possibility that the β subunit was associated with the endogenous *Xenopus* calcium channel (Hofmann et al., 1994).

In agreement with this criticism are the recent reports showing that recombinant cardiac calcium channels cannot be functionally phosphorylated in mammalian expression systems (Hofmann et al., 1994). Even when all putative phosphorylation sites were removed by mutagenesis the expressed currents do not differ from the currents induced by expression of wild type α_1 subunit (Mikala et al., 1995). Together with the finding that the recombinant currents can still be stimulated by intracellular perfusion of trypsin (Klöckner et al., 1995), i.e. in that respect recombinant cardiac calcium channels behave like native smooth muscle calcium channels (Klöckner, 1988; Obejero-Paz et al., 1991), it is suggested that an important factor is missing in the experiments which is present in native heart cells but not in smooth muscle cells. Experiments to identify this factor are underway.

REFERENCES

Biel, M., Ruth, P., Bosse, E., Hullin, R., Stühmer, W., Flockerzi, V. & Hofmann, F. (1990). Primary structure and functional expression of a high voltage activated calcium channel from rabbit lung. *FEBS Lett.* **269**, 409–412.

Bolton, T.B., MacKenzie, I. & Aaronson, P.I. (1988). Voltage dependent calcium channels in smooth muscle cells. *J. Cardiovasc. Pharmacol.* **12**, S3–S7

Bosse, E., Bottlender, R., Kleppisch, T., Hescheler, J., Welling, A., Hofmann, F. & Flockerzi, V. (1992). Stable and functional expression of the calcium channel alpha 1 subunit from smooth muscle in somatic cell lines. *EMBO J.* **11**(6), 2033–2038

Bourinet, E., Charnet, P., Tomlinson, W.J, Stea, A., Snutch, TP. & Nargeot, J. (1994). Voltage dependent facilitation of a neuronal α_{1C} L-type calcium channel. *EMBO J.* **13**, 5032–5039.

Fenwick, E.M., Marty, M. & Neher, E. (1982). Sodium and calcium channels in bovine chromaffin cells. *J. Physiol.* **331**, 599–635.

Feron, O., Octave, J.N., Christen, M.O. & Godfraind. T. (1994). Quantification of two splicing events in the L-type calcium channel alpha-1 subunit of intestinal smooth muscle and other tissues. *Eur. J. Biochem.* **222**, 195–202

Ganitkevich, V.Y. & Isenberg, G. (1990) Contribution of two types of calcium channels to membrane conductance of single myocytes from guinea pig coronary artery. *J. Physiol.* **426**, 19–42

Gollasch, M., Hescheler, J., Quayle, J.M., Patlak, J.B. & Nelson, M.T. (1992). Single calcium channel currents of arterial smooth muscle at physiological calcium concentrations. *Am. J. Physiol.* **263**(5 Pt 1), C948–952

Hofmann, F., Biel, M. & Flockerzi, V. (1994). Molecular basis for Ca^{2+} channel diversity. *Annu. Rev. Neurosci.* **17**, 399–418

Itagaki, K., Koch, W.J., Bodi, I., Klöckner, U., Slish, D.F. & Schwartz, A. (1992). Native-type DHP-sensitive calcium channel currents are produced by cloned rat aortic smooth muscle and cardiac alpha 1 subunits expressed in *Xenopus laevis* oocytes and are regulated by alpha 2- and beta-subunits. *FEBS Lett.* **297**(3), 221–225

Klöckner, U. (1988). Isolated coronary smooth muscle cells. Increase in the availability of L-type calcium channel current by intracellularly applied peptidases. *Pflügers Arch.* **412**, R82

Klöckner, U. & Isenberg, G. (1985). Action potentials and net membrane current of smooth muscle cells (urinary bladder of the guinea pig). *Pflügers Arch.* **405**, 329–339.

Klöckner, U. & Isenberg, G. (1991). Currents through single L-type Ca^{2+} channels studied at 2 mM $[Ca^{2+}]_o$ and 36°C in myocytes from the urinary bladder of the guinea pig). *J. Physiol.* **438**, 228P.

Klöckner, U., Schiefer, A. & Isenberg, G. (1990). L-type Ca-channels: similar Q10 of Ca-, Ba- and Na-conductance points to the importance of ion-channel interaction. *Pflügers Arch.* **415**(5), 638–641

Klöckner, U., Itagaki, K., Bodi, I. & Schwartz, A. (1992). Beta-subunit expression is required for cAMP-dependent increase of cloned cardiac and vascular calcium channel currents. *Pflügers Arch.* **420**(3–4), 413–415

Klöckner, U., Mikala, G., Varadi, M., Varadi, G. & Schwartz, A. (1995). The enhancement of Ca^{2+} channel activity by trypsin perfusion is due to partial removal of the C-terminal tail of the α_1 polypeptide. *Biophysical J.* **68**(2), A348

Koch, W.J., Ellinor, P.T. & Schwartz, A. (1990). cDNA cloning of a dihydropyridine-sensitive calcium channel from rat aorta. Evidence for the existence of alternatively spliced forms. *J. Biol. Chem.* **265**(29), 17786–17791

McDonald, T.F., Pelzer, S., Trautwein, W. & Pelzer, D.J. (1994). Regulation and modulation of calcium channels in cardiac, skeletal, and smooth muscle cells. *Physiol. Rev.* **74**(2), 365–507.

Mikala, G., Klöckner, U., Eisfeld, J., Varadi, M., Varadi, G. & Schwartz. A. (1995) cAMP-dependent phosphorylation sites are not required for activity of the recombinant cardiac L-type calcium channel. *Biophysical J.* **68**(2), A349

Mikami, A., Imoto, K., Tanabe, T., Niidome, T., Mori, Y., Takeshima, H., Narumiya, S. & Numa, S. (1989). Primary structure and functional expression of the cardiac dihydropyridine-sensitive calcium channel. *Nature* **340**, 230–233.

Nelson, M.T., Patlak, J.B., Worley, J.F. & Standen, N.B. (1990). Calcium channels, potassium channels, and voltage dependence of arterial smooth muscle tone. *Am. J. Physiol.* **259**, C3–C18.

Obejero-Paz, C.A., Jones, S.W. & Scarpa, A. (1991). Calcium currents in the A7r5 smooth muscle-derived cell line. Increase in current and selective removal of voltage-dependent inactivation by intracellular trypsin. *J. Gen. Physiol.* **98**, 1127–1140.

Perez-Reyes, E. & Schneider, T. (1994). Calcium channels: structure, function, and classification. *Drug Devel. Res.* **33**, 295–318.

Rose, W.C., Balke, C., Wier, W.G. & Marban, E. (1992). Macroscopic and unitary properties of physiological ion flux through L-type Ca^{2+} channels in guinea-pig heart cells. *J. Physiol. Lond.* **456**, 267–284.

Smirnov, S.V., Zholos, A.V. & Shuba, M.F. (1992). Potential-dependent inward currents in single isolated smooth muscle cells of the rat ileum. *J. Physiol.* **454**, 549–571.

Tang, S., Yatani, A., Bahinski, A., Mori, Y. & Schwartz, A. (1993). Molecular localization of regions in the L-type calcium channel critical for dihydropyridine action. *Neuron.* **11**, 1013–1021.

Tewari, K. & Simard, J.M. (1994). Protein kinase A increases availability of calcium channels in smooth muscle cells from guinea pig basilar artery. *Pflügers Arch.* **428**, 9–16.

Triggle, D.J. (1991) Calcium-channel drugs: structure-function relationships and selectivity of action. *J. Cardiovasc. Pharmacol.* **18**: S1–S6.

Welling, A., Kwan, Y.W., Bosse, E., Flockerzi, V., Hofmann, F. & Kass, R.S. (1993a). Subunit-dependent modulation of recombinant L-type calcium channels. Molecular basis for dihydropyridine tissue selectivity. *Circ. Res.* **73**, 974–980.

Welling, A., Bosse, E., Cavalie, A., Bottlender, R., Ludwig, A., Nastainczyk, W., Flockerzi, V. & Hofmann, F. (1993b). Stable co-expression of calcium channel α_1, β and α_2/δ subunits in a somatic cell line. *J. Physiol.* **417**, 749–765.

2

Multiple Open States of Calcium Channels and their Possible Kinetic Schemes

S. NAKAYAMA*
LORRAINE M. SMITH*
T. TOMITA***
ALISON F. BRADING**

*Department of Physiology,
School of Medicine, Nagoya University,
Nagoya, Japan

**Department of Pharmacology,
University of Oxford, UK

***Department of Physiology,
School of Health Sciences, Fujita Health University,
Toyoake, Aichi, Japan

Many smooth muscles are known to generate action potentials. From results obtained using ionic substitution, pharmacological tools and voltage clamp techniques, it is believed that the action potentials, especially spike activities of smooth muscle, are largely due to activation of voltage-sensitive Ca^{2+} channels. Also, sustained tension (tonic and/or slow contractions) is seen in many smooth muscles, either at the resting potential or during depolarizations. Most sustained tension is thought to depend on Ca^{2+} influx flowing through voltage-sensitive Ca^{2+} channels, because Ca^{2+} channel antagonists suppress, and agonists enhance, the tension developed. These facts suggest that in smooth muscle Ca^{2+} channels make a significant contribution to a wide range of physiological functions, from very transient to persistent Ca^{2+} movements.

In guinea pig urinary bladder cells (detrusor cells) large Ca^{2+} currents are seen. The peak amplitude of the currents sometimes exceeds 1 nA (Klöckner & Isenberg, 1985). These large Ca^{2+} currents provide an advantageous model for precise analyses. We thus investigated the properties of voltage-sensitive Ca^{2+} channels mainly in guinea pig urinary bladder cells. In some of our experiments we also measured Ca^{2+} currents in isolated cells from guinea pig stomach and taenia caeci.

SMOOTH MUSCLE EXCITATION
ISBN 0-12-112360-X

MEASUREMENT OF Ca²⁺ CHANNEL CURRENT

To measure whole-cell and unitary Ca^{2+} currents, standard whole-cell and cell-attached patch-clamp techniques were used. Enzymatically isolated guinea pig detrusor cells, and other smooth muscle cells were used (at room temperature). The composition of the 'normal' bathing solution is as follows (mM): NaCl, 125; KCl, 5.9; $CaCl_2$, 2.5; $MgCl_2$, 1.2; glucose, 11.8 and Hepes (*N*-2-hydroxyethylpiperazine-*N*-2-ethanesulphonic acid), 11.8. The pH of the solution was adjusted to 7.4 (25°C) with Tris base. The composition of the pipette solution was (mM): CsCl, 141; $MgCl_2$, 1.4; EGTA 2; Hepes/Tris, 10 (pH 7.2 at 25°C). In some experiments K^+ currents were more strongly depressed by adding TEA (7–10 mM) to the pipette solution and replacing extracellular K^+ with equimolar Cs^+. With this modification qualitatively similar results were obtained. In later experiments, 1 mM ATP and 0.1 mM GTP (guanosine 5′-triphosphate) were added in order to prevent rapid 'run down' of the Ca^{2+} channel activity. When Ca^{2+}-dependent inactivation was examined by application of neurotransmitters, the concentration of EGTA was reduced to 0.1 mM to demonstrate the inactivation clearly.

FORMATION OF SLOW DEACTIVATING TAIL CURRENTS

When we applied a series of depolarizing pulses (100–200 msec duration, from the holding potential of −60 mV) with variable amplitude to guinea pig urinary bladder smooth muscle cells (detrusor cells), the relationship between the test potential and the peak amplitude of the inward current evoked was similar to that observed previously in this and other smooth muscle preparations (the peak amplitude maximized at around −10 to 0 mV and reversed between +40 and +60 mV). In some of the experiments, we clearly observed slowly decaying inward tail currents after applying large depolarizing steps. Using the slow tail currents we assessed possible kinetic schemes for Ca^{2+} channels. Since Ca^{2+} channel currents were not inactivated at +80 mV, as described in the subsequent section of this chapter, this potential was used to induce slow tail currents.

As the duration of the large voltage step (at +80 mV) was increased, the amplitude of the tail current increased monotonically and saturated after 2–5 s depolarization. The decay time constant was about 10 to 15 ms (Nakayama & Brading, 1993a). To identify which channels were responsible for the slowly decaying inward tail currents, we performed the following experiments.

1. Conditioned and unconditioned inward currents were compared as shown in Figure 1. The current (a) was evoked by a simple depolarization (test

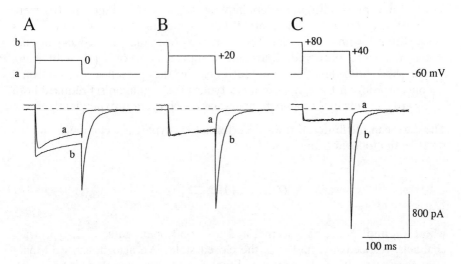

Figure 1 Comparison between conditioned (b) and unconditioned inward currents (a) in a guinea pig detrusor cell. The test step in (b) was preceded by a preconditioning positive polarization at +80 mV for 5 s). The potential of the test step was changed from 0mV (A) to +20 mV (B) and +40 mV (C). (Reproduced from Nakayama & Brading, 1993a.)

step) and the test step (depolarization) (b) was preceded by a large conditioning positive polarization to +80 mV for 5 s. In B, the test potential was increased from 0 to +20 mV, at which potential the degree of activation would be almost saturated. The inward currents seen at the test step were very similar, however, a slow inward tail current was induced only after a large conditioning positive polarization. The results suggest that the same ion channels are responsible for both inward currents seen in test and repolarizing steps, and the conformation of the ion channels are transferred from the normal to another open state during prolonged large depolarization.

2. At +80 mV we observed outward currents of several-hundred picoamps. After applying a large conditioning positive polarization at +80 mV (for 5 s) the cell membrane was transiently repolarized to −60 mV (5 ms). This protocol induced a slow tail current. During the decay time course of the tail current we returned the cell membrane to +80 mV. The amplitude of the subsequent outward current was almost the same as that seen before the transient repolarization. As the Cl^- concentrations of the pipette and bathing solutions are symmetrical, contribution of Cl^- conductances to the slow inward tail current would appear to be negligible. Also, in this experiment contribution from nonselective conductances can be ruled out.

3. The same preconditioning depolarizing steps used in Figure 1 (b) were repeated at 60–90 sec intervals. When extracellular Ca^{2+} (2.5 mM) was substituted with equimolar Ba^{2+}, similar test and slow decaying tail currents were observed. Subsequent replacement of Ba^{2+} with Mg^{2+} abolished both test and tail currents. In the presence of a normal concentration of Ca^{2+}, nifedipine (a typical Ca^{2+} antagonist) reduced both inward currents in the same manner, and concentration-dependently.

Thus, we can attribute all inward currents to L-type Ca^{2+} channels, and we propose the following kinetic scheme:

$$C \rightleftharpoons O_1 \rightleftharpoons O_2$$

where O_1 and O_2 are the normal and a second open states of L-type Ca^{2+} channels, respectively, and C is the closed state. We also describe O_2 as a long open state. It can be postulated that during large depolarization the O_1 to O_2 transition occurs, and that the transition from O_2 to O_1 is significantly slower than that from O_1 to C. The slow deactivating tail currents seen upon repolarization of the cell membrane are presumably due to the slow, O_2 to O_1 transition. Similar phenomena – long channel opening after large depolarization – have been reported in adrenal chromaffin cells (Hoshi & Smith, 1987) and cardiac myocytes (Pietrobon & Hess, 1990).

In smooth muscle cells isolated from guinea pig stomach and taenia caeci, slow deactivating tail currents were also observed after preconditioning depolarization. Thus, the long open state of the Ca^{2+} channel seems to be a common feature in smooth muscle. Also, the long channel opening in the second open state allowed us to measure directly the voltage dependence of the unit current amplitude of the Ca^{2+} channel by applying a ramp pulse after preconditioning positive polarization (with no Ca^{2+} agonist in the pipette, 50 mM Ba^{2+} as a charge carrier). The slope conductance was approximately 25 pS, which agreed with previous reports.

INACTIVATION INCORPORATING LONG OPEN STATE

We next assessed inactivation mechanisms taking the second open state into account. The degree of inactivation was measured at a test potential of 0 or +20 mV in guinea pig detrusor cells. The membrane potential was directly switched from preceding conditioning potentials to the test potential (no interpulse step between the conditioning and test steps) (Figures 1, 2 and 4 in Nakayama & Brading 1993b; Figure 1 in Nakayama & Brading, 1995b). When a wide range of conditioning potentials from −100 to +80 mV was applied (0.8 s duration), a fully U-shaped inactivation curve was obtained. The degree of inactivation was maximal at 0 mV and about 60%. The property of U-shaped inactivation is often used as evidence for Ca^{2+}-dependent inactivation, because Ca^{2+} entry and the degree of inactivation is maximal at the same potential.

When the duration of the conditioning step was prolonged to 5 s, maximum inactivation increased to 90% and still occurred at 0 mV. The conditioning potentials greater than +20 mV restored the amplitude of the test inward current as the potential increased, and again, a fully U-shaped inactivation curve was obtained. Because a conditioning duration of 5 s is considered to achieve steady-state inactivation, the U-shaped inactivation observed in our experiments is not explained solely by Ca^{2+}-dependent inactivation. This deduction is also supported by the fact that similar U-shaped inactivation curve is obtained even when Ba^{2+} was used as a charge carrier.

In the preceding section we proposed the presence of the second open state (O_2). If we assume that Ca^{2+} channels in the second, long open state do not inactivate at all or inactivate very slowly, we can predict a U-shaped inactivation curve (assuming Ca^{2+}-dependent inactivation plays a negligible role).

$$C \rightleftharpoons O_1 \rightleftharpoons O_2$$
$$\Updownarrow \qquad \Updownarrow$$
$$I_1 \qquad (I_2)$$

where O_1 and O_2 are the same as described in the initial scheme, and I_1 and I_2 are the corresponding inactivated states for O_1 and O_2. At around 0 mV Ca^{2+} channels are activated (to O_1), and then transferred to I_1 state. Also, conditioning potentials more positive than +20 mV progressively facilitate the O_1 to O_2 transition, and subsequently decrease the degree of inactivation.

How Ca^{2+}-dependent inactivation correlates with the inactivation kinetic scheme shown above was examined in the following experiments. (1) A prolonged simple depolarization to 0 mV was applied for 8 s. This depolarization is considered to mainly induce the normal open (O_1) state of Ca^{2+} channels. During the long depolarizing step extracellular Ca^{2+} was removed (replace with Mg^{2+}) for approximately 4 s, and inward Ca^{2+} current was completely suppressed. When Ca^{2+} was readmitted to the extracellular solution during the depolarization, the amplitude of the subsequently induced inward current was significantly larger than that predicted by fitting the decay of the inward current recorded before the removal of extracellular Ca^{2+}. This enhancement of the inward current upon readmission of extracellular Ca^{2+} can be explained as a recovery from Ca^{2+}-dependent inactivation during Ca^{2+} removal. Replacing Ba^{2+} with Ca^{2+} during a prolonged depolarization at 0 mV resulted in an immediate reduction in the amplitude of the inward current probably owing to Ca^{2+}-dependent inactivation. (2) To induce the long open state (O_2), a large conditioning positive polarization to +80 mV was applied for 5 s before a test step of 0 mV (100 ms). When carbachol (CCh) was rapidly applied by pressure ejection during the preconditioning polarization, the inward currents seen in the subsequent test and depolarizing steps were significantly reduced (compared with the preceding control in which inward currents were obtained without CCh) (Nakayama, 1993). In this tissue CCh is known to cause release Ca^{2+} from intracellular Ca^{2+} stores (sarcoplasmic reticulum). The reduction of the inward currents could be used as an evidence for Ca^{2+}-dependent inactivation of the Ca^{2+} channels in the O_2 state. Taken together, these experiments suggest that Ca^{2+}-dependent inactivation operates independently and separately from the inactivation kinetic scheme shown above.

NON-INACTIVATING Ca^{2+} CURRENT

When the cell membrane of smooth muscle is depolarized using voltage clamp techniques, the amplitude of Ca^{2+} current peaks at around 10 ms, and then declines to be a very small current after several seconds. This very small inward current observed at a steady state is termed the noninactivating Ca^{2+} channel current (I_{NI}), and is considered to be responsible for sustained Ca^{2+} influx during tonic and/or slow contractions in smooth muscle. The magnitude of this current could be expressed by a product of steady-state activation ($d_\infty(E)$) and inactivation ($f_\infty(E)$) of the Ca^{2+} channel at a certain potential (E):

$$I_{NI}(E) = d_\infty(E)\, f_\infty(E)\, I_{max}(E), \tag{1}$$

where $I_{max}(E)$ is voltage dependence of the maximal available Ca^{2+} current. $I_{max}(E)$ can be obtained by the following methods: (1) use of linear (ohmic) conductance or the Eyring model (Langton & Standen, 1993); or (2) direct measurement by switching the cell membrane to various repolarizing potentials after preconditioning with large depolarization (the slow deactivation in O_2 state makes it possible to estimate accurately the amplitude of the tail current: Nakayama & Brading, 1993a). $d_\infty(E)$ is estimated by fitting the (peak) current–voltage relationship of simple depolarizing steps (I–V curve) with combination of $I_{max}(E)$ and a sigmoidal function based on the Boltzmann distribution. Another method which may directly estimate $d_\infty(E)$ is to compare the amplitudes of unconditioned ($= d_\infty(E)\, I_{max}(E)$) and conditioned test inward currents ($= I_{max}(E)$) by changing the test potentials (assuming that the maximum available current is not changed by conversion of the Ca^{2+} channel conformation from O_1 to O_2: $I_{maxO_1} = I_{maxO_2}$) (Nakayama & Brading, 1995).

In our experiments using guinea pig detrusor cells, the inactivation curve is completely U-shaped even after conditioning steps of 5 s. The inactivation curve can be fitted with a sum of two Boltzmann equations (sigmoid curves). Leaving aside Ca^{2+}-dependent inactivation, it can be postulated that the descending phase of the U-shaped inactivation curve corresponds to the O_1 to I_1 transition (see the inactivation kinetic scheme), while the ascending phase is voltage-dependent development of O_2 state. Thus, in the model the noninactivating current may be simply divided into two components: so-called 'window' current and a persistent current brought about by the long open (O_2) state.

Window current is often used as a basis of noninactivating Ca^{2+} current model. In this model, the steady-state inactivation parameter is expressed as a single Boltzmann equation. However, since Ca^{2+} channel current in smooth muscle usually shows greater steady-state inactivation at more positive potentials, but does not fully inactivate at large depolarizing steps, the steady state inactivation parameter ($f_\infty(E)$) is sometimes expressed as a sum of Boltzmann equation and a constant component (e.g. Imaizumi et al., 1991). A simple interpretation for this constant component is that Ca^{2+} channels in the inactivation state (I_1) have a small conductance. We can also postulate an alternative explanation, applying our second open state model, that the constant component may correspond to premature development of the second, long open state (O_2) during conditioning steps (Nakayama & Brading, 1995).

When we fitted the U-shaped inactivation curve, the sum of two Boltzmann equations were used. The Boltzmann equation used for the descending phase of the inactivation curve corresponds to that used in conventional window current simulation, and also to the O_1 to I_1 transition shown in the inactivation kinetic scheme. The O_1 to I_1 transition, which occurs separately from Ca^{2+} dependent inactivation, may be alternatively classified as a voltage-dependent inactivation. There is abundant evidence that intracellular Ca^{2+} inactivates L-type Ca^{2+} channels, while the main evidence for voltage-dependent inactivation is the decay of Na^+ current flowing through Ca^{2+} channels during depolarization (reviewed by Pelzer et al., 1990). We also observed decay of Na^+ current in guinea pig detrusor cells. This result, however, only indicates that Ca^{2+} channels inactivate during depolarization with no Ca^{2+} entry. In accordance with other window current simulation, the O_1 to I_1 transition was, first of all, assumed to be voltage-dependent. Application of the Boltzmann distribution to inactivation kinetics, however, requires charge movement corresponding to the transition. At present there is no definite evidence that such a charge movement occurs.

Therefore, we may (alternatively) be able to postulate that the inactivation process is governed simply by a chemical equilibrium. Provided that K_1 and K_2 are the equilibrium constants of the O_1 to I_1 and O_2 to I_2 transitions, respectively, the peak of the simulated non-inactivating current would be greatly shifted (from approx. $+20$ to -20 mV) by changing the ratio of K_1 to K_2 (Nakayama & Brading, 1995b).

In smooth muscles, there is some discrepancy reported between simulated (based on window current theory) and direct measurements of non-inactivating Ca^{2+} current or measurements of sustained $[Ca^{2+}]_i$. Imaizumi *et al.* (1991) reported that in various smooth muscle preparations, the amplitude of the predicted window current is always larger than that of directly measured noninactivating current, but both of them are maximal in a similar voltage range (-10 to -15 mV). In rabbit ear artery, Aaronson *et al.*, (1988) have shown noninactivating Ca^{2+} current which is maximal at 0 mV and observed even at $+30$ mV. Ganitkevich & Isenberg (1991) have shown in guinea pig urinary bladder cells, that $[Ca^{2+}]_i$ at 0 mV is higher than that at -20 mV, at which potential the $[Ca^{2+}]_i$ predicted by window current should be maximal. Further investigation of noninactivating current (inactivation mechanisms) incorporating the long open state (O_2) may resolve these discrepancies.

INTERACTION OF LARGE POSITIVE POLARIZATION AND Ca^{2+} AGONIST

It is well known that dihydropyridine Ca^{2+} agonists, e.g. Bay K 8644, induce long channel opening of L-type Ca^{2+} channels and potentiation of Ca^{2+} current is often called 'mode 2 gating' (Hess *et al.*, 1984). In the preceding sections, we described the presence of a large depolarization-induced second open state in which Ca^{2+} channels hardly inactivate and deactivate slowly upon repolarization. In this section we describe experiments examining the interaction of these two factors which induce long channel opening (Nakayama & Brading, 1995a).

In normal solution, no large tail current was observed after simple depolarization (to 0 or $+20$ mV, 100–200 ms duration). When Bay K 8644 (100 nM) was applied to the bathing solution, the activation curve (estimated from the *I–V* curve obtained by simple depolarizing steps) was shifted in the hyperpolarizing direction, and tail currents of sizeable amplitude appeared. The time constant (3–5 ms) of the tail current in the presence of Bay K 8644 was significantly smaller than that (8 or 10–15 ms) observed after preconditioning large positive polarization (at $+80$ mV, 2–5 s) in normal solution. In the presence of Bay K 8644 preconditioning large positive polarization further slowed deactivation of the tail current. The tail current could be fitted with a sum of two exponential terms. The time constant of the slower decay component (τ_{slow}) was approximately 30–50 ms. As the duration of the large polarizing step (at +80 mV) was increased (from 200 to 1800 ms, by 400 ms increments), the amplitude of the tail current progressively increased. During the experiments the ratio of the amplitudes of the slow- to the fast-decaying component increased; the fast-decay time constant (τ_{fast}) was increased (from 4 to 10 ms), while τ_{slow} was relatively stable.

We have described three types of slow tail currents induced by combinations of large depolarization and Ca^{2+} agonists. Although many complicated models are possible, the formation of these three tail current components could be explained by a simple hypothesis that Ca^{2+} agonist-binding Ca^{2+} channels also have two open states: $C^*–O_1^*–O_2^*$ (* indicates channel states bound with Ca^{2+} agonists). The transition of the Ca^{2+} channel from O_1^* to C^* state is presumably slower than that from O_1 to C seen in normal solution, and subsequently, slow tail currents ($\tau = 3$–5 ms) are induced in the presence of Ca^{2+} channel agonists. Likewise, the O_2 to O_1 transition is slowed by binding Ca^{2+} agonists (the O_2^* to O_1^* transition corresponding to the slowest decay time constant (τ_{slow}), 30–50 ms). The increase in τ_{fast} as the duration of large depolarization increases, is probably due to the relative similarities of the time constants for the O_1^* to C^* (3–5 ms) and O_2 to O_1 transitions (10–15 ms). The two components of the tail currents can be fitted with a single exponential. (τ_{fast} would increase as the population of O_2 increases during large polarizations).

Interaction of Ca^{2+} agonist and antagonist was also examined. In the presence of Bay K 8644, a test potential of 0 mV preceded by large conditioning step (+80 mV, 5 s) was repeated. When nifedipine was added to the bathing solution, the amplitudes of the test and tail currents were reduced by proportionally the same degree. However, the decay time course (half decay time or τ_{slow}) was stable after application of nifedipine, despite the reduction in the amplitude. Taken together, we could explain all results by combining mode gating, which is often used to explain modulation of Ca current by Ca^{2+} agonists, and long open state induced by large depolarization (Figure 2): both mode 1 and mode 2 have a corresponding second open state; Ca^{2+} channels are transferred among the three modes with Ca^{2+} agonists and antagonists. As Bay K 8644 transferred the Ca^{2+} channels to mode 2, very slow deactivating tail current is induced after large depolarization due to O_2^* to O_1^* transition. Addition of nifedipine further transferred the Ca^{2+} channels to mode 0, but some channels remain in mode 2. Thus, only the magnitude of Ca^{2+} current is affected by nifedipine. In this model, it may be noteworthy that long channel opening induced by large depolarization is distinct from so-called 'mode gating' mechanism, and that these two mechanisms separately induce long opening of Ca^{2+} channels: i.e. there are four open states. Also, mode 1 and mode 2 may be divided into submodes: mode 1 ($C–O_1$ and $C–O_2$); mode 2 ($C^*–O^*_1$ and $C^*–O^*_2$).

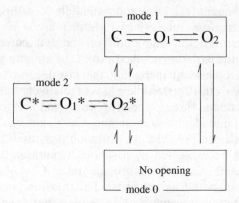

Figure 2 A possible kinetic scheme combining 'mode' gating and the second open state induced by a large positive polarization. There are three modes: mode 0 (null open mode, unavailable for opening) favoured by Ca^{2+} antagonists; mode 1 (normal open mode, brief opening); mode 2 (long-lasting channel opening) favoured by Ca^{2+} agonists. Both mode 1 and 2 have two open states. It is assumed that both of the transitions from O_2 to O_1 and from O_1 to C in mode 1 are faster than those in mode 2.

Single channel recording was undertaken to provide direct evidence for multiple open states of (L-type) Ca^{2+} channels. When no Ca^{2+} agonist was contained in the patch pipette (50 mM Ba^{2+} as a charge carrier), conditioned and unconditioned test pulses were alternately applied. Delayed closure of unitary Ca^{2+} channel current was observed only after preconditioning by a large positive polarization. With Bay K 8644 in the pipette, closure of Ca^{2+} channels was also delayed by a large preconditioning positive polarization. When the patch pipette contained more than 20 channels, the tail current of summation of unitary Ca^{2+} current was similar to that seen in whole-cell recording. The time constant obtained by fitting the summed unitary tail current seen after large positive polarization corresponded to the values for τ_{slow}.

POSSIBLE UNDERLYING MECHANISMS

Long channel opening induced by large positive polarization seems to be distinct from 'mode 2 gating'. What mechanism is responsible to the long open state (O_2)? In adrenal chromaffin cells it has been reported that voltage-dependent phosphorylation occurs during preconditioning large depolarizations and potentiates Ca^{2+} currents subsequently evoked (Artalejo *et al.*, 1992). We examined this possibility in our cells, guinea pig detrusor cells.

When the patch pipette contained ATP-γS, a nonhydrolysable ATP analogue, test depolarizing steps (0 mV, 100–200 ms) were repeated at 30 s intervals. In some experiments the test step was preceded by a preconditioning positive polarization (+80 mV, 5 s). After preconditioning by a large positive polarization, the slow deactivating tail currents were the same as seen when no ATP-γS was in the pipette. The Ca^{2+} current subsequently evoked by a simple test depolarization (30 s later) was not accompanied by slow tail current, suggesting that voltage-dependent phosphorylation is not a mechanism which induces the second open state during large depolarization. When a high concentration (100 μM) of H-7, which generally inhibits kinases, was applied to the bathing solution, a paired pulse protocol was applied: unconditioned and conditioned test depolarizations were repeated alternately. Even in the presence of H-7, slow tail currents were observed after preconditioning positive polarizations. In cardiac myocytes it has been reported that frequency-dependent potentiation of Ca^{2+} current is caused by cyclic AMP and Ca^{2+}-related phosphorylation mechanisms (Tiaho et al., 1994). The possibility that this mechanism may play a role in tail current formation was tested by reducing the interval between depolarizations (to 0.2 and 1Hz). However, only reduction of the inward Ca^{2+} current was seen in our cells (with no slow tail). Thus, the long open state does not appear to be caused by phosphorylation-like chemical reactions. The transition pathway from the normal to second open state is probably a feature of the physical structure of the Ca^{2+} channels themselves.

Molecular biology has revealed that α-subunits of voltage-sensitive Ca^{2+} channels have a fourfold internal repeat with positively charged amino acids in the S4 segment of each repeat. This charged region may act as an voltage sensor (summarized by Hille, 1992). In the Hodgkin & Huxley (HH) model (Hodgkin & Huxley, 1952), which is widely accepted as a standard description of channel current, each voltage sensor takes either an open or closed position. If we simply incorporate the findings of molecular biology into the HH model, we obtain a prediction of four closed states (which are based on a combination of open and closed positions of the four voltage sensors), but only one open state (all voltage sensors in the open position). Using classical theory, it seems difficult to account for the formation of multiple open states.

However, there is evidence of irregularities in the placing of the charged amino acids of the voltage sensors (Hille, 1992). Other parts of the channel protein, e.g. IS6 in the α-subunit and β-subunit itself, may also contribute to the irregularities. These irregularities may allow the voltage sensors to have another open state. An analogous situation is provided by nuclear magnetic resonance theory and the formation of magnetization by spinning nuclei in a magnetic field. Atoms in which charge is symmetrically distributed around the nucleus create only a simple magnetic dipole, whereas nuclei with nonuniformly distributed charge result in multi moments and consequently have more than two energy levels (Kemp, 1986). The voltage sensors in Ca^{2+} channels may behave as described in the latter case. Thus, the kinetic scheme of the Ca^{2+} channels might be expressed like an energy scheme (Figure 3).

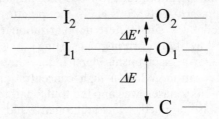

Figure 3 Possible energy levels of voltage sensors of Ca^{2+} channels. The population of the channel states could be expressed using a Boltzmann equation:

e.g. $O_2 (+ I_2) / O_1 (+ I_1) = \exp(-\Delta E'/kT)$.

In conclusion, we propose the presence of multiple open states of Ca^{2+} channels. Ordinary depolarizations transfer Ca^{2+} channels mainly to the normal open state (O_1). The second, long open state is induced by large positive polarizations. However, during ordinary depolarizations and even at resting potentials, a small number of channels may undertake a transition from O_1 to O_2 perhaps governed by the Boltzmann distribution. As smooth muscle commonly shows slow and/or tonic contractions, we can postulate that although the population of Ca^{2+} channels in the second open state is very small, the noninactivating characteristics of the open state may give an important physiological role in smooth muscle. Also, differences in the availability of multiple open states of the Ca^{2+} channels may be important in determining the varieties of contractile behaviour seen in different smooth muscles and under different physiological and pathophysiological conditions.

REFERENCES

Aaronson, P.I., Bolton, T.B., Lang, R.J. & MacKenzie, I. (1988). Calcium currents in single isolated smooth muscle cells from the rabbit ear artery in normal-calcium and high-barium solutions. *J. Physiol.* **405**, 57–75.

Artalejo, C.R., Rossie, S., Perlman, R.L. & Fox, A.P. (1992). Voltage-dependent phosphorylation may recruit Ca^{2+} current facilitation in chromaffin cells. *Nature* **358**, 63–66.

Ganitkevich, V.Ya. & Isenberg, G. (1991). Depolarization mediated intracellular calcium transients in isolated smooth muscle cells of guinea pig urinary bladder. *J. Physiol.* **435**, 187–205.

Hess, P., Lansman, J.B. & Tsien, R.W. (1984). Different modes of Ca channel gating behaviour favoured by dihydropyridine Ca agonists and antagonists. *Nature* **311**, 538–544.

Hille, B. (1992). *Ionic Channels of Excitable Membranes.* Sinauer Associates Inc., Sunderland, Massachusetts.

Hodgkin, A.L. & Huxley, A.F. (1952). A quantitative description of membrane current and its application of conduction and excitation in nerve. *J. Physiol.* **117**, 500–544.

Hoshi, T. & Smith, S.J. (1987). Large depolarization induces long openings of voltage-dependent calcium channels in adrenal chromaffin cells. *J. Neurosci.* **7**, 571–580.

Imaizumi, Y., Muraki, K. & Watanabe, M. (1991). Measurement of noninactivating Ca current in smooth muscle cells. *Methods Neurosci.* **4**, 44–60.

Kemp, W. (1986). The fundamental basis of magnetic resonance. In *NMR in Chemistry: A Multinuclear Introduction*, pp. 14–28. The Macmillan Press, London.

Klöckner, U. & Isenberg, G. (1985). Calcium currents of cesium loaded isolated smooth muscle cells (urinary bladder of guinea pig). *Pflügers Arch.* **405**, 340–348.

Langton, P.D. & Standen, N.B. (1993). Calcium currents elicited by voltage steps and steady voltages in myocytes isolated from the rat basilar artery. *J. Physiol.* **469**, 535–548.

Nakayama, S. (1993). Effects of excitatory neurotransmitters on Ca^{2+} channel current in smooth muscle cells isolated from guinea pig urinary bladder. *Br. J. Pharmacol.* **110**, 317–325.

Nakayama, S. & Brading., A.F. (1993a). Evidence for multiple open states of the Ca^{2+} channels in smooth muscle cells isolated from the guinea pig detrusor. *J. Physiol.* **471**, 87–105.

Nakayama, S., & Brading, A.F. (1993b). Inactivation of the voltage-dependent Ca^{2+} channel current in smooth muscle cells isolated from the guinea pig detrusor. *J. Physiol.* **471**, 107–127.

Nakayama, S. & Brading, A.F. (1995a). Interaction of Ca^{2+} agonist and depolarization on Ca^{2+} channel current in guinea pig detrusor cells. *J. Gen. Physiol.* **106**, 1211–1224.

Nakayama, S. & Brading, A.F. (1995b). Possible contribution of a long channel open state to non-inactivating Ca^{2+} current in detrusor cells. *Am. J. Physiol.* **269**, C48–54.

Pelzer, D., Pelzer, S. & McDonald, T.F. (1990). Properties and regulation of calcium channels in muscle cells. *Rev. Physiol. Biochem. Pharmacol.* **114**, 107–207.

Pietrobon, D & Hess, P. (1990). Novel mechanism of voltage-dependent gating in L-type calcium channels. *Nature* **346**, 651–655.

Tiaho, F., Piot, C., Nargeot, J. & Richard, S. (1994). Regulation of the frequency-dependent facilitation of L-type Ca^{2+} currents in rat ventricular myocytes. *J. Physiol.* **477**: 237–252.

3

Noradrenaline-induced Ca-channel Current Modulation in Smooth Muscles

M. WATANABE*
Y. IMAIZUMI*
K. MURAKI*
T. B. BOLTON**

*Department of Chemical Pharmacology,
Faculty of Pharmaceutical Sciences,
Nagoya City University, Nagoya, Japan

**Department of Pharmacology and Clinical Pharmacology,
St. George's Hospital Medical School,
London, UK

INTRODUCTION

Voltage-dependent Ca channel activity can be regulated by neuro-transmitters and hormones (Hofmann *et al.*, 1987; Dolphin, 1990). Although the modulation of Ca channel activity by noradrenaline (NA) has been studied in several smooth muscle cells, the effects vary widely depending on the tissue and species employed. In this article, modulations of voltage-dependent Ca channel current by NA in guinea pig (g.p.) vas deferens, ureter and taenia caeci cells are highlighted and compared with those by NA and other substances in vascular and other visceral smooth muscle cells.

METHODS

Single g.p. vas deferens, ureter and taenia caeci cells were dispersed using collagenase as previously described (Imaizumi *et al.*, 1989, 1991). Membrane currents were recorded with standard whole-cell voltage-clamp method. Experiments were carried out at $23 \pm 2°C$ in a physiological salt solution. To record Ba current the through Ca channel, external Ca^{2+} was replaced with equimolar Ba^{2+}. Pipette solution contained mainly 140 mM CsCl and 4 to 5 mM EGTA unless stated otherwise.

SMOOTH MUSCLE EXCITATION
ISBN 0-12-112360-X

RESULTS AND DISCUSSION

Inhibition of voltage-dependent Ca channel current by NA

It has been reported that some excitatory substances, such as NA, histamine (His), ATP and carbachol (CCh) inhibit voltage-dependent Ca channel current (I_{Ca}) in some smooth muscle cells (rabbit ear artery, Droogmans *et al.*, 1987; rabbit portal vein, Xiong *et al.*, 1991; g.p. ileum, Beech, 1993, Unno *et al.*, 1995; g.p. urinary bladder, Nakayama, 1993). NA can also reduce I_{Ca} in g.p. vas deferens smooth muscle cells (Figure 1, Imaizumi *et al.*, 1991). The cell was depolarized every 2 s from the holding potential of -60 to $+20$ mV for 50 ms. The peak inward currents are denoted by dots. The application of 10 μM NA decreased I_{Ca} and induced a phasic inward current.

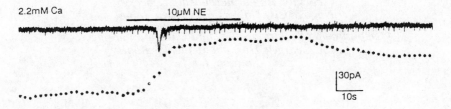

Figure 1 Effect of 10 μM NA on I_{Ca} in single smooth muscle cells isolated from vas deferens of the guinea pig in solution containing 2.2 mM Ca. (From Imaizumi *et al.*, 1991, with permission of the American Physiological Society).

Inhibitory mechanisms can be divided into Ca-dependent and Ca-independent types. In g.p. ileal cells, a rapid and transient suppression of I_{Ca} by His and CCh was followed by a sustained suppression (Beech, 1993; Unno *et al.*, 1995). The transient inhibition of I_{Ca} was Ca-dependent and could be caused by Ca-dependent Ca channel inactivation via IP_3(inositol, 1,4,5 trisphosphate)-induced Ca release (Komori & Bolton, 1991). The following observations support this view: heparin, which inhibits the interaction between IP_3 and its receptor, blocked the transient inhibition (Beech, 1993; Unno *et al.*, 1995); flash photolysis of caged IP_3 induced a transient inhibition of I_{Ca} in rabbit jejunum cell (Komori & Bolton, 1991). The sustained inhibitions of I_{Ca} in g.p. ileal cells by His and CCh were also Ca-dependent as strong buffering of intracellular Ca concentration by EGTA or BAPTA abolished the inhibitory effect (Beech, 1993; Unno *et al.*, 1995). However, the sustained inhibition was heparin-resistant, suggesting that IP_3 is not involved in the response (Beech, 1993; Unno *et al.*, 1995). Sustained ATP-induced inhibition of I_{Ca} in rabbit portal vein exhibited some Ca-dependence; suppression was reduced in the presence of a high concentration of EGTA

(20 mM) in the pipette solution (Xiong *et al.*, 1991). A part of the suppression of I_{Ca} by NA observed in g.p. vas deferens was Ca-mediated because the inhibition of Ba current through Ca channel (I_{Ba}) was smaller than that of I_{Ca}. As shown in Figure 2, decrease of I_{Ca} in the presence of NA was significantly different from that of I_{Ba} (first versus second column, $P < 0.01$; Imaizumi *et al.*, 1991). Transient Ca-mediated inhibition of I_{Ca} by NA via IP$_3$-formation might be also present in g.p. vas deferens although systematical investigations have not been carried out. A large part of the inhibition of I_{Ca} by NA in g.p. vas deferens was, however, Ca-independent because I_{Ba} was also decreased during the application of NA (Figure 2, second column); 20 mM EGTA in the pipette solution had little effect on the I_{Ba} suppression. Conversely, in g.p. ureter smooth muscle cells, I_{Ca} which was recorded using a pipette solution of pCa 7.5 was decreased by application of NA (Muraki *et al.*, 1994b). The inhibition was, however, totally heparin-sensitive and Ca-dependent, suggesting that Ca^{2+}, which is released from the sarcoplasmic reticulum (SR) by IP$_3$-formation through adrenoceptor activation, inactivates Ca channel activity.

There are several observations that support the view that some GTP-binding protein (G-protein) is necessary for the inhibition of I_{Ca} by these substances (see Figure 2; Droogmans *et al.*, 1987; Imaizumi *et al.*, 1991; Xiong *et al.*, 1991; Beech, 1993; Unno *et al.*, 1995); perfusion of GDP-βS in the pipette almost abolished the NA, His, ATP or CCh-induced I_{Ca} inhibition; intracellular GTP-γS or Gpp(NH)p induced an irreversible suppression of I_{Ca}. Figure 2 shows the summarized data about the effects of

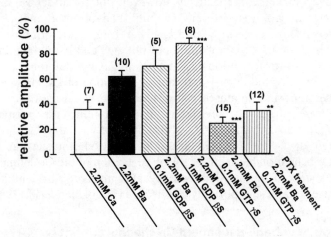

Figure 2 Summarized data on effects of NA on I_{Ca} and I_{Ba} obtained in g.p. vas deferens under various experimental conditions. Ordinate: relative amplitude of I_{Ca} or I_{Ba} after treatment with 10 µM NA vs. that before the treatment; ** and *** indicate statistical significance versus closed column (2.2 mM Ba) at levels of $P < 0.01$ and $P < 0.001$, respectively. (From Imaizumi *et al.*, 1991, with permission of the American Physiological Society).

NA on I_{Ca} and I_{Ba} under various conditions in g.p. vas deferens smooth muscle cells (Imaizumi et al., 1991). The I_{Ca} and I_{Ba} were elicited upon depolarization from -60 to $0\,mV$ at 0.067 Hz. Internal application of GDP-βS or GTP-γS prevented I_{Ba} suppression by NA (second versus third and fourth columns) and caused more potent inhibition of I_{Ba}, respectively (second versus fifth column). In addition, the effects of pertussis toxin (PTX), which ADP-ribosylates the α-subunit of some G-proteins and makes them inactive in signal transduction (Gilman, 1987), were examined. PTX treatment had no significant effect on I_{Ba} inhibition by NA (fifth versus sixth column). The inhibition of I_{Ba} by CCh in g.p. ileum was also PTX-resistant (Unno et al., 1995). In rabbit portal vein, 40 to 50 % I_{Ba} suppression by ATP was, however, PTX-sensitive. To identify how many G-proteins are involved in I_{Ca} inhibition and which processes intervene between receptor activation and Ca channel inhibition, including G-protein activation (direct or indirect regulation by G-protein; Yatani & Brown, 1989), further investigation is required.

It is well known that $α_1$-adrenoceptor stimulation activates not only phospholipase C (PLC) but also phospholipase A_2 which liberates arachidonic acid (AA) from membrane lipid. Therefore, AA and its metabolites are candidates for second messengers involved in the I_{Ca} inhibition by NA in g.p. vas deferens. It has been also reported that AA inhibits I_{Ca} in rabbit intestinal smooth muscle cells (Shimada & Somlyo, 1992). Pretreatment with cyclo-oxygenase and lipo-oxygenase inhibitors, such as indomethacin, and mepacrine, nordihydroguaiaretic acid and p-bromophenacyl bromide, respectively, however, did not affect the inhibition of I_{Ca} by NA in g.p. vas deferens (unpublished observations). In rabbit intestine, AA itself decreased I_{Ca} and I_{Ba}. Therefore, a role of phospholipase A_2 in the inhibition of I_{Ca} is not ruled out but AA and its metabolites seem unlikely mediators for inhibition of I_{Ca} by NA in g.p. vas deferens.

The receptor activated by NA and causing inhibition of Ca channel current in g.p. vas deferens smooth muscle cell was mainly an $α_1$-adrenoceptor because prazosin (Praz) effectively prevented the inhibition and phenylephrine decreased I_{Ba} (Imaizumi et al., 1991). Application of yohimbin had little effect on inhibition of I_{Ca} by NA (Imaizumi et al., 1991), suggesting that $α_2$-adrenoceptor activation has a minor role in regulation of the Ca channel in g.p. vas deferens smooth muscle. The adrenoceptor involved in I_{Ca} inhibition in rabbit ear artery was also reportedly $α_1$-selective (Droogmans et al., 1987).

Potentiation of voltage-dependent Ca channel current by NA

Potentiation of Ca channel current by NA has been observed in several types of smooth muscle cells (rat portal vein, Loirand et al., 1990, Leprêtre & Mironneau, 1994; rabbit mesenteric artery, Nelson et al., 1988; rabbit ear artery, Benham & Tsien, 1988; rabbit saphenous artery, Oike et al., 1992; g.p.

taenia caeci, Muraki *et al.*, 1993; g.p. ureter, Muraki *et al.*, 1994b). Figure 3 shows the effects of NA on I_{Ba} in g.p. ureter smooth muscle cell. The cell was depolarized every 15 s from -60 to $+30\,mV$ using a ramp pulse protocol of $91\,mV\,s^{-1}$. External 2.2 mM Ca^{2+} was replaced with equimolar Ba^{2+}. Application of 10 μM NA potentiated the I_{Ba} by 35.5 ± 3.9 % ($n = 4$, Figure 3, left panel, ●). The increase in I_{Ba} at 0 mV was almost removed by washout of NA (Figure 3, left panel, ○). The response is mediated by activation of α_1-adrenoceptor since phenylephrine also increased the I_{Ba} (Figure 3, right panel, ●) and a large part of the potentiation of I_{Ba} by NA ($\sim$80 %) was abolished in the presence of Praz. NA-induced I_{Ba} potentiation in rat portal vein was also Praz-sensitive, indicating that an α_1-adrenoceptor is involved in the response (Loirand *et al.*, 1990). A recent study, however, indicates that clonidine, an α_2-selective agonist, also activates I_{Ba} in rat portal vein (Leprêtre & Mironneau, 1994).

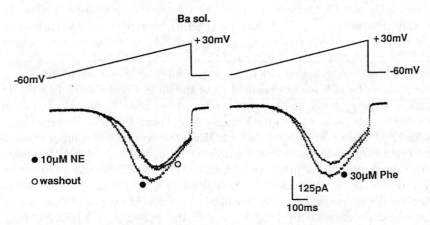

Figure 3   Effects of 10 μM NA (left) and 30 μM Phe (right) on I_{Ba} in ureter smooth muscle cells. Current traces before and during (●) application of NA and Phe, and after washout of NA (○) were superimposed.

The potentiation of I_{Ba} observed in g.p. ureter was abolished by intracellular perfusion of GDP-βS, suggesting that some G-protein is involved in the response (Muraki *et al.*, 1994b). Similar block in the presence of internal GDP-βS of the potentiation of Ca channel current by various substances has been reported in several smooth muscles (Loirand *et al.*, 1990; Ohya & Sperelakis, 1991; Oike *et al.*, 1992; Welling *et al.*, 1992; Muraki *et al.*, 1994b). The potentiation of I_{Ba} by NA via α_1-adrenoceptor, angiotensin II (Ang II) and His observed in rat and g.p. portal vein, and rabbit saphenous artery, respectively, were all PTX-insensitive. However, the effects of GTP-γS on the potentiation of Ca channel current are complicated. In g.p. ureter and bovine trachea, sustained potentiation of I_{Ba} and I_{Ca} even after washout of NA or isoprenaline (Iso) was observed in the presence of GTP-γS (Welling *et al.*, 1992; Muraki *et al.*, 1994b). After internal perfusion of GTP-γS, the potentiation of I_{Ba} by His in rabbit saphenous artery was converted to an inhibition (Oike *et al.*, 1992). Increase in I_{Ba} by NA and Ang II observed in rat and g.p. portal vein, respectively, was attenuated depending on the concentration of GTP-γS and almost abolished in the presence of 1 mM GTP-γS. These results show that several types of G-protein are involved in I_{Ca}-modulations.

Stimulation of α_1-adrenoceptor results in the hydrolysis of a membrane phospholipid, phosphatidylinositol 4,5-bisphosphate, by PLC with the consequent generation of two second-messengers; IP_3 and diacylglycerol (DAG). The IP_3 can release Ca^{2+} from SR and subsequently the Ca ions inactivate Ca channel activity (Komori & Bolton, 1991). Therefore, protein kinase C (PKC) which is activated by DAG is a candidate for NA-induced potentiation of Ca channel current. In rat portal vein, increases in I_{Ba} produced by phorbol 12, 13-dibutyrate (PDBu), an exogenous PKC activator, and by NA were not additive, indicating that PKC is the second messenger mediating the NA-induced I_{Ba} potentiation (Loirand *et al.*, 1990). In g.p. ureter, however, whether PKC is a second messenger involved in I_{Ba} potentiation by NA is not conclusive. As shown in Figure 4, 0.3 μM PDBu increased the I_{Ba} by 17.8±4.8 % in four out of five cells. I_{Ba} was elicited upon depolarization from -60 to 0 mV every 15 s. Three series of current traces before and during the application of PDBu were averaged and superimposed in Figure 4a. I_{Ba} potentiation was not removed by washout of PDBu (Figure 4b). Conversely, in the presence of 1 mM GDP-βS, PDBu had no effect on I_{Ba} (101.2 ± 0.8 % of control, $n = 5$). If PKC is a final second messenger to mediate the I_{Ba} potentiation by NA in g.p. ureter as in rat portal vein, the I_{Ba} should be potentiated by PDBu, even in the presence of GDP-βS. Both stimulatory and inhibitory effects of PKC on Ca channel activity have been reported in smooth muscle cells (Fish *et al.*, 1988, Loirand *et al.*, 1990; Oike *et al.*, 1992; Obara & Yabu, 1993). PKC is a modulator of Ca channel activity which is involved in the signal transduction pathway when PLC is activated by stimulating some receptors including α_1-adrenoceptors.

When the potentiation of Ca channel current by several substances has been examined, most previous studies were carried out under unphysiological conditions; the pipette solution contained a high concentration of EGTA; external Ca was replaced with Ba. In our recent approach to elucidate the mechanisms of Ca channel modulation by NA in g.p. ureter, the pipette solution was adjusted to pCa 7.5 using 1.78 mM EGTA and 0.5 mM Ca (Muraki *et al.*, 1994b). Under these conditions, I_{Ca} recorded upon depolarization from -50 to 0 mV was transiently inhibited by application of NA. In contrast, when cells were perfused internally with

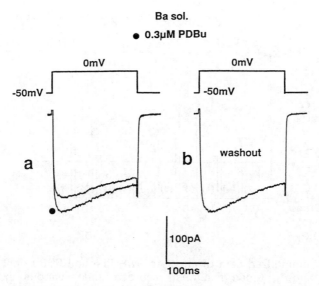

Figure 4 Effects of PDBu on I_{Ba} recorded from ureter smooth muscle cell. Three series of current traces before and during (●) application of 0.3 μM PDBu (a), and after washout of PDBu (b) were averaged and are shown.

3 mg ml^{-1} heparin, inhibition of I_{Ca} by 10 μM NA was converted to potentiation. In Figure 5, effects of NA, Phe and PDBu on I_{Ca} and I_{Ba} obtained from g.p. ureter cells under various experimental conditions are summarized. NA increased I_{Ba} in concentration-dependent manner (columns 1–3). Although I_{Ca} obtained under conditions without heparin was inhibited by NA, transiently (27.3±5.0% decrease, $n = 4$, P) and sustainedly (17.8±8.4% decrease, $n = 4$, S), NA slightly potentiated I_{Ca} in the presence of 3 mg ml^{-1} heparin (8.0 ± 2.4% increase, $n = 4$). Internal perfusion with heparin had a tendency to increase the potentiation of I_{Ba} by NA but the response varied widely from cell to cell (189±43 % of control, $n = 3$, column 4). Two mechanisms (inhibition and potentiation), therefore, are involved in the regulation of Ca channel activity by NA in ureter smooth muscle cells. Both mechanisms may be functional in Ca channel regulation under physiological conditions in ureter cells since Ca-dependent Ca channel inactivation is minor compared with other types of smooth muscle cell (Imaizumi et al., 1989; Lang, 1990). A similar dual regulation of Ca channel activity by NA has been reported in rat portal vein cells (Pacaud et al., 1987; Loirand et al., 1990). In rat portal vein, although Ca-dependent Ca channel inactivation is dominant under physiological conditions (Pacaud et al., 1987; Loirand et al., 1989), Ca channel activity may be increased under conditions in which the potentiation of I_{Ba} is observed; to clarify the physiological significance of the dual regulation of I_{Ca}, further investigations are necessary.

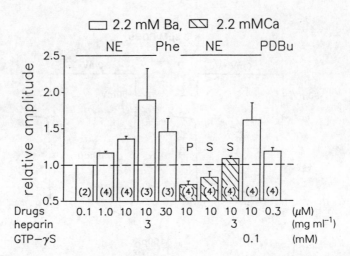

Figure 5 Summarized data of effects of NA, Phe and PDBu on I_{Ca} (hatched colummns) and I_{Ba} (open columns) recorded under various experimental conditions. I_{Ca} and I_{Ba} were elicited upon depolarization to 0 mV. The pCa in the pipette solution was adjusted to 7.5 using 1.78 mM EGTA and 0.5 mM $CaCl_2$. 'P' and 'S' indicate the phasic and sustained inhibition component of I_{Ca}. ordinate: relative amplitude of I_{Ba} and I_{Ca} before and after application of NA, Phe and PDBu. Numbers in parentheses show the number of cells examined. (Muraki *et al.*, 1994b, with permission of The Physiological Society).

Ca channel modulation mediated by an atypical adrenoceptor

Since Ahlquist's division of adrenoceptors into α and β groups, adrenoceptors have been further subdivided into α_1 and α_2, and β_1, β_2 and β_3 varieties (Ahlquist, 1948). These subclassifications have been carried out using the selective novel agonists and antagonists, and molecular biological techniques. It is well known that these adrenoceptors are functionally expressed on smooth muscles. However, some atypical responses mediating by adrenoceptors which do not belong to conventional classifications have been revealed. A γ-receptor was proposed by Hirst & Nield (1980) as an atypical adrenoceptor at the neuromuscular junctional region of post-sympathetic nerve. Modulation of Ca channel current by atypical adreno-ceptor activation has been found in rabbit ear artery, rat aorta and g.p. taenia caeci (Benham & Tsien, 1988; Serebryakov & Takeda, 1992; Muraki *et al.*, 1993, 1994a). I_{Ba} obtained from rabbit ear artery was augmented by NA (Benham & Tsien, 1988). The potentiation, however, was phentolamine (Phent), Praz and propranolol (Prop) resistant. Adrenaline (Adr) also produced an increase in I_{Ba} but Phe was not effective. In rat aortic smooth muscle cells, NA and Adr but not Phe caused a decrease in the transient type

Ca channel current (I_{Ca-T}) (Serebryakov & Takeda, 1992). Neither Phent, Praz nor Prop had any effect on the I_{Ca-T} inhibition by NA.

I_{Ca} recorded from g.p. taenia caeci cells was potentiated by NA, Adr and Iso (Muraki et al., 1994a). The EC_{50} values for NA, Adr and Iso to potentiate I_{Ca} were calculated to be 24, 58 and 42 nM, respectively, and these were not significantly different ($P > 0.05$). The structure–activity relationship was systematically investigated and is shown in Table 1. Two isomers (−) and (+), and racemic mixtures (±) of NA, Adr and Iso were all equipotent. Further observations showed the importance of the 3-OH, 4-OH catechol nucleus for activity, that the N-substitute on the molecule was not important and that the β-OH group and substitution of a group for hydrogen on the α-carbon were not important. Finally, catechol (3,4, dihydroxybenzene) was active at this receptor and it was found that catechol and catecholamines

Table 1 Relative potencies of various sympathomimetics and related compounds to potentiate voltage-dependent Ca current in g.p. taenia caeci cells. Relative potencies were obtained by application of equal concentrations to the same cell of the drug and (-) or (±)Iso. [Muraki et al., 1994a, with permission of Macmillan Press Limited]

4	3	β	α	NH			Relative potency
OH	OH	OH	H	CH(CH₃)₂	(−)	Isoprenaline β	1.00
					(±)	Isoprenaline β	1.00
					(+)	Isoprenaline β	1.2±0.11
OH	OH	OH	H	CH₃	(−)	Adrenaline αβ	1.1±0.11
					(±)	Adrenaline αβ	0.91±0.06
OH	OH	OH	H	H	(−)	Noradrenaline αβ₁	0.91±0.13
					(±)	Noradrenaline αβ₁	0.88±0.03
OH	OH	H	H	H		Dopamine	1.0±0.09
OH	OH	OH	CH₂CH₃	CH(CH₃)₂	(±)	Isoetharine β	1.0±0.07
OH	OH	H	COOH	H		L-Dopa	1.2±0.18
OH	OH	–	–	–		Catechol	0.96±0.11
H	OH	OH	H	CH₃	(−)	Phenylephrine α	>>0.001
5OCH₃	2OCH₃	OH	CH₃	H	(±)	Methoxamine α	>>0.001
5OH	OH	OH	H	C(CH₃)₃	(±)	Terbutaline β₂	>>0.001
OH	CH₂OH	OH	H	C(CH₃)₃	(±)	Salbutamol β₂	0.1–0.01§
OH	Ring	OH	C₂H₅	CH(CH₃)₂	(±)	Procaterol β₂	0.03–0.001§
H	Cl	OH	H	Complex	(±)	BRL 37344 β₃	0.0003
H	H	Complex				ICI 215001 β₃	0.0003
OH	H	H	H	H		Tyramine	>>0.001

§ Partial agonists.

were equipotent and, in maximally effective concentrations, the effects of catechol and Iso to potentiate I_{Ca} were not additive. Various adrenoceptor blocking agents were tested for their antagonism at this receptor. ($\pm$) and ($-$) Prop, atenolol, Phent, CGP 20712A, ICI 118551 and dihydroergotamine were all ineffective. The increase in I_{Ca} produced by dopamine or Iso was also unaffected by dopamine receptor antagonists, haloperidol and flupenthixol. The inability of Phe to increase I_{Ca} and lack of effects of various antagonists on NA-induced I_{Ca} potentiation in g.p. taenia caeci suggest that a similar type of receptor to that in rabbit ear artery and rat aorta might be involved in the response. The physiological significance of this receptor is not clear. It has been reported that collagenase treatment eliminates the electrical responses of g.p. taenia caeci to catecholamines (Tokuno & Tomita, 1987), therefore, intrinsic receptors or Ca channels on smooth muscles may be modified by enzymes and a molecular site may be revealed which can interact with some agonists but which is not accessible for antagonists.

CONCLUSION

The inhibition of I_{Ca} by NA observed in g.p. vas deferens was mediated via some PTX-insensitive G-protein and was mostly Ca-insensitive. Similar I_{Ca} inhibition mediated by G-protein was observed in g.p. ileum, rabbit portal vein and ear artery when His, CCh, ATP and NA were applied, respectively (Droogmans *et al.*, 1987; Xiong *et al.*, 1991; Beech, 1993; Unno *et al.*, 1995,). The precise mechanism and the second messengers involved, or channels and G-protein directly coupled, however, have not been identified. The mechanism of the potentiation of I_{Ba} by NA in g.p. ureter has also not been determined, although activation of some G-protein is involved in the mechanism. As indicated in rat portal vein myocytes (Loirand *et al.*, 1990), a PKC cannot be ruled out as the candidate for the final second-messenger to potentiate I_{Ba} in ureter cell. Ca^{2+} released from SR by IP_3 via activation of adrenoceptor by NA in g.p. ureter partially inactivates Ca channel activity and subsequently I_{Ca} is transiently inhibited in the presence of NA. This dual (stimulatory and inhibitory) regulation of Ca channels by a neurotransmitter is important as a positive and negative feedback system to control cell-excitability. The potentiation of I_{Ca} in g.p. taenia caeci by some catecholamines, including catechol, might be mediated via an atypical adrenoceptor. To clarify its physiological function and the mechanism of the potentiation, further studies are necessary.

It has been shown that the modulation of voltage-dependent Ca channel current by NA varied widely depending upon the smooth muscle tissue and upon the experimental conditions. To understand how I_{Ca} is functionally regulated by NA and neurotransmitters, it is important to maintain physiological conditions. Therefore, a weak buffering system in the pipette solution, or a nondialysis technique such as perforated patch-clamp, was used along with the perfusion of physiological salt solution. These conditions are suitable to study regulation of the ion channel by neurotransmitters.

ACKNOWLEDGMENTS

This work was supported by a grant from the Fujisawa Foundation, the Japanese Ministry of Education, Science and Culture, the Japanese Society for the Promotion of Science and the British MRC for M.W., Y.I., K.M. and T.B.B., respectively.

REFERENCES

Ahlquist, R.P. (1948). A study of the adrenotropic receptors. *Am. J. Physiol.* **153**, 586–600.

Beech, D.J. (1993). Inhibitory effects of histamine and bradykinin on calcium current in smooth muscle cells isolated from guinea pig ileum. *J. Physiol.* **463**, 565–583.

Benham, C.D. & Tsien, R.W. (1988). Noradrenaline modulation of calcium channels in single smooth muscle cells from rabbit ear artery. *J. Physiol.* **404**, 767–784.

Dolphin, A.C. (1990). G protein modulation of calcium currents in neurons. *Annu. Rev. Physiol.* **52**, 243–255.

Droogmans, G., Declerck, I. & Casteels, R. (1987). Effect of adrenergic agonists on Ca^{2+}-channel currents in single vascular smooth muscle cells. *Pflügers Archiv.* **409**, 7–12.

Fish, R.D., Sperti, G., Colucci, W.S. & Clapham, D.E. (1988). Phorbol ester increases the dihydropyridine-sensitive calcium conductance in a vascular smooth muscle cell line. *Circ. Res.* **62**, 1049–1054.

Gilman, A.G. (1987). G proteins: transducers of receptor-generated signals. *Annu. Rev. Biochem.* **56**, 615–649.

Hirst, G.D.S. & Nield, T.O. (1980). Evidence for two populations of excitatory receptors for noradrenaline on arteriolar smooth muscle. *Nature* **283**, 767–768.

Hofmann, F., Nastainczyk, W., Rohrkasten, A. & Schneider, T. (1987). Regulation of the L-type calcium channel. *Trends Pharmacolog. Sci.* **8**, 393–398.

Imaizumi, Y., Muraki, K. & Watanabe, M. (1989). Ionic currents in single smooth muscle cells from the ureter of the guinea pig. *J. Physiol.* **411**, 131–159.

Imaizumi, Y., Takeda, M., Muraki, K. & Watanabe, M. (1991). Mechanisms of NE-induced reduction of Ca current in single smooth muscle cells from guinea pig vas deferens. *Am. J. Physiol.* **260**, C17–C25.

Komori, S. & Bolton, T.B. (1991). Inositol trisphosphate releases stored calcium to block voltage-dependent calcium channels in single smooth muscle cells. *Pflügers Archiv.* **418**, 437–441.

Lang, R.J. (1990). The whole-cell Ca^{2+} channel current in single smooth muscle cells of the guinea pig ureter. *J. Physiol.* **423**, 453–473.

Leprêtre, N. and Mirroneau, J. (1994). α_2-Adrenoceptors activate dihydropyridine-sensitive calcium channels via Gi-proteins and protein C in rat portal vein myocites. *Pflügers Archiv.* **429**, 253–261.

Loirand, G., Mironneau, C. & Mironneau, J. & Pacaud, P. (1989). Two types of calcium currents in single smooth muscle cells from rat portal vein. *J. Physiol.* **412**, 333–340.

Loirand, G., Pacaud, P., Mironneau, C. & Mironneau, J. (1990). GTP-binding proteins mediate noradrenaline effects on calcium and chloride currents in rat portal vein myocytes. *J. Physiol.* **428**, 517–529.

Muraki, K., Bolton, T.B., Imaizumi, Y. & Watanabe, M. (1993). Effect of isoprenaline on Ca channel current in single smooth muscle cells isolated from taenia of the guinea pig caecum. *J. Physiol.* **471**, 563–582.

Muraki, K., Bolton, T.B., Imaizumi, Y. & Watanabe, M. (1994a). Receptor for catecholamines responding to catechol which potentiates voltage-dependent calcium current in single cells from guinea pig taenia caeci. *Br. J. Pharmacol.* **111**, 1154–1162.

Muraki, K., Imaizumi, Y. & Watanabe, M. (1994b). Effects of noradrenaline on membrane currents and action potential shape in smooth muscle cells from guinea pig ureter. *J. Physiol.* **481.3**, 617–627.

Nakayama, S. (1993). Effects of excitatory neurotransmitters on Ca channel current in smooth muscle cells isolated from guinea pig urinary bladder. *Br. J. Pharmacol.* **110**, 317–325.

Nelson, M.T., Standen, N.B., Brayden, J.E. & Worley, J.F. (1988). Noradrenaline contracts arteries by activating voltage-dependent calcium channels. *Nature* **336**, 382–385.

Obara, K. & Yabu, H. (1993). Dual effect of phosphatase inhibitors on calcium channels in intestinal smooth muscle cells. *Am. J. Physiol.* **264**, C296–C301.

Ohya, Y. & Sperelakis, N. (1991). Involvement of a GTP-binding protein in stimulating action of angiotensin II on calcium channels in vascular smooth muscle cells. *Circ. Res.* **68**, 763–771.

Oike, M., Kitamura, K. & Kuriyama, H. (1992). Histamine H_3-receptor activation augments voltage-dependent Ca^{2+} current via GTP hydrolysis in rabbit saphenous artery. *J. Physiol.* **448**, 133–152.

Pacaud, P., Loirand, G., Mironneau, C. & Mironneau, J. (1987). Opposing effects of noradrenaline on the two classes of voltage-dependent calcium channels of single vascular smooth muscle cells in short-term primary culture. *Pflügers Archiv.* **410**, 557–559.

Serebryakov, V. & Takeda, K. (1992). Voltage-dependent calcium current and the effects of adrenergic modulation in rat aortic smooth muscle cells. *Phil. Trans. R. Soc. Lond. B.* **337**, 37-47.

Shimada, T. & Somlyo, A.P. (1992). Modulation of voltage-dependent Ca channel current by arachidonic acid and other long-chain fatty acids in rabbit intestinal smooth muscle. *J. Gen. Physiol.* **100**, 27–44.

Tokuno, H. & Tomita, T. (1987). Collagenase eliminates the electrical responses of smooth muscle to catecholamines. *Eur. J. Pharmacol.* **141**, 131–133.

Unno, T., Komori, S. & Ohashi, H. (1995). Inhibitory effect of muscarinic receptor activation on Ca^{2+} channel current in smooth muscle cells of guinea pig ileum. *J. Physiol.* **484**, 567–581.

Welling, A., Feibel, J., Peper, K. & Hofmann, F. (1992). Hormonal regulation of calcium current in freshly isolated airway smooth muscle cells. *Am. J. Physiol.* **262**, L351–L359.

Xiong, Z., Kitamura, K. & Kuriyama, H. (1991). ATP activates cationic currents and modulates the calcium current through GTP-binding protein in rabbit portal vein. *J. Physiol.* **440**, 143–165.

Yatani, A. & Brown, A.M. (1989). Rapid beta-adrenergic modulation of cardiac calcium channel currents by a fast G protein pathway. *Science* **245**, 71–74.

4

Regulation of the Opening of Voltage-gated Ca Channels in Smooth Muscle Cells

D. J. BEECH
D. McHUGH

Department of Pharmacology,
University of Leeds,
Leeds, UK.

The intracellular Ca^{2+} concentration, the primary determinant of the contractile state of smooth muscle cells, is dependent on a balance between Ca^{2+}-release from intracellular stores and Ca^{2+}-influx and Ca^{2+}-efflux across the plasma membrane (reviewed by Missiaen *et al.*, 1992). This review focuses on one mechanism which controls Ca^{2+}-flux across the membrane, the voltage-gated Ca channel; other mechanisms include the Ca^{2+}-ATPase, Na^{+}–Ca^{2+} exchanger, ATP-gated cation channel and a Ca^{2+}-store refilling pathway. Voltage-gated Ca channels enable Ca^{2+}-influx to increase on depolarization, despite the decrease in driving force on Ca^{2+} ions into the cell, and permit a multitude of other proteins which simply regulate the membrane potential to modify Ca^{2+}-entry indirectly. Like many other cell types, smooth muscle cells have low- (LVA) and high- (HVA) voltage-activated Ca channel current components. The HVA current component is present in all smooth muscles investigated to date and there is good evidence that it is carried largely by L-type Ca channels; those that are blocked by nanomolar concentrations of dihydropyridine Ca-antagonists. The central – pore-forming – protein component of the L-type Ca channel appears to be the cloned α_{1C} (CaCh2b) protein (reviewed by Hofmann *et al.*, 1994). In some smooth muscle cells, for example those from coronary artery, there is an LVA current component which is similar to T-type Ca^{2+}-current described in sensory neurones (Ganitkevich & Isenberg, 1991), in others there is a less well defined L/T-intermediate form (Simard, 1991), and in others the LVA

SMOOTH MUSCLE EXCITATION
ISBN 0-12-112360-X

current component is absent (Inoue *et al.*, 1989). We will consider almost exclusively the L-type Ca channel and physiological factors which regulate its opening in the short term.

The cardiac and smooth muscle cell HVA current is blocked by dihydropyridine Ca antagonists, which suggests that both cells express L-type Ca channels. However, although the α_1 proteins of the channels are encoded by the same gene and are 95% identical in primary amino acid sequence, they represent different splice variants (Hofmann *et al.*, 1994). There is accumulating evidence that this alternative splicing affects the channel function. For example, the smooth muscle L-type Ca channels are more sensitive to inhibition by Ca antagonists (Welling *et al.*, 1993a, and references therein). In addition, the regulatory β-subunit (see Membrane Potential section) appears to be different in cardiac and smooth muscles (Hofmann *et al.*, 1994). It is thus not surprising that patch-clamp studies of isolated smooth muscle cells are revealing similarities and differences between the ways in which the openings of the cardiac and smooth muscle channels are regulated. Many regulators have been identified in various smooth muscles which will be loosely categorised under the headings membrane potential, Ca^{2+}, protons, kinases, ATP, and G-proteins. Only selected references have been included and there is emphasis on our findings, in particular on G-protein-coupled receptor mechanisms.

MEMBRANE POTENTIAL

Voltage-gated Ca channels are regulated by the membrane potential, becoming permeable to Ca^{2+} ions in response to depolarization. In smooth muscle cells with HVA but not LVA Ca^{2+}-current, a clear Ca^{2+}-current (I_{Ca}) is elicited when the membrane potential is depolarized to positive of $-40\,mV$. There is no sharp threshold for activation, however, and very low Ca channel opening probabilities in the region of -40 to $-50\,mV$ may be crucial for the Ca^{2+}-influx which underlies arterial myogenic tone (Gollasch *et al.*, 1992). Ca channels switch off on repolarization and also because of voltage-dependent inactivation. Both fast ($t = 0.1$ to $0.15\,s$) and slow ($t = 3$ to $14\,s$) types of voltage-dependent inactivation have been identified in rabbit portal vein cells (Nilius *et al.*, 1994).

Molecular studies have indicated that voltage-dependence is an intrinsic property of the α_1-protein of Ca channels. This protein is thought to be composed of four homologous repeats of six membrane-spanning α-helical domains. On the basis of analogies with other voltage-gated ion channels, it would appear that the fourth membrane-spanning domain of each repeat comprises a voltage-sensor which has positively charged amino acid residues at each turn of the helix moving in the extracellular direction on depolarization (Catterall, 1988). Voltage-dependent inactivation has been suggested to result from a structural rearrangement of amino acid residues in the sixth membrane-spanning domain of the first repeat (Zhang *et al.*, 1994). Auxiliary proteins affect the voltage-dependence of the α_1-protein. The β-subunit (β_3 in smooth muscle) causes a hyperpolarizing shift of activation and inactivation curves and accelerates current kinetics; the α_2/γ-subunit has similar effects, but only on inactivation (Welling *et al.*, 1993b). The β-subunit appears to be a cytoplasmic cytoskeleton-binding protein which interacts directly with a conserved linker region between repeats 1 and 2 of the α_1-protein (Pragnell *et al.*, 1994).

CALCIUM

Inactivation

L-type Ca channels show a current-dependent inactivation, which generally occurs more rapidly than voltage-dependent inactivation (Ganitkevich *et al.*, 1987; Vogalis *et al.*, 1992). The molecular processes underlying the two types of inactivation are separate because, for example, intracellular dialysis with trypsin removes the voltage- but not the current-dependent effect (Obejero-Paz *et al.*, 1991). Current-dependent inactivation reaches a maximum at the peak of the whole-cell I_{Ca}/voltage relationship and is less pronounced if Ba^{2+} or Na^+ ions replace Ca^{2+} as the charge carrier. The inactivation is, therefore, caused by the Ca^{2+} ion itself. The Ca^{2+} ions appear to act at a site very near to the Ca channel protein, perhaps within the pore, because high intracellular concentrations of the Ca^{2+}-chelators BAPTA or EGTA are not very effective at preventing current-dependent inactivation (Obejero-Paz *et al.*, 1991; Vogalis *et al.*, 1992). It has been suggested that Ca^{2+} induces inactivation in Ca channels by activating calcineurin which dephosphorylates the channel (reviewed by Armstrong, 1989). However, the role of phosphorylation in Ca^{2+}-induced inactivation has been questioned (Johnson & Byerly, 1993) and the issue has not been addressed in detail in smooth muscle cells.

L-type Ca channels are also inhibited by Ca^{2+} ions which do not enter via the channel pore. Intracellular perfusion experiments with different concentrations of Ca^{2+} buffered with EGTA suggest that the resting level of Ca^{2+} causes a tonic inhibition of smooth muscle Ca channel activity (Ohya *et al.*, 1988). Indeed, I_{Ca} increases when the concentration of EGTA in the whole-cell pipette is raised above 0.1 mM (Schneider *et al.*, 1991; Vogalis *et al.*, 1992; Beech, 1993; Unno *et al.*, 1995). Ca^{2+} ions released from intracellular stores by IP_3 or caffeine have an even more striking effect, often abolishing I_{Ca} (Komori & Bolton, 1991). It is not yet established whether Ca^{2+} released from intracellular stores acts via the same mechanism as Ca^{2+} entering via the Ca channel pore.

Facilitation

Increased $[Ca^{2+}]_i$ can also stimulate Ca channel activity, and in this case there is evidence that Ca^{2+} acts via a protein kinase. In toad, stomach smooth muscle cells, McCarron et al. (1992) found that I_{Ca} was potentiated after a transient loading of the cell with Ca^{2+} by a train of short depolarizing pulses. A high intracellular concentration of the Ca^{2+}-chelator BAPTA prevented the effect, as did peptide inhibitors of calmodulin and calmodulin-dependent protein kinase II, suggesting phosphorylation of Ca channels by this calmodulin-dependent kinase increases their activity. This effect has not been reported for other smooth muscles (Ganitkevich & Isenberg, 1991), perhaps because of a dominating effect of Ca^{2+}-induced inactivation. Kleppisch et al. (1994) observed facilitation in smooth muscle α_{1C} proteins but this effect appeared to be Ca^{2+}-independent. Facilitation of T-type I_{Ca} in coronary artery smooth muscle cells was Ca^{2+}-independent and could be accounted for by removal of voltage-dependent inactivation (Ganitkevich & Isenberg, 1991).

PROTONS

Acidosis-induced vasodilation may in part be mediated by an effect on Ca channels in vascular smooth muscle cells. Early indications that pH has a strong effect on Ca channels came from work on cardiac muscle cells, where extracellular and particularly intracellular protons inhibit I_{Ca}. Irisawa & Sato (1986) found that quite strong external acidification (below pH 6.5) was needed to inhibit I_{Ca} when internal pH was strongly buffered with 50 mM HEPES. In contrast, provided that Na^+-H^+ exchange was blocked, I_{Ca} was reduced by > 50% when internal pH was reduced from only 7.2 to 6.8 while pH 6.0 irreversibly abolished the current. Recent studies suggest that the smooth muscle L-type Ca channel is affected similarly. An external pH fall from 7.4 to 6.4 caused about 50% reduction of current in cerebral and coronary arterial cells (West et al., 1992; Klöckner & Isenberg, 1994b). Klöckner & Isenberg (1994b) also observed a +10 mV shift in the voltage-dependence of activation and inactivation for a 1 unit fall in pH, an effect which may be explained by a shielding of surface charges. Changes in intracellular pH may also have occurred in these experiments. Intracellular acidification inhibits Ca channel current in arterial smooth muscle cells, but does not affect its voltage-dependence. A change from pH 7.2 to 6.0 at the intracellular side of the membrane abolished Ca channel activity in inside-out patches (Klöckner & Isenberg, 1994a).

The histidine-specific reagent diethylpyrocarbonate prevented effects of intracellular alkalinisation on HVA Ca channel current in sensory neurones (Mironov & Lux, 1991), suggesting that protons may act via histidine residues in the Ca channel or an associated protein. However, as the physiologically relevant pK for histidine is 6, the apparent pK values of 6.9 for external pH effects on the smooth muscle Ca channel (West et al., 1992; Klöckner & Isenberg, 1994a) and 7.5 on the cardiac channel (Prod'hom et al., 1987) indicate that other amino acid residues are also involved.

KINASES

Cyclic AMP- and cyclic GMP-dependent protein kinases (PKA and PKG)

In contrast to studies on cardiac muscle (reviewed by Hartzell, 1988), a stimulatory effect of cAMP on smooth muscle Ca channels has often proved difficult to demonstrate. Cyclic AMP appears to have no effect on the I_{Ca} in intestinal or tracheal smooth muscle cells (Ohya et al., 1987; Welling et al., 1992; Muraki et al., 1993) and in some studies where a stimulatory effect of β-adrenoceptor agonists has been observed the effect appeared not to be mediated by cAMP (see section on GTP-binding proteins). Cyclic AMP also has no effect on the cloned smooth muscle α_{1C}-protein (Klöckner et al., 1992; Kleppisch et al., 1994), which has the same consensus PKA phosphorylation sites as the cardiac protein. Co-expression of the smooth muscle α_{1C}-protein with skeletal muscle β-subunit, however, conferred sensitivity to cAMP, perhaps indicating that auxiliary proteins are required for cAMP to be effective (Klöckner et al., 1992).

Effects of cAMP have, nevertheless, been observed on vascular smooth muscle Ca channels. Fukumitsu et al. (1990) found that the β-adrenoceptor agonist isoprenaline stimulated Ca channels in porcine coronary artery cells and the effect was mimicked by forskolin (an activator of adenylyl cyclase), suggesting that it may have been mediated by cAMP. Ishikawa et al. (1993) found small stimulatory effects of low concentrations of forskolin (1 μM) and 8-bromo-cAMP (0.1 mM) in rabbit portal vein cells. However, in the same cells, Xiong et al. (1994b) observed that the nonspecific protein kinase inhibitor H-7 did not block isoprenaline-induced stimulation of Ca channel activity and reported inhibition, not stimulation, of the current on intracellular perfusion with the catalytic subunit of PKA. A striking effect of PKA-dependent phosphorylation was observed in inside-out patches from guinea pig basilar artery cells (Tewari & Simard, 1994). Excision of patches into a solution containing cAMP, Mg.ATP and the catalytic subunit of PKA prevented the rapid run-down of channel activity observed in the absence of the catalytic subunit. Such a strong effect contrasts with the small stimulation of whole-cell current induced by isoprenaline or forskolin reported in the same smooth muscle cells (Simard et al., 1991). A hypothesis which could explain these various observations is that phosphorylation by PKA stimulates smooth muscle

Ca channels, perhaps via a β-subunit, and that these phosphorylation sites are maximally phosphorylated in many studies, especially in whole-cell recordings from intestinal smooth muscle cells. In inside-out patches, there may be rapid dephosphorylation, causing channel activity to decline quickly, thus allowing stimulatory effects of PKA to be observed.

High concentrations of isoprenaline (10 μM), forskolin (10 μM) or 8-bromo-cAMP (1 mM) inhibited Ca channel current, increased the rate of inactivation and induced a negative shift in the steady-state inactivation curve in rabbit portal vein cells (Ishikawa et al., 1993; Xiong et al., 1994a,b). This inhibitory effect was prevented by H-7, suggesting the involvement of a protein kinase (Xiong et al., 1994a,b). The identity of this kinase has not been established but the observations that 8-bromo-cGMP (0.1 mM) and sodium nitroprusside (an activator of guanylyl cyclase) mimic the effect (Clapp & Gurney, 1991; Blatter & Wier, 1994) indicate that it may be PKG.

Protein kinase C (PKC)

There has been some controversy over the role of PKC in the regulation of Ca channel activity as phorbol esters (the commonly used stimulators of PKC) appear to be able to affect Ca channels by PKC-dependent and -independent mechanisms (Reeve et al., 1995, and references therein). Nevertheless, patch-clamp studies on single smooth muscle cells and the observation that there are numerous consensus PKC phosphorylation sites, for example, on the Ca channel β_3-subunit indicate that PKC-dependent phosphorylation may be important for Ca channel activity in smooth muscle cells. Loirand et al. (1990) have observed that phorbol dibutyrate, an activator of PKC, stimulated Ca channel current in rat portal vein cells, whereas the related compound phorbol 12, 13 diacetate, which does not activate PKC, had no effect. This effect also occurs in rabbit saphenous vein and guinea pig ileum cells (Oike et al., 1992; Unno et al., 1995). Similarly, diC_8 (a diacylglycerol analogue) stimulated I_{Ca} in toad stomach smooth muscle cells and derivatives which do not stimulate PKC had no effect (Vivaudou et al., 1988). Therefore, it appears likely that PKC-dependent phosphorylation does enhance smooth muscle Ca channel activity and may play a role in the action of G-protein-coupled receptors (see section on GTP-binding proteins).

ATP

In some cell types, intracellular ATP stimulates L-type Ca channels and may be required for their activity (reviewed by McDonald et al., 1994). Indeed, ATP and its stable analogues stimulate I_{Ca} of cardiac muscle cells (O'Rourke *et al.*, 1992), and ATP appears to prevent run-down of Ca channels in excised membrane patches via a cytoskeletal mechanism in snail neurones (Johnson & Byerly, 1993). In smooth muscle cells, raising the concentration of intracellular ATP above 0.1 mM has been observed to increase I_{Ca} in rabbit ileum and guinea pig mesenteric artery cells and I_{Ca} was abolished by metabolic poisons unless ATP was in the recording pipette (Ohya *et al.*, 1987; Ohya & Sperelakis, 1989a). ATP (5 mM) also slowed run-down of Ca channel activity in cell-attached patches on permeabilized cells (Ohya & Sperelakis, 1989b). Thus, high concentrations of ATP are thought to be required for opening of the smooth muscle Ca channel. It appears unlikely that the effect occurred via PKA-dependent phosphorylation because this had no effect on I_{Ca} in rabbit ileum cells (Ohya *et al.*, 1987; also see section on PKA). Indeed, the mechanism of action of ATP in these experiments is still not resolved.

Furthermore, the effect does not appear to occur consistently in all smooth muscle cells (Figure 1). Although Okashiro *et al.* (1992) found that ATP stimulated I_{Ca} of guinea pig portal vein cells its effect was not always observed and in many cells I_{Ca} was maintained without ATP in the recording

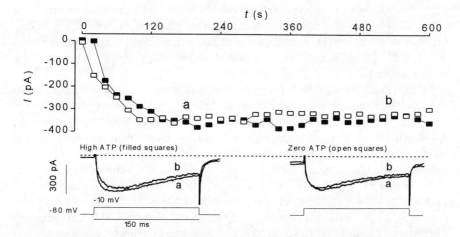

Figure 1   Typical Ca channel current amplitudes in guinea pig basilar artery smooth muscle cells recorded with a CsCl pipette solution which included (■) or excluded (□): 9 mM Na$_2$.ATP, 2.8 mM MgCl$_2$, PKA catalytic subunit, 8-bromo-cAMP and calyculin A. Time zero is the time when access to the whole-cell was achieved. The PKA inhibitors H-89 and PKI$_{(6-22)}$ were also included in the zero ATP pipette, and 2,4-dinitrophenol and 2-deoxyglucose were present in the bath throughout the recordings. The bath solution was divalent cation-free and so the currents, which were abolished by 1 μM nicardipine, were carried mostly by Na$^+$. The holding potential was −80 mV and voltage steps to −10 mV were applied every 20 s. The measured series resistance and capacitance values were 5 and 11 MΩ, and 15 and 9.5 pF, respectively, for the two recordings.

pipette; also, ATP did not prevent run-down of Ca channel activity in excised patches from basilar artery cells (Tewari & Simard, 1994). In recent experiments, we found that Ca channel activity was well maintained in basilar artery cells even when intracellular ATP and Mg^{2+} levels were severely lowered and PKA activity inhibited (Figure 1).

GTP-BINDING PROTEINS

Inhibitory effects in guinea pig ileum smooth muscle cells

Agonists at histamine H_1, muscarinic, bradykinin or tachykinin receptors suppress I_{Ca} in guinea pig ileum cells. The suppression occurs in the context of several excitatory effects. Stimulation of H_1 receptors, for example, causes Ca^{2+} release from intracellular stores via IP_3 (Jafferji & Michell, 1975; Pacaud & Bolton, 1991) and activation of nonselective monovalent cation channels (Komori et al., 1992) which leads to depolarization (Bolton et al., 1981). Inhibition of Ca channel activity will have a relaxant effect, and it thus may underlie histamine-induced relaxation of high KCl-induced contraction (Bolton et al., 1981) and desensitisation to the effects of acetylcholine (Himpens et al., 1991). Whether Ca channel inhibition occurs purely as a mechanism for desensitization or for additional reasons is unknown (see Beech, 1993; Unno et al., 1995).

In this discussion we will focus on the action of histamine as there is no evidence that muscarinic, bradykinin and tachykinin receptors couple to Ca channels via different mechanisms. Histamine has two inhibitory effects on I_{Ca} which are most readily distinguished on the basis of time-course; one is transient and the other sustained (Beech, 1993; Figure 2). The sustained inhibition is not accompanied by any change in the kinetics or voltage-dependence of I_{Ca} (Beech, 1993); whether this is also true for the transient effect is unknown. Both effects are abolished by mepyramine, suggesting a common origin at the H_1 receptor, and by intracellular GDP-β-S, suggesting G-protein-coupling. It is our working hypothesis that both effects occur via divergent pathways from a common initiation point.

Transient inhibition occurs via IP_3-induced Ca^{2+} release from intracellular stores. There are numerous observations which support this statement. Histamine induces the production of IP_3 in the guinea pig ileum (Jafferji & Michell, 1975). Heparin, which prevents IP_3 from stimulating its receptor, and caffeine, which empties the sarcoplasmic reticulum of Ca^{2+}, prevent transient inhibition (Beech, 1993). Flash photolysis of caged IP_3, which releases free IP_3 inside rabbit jejunum cells mimics transient inhibition (Komori & Bolton, 1991). The use of intracellular indo-1 (Pacaud & Bolton, 1991) or Ca^{2+}-dependent K^+ currents to indicate changes in $[Ca^{2+}]_i$ have shown that histamine causes a transient increase in $[Ca^{2+}]_i$, and strong buffering of $[Ca^{2+}]_i$ with EGTA or BAPTA prevents transient inhibition (Beech, 1993).

Sustained inhibition does not occur via IP_3-induced Ca^{2+}-release from stores because it is not prevented by heparin or caffeine (Beech, 1993). However, the underlying mechanism does, for some reason, depend on $[Ca^{2+}]_i$ in such a way that it ceases to function if $[Ca^{2+}]_i$ is reduced below the resting level. It is prevented if $[Ca^{2+}]_i$ is lowered by high concentrations of intracellular EGTA or BAPTA but not if $[Ca^{2+}]_i$ is strongly buffered near the resting level by a mixture of BAPTA and Ca^{2+} (Beech, 1993). The molecular components necessary for sustained inhibition are unknown but there are four observations which support the supposition that a phospholipase C-type mechanism is involved. Agonists at H_1, muscarinic, bradykinin and tachykinin receptors all increase phosphatidylinositol hydrolysis in ileal smooth muscle and all inhibit I_{Ca} (see Beech, 1993 and references therein). The G-protein which mediates sustained inhibition is not sensitive to pertussis toxin (Figure 2; Unno et al., 1995). This rules out the involvement of G_i/G_o proteins and allows for the possibility that the G-protein is G_q, which couples to some isoforms of phospholipase C in smooth muscle and other cell

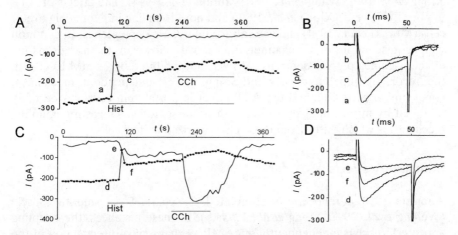

Figure 2 Pertussis toxin (PTX) does not inhibit transient or sustained inhibition of I_{Ca}. Longitudinal muscle from guinea pig ileum was maintained for 24 h in a 5% CO_2 / 37°C incubator in minimum essential medium (Gibco) which included 200 ng ml^{-1} PTX (A, B) or 200 ng/ml heat-inactivated PTX (C, D). Following this incubation, single cells were isolated and whole-cell recordings made at 25°C. The two plots on the left (A, C) show the holding current at −60 mV (continuous line) and the peak leak-subtracted amplitude of I_{Ca} measured every 5 s on depolarization to 0 mV. Actual currents are on the right. Histamine (10 μM) and carbachol (10 μM) were bath-applied. I_{Ca} inhibition was unaffected by PTX but the cation current seen at −60 mV was prevented.

types (Smrcka *et al.*, 1991; Leprêtre *et al.*, 1994). Inclusion of the phospholipase C inhibitor D609 (Müller-Decker, 1989) in the whole-cell recording pipette prevents histamine-, bradykinin- and carbachol-induced transient and sustained inhibitions of I_{Ca} (D.J.B., unpublished). Finally, sustained inhibition is Ca^{2+}-dependent, as is phospholipase C (reviewed by Meldrum *et al.*, 1991). Despite these indications that phospholipase C may be involved there is no experimental evidence to support the involvement of IP_3 or PKC. IP_3 did not inhibit I_{Ca} when it was prevented from activating IP_3 receptors by heparin (Komori & Bolton, 1991). Phorbol esters did not inhibit I_{Ca} in guinea pig ileal cells (Unno *et al.*, 1995) or affect high KCl-induced contractions in the whole tissue (Baraban *et al.*, 1985), and the protein kinase inhibitor H-7 did not affect sustained carbachol-induced I_{Ca} inhibition (Unno *et al.*, 1995). It is, however, possible that diacylglycerol acts independently of PKC.

Inhibitory effects in other smooth muscles

Noradrenaline, ATP and parathyroid hormone have also been observed to inhibit Ca channel activity in smooth muscle cells (Imaizumi *et al.*, 1991; Xiong *et al.*, 1991; Wang *et al.*, 1991; Muraki *et al.*, 1994). The effects of ATP in portal vein cells (Xiong *et al.*, 1991) and noradrenaline in guinea pig ureter cells (Muraki *et al.*, 1994) showed intracellular Ca^{2+}-dependence, in common with agonist actions on Ca channels in ileal cells. However, the noradrenaline effect in guinea pig vas deferens cells was not inhibited by 20 mM EGTA in the recording pipette, clearly indicating a Ca^{2+}-independent mechanism (Imaizumi *et al.*, 1991), and the ATP effect in portal vein cells was partially inhibited by intracellular perfusion with pertussis toxin, suggesting coupling mechanisms which differ from those characterized in ileal cells.

Stimulatory effects

Agonists at β_2-adrenoceptors stimulated Ca channels in smooth muscle (Welling *et al.*, 1992; Xiong *et al.*, 1994a,b). In these instances, the coupling appeared to occur independently of cAMP, perhaps via a direct action of the α-subunit of the G_s-protein, as was originally suggested to occur in cardiac muscle cells (Yatani & Brown, 1989; but see Hartzell & Fischmeister, 1992). A 2.6-fold increase in I_{Ca} caused by β-adrenoceptor agonists in bovine tracheal smooth muscle cells was not mimicked by intracellular perfusion with cAMP, cAMP analogues or the catalytic subunit of PKA, and yet it was prevented by intracellular GDP-β-S and mimicked by GTP-γ-S (Welling *et al.*, 1992). Xiong *et al.* (1994a,b) also found no stimulatory effect of 8-bromo-cAMP or forskolin in rabbit portal vein cells and the stimulatory action of isoprenaline was not inhibited by the protein kinase inhibitor H-7. These data indicate that cAMP and PKA are not involved, but whether G_S acts directly on the Ca channel protein remains unresolved.

Noradrenaline acting at α-adrenoceptors and thrombin acting at the thrombin receptor stimulate Ca channels in rat portal vein cells via a pertussis toxin insensitive G-protein (Loirand *et al.*, 1990; Baron *et al.*, 1993). As phorbol esters mimic and occlude their effects, and antiphosphatidylinositide antibodies prevent them, it is plausible that PKC is involved in the receptor-channel coupling mechanism (Loirand *et al.*, 1992; Baron *et al.*, 1993). Agonists at endothelin, angiotensin II, neuropeptide Y, histamine H_1 and H_3, and 5HT receptors have also been reported to stimulate smooth muscle Ca channels. Whether these effects also occur via protein kinase C remains to be determined.

SUMMARY

Openings of the smooth muscle L-type voltage-gated Ca channel are subject to the influence of a variety of regulators which are outlined in Figure 3. The most fundamental of these are the membrane potential, Ca^{2+} ions and protons, but a variety of other modulators play important roles. Phosphorylation of the channel core (or a regulatory subunit) by a variety of serine/threonine kinases affects opening. PKA, however, is not a dominant

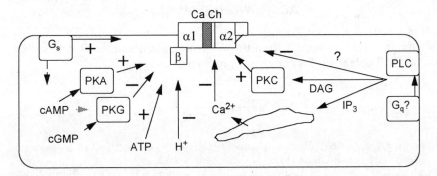

Figure 3 Mechanisms for the regulation of smooth muscle L-type voltage-gated Ca channels. The significance of these mechanisms may vary between smooth muscles, and details of some of the mechanisms are controversial (see text). Abbreviations: G_S, cholera toxin-sensitive G-protein which stimulates adenylyl cyclase; G_q, a pertussis toxin-insensitive G-protein which couples receptors to phospholipase C (PLC); PKA, cAMP-dependent protein kinase ; PKG, cGMP-dependent protein kinase; PKC, protein kinase C; DAG, diacylglycerol; IP_3, inositol 1,4,5-trisphosphate; α_1, α_2 (δ attached) and β are subunits of the Ca channel.

regulator, which is surprising considering the closely related cardiac channel is so strongly stimulated by cAMP, but not surprising considering cAMP is a smooth muscle relaxant. (It remains to be determined how the smooth muscle channel avoids a strong stimulatory effect of cAMP when its α_1-protein has the same consensus PKA phosphorylation sites as the cardiac α_1-protein; perhaps the expression of a different β-subunit in the two cells is the key to the difference). In smooth muscle cells, an inhibitory effect of cGMP via PKG may be of greater significance than any effect of cAMP, and could be a major contributor to the relaxant effect of nitro-vasodilators. G-protein-coupled receptors may affect Ca channel opening via protein kinases but they also affect the channels by additional mechanisms. There is evidence that the G_S protein couples to the Ca channel via a kinase-independent mechanism, and a pertussis toxin-resistant G-protein (possibly G_q) may couple to Ca channels via phospholipases. In contrast to Ca channel regulation in neurones (reviewed in Hille, 1994), there is no evidence for membrane-delimited coupling of pertussis toxin-sensitive G proteins to smooth muscle Ca channels, perhaps because the G_o protein is absent from smooth muscle. Finally, if the degree of regulation of a channel correlates directly with its functional importance then we can expect that the list of regulators will increase still further, perhaps to arachidonic acid and its metabolites (Shimada & Somlyo, 1992), tyrosine kinase (Wijetunge et al., 1992) and cell volume (Langton, 1993).

ACKNOWLEDGEMENTS

We are grateful for support from the Wellcome Trust and the Royal Society, and to Dr. H. Pearson for comments on the manuscript.

REFERENCES

Armstrong, D.L. (1989). Calcium channel regulation by calcineurin, a Ca^{2+}-activated phosphatase in mammalian brain. *Trends Neurosci.* **12**, 117–122.

Baraban, J.M., Gould, R.J., Peroutka, S.J. & Snyder, S.H. (1985). Phorbol ester effects on neurotransmission: interactions with neurotransmitters and calcium in smooth muscle. *Proc. Natl Acad. Sci. USA* **82**, 604–608.

Baron, A., Loirand, G., Mironneau, C. & Mironneau, J. (1993). Dual effect of thrombin on voltage-dependent Ca^{2+} channels of portal vein smooth muscle cells. *Circ. Res.* **72**, 1317–1325.

Beech, D.J. (1993). Inhibitory effects of histamine and bradykinin on calcium current in smooth muscle cells isolated from guinea pig ileum. *J. Physiol.* **463**, 565–583.

Blatter, L.A. & Weir, W.G. (1994). Nitric oxide decreases $[Ca^{2+}]_i$ in vascular smooth muscle by inhibition of the calcium current. *Cell Calcium* **15**, 122–131.

Bolton, T.B., Clark, J.P., Kitamura, K. & Lang. R.J. (1981). Evidence that histamine and carbachol may open the same ion channels in longitudinal smooth muscle of the guinea pig ileum. *J. Physiol.* **320**, 363–379.

Catterall, W.A. (1988). Structure and function of voltage-sensitive ion channels. *Science* **242**, 50–61.

Clapp, L.H. & Gurney, A.M. (1991). Modulation of calcium movements by nitroprusside in isolated vascular smooth cells. *Pflügers Arch.* **418**, 462–470.

Fukumitsu, T., Hayashi, H., Tokuno, H. & Tomita, T. (1990). Increase in calcium channel current by β-adrenoceptor agonists in single smooth muscle cells isolated from porcine coronary artery. *Br. J. Pharmacol.* **100**, 593–599.

Ganitkevich, V.Y. & Isenberg, G. (1991). Stimulation-induced potentiation of T-type Ca^{2+} channel currents in myocytes from guinea pig coronary artery. *J. Physiol.* **443**, 703–725.

Ganitkevich, V.Y., Shuba, M.F. & Smirnov, S.V. (1987). Calcium-dependent inactivation of potential-dependent calcium inward current in an isolated guinea pig smooth muscle cell. *J. Physiol.* **392**, 431–449.

Gollasch, M., Hescheler, J., Quayle, J.M., Patlak, J.B. & Nelson, M.T. (1992). Single calcium channel currents of arterial smooth muscle at physiological calcium concentrations. *Am. J. Physiol.* **263**, C948–952.

Hartzell, H.C. (1988). Regulation of cardiac ion channels by catecholamines, acetylcholine and second messenger systems. *Prog. Biophys. Molec. Biol.* **52**, 165–247.

Hartzell, H.C. & Fischmeister, R. (1992). Direct regulation of cardiac Ca^{2+} channels by G proteins: neither proven nor necessary? *Trends Pharmacolo. Sci.* **13**, 380–385.

Hille, B. (1994). Modulation of ion-channel function by G-protein-coupled receptors. *Trends Neurosci.* **17**, 531–536.

Himpens, B. Droogmans, G. & Casteels, R. (1991). Carbachol-induced nonspecific desensitization in guinea pig ileum. *Naunyn-Schmiedberg's Arch. Pharmacol.* **343**, 580–587.

Hofmann, F., Biel, M. & Flockerzi, V. (1994). Molecular basis for Ca^{2+} channel diversity. *Annu. Rev. Neurosci.* **17**, 399–418.

Imaizumi, Y., Takeda, M., Muraki, K. & Watanabe, M. (1991). Mechanisms of NE-induced reduction of Ca current in single smooth muscle cells from guinea pig vas deferens. *Am. J. Physiol.* **260**, C17–C25.

Inoue, Y., Xiong, Z., Kitamura, K. and Kuriyama, H. (1989). Modulation produced by nifedipine of the unitary Ba current of dispersed smooth muscle cells of the rabbit ileum. *Pflügers Arch.* **414**, 534–542.

Irisawa, H. & Sato, R. (1986). Intra- and extracellular actions of proton on the calcium current of isolated guinea pig ventricular cells. *Circ. Res.* **59**, 348–355.

Ishikawa, T., Hume, J.R. & Keef, K.D. (1993). Regulation of Ca^{2+} channels by cAMP and cGMP in vascular smooth muscle cells. *Circ. Res.* **73**, 1128–1137.

Jafferji, S.S. & Michell, R.H. (1975). Stimulation of phosphatidylinositol turnover by histamine, 5-hydroxytryptamine and adrenaline in the longitudinal muscle of the guinea pig ileum. *Biochem. Pharmacol.* **25**, 1429–1430.

Johnson, B.D. & Byerly, L. (1993). A cytoskeletal mechanism for Ca^{2+} channel metabolic dependence and inactivation by intracellular Ca^{2+}. *Neuron* **10**, 797–804.

Kleppisch, T., Pederson, K., Strübing, C., Bosse-Doenecke, E., Flockerzi, V., Hofmann, F. & Hescheler, J. (1994). Double-pulse facilitation of smooth muscle α_1-subunit Ca^{2+}-channels expressed in CHO cells. *EMBO J.* **13**, 2502–2507.

Klöckner, U. & Isenberg, G. (1994a). Intracellular pH modulates the availability of vascular L-type Ca^{2+} channels. *J. Gen. Physiol.* **103**, 647–663.

Klöckner, U. & Isenberg, G. (1994b). Calcium channel current of vascular smooth muscle cells: extracellular protons modulate gating and single channel conductance. *J. Gen. Physiol.* **103**, 665–678.

Klöckner, U., Itagaki, K., Bodi, I. & Sschwartz, A. (1992). β-Subunit expression is required for cAMP-dependent increase of cloned cardiac and vascular calcium channel currents. *Pflügers Arch.* **420**, 413–415.

Komori, S. & Bolton, T.B. (1991). Inositol trisphosphate releases stored calcium to block voltage-dependent calcium channels in single smooth muscle cells. *Pflügers Arch.* **418**, 437–441.

Komori, S., Kawai, M., Takewaki, T. & Ohashi, H. (1992). GTP-binding protein involvement in membrane currents evoked by carbachol and histamine in guinea pig ileal muscle. *J. Physiol.* **450**, 105–126.

Langton, P.D. (1993). Calcium channel currents recorded from isolated myocytes of rat basilar artery are stretch sensitive. *J. Physiol.* **471**, 1–11.

Leprêtre, N., Mironneau, J., Arnaudeu, S., Tanfin, Z., Harbon, S., Guillon & Ibarrondo, J. (1994). Activation of alpha-1A adrenoceptors mobilizes calcium from intracellular stores in myocytes from rat portal vein. *J. Pharmacol. Exp. Therap.* **268**, 167–174.

Loirand, G., Pacaud, P., Mironneau, C., & Mironneau, J. (1990). GTP-binding proteins mediate noradrenaline effects on calcium and chloride currents in rat portal vein myocytes. *J. Physiol.* **428**, 517–529.

Loirand, G., Faiderbe, S., Baron, A., Geffard, M. & Mironneau, J. (1992). Autoanti-phosphatidylinositide antibodies specifically inhibit noradrenaline effects on Ca^{2+} and Cl^- channels in rat portal vein myocytes. *J. Biol. Chem.* **267**, 4312–4316.

McCarron, J.G., McGeown, J.G., Reardon, S., Ikebe, M., Fay, F.S. & Walsh JR, J.V. (1992). Calcium-dependent enhancement of calcium current in smooth muscle by calmodulin-dependent protein kinase II. *Nature* **357**, 74–77.

McDonald, T.F., Pelzer, S., Trautwein, W. & Pelzer, D. (1994). Regulation and modulation of calcium channels in cardiac, skeletal, and smooth muscle cells. *Physiol. Rev.* **74**, 365–507.

Meldrum, E., Parker, P.J. & Carozzi, A. (1991) The PtdIns-PLC superfamily and signal transduction. *Biochim. Biophys. Acta* **1092**, 49–71.

Mironov, S.L. & Lux, H.D. (1991). Cytoplasmic alkalinization increases high-threshold calcium current in chick dorsal root ganglion neurones. *Pflügers Arch.* **419**, 138–143.

Missiaen, L., DE Smedt, H., Droogmans, G., Himpens, B. & Casteels, R. (1992). Calcium ion homeostasis in smooth muscle. *Pharmac. Ther.* **56**, 191–231.

Müller-Decker, K. (1989). Interuption of TPA-induced signals by an antiviral and antitumoral xanthate compound: inhibition of a phospholipase C-type reaction. *Biochem. Biophys. Res. Commun.* **162**, 198–205.

Muraki, K., Bolton, T., Imaizumi, Y. & Watanabe, M. (1993). Effect of isoprenaline on Ca^{2+} channel current in single smooth muscle cells isolated from taenia of the guinea pig caecum. *J. Physiol.* **471**, 563–582.

Muraki, K., Imaizumi, Y. & Watanabe, M. (1994). Effects of noradrenaline on membrane currents and action potential shape in smooth muscle cells from guinea pig ureter. *J. Physiol.* **481**, 617–627.

Nilius, B., Kitamura, K. & Kuriyama, H. (1994). Properties of inactivation of calcium channel currents in smooth muscle cells of rabbit portal vein. *Pflügers Arch.* **426**, 239–246.

Obejero-Paz, C. A., Jones, S.W. & Scarpa, A. (1991). Calcium currents in the A7r5 smooth muscle-derived cell line. *J. Gen. Physiol.* **98**, 1127–1140.

Ohya, Y. & Sperelakis, N. (1989a). ATP regulation of the slow calcium channels in vascular smooth muscle cells of guinea pig mesenteric artery. *Circ. Res.* **64**, 145–154.

Ohya, Y. & Sperelakis, N. (1989b). Modulation of single slow (L-type) calcium channels by intracellular ATP in vascular smooth muscle cells. *Pflügers Arch.* **414**, 257–264.

Ohya, Y., Kitamura, K. & Kuriyama, H. (1987). Modulation of ionic currents in smooth muscle balls of the rabbit intestine by intracellularly perfused ATP and cyclic AMP. *Pflügers Arch.* **408**, 465–473.

Ohya, Y., Kitamura, K. & Kuriyama, H. (1988). Regulation of calcium current by intracellular calcium in smooth muscle cells of rabbit portal vein. *Circ. Res.* **62**, 375–383.

Oike, M., Kitamura, K. & Kuriyama, H. (1992). Histamine H_3-receptor activation auguments voltage-dependent Ca^{2+} current via GTP hydrolysis in rabbit saphenous artery. *J. Physiol.* **448**, 133–152.

Okashiro, T., Tokuno, H., Hayashi, H. & Tomita, T. (1992). Effects of intracellular ATP on calcium current in freshly dispersed single cells of guinea pig portal vein. *Exp. Physiol.* **77**, 719–731.

O'Rourke, B., Backx, P.H. & Marban, E. (1992). Phosphorylation-independent modulation of L-type calcium channels by magnesium-nucleotide complexes. *Science* **257**, 245–248.

Pacaud, P. & Bolton, T.B. (1991). Relation between muscarinic receptor cationic current and internal calcium in guinea pig jejunal smooth muscle cells. *J. Physiol.* **441**, 477–499.

Pragnell, M., de Waard, M., Mori, Y., Tanabe,T., Snutch, T.P. & Campbell, K.P. (1994). Calcium channel β-subunit binds to a conserved motif in the I–II cytoplasmic linker of the α_1-subunit. *Nature* **368**, 67–70.

Prod'hom, B., Pietrobon, D. & Hess, P. (1987). Direct measurement of proton transfer rates to a group controlling the dihydropyridine-sensitive Ca^{2+} channel. *Nature* **329**, 243–246.

Reeve, H.L., Vaughan, P.T. & Peers, C. (1995). Enhancement of Ca^{2+} channel currents in human neuroblastoma (SH-SY5Y) cells by phorbol esters. *Pflügers Arch* **429**, 729–737.

Schneider, P., Hopp, H.H. & Isenberg, G. (1991). Ca^{2+} influx through ATP-gated channels increments $[Ca^{2+}]i$ and inactivates I_{Ca} in myocytes from guinea pig urinary bladder. *J. Physiol.* **440**, 479–496.

Shimada, T. & Somlyo, A.P. (1992). Modulation of voltage-dependent Ca channel current by arachidonic acid and other long-chain fatty acids in rabbit intestinal smooth muscle. *J. Gen. Physiol.* **100**, 27–44.

Simard, J.M. (1991). Calcium channel currents in isolated smooth muscle cells from the basilar artery of the guinea pig. *Pflügers Arch.* **417**, 528–536.

Simard, J.M., Kent, T.A., Sandleback, B. & Leppla, D. (1991). L-type calcium current in basilar artery cells is transiently increased by isoproterenol, forskolin and cAMP. *J. Cerebral Blood Flow .Metab.* **11**(Suppl. 2), S253.

Smrcka, A.V., Hepler, J.R., Brown, O.K. & Sternweis, P.C. (1991). Regulation of polyphosphoinositide-specific phospholipase C activity by purified G_q. *Science* **251**, 804–807.

Tewari, K. & Simard, J.M. (1994). Protein kinase A increases availability of calcium channels in smooth muscle cells from guinea pig basilar artery. *Pflügers Arch.* **428**, 9–16.

Unno, T., Komori, S. & Ohashi, H. (1995). Inhibitory effect of muscarinic receptor activation on Ca^{2+} channel current in smooth muscle cells of guinea pig ileum. *J.*

Physiol. **484**, 567–581.

Vivaudou, M.B., Clapp, L.C., Wwalsh, JR, J.V. & Singer, J.J. (1988). Regulation of one type of Ca^{2+} current in smooth muscle cells by diacylglycerol and acetylcholine. *FASEB J.* **2**, 2497–2504.

Vogalis, F., Publicover, N.G. & Sanders, K.M. (1992). Regulation of calcium current by voltage and cytoplasmic calcium in canine gastric smooth muscle. *Am. J. Physiol.* **262**, C691–C700.

Wang, R., Karpinski, E. & Pang, P.K. (1991). Parathyroid hormone selectively inhibits L-type calcium channels in single vascular smooth muscle cells of the rat. *J. Physiol.* **441**, 325–346.

Welling, A. Felbel, J., Peper, K. & Hofmann, F. (1992). Hormonal regulation of calcium current in freshly isolated airway smooth muscle cells. *Am. J. Physiol.* **262**, L351–L359.

Welling, A., Kwan, Y.W., Bosse, E., Flockerzi, V., Hofmann, F. & Kass, R.S. (1993a). Subunit-dependent modulation of recombinant L-type calcium channels; molecular basis for dihydropyridine tissue sensitivity. *Circ. Res.* **73**, 974–980.

Welling, A., Bosse, E., Cavalié, A., Bottlender, R., Ludwig, A., Nastainczyk, W., Flockerzi, V. & Hofmann, F. (1993b). Stable co-expression of calcium channel α_1, β and α_2/δ subunits in a somatic cell line. *J. Physiol.* **471**, 749–765.

West, G.A., Leppla, D.C. & Simard, J.M. (1992). Effects of external pH on ionic currents in smooth muscle cells from the basilar artery of the guinea pig. *Circ. Res.* **71**, 201–209.

Wijetunge, S., Aalkjaer, C., Schaeter, M. & Hughes, A. (1992). Tyrosine kinase inhibitors block calcium channel currents in vascular smooth muscle cells. *Biochem. Biophys. Res. Comm.* **189**, 1620–1623.

Xiong, Z., Kitamura, K. & Kuriyama, H. (1991). ATP activates cationic currents and modulates the calcium current through GTP-binding protein in rabbit portal vein. *J. Physiol.* **440**, 143–165.

Xiong, Z., Sperelakis, N. & Fenoglio-Preiser, C. (1994a). Regulation of L-type calcium channels by cyclic nucleotides and phosphorylation in smooth muscle cells from rabbit portal vein. *J. Vascular Res.* **31**, 271–279.

Xiong, Z., Sperelakis, N. & Fenoglio-Preiser, C. (1994b). Isoproterenol modulates the calcium channels through two different mechanisms in smooth-muscle from rabbit portal vein. *Pflügers Arch.* **428**, 105–113.

Yatani, A. and Brown, A.M. (1989). Rapid β-adrenergic modulation of cardiac calcium channel currents by a fast G protein pathway. *Science* **245**, 71–74.

Zhang, J., Ellinor, P.T., Aldrich, R.W. & Tsien, R.W. (1994). Molecular determinants of voltage-dependent inactivation in calcium channels. *Nature* **372**, 97–100.

5

Mechanisms of Ca^{2+} Entry into Smooth Muscle after Ca^{2+} Store Depletion

P. PACAUD
G. GRÉGOIRE
G. LOIRAND

*Institut de Pharmacologie
Moléculaire et Cellulaire,
CNRS UPR 411,
Valbonne, France*

INTRODUCTION

The concentration of cytosolic Ca^{2+} ([Ca^{2+}]$_i$) plays an essential role in regulating force generation in smooth muscle cells. Changes in [Ca^{2+}]$_i$ are dependent, in part, on the opening and closing of Ca^{2+} permeable channels located in the smooth muscle cell membrane. The best known members of this family of channels are the voltage-dependent Ca^{2+} channels, found in all smooth muscle cells examined. However, in addition to electrophysiological studies, the development of experimental approaches to measure [Ca^{2+}]$_i$, such as the use of Ca^{2+}-sensitive fluorescent dyes (fura 2, indo 1) have provided informations about other types of Ca^{2+} permeable channels.

It is now obvious that voltage-independent Ca^{2+} channels exist in many cell types, including smooth muscle cells. The first direct measurements of a Ca^{2+}-permeable ligand-gated channel were made in vascular smooth muscle cells stimulated with ATP (Benham & Tsien, 1987). In addition to receptor-operated Ca^{2+} entry, another mechanism of voltage-independent Ca^{2+} influx has been identified in a large number of nonexcitable cells following Ca^{2+} store depletion. Putney (1986) proposed that the emptying of intracellular Ca^{2+} store activates a Ca^{2+} entry pathway in the plasma membrane called 'capacitative Ca^{2+} entry'. However, the mechanism by which Ca^{2+} level in the store controls plasma membrane permeability is not known. This mechanism probably involves a diffusible messenger and the major candidates that have

SMOOTH MUSCLE EXCITATION
ISBN 0-12-112360-X

been proposed include: inositol 1,3,4,5-tetrakisphosphate ($InsP_4$) (Irvine, 1992) ; a product of cytochrome P-450 activity (Alvarez et al., 1991); an anionic, phosphate-containing message named CIF (Ca^{2+}-influx factor) (Randriamampita & Tsien, 1993); a small G protein (Fasolato et al., 1993) and cGMP (Pandol & Schoeffield-Payne, 1990; Bahnson et al., 1993).

We describe in the present article some properties of the Ca^{2+} influx activated following Ca^{2+} store depletion in smooth muscle cells, and some data on its mechanism of regulation.

STORE-DEPENDENT Ca^{2+} INFLUX INTO SMOOTH MUSCLE CELLS

As early as 1981, Casteels and Droogmans hypothesized, on the basis of indirect evidence, that agonist-induced Ca^{2+} entry into arterial myocytes was controlled by the depletion of a limited Ca^{2+} pool. This hypothesis was not followed up for several years, until recent work using $[Ca^{2+}]_i$ measurements demonstrated depletion-activated Ca^{2+} influx in visceral and in vascular smooth muscle cells. In intestinal smooth muscle cells stimulated by caffeine or carbachol (Pacaud & Bolton, 1991), tracheal smooth muscle cells stimulated by histamine or bradykinin (Murray & Kotlikoff, 1991; Murray et al., 1993) and portal vein myocytes stimulated by noradrenaline (NA) (Pacaud et al., 1992, 1993), the transient $[Ca^{2+}]_i$ rise due to Ca^{2+} store release is followed by a maintained increase in $[Ca^{2+}]_i$ until these drugs are washed off the cells. In portal vein myocytes, contrary to that observed in intestinal myocytes, Ca^{2+} store depletion induced by caffeine or ryanodine is not followed by a maintained rise in $[Ca^{2+}]_i$. This maintained increase in $[Ca^{2+}]_i$ is enhanced by increasing the driving force for Ca^{2+}, i.e. by membrane hyperpolarization (Pacaud & Bolton, 1991; Pacaud et al., 1992) or by increasing the external Ca^{2+} concentration (Figure 1). This phase is insensitive to organic blockers of voltage-dependent Ca^{2+} channels but is inhibited by polyvalent cations (Mn^{2+}, Ni^{2+}) (Pacaud & Bolton, 1991; Murray & Kotlikoff, 1991; Murray et al., 1993; Pacaud et al., 1993). Contrary to that observed in a large number of nonexcitable cells, the Ca^{2+} entry pathway involved in the agonist-induced maintained $[Ca^{2+}]_i$ rise in smooth muscle cells does not appear to be permeable to Mn^{2+}. Although membrane currents and $[Ca^{2+}]_i$ have been simultaneously recorded (Pacaud & Bolton, 1991; Pacaud et al., 1992), the maintained rise in $[Ca^{2+}]_i$ recorded with 2 mM external Ca^{2+} is not accompanied by a detectable change in the whole-cell membrane current. All these data suggest that this agonist-induced maintained $[Ca^{2+}]_i$ rise is due to Ca^{2+} entry through a membrane pathway which is not gated by membrane potential and seems to be highly selective for Ca^{2+} ions.

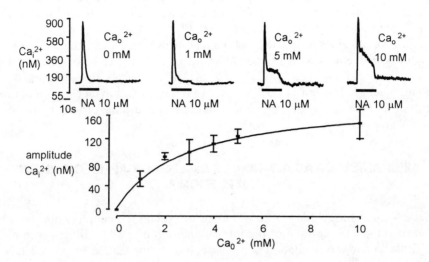

Figure 1 Effect of the external Ca^{2+} concentration on the amplitude of the maintained component of the noradrenaline (NA)-induced [Ca^{2+}]$_i$ rise in portal vein myocytes. The amplitude of the maintained [Ca^{2+}]$_i$ rise induced by 10 μM NA was plotted against the external Ca^{2+} concentration in the range 0–10 mM. Each point represents the mean value recorded in 5–36 cells $\pm$ s.e.m. Typical traces obtained in the presence of 0, 1, 5 and 10 mM Ca^{2+} are shown above the curve. See Pacaud *et al.* (1992, 1993) for further details about the experimental conditions.

CHARACTERIZATION OF THE Ca^{2+} STORE DEPLETION-ACTIVATED Ca^{2+} CURRENT

The first clear-cut demonstration that depletion of intracellular stores leads to the activation of a Ca^{2+} current was obtained in mast cells by Hoth & Penner (1992). They named this current I_{CRAC} (Ca^{2+} release-activated Ca^{2+} current). They recorded the activation of I_{CRAC} upon establishment of the whole-cell configuration with a patch pipette containing high concentration of Ca^{2+} buffers (EGTA or BAPTA) and inositol 1,4,5-trisphosphate (InsP$_3$) which produce Ca^{2+} store depletion.

By using a similar approach, the existence of I_{CRAC}-type current has been recently demonstrated in aortic smooth muscle cell line A7r5 (van Renterghem & Lazdunski, 1994) in which previous studies have shown that Ca^{2+} entry is increased after depletion of the agonist-sensitive store (Missiaen *et al.*, 1990). This current has a very low amplitude (-18 ± 2 pA, $n = 50$ at -61 mV in 110 mM external Ca^{2+}) and the absence of observable noise on the current trace suggests that the single channel conductance is very small.

The properties of this I_{CRAC}-like current recorded in A7r5 cells are similar to those of the maintained $[Ca^{2+}]_i$ rise described above, i.e. (1) is activated by an $InsP_3$-generating agonist (vasopressin), (2) is not voltage-gated, (3) is insensitive to organic blockers of voltage-dependent Ca^{2+} channel, (4) is highly selective for Ca^{2+} and poorly permeable to Mn^{2+}, and (5) is blocked by polyvalent cations (La^{3+}, Cd^{2+}, Co^{2+}, Ni^{2+}, Mn^{2+}). In addition, van Renterghem & Lazdunski (1994) report that the activation mechanism of this current is rapidly lost during whole-cell dialysis and thus, probably involves soluble messengers.

MECHANISM OF ACTIVATION OF Ca²⁺ INFLUX AFTER Ca²⁺ STORE DEPLETION

Several mechanisms have been proposed to explain the coupling mechanism between the Ca^{2+} content of the intracellular store (mainly the sarcoplasmic reticulum) and the regulation of a plasma membrane Ca^{2+} channel. We have used various pharmacological agents to test the involvement of these mechanisms in the activation of the maintained Ca^{2+} rise induced by NA in venous myocytes. The main results are summarized in Table 1.

Table 1   Effect of various pharmacological agents on the basal $[Ca^{2+}]_i$, the transient and the maintained rise in $[Ca^{2+}]_i$ induced by 10 μM NA in portal vein myocytes.

	Basal $[Ca^{2+}]_i$ (%)	Transient $[Ca^{2+}]_i$ (%)	Maintained $[Ca^{2+}]_i$ (%)	n
Control	100	100	100	5–14
Doxorubicin 10 μM	90 ± 6	96 ± 14	95 ± 19	7
Econazole 5 μM				
2 min	80 ± 5	106 ± 12	101 ± 7	4
20 min	115 ± 11	38 ± 2¶	13 ± 5¶	15
Genistein				
10 μM	104 ± 7	57 ± 6*	71 ± 8*	9
50 μM	98 ± 2	49 ± 7*	63 ± 4†	6
100 μM	96 ± 5	—	—	10
LY 83583 25 μM	92 ± 6	88 ± 13	19 ± 7¶	16
+ DB-cGMP 0.5–1 mM	95 ± 6	84 ± 10	96 ± 12	7
Okadaic acid 100 nM	128 ± 6	105 ± 11	216 ± 23‡	17

$[Ca^{2+}]_i$ was estimated by indo 1 signal in single cells of rat portal vein. See Pacaud *et al.* (1992, 1993) for further details. Values represent means ± S.E.M., n is the number of experiments. *$p < 0.05$; †$p < 0.01$; ‡$p < 0.001$; ¶$p < 0.0001$.

InsP₄

The maintained Ca^{2+} rise induced by NA was abolished when cells were intracellularly perfused with heparin (Pacaud *et al.*, 1993). This effect seems to be due to inhibition of the Ca^{2+} store release rather than to the inhibitory action of heparin on the $InsP_3$ 3-kinase. Doxorubicin, which specifically inhibits this enzyme and thus prevents the generation of $InsP_4$ (da Silva *et al.*, 1994), does not affect the maintained phase of the NA-induced $[Ca^{2+}]_i$ rise, suggesting that $InsP_4$ is not involved.

Tyrosine phosphorylation

Because tyrosine phosphorylation has also been proposed to play a role in regulating Ca^{2+} influx pathway induced by depletion of intracellular store (Vostal *et al.*, 1991; Lee *et al.*, 1993), the effect of the tyrosine kinase inhibitor genistein was investigated. In cells treated with genistein, both the release and the Ca^{2+} entry component of the NA-induced $[Ca^{2+}]_i$ rise are inhibited (Table 1). At 100 μM genistein, the NA-induced $[Ca^{2+}]_i$ rise is completely abolished. These results suggest that genistein does not act specifically on the Ca^{2+} entry mechanism activated after Ca^{2+} store depletion in portal vein myocytes.

Cytochrome P450

A product of cytochrome P450 activity has also been proposed as the missing link between the Ca^{2+} store and plasma membrane channels. Treatment with inhibitors of this enzyme, such as econazole for 2 min, has been shown to block the Ca^{2+} store depletion-induced Ca^{2+} influx in thymocytes (Alvarez *et al.*, 1991). A similar treatment is totally ineffective in portal vein cells and a prolonged treatment inhibits both components of the NA-induced $[Ca^{2+}]_i$ rise (Table 1) probably via a nonspecific action as voltage-dependent Ca^{2+} channels and K^+ channels are also blocked.

cGMP

In pancreatic acinar cells, cGMP has been suggested to activate I_{CRAC} (Banhson *et al.*, 1993). We used the inhibitor of guanylate cyclase LY-83583 to investigate the role of cGMP in the NA-induced $[Ca^{2+}]_i$ entry. LY-83583 (25 μM) inhibits the Ca^{2+} entry component of the NA-induced Ca^{2+} rise without affecting the release component. This effect was reversed by addition to the bath of 0.5–1 mM of the membrane permeant analogue of cGMP, dibutyryl cGMP (DB-cGMP, Table 1, Figure 2) although the application of

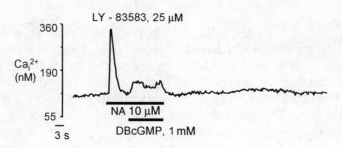

Figure 2 Effect of the addition of DB-cGMP (1 mM) during NA (10 μM) application in the presence of the guanylate cyclase inhibitor LY-83583 (25 μM). $[Ca^{2+}]_i$ was estimated by indo 1 signal in single cells of rat portal vein. See Pacaud *et al.* (1992, 1993) for further details about the experimental conditions.

cGMP alone under control conditions (i.e. with a full Ca^{2+} store) does not activate Ca^{2+} influx. This result suggests that cGMP is involved in the activation of Ca^{2+} entry after NA-induced Ca^{2+} store depletion.

Our results thus suggest that both Ca^{2+} store depletion and cGMP were necessary for the activation of Ca^{2+} entry pathway. Protein phosphorylation also seems to be involved in the activation of the Ca^{2+} influx as the maintained $[Ca^{2+}]_i$ rise induced by NA is increased to 216 ± 26% of control ($n = 17, p < 0.001$) by treatment of the cell with the inhibitor of phosphatase 1 and 2A, okadaic acid (100 nM). The reversible blockade of the NA-induced maintained $[Ca^{2+}]_i$ rise by the inhibitors of cGMP-dependent protein kinase (PKG), KT-5823 (0.5 μM) and H-8 (300 μM) suggests that a PKG-mediated phosphorylation is involved in the coupling system between the Ca^{2+} store depletion and the plasma membrane Ca^{2+} channel activation.

CONCLUSION

Our results obtained in venous myocytes suggest that the activation of Ca^{2+} entry across the plasma membrane following NA-induced Ca^{2+} store depletion involves cGMP. Neither the depletion of Ca^{2+} store nor cGMP alone are sufficient to activate Ca^{2+} influx but rather, the combination of both factors is required. This is an unexpected role for cGMP as, in vascular smooth muscle cells, increased cGMP levels are commonly associated to a decrease in $[Ca^{2+}]_i$ and a vasorelaxing effects. However, whether NA increases cGMP levels in venous myocytes is not known.

The physiological role of such a Ca^{2+} entry in smooth muscle cells also remains to be elucidated as, contrary to nonexcitable cells, this pathway is not the major mechanism of Ca^{2+} entry. Its involvement in the regulation of muscular tone appears to differ, depending on the smooth muscle type. Ca^{2+} that enters the cell through this pathway does not activate contractile proteins in the portal vein whereas it produces a contractile response in the main pulmonary artery (Gonzales de la Fuente *et al.*, 1995). This difference could be linked to the existence of phasic (such as portal vein) and tonic (such as pulmonary artery) smooth muscles. Morphological specializations of the sarcoplasmic reticulum and its distribution (central or peripheral) in different smooth muscles could be responsible for the different use of this Ca^{2+} (Nixon *et al.*, 1994). In phasic smooth muscle, the main role of this Ca^{2+} appears to be the refilling of the Ca^{2+} stores.

REFERENCES

Alvarez, J., Montero, M. & Garcia-Sancho, J. (1991). Cytochrome P-450 may link intracellular Ca^{2+} stores with plasma membrane Ca^{2+} influx. *Biochem. J.* **274,** 193–197.

Bahnson, T.D., Pandol, S.J. & Dionne, V.E. (1993). Cyclic GMP modulates depletion-activated Ca^{2+} entry in pancreatic acinar cells. *J. Biolog. Chem.* **268,** 10808–10812.

Benham, C.D. & Tsien, R.W. (1987). A novel receptor-operated Ca^{2+} permeable channel activated by ATP in smooth muscle. *Nature* **328,** 275–278.

Casteels, R. & Droogmans, G. (1981). Exchange characteristics of the noradrenaline-sensitive calcium store in vascular smooth muscle of rabbit ear artery. *J. Physiol. (London)* **317,** 263–279.

Fasolato, C., Hoth, M. & Penner, R. (1993). A GTP-dependent step in the activation mechanism of capacitive calcium influx. *J. Biolog. Chem.* **268,** 20737–20740.

Gonzalez De La Fuente, P., Savineau, J.P. & Marthan, R. (1995). Control of pulmonary vascular smooth muscle tone by sarcoplasmic reticulum Ca^{2+} pump blockers: thapsigargin and cyclopiazonic acid. *Pflügers Arch.* **429,** 617–624.

Hoth, M. & Penner, R. (1992). Depletion of intracellular calcium stores activates a calcium current in mast cells. *Nature* **355,** 353–355.

Irvine, R.F. (1992). Inositol phosphates and Ca^{2+} entry: toward a proliferation or a simplification. *FASEB J.* **6,** 3085-3091.

Lee, K.M., Toscas, K. & Villereal, M.L. (1993). Inhibition of bradykinin- and thapsigargin-induced Ca^{2+} entry by tyrosine kinase inhibitors. *J. Biolog. Chem.* **268,** 9945–9948.

Missiaen, L., Declerck, I., Droogmans, G., Plessers, L., De Smedt, H., Raeymaekers & Casteels, R. (1990). Agonist-dependent Ca^{2+} and Mn^{2+} entry dependent on state of filling of Ca^{2+} stores in aortic smooth muscle cells of the rat. *J. Physiol. (London)* **427,** 171–186.

Murray, R.K. & Kotlikoff, M.I. (1991). Receptor-activated calcium influx in human airway smooth muscle cells. *J. Physiol. (London)* **435,** 123–144.

Murray, R.K., Fleischmann, B.K. & Kotlikoff, M.I. (1993). Receptor-activated Ca influx in human airway smooth muscle: use of Ca imaging and perforated patch-clamp techniques. *Am. J. Physiol.* **264,** C485–C490.

Nixon, G.F., Mignery, G.A. & Somlyo, A.V. (1994). Immunogold localization of inositol 1,4,5-trisphosphate receptors and characterization of ultrastructural features of the sarcoplasmic reticulum in phasic and tonic smooth muscle. *J. Muscle Res. Cell Motil.* **15**, 682–700.

Pacaud P. & Bolton, T.B. (1991). Relation between muscarinic receptor cationic current and internal calcium in guinea pig jejunal smooth muscle cells. *J.Physiol. (London)* **441**, 477–499.

Pacaud, P., Loirand, G., Bolton, T.B., Mironneau, C. & Mironneau, J. (1992). Intracellular cations modulate noradrenaline-stimulated calcium entry into smooth muscle cells of rat portal vein. *J. Physiol. (London)* **456**, 541–556.

Pacaud, P., Loirand, G., Grégoire, G., Mironneau, C. & Mironneau, J. (1993). Noradrenaline-activated heparin-sensitive Ca^{2+} entry after depletion of intracellular Ca^{2+} store in portal vein smooth muscle cells. *J. Biolog. Chem.* **268**, 3866–3872.

Pandol, S.J. & Schoeffield-Payne, M.S. (1990). Cyclic GMP mediates the agonist-stimulated increase in plasma membrane calcium entry in the pancreatic acinar cell. *J. Biolog. Chem.* **265**, 12846–12853.

Putney, Jr. J.W. (1986). A model for receptor-regulated calcium entry. *Cell Calcium* **7**, 1–12.

Randriamampita, C. & Tsien, R.Y. (1993). Emptying of intracellular Ca^{2+} stores releases a novel small messenger that stimulates Ca^{2+} influx. *Nature* **364**, 809–814.

van Renterghem, C. & Lazdunski, M. (1994). Identification of the Ca^{2+} current activated by vasoconstrictors in vascular smooth muscle cells. *Pflügers Arch.* **429**, 1–6.

da Silva, C.P., Emmrich, F. & Guse, A.H. (1994). Adriamycin inhibits inositol 1,4,5-trisphosphate 3-kinase activity *in vitro* and blocks formation of inositol 1,3,4,5-tetrakisphosphate in stimulated jurkat T-lymphocytes. *J. Biolog. Chem.* **269**, 12521–12526.

Vostal, J.G., Jackson, W.L. & Shulman, N.R. (1991). Cytosolic and stored calcium antagonistically control tyrosine phosphorylation of specific platelet proteins. *J. Biolog. Chem.* **266**, 16911–16916.

6

Regulation of Voltage-gated K⁺ Channels in Vascular Smooth Muscle Cells

PHILIP I. AARONSON
SERGEY V. SMIRNOV

Department of Pharmacology,
United Medical and Dental Schools of Guy's and
St Thomas's Hospitals, London, UK

Three types of macroscopic voltage-gated K⁺ channels have been demonstrated in vascular smooth muscle cells (VSMCs). These include the ubiquitous delayed rectifier current (Beech & Bolton, 1989b), the A- or A-like current (Beech & Bolton, 1989a), and the inward rectifier (Edwards *et al.*, 1988). It seems likely that the primary function of these voltage-gated K⁺ channels is to set the resting membrane potential (E_m). Pharmacological blockade of the delayed rectifier, for example, causes membrane depolarization (Gelband *et al.*, 1993; Smirnov *et al.*, 1994), and small changes in the extracellular K⁺ concentration shift the activation of the inward rectifier, thereby altering E_m in rat cerebral arterioles (Edwards *et al.*, 1988).

The putative involvement of the delayed rectifier K⁺ channel in setting the resting potential suggests that modulation of the activity of this channel would provide VSMCs a mechanism for altering E_m. Indeed, much interest has recently been generated by evidence that alterations in cell redox state might affect membrane potential via direct or indirect modulation of K⁺ voltage-gated currents in pulmonary arterial VSMCs. Recent work suggests that interventions which should result in cell reduction (e.g. hypoxia, application of reduced glutathione) cause K⁺ current inhibition, while oxidizing agents such as oxidized glutathione and H_2O_2 have the opposite effect (Post *et al.*, 1992; Weir & Archer, 1995; Yuan *et al.*, 1993, 1994). Similar findings have been reported for transient K⁺ currents in type I cells of the carotid body (Ganfornina & López-Barneo, 1992), and compelling evidence has been presented that the redox state of a cysteine residue located within a distinct sequence present near the amino-terminal end of

SMOOTH MUSCLE EXCITATION
ISBN 0-12-112360-X

several types of cloned voltage-gated K^+ channels determines the nature of current inactivation (Ruppersberg *et al.*, 1991).

Except for these observations, relatively little is known about other types of regulation of voltage-gated K^+ currents in vascular smooth muscle. Aiello *et al.*, (1995) have recently demonstrated that the delayed rectifier K^+ current in rabbit portal vein VSMCs is potentiated by isoprenaline and forskolin, and that the effect of isoprenaline is suppressed if cells are dialysed with a peptide inhibitor of protein kinase A. The existence of I_K regulation by other second messenger systems has not been confirmed, although it is clear that voltage-gated K^+ channels are regulated by protein kinases in many other types of cell (Walsh & Kass, 1991; Busch *et al.*, 1992; Payett & Dupuis, 1992; Varnum *et al.*, 1993). It is also noteworthy that a $K_v1.5$ delayed rectifier K^+ current abundantly expressed in canine vascular smooth muscles contains consensus sites for protein kinase C-mediated phosphorylation (Overturf *et al.*, 1994).

Here, we describe observations which have resulted from our recent studies of the regulation of the delayed rectifier K^+ current (I_K), mostly in VSMCs isolated from the rat pulmonary artery (RPA). We have previously demonstrated that the blockade of this current with 4-aminopyridine (4-AP) causes a marked depolarization in cells held in current clamp, which does not occur when the smaller Ca^{2+}-activated K^+ current is inhibited with tetraethylammonium (TEA). The importance of this current in setting the resting potential is also suggested by our observation that pulmonary arterial myocytes isolated from chronically hypoxic rats demonstrate both a depolarization of the resting potential, and a reduction of I_K amplitude, compared with similar cells from normoxic rats (Smirnov *et al.*, 1994).

METHODS AND RESULTS

Whole-cell K^+ currents were examined in rat and human arterial VSMCs using the conventional whole-cell patch-clamp technique at room temperature. Cells were isolated using a combination of papain and collagenase in low Ca^{2+} solution, and currents were measured and analysed as described in detail previously (Smirnov & Aaronson, 1992; Smirnov *et al.*, 1994). The Ca^{2+}-activated K^+ current was suppressed by using a highly Ca^{2+}-buffered pipette solution containing 10 mM EGTA and 0.5 mM Ca^{2+}, such that the calculated Ca^{2+} concentration was 8 nM at pH 7.2. The inclusion of 5 mM ATP in the pipette solution, and also the exclusion of any added nucleotide diphosphates, would be expected to minimize any current flowing through glibenclamide-sensitive K^+ channels.

Figure 1 compares the whole-cell K^+ currents from cells described above with those observed in rat and human pulmonary and mesenteric arteries.

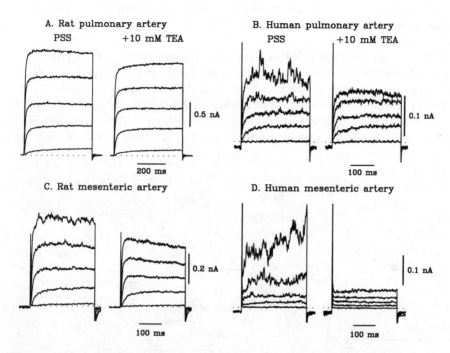

A. Rat pulmonary artery
PSS   +10 mM TEA

0.5 nA

200 ms

B. Human pulmonary artery
PSS   +10 mM TEA

0.1 nA

100 ms

C. Rat mesenteric artery

0.2 nA

100 ms

D. Human mesenteric artery

0.1 nA

100 ms

Figure 1 Comparison of K⁺ currents in myocytes from: A, rat pulmonary artery; B, human pulmonary artery; C, rat mesenteric artery; and D, human mesenteric artery. Cells were stepped to −20, 0, +20, +40, and +60 mV from a holding potential of −60 mV in the absence and presence of 10 mM tetraethyl ammonium (TEA). The dotted line indicates the zero current level in this and following figures.

Currents were elicited under control conditions, and in the presence of TEA (10 mM), which blocks the Ca^{2+}-activated but not voltage-gated K⁺ currents. Figure 1 illustrates that the voltage-gated (TEA-insensitive) K⁺ current was especially prominent in the RPA, compared with the other myocytes examined. This observation appears consistent with the apparent importance of this current in setting the resting potential in these cells. The TEA-insensitive current also showed similar kinetics in both types of rat myocytes, and in those from the human pulmonary artery. Conversely, the TEA-insensitive current in the human mesenteric artery VSMCs demonstrated an initial rapid decay. We have presented evidence that the voltage-gated K⁺ current in these cells is composed of two components which can be distinguished on the basis of differing sensitivities to conditioning potential, and to extracellular divalent cations (Smirnov & Aaronson, 1992).

Effects of pharmacological modulators of the cyclic AMP second messenger system

Figure 2 illustrates the effect of forskolin, an agent which directly stimulates adenylyl cyclase activity, on I_K in RPA myocytes. Forskolin caused a dose-dependent reduction in the amplitude of I_K, with an IC_{50} of 98 μM (Figure 2A,B,C). The involvement of cyclic AMP in this effect was suggested by the observation that inclusion of H-7 (10μM), an inhibitor of protein kinases A and C, in the pipette solution significantly attenuated the effect of forskolin

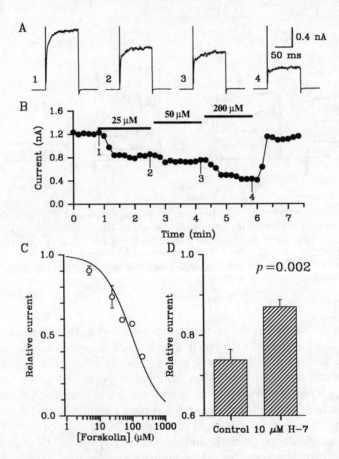

Figure 2   Effect in an RPA myocyte of several concentrations of forskolin on I_K kinetics (A) and amplitude after 100 ms depolarization (B), measured at +60 mV; C, the concentration–response relationship for inhibition of I_K in several cells ($n = 1$–8), and D, inhibition of I_K by forskolin (25 μM) in the absence ($n = 8$) and presence ($n = 6$) of the protein kinase inhibitor H-7 (10 μM) in the pipette solution.

(Figure 2D); H-7 itself had no effect on the current. Conversely, 8-bromo cyclic AMP (400 μM), a membrane-permeable analogue of cyclic AMP, had no obvious effect on I_K.

Effects of pharmacological modulators of protein kinase C

Protein kinase C activity may be stimulated by using phorbol esters, which mimic the effects of diacylglycerol. Figure 3A shows that 4-β-phorbol 12,13 dibutyrate (4-β-PDBu) reduced the amplitude of I_K in RPA myocytes (measured at the end of the 100 ms depolarizing step); the IC_{50} for this effect was approximately 25 μM. Figure 3B illustrates that at a concentration of

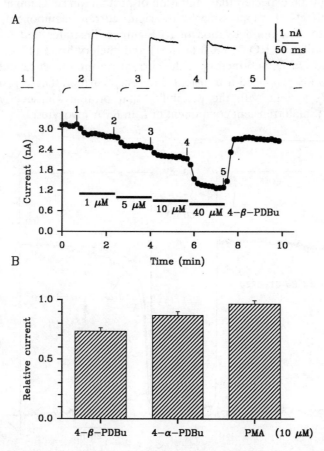

Figure 3 A, Effect of several concentrations of 4-β-PDBu on I_K at +60 mV in one RPA myocyte, B, the effects of 4-β-PDBu, 4-α-PDBu, and PMA (all 10 μM) on I_K amplitude in several cells.

10 μM 4-β-PDBU was significantly more effective than the inactive phorbol ester 4-α-phorbol dibutyrate in reducing I_K amplitude. Conversely, however, the active phorbol 12 myristate 13-acetate (PMA, 10 μM) had no significant effect on current amplitude. It was unclear, therefore, whether the inhibitory effects of 4-β-PDBU resulted from an effect on protein kinase C which was for some reason not mimicked by PMA, or whether the 4-β-PDBU was acting to reduce I_K by a protein kinase C-independent mechanism.

It is interesting, however, that the diminution of I_K caused by 4-β-PDBU was associated with a change in the kinetics of I_K, such that an initial transient component of current became prominent (Figure 3A, 10 and 40 μM). A possible explanation of this result was that 4-β-PDBU enhanced a transient component of current that was normally too small to observe clearly. In this case, it might be expected that inhibition of protein kinase C might have the opposite effect of suppressing a transient current component, thereby appearing to slow the activation of I_K. Figure 4 illustrates that the protein kinase C inhibitors RO 31-8820 (10 μM) and chelerythrine (10 μM) slowed the activation of I_K. Subtraction of the currents in the presence and absence of these agents produced a transient difference current. These results were therefore consistent with the possibility that protein kinase C might be regulating a small transient component of I_K in RPA myocytes.

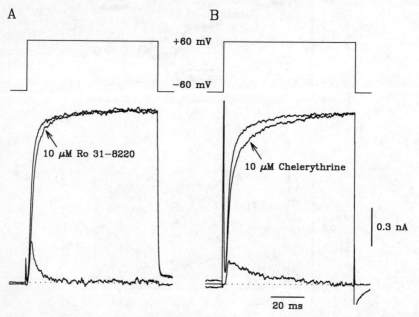

Figure 4   Effects of A, RO 31-8220, and B, chelerythrine (both 10 μM) on I_K in two RPA myocytes. The difference currents obtained by subtracting the current traces in the presence and absence of drugs are also shown.

Effects of pharmacological modulators of tyrosine kinases

We recently evaluated the effects of several pharmacological inhibitors of tyrosine kinases upon I_K in rat and rabbit pulmonary arteries (Smirnov & Aaronson, 1995). The effects of these agents were diverse. In RPA myocytes, tyrphostin 23 (100 μM) had no effect on I_K. Genistein (100 μM) reduced the amplitude of the current by about a half and slowed current activation. ST 638 (10 μM) reduced the amplitude of I_K by more than 90%, and also produced a striking change in current kinetics (Figure 5). The current, which usually showed minimal inactivation over several-hundred ms, decayed to a very low level with a time constant of 15.8 ± 0.8 ms if ST 638 was present (mean ± SEM, $n=15$).

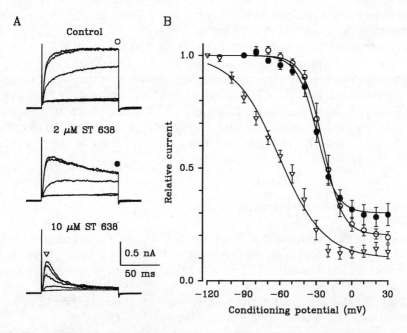

Figure 5   A, Effects of 30 s conditioning potentials (−90, −60, −30, 0, +30, +60) on I_K in RPA myocytes at +60 mV, under control conditions (upper traces), and in the presence of 2 μM (middle traces) and 10 μM (lower traces) ST 638. B, The relationship between conditioning potential and current availability at the end of a 300 ms pulse in the absence of drug, (o, $n = 7$) in the presence of 2 μM ST 638 (●, $n = 6$), and 4-6 ms after depolarization in the presence of 10 μM ST 638 (∇, $n = 7$). Solid lines were drawn according to the Boltzmann function with half-inactivation potentials of −24.4, −29.5 and −60.8 mV, and slope factors of 8.3, 8.3 and 18.8 mV for control, 2 and 10 μM ST 638, respectively.

The effects of genistein and ST 638 did not appear to be mediated by tyrosine kinase inhibition, as they were not modified when ATP was omitted from the patch pipette, or when it was replaced by the poor tyrosine kinase substrate ATPγS (both under glucose free conditions). Similarly, the effects of these drugs were unaltered by including the tyrosine phosphatase inhibitor orthovanadate in the pipette or bathing solution.

Two observations suggested that the effects of ST 638 might be attributed to the presence of two components of current, a transient component which was ST 638 resistant, and a sustained component which was relatively ST 638 sensitive. First, as illustrated in Figure 5, the inactivation–potential relationship of the ST 638-resistant current in RPA myocytes was significantly more negative than that of the sustained current, measured in the absence of any drug, or in the presence of a concentration of ST 638 which caused marked inhibition. Second, evaluation of the effects of ST 638 in rabbit pulmonary arteries, which exhibit a prominent A-like current under control conditions, revealed that ST 638 had no effect on this transient current, but greatly reduced the sustained current (Smirnov & Aaronson, 1995).

These results provided little information about the regulation of I_K by tyrosine kinases, but emphasized the dangers inherent in the use of 'selective' pharmacological inhibitors. It was interesting, however, that the effects of ST 638 echoed those of the protein kinase C modulators in implying that separate transient and sustained components of I_K existed in the RPA myocytes, although no such distinction was apparent kinetically under control conditions.

Modification of I_K by arachidonic acid

Bath application of arachidonic acid (1–50 μM) caused marked effects upon I_K in RPA myocytes which are illustrated in Figure 6A. The activation of the current was accelerated and there was an increase in the amplitude of early current. The current then decayed rapidly to a low level. Similar effects were exerted by linoleic acid which is also polyunsaturated; the unsaturated myristic acid had a much smaller inhibitory effect on I_K.

The amplitude of the inhibitory effect of arachidonic acid (AA) appeared to be concentration dependent, although this could be attributed in part to the fact that the rate of development of inhibition was also concentration dependent. Thus, for example, current inhibition by 50 μM AA stabilized at approximately 78% within 2 min of application, but was still progressively decreasing beyond 50% 4 min after 3 μM AA was applied. The increase in the peak current showed little sign of concentration dependency between 1 and 50 μM AA, possibly because the amplitude of the current peak was affected by the acceleration of both I_K activation and inactivation.

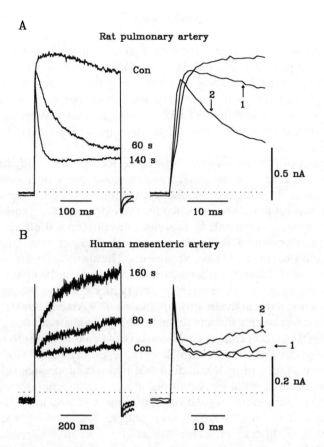

Figure 6 Effects of 50 μM arachidonic acid on I_K at +60 mV in myocytes from A, rat pulmonary artery; B, human mesenteric artery. Traces on the right are displayed at an expanded time scale to illustrate the effects on the early current.

The inhibitory effects of AA were not suppressed by the cyclo-oxygenase inhibitor indomethacin (20 μM, 5–8 min incubation) or by the lipoxygenase inhibitor nordihydroguaiaretic acid (20 μM, 6–8 min incubation), suggesting that the production of prostaglandins or leukotrienes was not involved in this response. However, the cytochrome P-450 metabolite 11,12-epoxy-(5Z,11Z,14Z)-eicosatrienoic acid did cause inhibition of the current at 0.8 and 3.0 μM ($n = 3$ and 2 cells, respectively).

The effect of 50 μM AA on I_K in human mesenteric arterial myocytes was quite different from that seen in the RPA. Figure 6B shows that AA greatly enhanced the sustained K+ current in the mesenteric arterial cells. The initial transient component of this current, illustrated on the right was, however, not obviously affected by AA.

DISCUSSION

The results presented above indicate that a number of pharmacological modulators of protein kinases exert marked effects on I_K in RPA myocytes. It is not at all clear, unfortunately, to what extent these effects can be ascribed to alterations in kinase activity. In particular, an examination of the effects of the tyrosine kinases inhibitors ST 638 and genistein on I_K suggested that they resulted from direct action on the K^+ channels rather than from kinase inhibition.

The results of the studies with 4-β-PBDu, RO-31 8820, and chelerythrine suggested, however, that an initial transient component of I_K exists in RPA myocytes, and is enhanced by the activation of protein kinase C. This possibility was supported by evidence for the existence of a transient ST 638-resistant current component. In this case, the differential effects of AA on the early and sustained K^+ current might also reflect separate effects on transient and sustained current components. The stimulatory effect of AA on the early current, taken together with the effects of the PKC modulators on the early current, might be connected observations, in that unsaturated fatty acids are known to activate protein kinase C (Asaoka *et al.,* 1992). At present, however, such a linkage remains highly speculative.

The possible heterogeneous distribution between blood vessels of subtypes of voltage-gated K^+ channels which may be differentially modulated has already been suggested by the finding that hypoxia suppresses voltage-gated currents in cultured pulmonary, but not mesenteric arterial myocytes (Yuan *et al.,* 1993). Differential regulation may, however, not be limited to that exerted by cell redox state. As shown above, AA enhances the sustained current in I_K in human mesenteric arterial myocytes while inhibiting the sustained K^+ current in rat pulmonary arterial myocytes. The possibility that AA and other second messengers might have artery-specific effects on membrane potential depend, at least in part, on the presence of specific types of voltage-gated K^+ channels is especially interesting in that hypoxia has been demonstrated to activate phospholipase A. The ongoing classification of vascular K^+ channels, both on functional and molecular biological criteria, is likely to continue to provide new insights into how diverse blood vessels are differentially controlled by various stimuli.

REFERENCES

Aiello, E.A., Walsh, M.P. & Cole, W.C. (1995). Phosphorylation by protein kinase A enhances delayed rectifier K^+ current in rabbit vascular smooth muscle cells. *Am. J. Physiol.* **268,** H926–H934.

Asaoka, Y., Nakamura, S., Yoshida, K. & Nishizuka, Y. (1992). Protein kinase C, calcium and phospholipid degradation. *Trends Biochem. Sci.* **17**, 414–417.

Beech, D.J. & Bolton, T.B. (1989a). A voltage-dependent outward current with fast kinetics in single smooth muscle cells isolated from rabbit portal vein. *J. Physiol.* **412**, 397–414.

Beech, D.J. & Bolton, T.B. (1989b). Two components of potassium current activated by depolarisation of single smooth muscle cells from the rabbit portal vein. *J. Physiol.* **418**, 293–309.

Busch, A.E., Varnum, M.D., North, J.P. & Adelman, J.P. (1992). An amino acid mutation in a potassium channel that prevents inhibition by protein kinase C. *Science* **255**, 1705–1707.

Edwards, F.R., Hirst, G.D.S. & Silverberg, G.D. (1988). Inward rectification in rat cerebral arterioles; involvement of potassium ions in autoregulation. *J. Physiol.* **404**, 455–466.

Ganfornina, M.D. & López-Barneo, J. (1992). Potassium channel types in arterial chemoreceptor cells and their selective modulation by oxygen. *J. Gen. Physiol.* **100**, 401–426.

Overturf, K.E., Russell, S.N., Carl, A., Vogalis, F., Hart, P.J., Hume, J.R., Sanders, K.M., Horowitz, B. (1994). Cloning and characterization of a $K_v1.5$ delayed rectifier K+ channel from vascular and visceral smooth muscles. *Am. J. Physiol.* **267**, C1231–C1238.

Payett, M.D. & Dupuis, G. (1992). Dual regulation of the *n* type K+ channel in Jurkat T lymphocytes by protein kinases A and C. *J. Biolog. Chem.* **267**, 18270–18273.

Post, J., Hume, J., Archer, S. & Weir, E. (1992). Direct role for potassium channel inhibition in hypoxic pulmonary vasoconstriction. *Am. J. Physiol.* **262**, C882–C890.

Ruppersberg, J.P., Stocker, M., Pongs, O., Heinemann, S.H., Frank, R. & Koenen, M. (1991). Regulation of fast inactivation of cloned mammalian $I_k(A)$ channels by cysteine oxidation. *Nature* **352**, 711-714.

Smirnov, S.V. & Aaronson, P.I. (1992). Ca^{2+}-activated and voltage-gated K+ currents in smooth muscle cells isolated from human mesenteric arteries. *J. Physiol.* **457**, 431–454.

Smirnov. S.V. & Aaronson, P.I. (1995). Inhibition of vascular smooth muscle cell K+ currents by tyrosine kinase inhibitors genistein and ST 638. *Circ. Res.* **76**, 310–316.

Smirnov, S.V., Robertson, T.P., Ward, J.P.T. & Aaronson, P.I. (1994). Chronic hypoxia is associated with reduced delayed rectifier K+ current in rat pulmonary artery muscle cells. *Am. J. Physiol.* **266**, H365–H370.

Varnum, M.D., Busch, A.E., Bond, C.T., Maylie, J. & Adelman, J.P. (1993). The min K channel underlies the cardiac potassium current I_{Ks} and mediates species-specific responses to protein kinase C. *Proc. Natl Acad. Sci. USA* **90**, 11528–11532.

Walsh, K.B. & Kass, R.S. (1991). Distinct voltage-dependent regulation of a heart-delayed I_K by protein kinases A and C. *Am. J. Physiol.* **261**, C1081–C1090.

Weir, E.K. & Archer, S.G. (1995). The mechanism of acute hypoxic pulmonary vasoconstriction: the tale of two channels. *FASEB J.* **9**, 183–189.

Yuan, X-J., Goldman, W., Tod, M., Rubin, L. & Blaustein, M. (1993). Hypoxia reduces potassium currents in cultured rat pulmonary but not mesenteric arterial myocytes. *Am. J. Physiol.* **264**, L116–L123.

Yuan, X-J., Tod, M., Rubin, L. & Blaustein, M. (1994). Deoxyglucose and reduced glutathione mimic effects of hypoxia on K+ and Ca^{2+} conductances in pulmonary artery cells. *Am. J. Physiol.* **267**, L52–L63.

7

Glibenclamide-sensitive Potassium Channels in Smooth Muscle

K. KITAMURA*
R. OGATA**
M. KAMOUCHI**
K. TSURUDA*
M. SHIBATA*
T. OHKUBO*
H. KURIYAMA**

*Department of Dental Pharmacology,
Fukuoka Dental College,
Fukuoka, Japan

**Departments of Internal Medicine and Pharmacology,
Faculty of Medicine,
Kyushu University,
Fukuoka, Japan

The presence of ATP-sensitive K^+ channels has now been confirmed in various cells including smooth muscle cells (Noma, 1983; Ashcroft, 1988; Standen et al., 1989; Kajioka et al., 1991). The channel was called the ATP-sensitive K^+ channel as submillimolar concentrations of intracellular ATP ($[ATP]_i$) could block channel activity. However, for activation of the channel a small amount of ATP with Mg^{2+} or other nucleotide is also required. Another important feature of the ATP-sensitive K^+ channel is its inhibition by glibenclamide. To date, all ATP-sensitive K^+ channels observed in various cells have been reported to be sensitive to glibenclamide or other sulphonylurea derivatives. In the rabbit portal vein, K^+ channel openers produced marked hyperpolarization and glibenclamide attenuated this hyperpolarization. However, glibenclamide alone did not depolarize the membrane, suggesting that this K^+ channel did not contribute to the resting membrane potential in this vascular cell. Other K^+ channel blockers, such as tetraethylammonium (TEA) or 4-aminopyridine (4AP) also partly inhibited the glibenclamide-sensitive current in smooth muscle cells. Much higher

SMOOTH MUSCLE EXCITATION
ISBN 0-12-112360-X

concentrations of TEA and 4AP (10 mM) than glibenclamide (3–10 µM) were required to inhibit the pinacidil-induced outward current. Reduction of Ca^{2+} concentration in the cell and/or superfusate did not change the channel activity of the ATP-sensitive K^+ channel in rabbit portal vein or mesenteric and basilar arteries. However, several Ca^{2+}-dependent K^+ channels recorded in smooth muscle cells are also inhibited by glibenclamide and intracellular ATP. In smooth muscle cells, several results indicate that K^+ channel openers open different K^+ channels. In guinea pig mesenteric vein the hyperpolarization induced by nicorandil and cromakalim was classified into fast and slow components by their Ca^{2+} sensitivity (Nakao *et al.*, 1988). Conversely, a glibenclamide-sensitive outward current in the rabbit portal vein induced by pinacidil and LP 805 was classified as a Ca^{2+}-independent current, because the amplitude of the outward current induced by K^+ channel openers was not attenuated by removal of $[Ca^{2+}]_o$ or by addition of a high concentration of EGTA in the cell (Kamouchi *et al.*, 1993). However, in the rat portal vein and porcine coronary artery a glibenclamide-sensitive outward current produced by nicorandil or cromakalim was sensitive to $[Ca^{2+}]_o$ (Okabe *et al.*, 1990; Inoue *et al.*, 1990).

Single channel current recording also revealed that K^+ channel openers activate several different types of K^+ channel in smooth muscle cells. Kusano *et al.* (1987) first reported that cromakalim opens a large conductance Ca^{2+}-dependent K^+ channel in cultured cells of bovine and rabbit aorta (200 pS with symmetrical high K^+ solution). High concentrations of TEA could block this K^+ channel current. Gelband *et al.* (1989) demonstrated that cromakalim increased the open probability of the maxi-K^+ channel in the rabbit thoracic aorta by reducing the closed time of the slow component. Gelband *et al.* (1991) also reported that cromakalim and also lemakalim, an active isomer of cromakalim, increased the open probability of the large conductance Ca^{2+}-dependent K^+ channel (maxi-K^+ channel), which was very sensitive to the external application of low concentrations of TEA, in the canine colon and renal and coronary arteries. They also reported that glibenclamide reduced the open probability of the maxi-K^+ channel induced by K^+ channel openers in the inside-out membrane patch. Similarly, Hermsmeyer (1991) demonstrated that ChTX could partly inhibit the outward current induced by pinacidil, but he also noted that an ATP-sensitive K^+ channel was distributed in the same rat azygos veins, with unitary conductance of 50 pS. It is interesting that lemakalim had no action on the maxi-K^+ channel pretreated by TEA (Gelband *et al.*, 1991). It might be suggested that a binding site for TEA on the maxi-K^+ channel is situated at the outer mouth of the channel, whereas lemakalim probably binds to the channel via a hydrophobic pathway. The gating mechanism of the maxi-K^+ channel is modulated by cAMP and cGMP or other metabolic processes, but activation of the maxi-K^+ channel by cromakalim is not related to such metabolic pathways, as lemakalim is reported to increase neither cAMP nor cGMP content (Coldwell & Howlett, 1987). Therefore, we may expect that lemakalim activates the channel in a direct way rather than by a known second messenger system and that binding of TEA in the channel leads to a kinetic change of the open gate regulated by K+ channel openers in the maxi-K+ channel. However, contribution of the maxi-K+ channel to K+ channel opener-induced current was probably small, and evidence has now accumulated against the maxi-K+ channel being the target for K+ channel openers. For example, in cell-attached patches of the rabbit portal vein the maxi-K+ channel spontaneously opened and glibenclamide did not block the activity of this channel. Furthermore, in the presence of pinacidil, a small conductance K+ chanel current (15 pS; ATP-sensitive K+ channel) was also activated, while the frequency of channel opening of the maxi-K+ current was not modified by pinacidil.

Standen et al. (1989) first reported that a ATP-sensitive K+ channel similar to those in cardiac and pancreatic β-cells is present in smooth muscle cells of the rabbit mesenteric artery. The unitary conductance of this ATP-sensitive K+ channel is larger than those in cardiac, pancreatic β-cells and rabbit portal vein but similar to that of the maxi-K+ channel (135 pS). However, pharmacological properties of the ATP-sensitive K+ channel in the mesenteric artery resemble those in cardiac and pancreatic β-cells, in being Ca^{2+}-insensitive, ChTX-insensitive, TEA-resistant and glibenclamide-sensitive. In rabbit portal vein, an ATP-sensitive K+ channel with smaller unitary conductance than in the rabbit mesenteric artery was reported to be present, but the pharmacological properties of the channel are very similar (Kajioka et al., 1991). In rat portal vein, a different type of ATP-sensitive K+ channel was activated by K+ channel openers (Kajioka et al., 1990; Okabe et al., 1990). The outward current induced by cromakalim or nicorandil was attenuated by removal of $[Ca^{2+}]_o$ and the unitary current (10 pS in asymmetrical K+ concentrations) was sensitive to $[ATP]_i$, $[Ca^{2+}]_i$ and glibenclamide, but not sensitive to apamin and ChTX. Noack et al. (1992) also estimated that in the same cells (rat portal vein) lemakalim opened a small conductance K+ channel (17 pS), which was sensitive to glibenclamide, but insensitive to $[Ca^{2+}]_o$. This discrepancy might be due to the presence of more than one glibenclamide-sensitive K+ channel in rat portal vein. In guinea pig mesenteric vein, K+ channel openers produce hyperpolarization with transient Ca^{2+}-resistant and slow Ca^{2+}-sensitive components, while in guinea pig mesenteric artery only Ca^{2+}-resistant, transient hyperpolarization was seen by application of a K+ channel opener (Nakao et al., 1988). Furthermore, Okabe et al. (1990) demonstrated that cromakalim still produced an outward current even in the presence of Mn^{2+}, although a major part of the outward current was inhibited by removal of Ca^{2+}. Conversely, Noack et al. (1992) speculated that the difference in sensitivity to $[Ca^{2+}]$ may be due to interference of the channel by Mn^{2+} because we always used Mn^{2+} as a Ca^{2+} substitute.

Although glibenclamide-sensitive K^+ channels recorded in the rat portal vein and guinea pig mesenteric vein were also classified as Ca^{2+}-dependent K^+ channels from their Ca^{2+} sensitivity, these channels clearly differed from the maxi-K^+ channel. No effect of charybdotoxin on the K^+ channel current induced by various K^+ channel openers was seen in the rabbit portal vein, indicating that the maxi-K^+ channel is not the target for these K^+ channel openers. The observation that pinacidil produced an outward current in the presence of 4 mM EGTA in the pipette or without Ca^{2+} in the bath, also supports the idea that K^+ channel openers open a Ca^{2+}-resistant K^+ channel in smooth muscle cells except in rat portal vein and in pig coronary artery (Inoue *et al.*, 1990; Okabe *et al.*, 1990).

Pinacidil also inhibited the Ca^{2+}-dependent K^+ channel current, possibly acting on the Ca^{2+} release-uptake mechanism of the Ca^{2+} store sites. Indeed, pinacidil at high concentrations partly inhibited the high-K^+-induced contraction of vascular muscle. Although other K^+ channel openers had no such action, nicorandil is known to activate guanylate cyclase and cromakalim had inhibitory effects on the voltage-dependent Ca^{2+} channels in rat portal vein. In the rat portal vein, cromakalim, nicorandil and pinacidil linearly increased the membrane conductance at negative membrane potentials. However, at positive membrane potentials, these K^+ channel openers did not increase the conductance but in some cases inhibited the outward current. This inhibition of the outward current at positive membrane potentials was still seen in the absence of Ca^{2+}. We simply concluded that K^+ channel openers also had an inhibitory action on the delayed K^+ current (Okabe *et al.*, 1990). In hippocampal CA1 neurone of the rat, cromakalim was also reported to inhibit the delayed K current (Erdemli & Krnjevic, 1994).

Glibenclamide and other sulphonylurea derivatives are thought to be specific blockers of the ATP-sensitive K^+ channel in many cells (Sanguinetti *et al.*, 1988; de Weille *et al.*, 1989; Nelson *et al.*, 1990; Kajioka *et al.*, 1990, 1991; Ciampolillo *et al.*, 1992). However, glibenclamide has been reported to inhibit other K^+ channels in several preparations; For example, glibenclamide (1–20 μM) produces a voltage-independent but time-dependent inhibition of the K^+ channel, which is insensitive to $[ATP]_i$ and $[Ca^{2+}]_o$ in the human neuroblastoma cell line (SH-SY5Y) (Reeve *et al.*, 1992). Glibenclamide was also reported to inhibit the maxi-K^+ channel in smooth muscle cell-attached patches (Gelband, 1991). However, we observed that glibenclamide had no effect on the maxi-K^+ channel in the rabbit portal vein in isolated patches (Kajioka *et al.*, 1991; Xiong *et al.*, 1992). As glibenclamide inhibited the ryanodine-sensitive outward current, glibenclamide possibly inhibited the maxi-K^+ channel through acting on the Ca^{2+}-induced Ca^{2+} release mechanism (Xiong *et al.*, 1991).

Binding experiments showed that there were two binding sites for glibenclamide (high- and low-affinity sites) in brain, β-cells, cardiac and smooth muscle cells (Geisen et al., 1985; Niki et al., 1989; Gopalakrishnan et al., 1991). Electrophysiological experiments also revealed more than one binding site for glibenclamide, as glibenclamide inhibited the ATP-sensitive K+ channel with a Hill coefficient of 1.26 in guinea pig ventricular cells (Findlay, 1992). However, it is interesting that K+ channel openers, such as cromakalim, lemakalim, pinacidil, minoxidil and nicorandil, are reported not to interact with the glyburide-binding site, suggesting different binding sites for K+ channel openers and sulfonylurea (Gopalakrishnan et al., 1991).

The 'run down' phenomenon is a interesting feature of the ATP-sensitive K+ channel in the rabbit portal vein. The activity of the ATP-sensitive K+ channel was reduced within 1 min after excision of the membrane in ATP-free solution (Findlay & Dunne, 1986; Ohno-Shosaku et al., 1987; Standen et al., 1989; Kajioka et al., 1991; Kamouchi & Kitamura, 1994). Channel life time (the period until final appearance of the channel opening) depended on the absence or presence of $MgCl_2$. In inside-out patch of the rabbit portal vein the ATP-sensitive K+ channel current was abolished within 1 min, when $MgCl_2$ was omitted from the intracellular solution. However, the current appeared for more than 3 min in the presence of 1–2 mM Mg^{2+}. The 'run down' probably occurs through channel de-phosphorylation by depletion of ATP inside the membrane, because re-administration of low concentrations of ATP or withdrawal of high concentrations of ATP activate the ATP-sensitive K+ channel in various cells (Findlay & Dunne, 1986; Ohno-Shosaku et al., 1987; Ribalet et al., 1989). In the rabbit portal vein, when $MgCl_2$ was present in the bath, the ATP-sensitive K+ channel current was transiently augmented by excision of the membrane, then gradually inactivated. This was not caused by a change in the drug concentration because no enhancement of the current activity was seen upon membrane excision in the absence of $MgCl_2$. In the presence of a K+ channel opener and Mg^{2+}, ATP activated the ATP-sensitive K+ channel and withdrawal of ATP further enhanced the channel activity in the rabbit portal vein. However, in the absence of Mg^{2+}, simultaneous presence of the K+ channel opener and ATP barely activate the channel. Therefore, we could speculate that membrane excision immediately changes cytosolic circumstances especially Mg^{2+}-ATP content which modulate channel activity. Ribalet et al. (1989) reported, in insulin-secreting cells, that cAMP-dependent protein kinase or cAMP also enhanced the channel activity and a specific inhibitor of the cAMP-dependent protein kinase inhibited the activity. It is not yet clear that Mg^{2+}-ATP-dependent channel reactivation is related to channel phosphorylation with cAMP-dependent protein kinase in the rabbit portal vein. However, we may conclude that channel phosphorylation by cAMP-dependent protein kinase or other kinases might be involved in the activation mechanisms of the

ATP-sensitive K$^+$ channel. Evidence that reactivation of the channel by ATP required Mg^{2+} (Kamouchi & Kitamura, 1994) and that nonhydrolysable ATP analogues (such as AMP-PNP, AMP-PCP, ATPγS and ADPβS) had little or no effect on the channel reactivation; (Ohno-Shosaku *et al.*, 1987; Dunne & Petersen, 1986a; Takano *et al.*, 1990), also indicate involvement of channel phosphorylation in the reactivation mechanisms.

In insulin-secreting cells, GTP and its analogues (GTPγS, GDP and GDPβS) have been reported to activate the channel, when Mg^{2+} was simultaneously present (Dunne & Petersen, 1986b). Tung & Kurachi (1991) also reported that, in guinea pig ventricular cells, various nucleotide diphosphates could activate the ATP-sensitive K$^+$ channel in the de-phosphorylated condition. However, they did not see any action of triphosphate and monophosphate forms of nucleotide on the K$^+$ channel.

Kajioka *et al.* (1991) demonstrated that in the smooth muscle cells of rabbit portal vein K$^+$ channel openers only opened the ATP-sensitive K$^+$ channel when GDP or GTP was present in the cell. However, GTPγS had no action on the channel activity and GDPβS reduced it. GTP-binding protein was not involved in channel reactivation since GTPγS did not mimic GTP action in the smooth muscle cells nor did GDPβS antagonize GTP action in insulin secreting cells. Mg^{2+} is essential for reactivation of the channel by nucleotide diphosphate in cardiac cells, but not in smooth muscle cells (Kajioka *et al.*, 1991; Tung & Kurachi, 1991). In rabbit portal vein in the presence of K$^+$ channel opener, GDP opened ATP-sensitive K$^+$ channels even in the absence of Mg^{2+}. However, addition of Mg^{2+} augmented channel opening. Under our experimental conditions, the ATP-sensitive K$^+$ channel opened only when nucleotide and K$^+$ channel opener were simultaneously present. These results indicate that the intracellular mechanism of channel activation involves Mg^{2+}- and nucleotide-requiring systems in the rabbit portal vein. At present, it is not clear whether Mg^{2+}- and nucleotide-requiring systems are related to channel phosphorylation-dephosphorylation. It is possible that intracellular Mg^{2+}-ATP and GDP, or other nucleotide diphosphate, shift the channel to an operative state through channel phosphorylation or some other unknown mechanism. K$^+$ channel openers open the channel gate when the ATP-sensitive K$^+$ channel is in an operative state.

REFERENCES:

Ashcroft, F.M. (1988). Adenosine 5'-triphosphate-sensitive potassium channels. *Annu. Rev. Neurosci.* **11**, 97–118.

Ciampolillo, F., Tung, D.E. & Cameron, J.S. (1992). Effects of diazoxide and glyburide on ATP-sensitive K$^+$ channels from hypertrophied ventricular myocytes. *J. Pharmacol. Exp. Therap.* **260**, 254–260,.

Coldwell, M.C. & Howlett, D.R. (1987). Specificity of action of the novel antihypertensive agent, BRL 34915, as a potassium channel activator. Comparison with nicorandil. *Biochem. Pharmacol.* **36**, 3663–3669.

Dunne, M.J. & Petersen, O.H. (1986a). Intracellular ADP activates K+ channels that are inhibited by ATP in an insulin-secreting cell line. *FEBS Lett.* **208**, 59–62.

Dunne, M.J. & Petersen, O.H. (1986b). GTP and GDP activation of K+ channels that can be inhibited by ATP. *Pflügers Arch. Eur. J. Physiol.* **407**, 564–565.

Erdemli, G. & Krnjevic, K. (1994). Actions of cromakalim on outward currents of CA1 neurones in hyppocampal slices. *Br. J. Pharmacol.* **113**, 411–418.

Findlay, I. (1992). Inhibition of ATP-sensitive K+ channels in cardiac muscle by the sulphonylurea drug glibenclamide. *J. Pharmacol. Exp. Therap.* **261**, 540–545.

Findlay, I. & Dunne, M.J. (1986). ATP maintains ATP-inhibited K+ channels in an operational state. *Pflügers Arch. Eur. J. Physiol.* **407**, 238–240.

Geisen, K., Hetzel, V., Ökomomopoulos, R., Pünter, J., Weyer, R. & Summ, H.D. (1985). Inhibition of [³H]glibenclamide binding to sulfonylurea receptors by oral antidiabetics. *Arzneimitt. Forsch.* **35**, 707–712.

Gelband, C.H., Lodge, N.J. & Van Breemen, C. (1989). A Ca²⁺-activated K+ channel from rabbit aorta, modulation by cromakalim. *Eur. J. Pharmacol.* **167**, 201–210.

Gelband, C.H., Carl, A., Post, J.M., Bowen, S.M., Ishikawa, T., Keef, K.D., Sanders, K.M. & Hume, J.R. (1991). Effects of cromakalim and lemakalim on whole-cell and single-channel K+ currents in canine colonic, renal and coronary smooth muscle cells. In *Ion Channels of Vascular Smooth Muscle Cells and Endothelial Cells* (Sperelakis, N. & Kuriyama, H., eds), pp. 125–138. Elsevier, New York.

Gopalakrishnan, M., Johnson, D.E., Janis, R.A. & Triggle, D.J. (1991). Characterization of binding of the ATP-sensitive potassium channel ligand, [³H]glyburide, to neuronal and muscle preparations. *J. Pharmacol. Exp. Therap.* **257**, 1162–1171.

Hermsmeyer, K. (1991). Potassium channel currents of vascular muscle. In *Ion Channels of Vascular Smooth Muscle Cells and Endothelial Cells* (Sperelakis, N. & Kuriyama, H., eds), pp. 107–110. Elsevier, New York.

Inoue, I., Nakaya, S. & Nakaya, Y. (1990). An ATP-sensitive K+ channel activated by extracellular Ca²⁺ and Mg²⁺ in primary cultured arterial smooth muscle cells. *J. Physiol. (London)* **430**, 132P.

Kajioka, S., Oike, M. & Kitamura, K. (1990). Nicorandil opens a calcium-dependent potassium channel in smooth muscle cells of the rat portal vein. *J. Pharmacol. Exp. Therap.* **254**, 905–913.

Kajioka, S., Kitamura, K. & Kuriyama, H. (1991). Guanosine diphosphate activates an adenosine-5'-triphosphate-sensitive K+ channel in the rabbit portal vein. *J. Physiol. (London)* **444**, 397–418.

Kamouchi, M. & Kitamura, K. (1994). Regulation of ATP-sensitive K+ channels by ATP and nucleotide diphosphate in rabbit portal vein. *Am. J. Physiol.* **266**, H1687–H1698.

Kamouchi, M., Kajioka, S., Sakai, T., Kitamura, K. & Kuriyama, H. (1993). A target K+ channel for the LP-805-induced hyperpolarization in smooth muscle cells of the rabbit portal vein. *Naunyn-Schmiedeberg's Arch. Pharmacol.* **347**, 329–335.

Kusano, K., Barros, F., Katz, G.M., Roy-Contancin, L. & Reuben, J.P. (1987). Modulation of K channel activity in aortic smooth muscle by BRL 34915 and scorpion toxin. *Biophys. J.* **51**, 55a.

Nakao, K., Okabe, K., Kitamura, K., Kuriyama, H. & Weston, A.H. (1988). Characteristics of cromakalim-induced relaxations in the smooth muscle cells of guinea pig mesenteric artery and vein. *Br. J. Pharmacol.* **95**, 795–804.

Nelson, M.T., Huang, Y., Brayden, J.E., Hesceler, J. & Standen, N.B. (1990). Arterial dilations in response to calcitonin gene-related peptide involve activation of K^+ channels. *Nature* **344**, 770–773.

Niki, I., Kelly, R.P., Ashcroft, S.J.H. & Ashcroft, F.M. (1989). ATP-sensitive K-channels in HIT T15b cells studied by patch clamp methods, $^{86}Rb^+$ efflux and glibenclamide binding. *Pflügers Arch. Eur. J. Physiol.* **415**, 47–55.

Noack, T., Deitmer, P., Edwards, G. & Weston, A.H. (1992). Characterization of potassium currents modulated by BRL 38227 in rat portal vein. *Br. J. Pharmacol.* **106**, 717–726.

Noma, A. ATP-regulated K^+ channels in cardiac cells. *Nature* **305**, 147–148, 1983.

Ohno-Shosaku, T., Zünkler, B.J. & Trube, G. (1987). Dual effects of ATP on K^+ currents of mouse pancreatic b-cells. *Pflügers Arch. Eur. J. Physiol.* **408**, 133–138.

Okabe, K., Kajioka, S., Nakao, K., Kitamura, K., Kuriyama, H. & Weston, A.H. (1990). Actions of cromakalim on ionic currents recorded from single smooth muscle cells of the rat portal vein. *J. Pharmacol. Exp. Therap.* **250**, 832–839.

Reeve, H.L., Vaugham, P.F.T. & Peers, C. (1992). Glibenclamide inhibits a voltage-gated K^+ current in the human neuroblastoma cell line SH-SY5Y. *Neurosci. Lett.* **135**, 37–40.

Ribalet, B., Ciani, S. & Eddlestone, G.T. (1989). ATP mediates both activation and inhibition of K(ATP) channel activity via cAMP-dependent protein kinase in insulin-secreting cell lines. *J. Gen. Physiol.* **94**, 693–717.

Sanguinetti, M.C., Scott, A.L., Zingaro, G.J. & Siegel, P.K. (1988). BRL 34915 (cromakalim) activates ATP-sensitive K^+ current in cardiac muscle. *Proc. Natl Acad. Sci. USA* **85**, 8360–8364.

Standen, N.B., Quayle, J.M., Davies, N.W., Brayden, J.E., Huang, Y. & Nelson, M.T. (1989). Hyperpolarizing vasodilators activate ATP-sensitive K^+ channels in arterial smooth muscle. *Science* **245**, 177–180.

Takano, M., Qin, D. & Noma, A. (1990). ATP-dependent decay and recovery of K^+ channels in guinea pig cardiac myocytes. *Am. J. Physiol.* **258**, H45–50.

Tung, R.T. & Kurachi, Y. (1991). On the mechanism of nucleotide diphosphate activation of the ATP-sensitive K^+ channel in ventricular cell of guinea pig. *J. Physiol. (London)*.

de Weille, J.R., Fosset, M., Mourre, C., Schmid-Antomarchi, H., Bernardi, H. & Lazdunski, M. (1989). Pharmacology and regulation of ATP-sensitive K^+ channels. *Pflügers Arch. Eur. J. Physiol.* **414** (Suppl. 1), S80–87.

Xiong, Z., Kajioka, S., Sakai, T., Kitamura, K. & Kuriyama, H. (1991). Pinacidil inhibits the ryanodine-sensitive outward current and glibenclamide antagonizes its action in cells from the rabbit portal vein. *Br. J. Pharmacol.* **102**, 788–790.

Xiong, Z., Kitamura, K. & Kuriyama. H. (1992). Evidence for contribution of Ca^{2+} storage sites on unitary K^+ channel currents in inside-out membrane of rabbit portal vein. *Pflügers Arch. Eur. J. Physiol.* **420**, 112–114.

8

Inward Rectifier and ATP-sensitive Potassium Channels in Arterial Smooth Muscle

J. M. QUAYLE**
A. D. BONEV*
J. G. McCARRON*
J. E. BRAYDEN*
M. T. NELSON*

*Department of Pharmacology,
University of Vermont,
Colchester, Vermont, USA

**Department of Cell Physiology and Pharmacology,
University of Leicester,
Leicester, UK

SUMMARY

1. Whole-cell currents through inward rectifier potassium channels and through ATP-sensitive potassium channels were recorded in single smooth muscle cells enzymatically isolated from arteries.
2. The properties of the inward rectifier potassium channel were investigated in the posterior cerebral artery of rat. The channel was inhibited by extracellular barium and caesium ions, with half-inhibition constants at $-60\,\text{mV}$ of around $2\,\mu\text{M}$ for barium and $1000\,\mu\text{M}$ for caesium. Inhibition by both caesium and barium was voltage-dependent, increasing with membrane hyperpolarization. The properties of the channel are discussed in relation to the hypothesis that activation of this channel underlies the metabolic vasodilation seen in response to potassium ions in several vascular beds.
3. Currents through the ATP-sensitive potassium channel in single cells from rabbit mesenteric artery were activated by the vasodilator calcitonin gene-related peptide (CGRP). The second-messenger system underlying

SMOOTH MUSCLE EXCITATION
ISBN 0-12-112360-X

activation of the channel by CGRP involves adenylate cyclase, cAMP, and cAMP-dependent protein kinase. The relevance of these results to regulation of ATP-sensitive potassium channels, and arterial tone, by other vasodilators is discussed.

INTRODUCTION

Several types of potassium channels have been identified in the plasma membrane of arterial smooth muscle cells. These include inward rectifier potassium (K_{IR}) channels, ATP-sensitive potassium (K_{ATP}) channels, voltage-activated potassium (K_V) channels, and calcium-activated (K_{Ca}) potassium channels. Regulation of these channels, for example by vasoactive factors, membrane potential, or intracellular calcium, influences arterial diameter. At physiological potassium concentrations and membrane potentials there is a driving force for potassium ions to leave the smooth muscle cell. Activation of a potassium channel will therefore result in potassium efflux from the cell. The resulting membrane hyperpolarisation will cause smooth muscle relaxation (Nelson *et al.*, 1990a). Conversely, closure of a potassium channel will cause membrane depolarization and smooth muscle contraction. In this chapter we review some recent work on inward rectifier potassium channels and on ATP-sensitive potassium channels in arterial smooth muscle. In particular, we review the evidence that activation of these channels may underlie the vascular relaxation which is seen in response to certain vasodilators.

Inward rectifier potassium (K_{IR}) channels

Inward rectifier potassium channels are present in small diameter cerebral, coronary, and mesenteric arteries (Bonev *et al.*, 1994; Edwards *et al.*, 1988; Edwards & Hirst, 1988; Hirst & Edwards, 1989; Quayle *et al.*, 1993). This type of channel allows movement of potassium ions in one direction (into the cell) more easily than the other direction (out of the cell). However, in physiological situations the cell membrane potential is positive to the potassium equilibrium potential, providing an electrochemical gradient for potassium ions to leave the cell. The inward rectifier will therefore normally conduct an outward and hyperpolarizing membrane current. K_{IR} channels may be preferentially expressed in small or resistance-sized arteries, which have an important role in regulating blood pressure and local blood flow (Quayle *et al.*, 1993).

K_{IR} channels may be involved in the metabolic vasodilation which occurs in response to extracellular potassium ion ($[K^+]_o$) accumulation in several vascular beds. Blood flow within many organs is linked to metabolic demand,

and this is a consequence of the release of vasodilator metabolites from surrounding tissue. These vasodilators include protons, adenosine, and potassium ions, and the relative importance of an individual dilator will depend on the vascular bed. An increase in the extracellular potassium concentration causes small cerebral arteries to dilate, and potassium ions released during neuronal activity may be one of the factors that increase local blood flow in response to metabolic demand (Kuschinsky et al., 1972). An increase in $[K^+]_o$ at the arterial wall may be aided by 'potassium siphoning' through glial cells. Glial endfeet, which lie close to the arterial wall, have a higher potassium conductance than other areas of the cell. Glial cell depolarization following the increase in $[K^+]_o$ which occurs during neuronal activity will therefore result in dumping of potassium ions onto the arterial wall (Newman, 1986).

Extracellular potassium dilates arteries by at least two mechanisms; activation of the electrogenic Na/K pump and activation of inward rectifier potassium channels. The role of the K_{IR} channel in potassium induced dilations was first proposed in the cerebral circulation by Edwards, Hirst, & Silverberg. Increasing extracellular potassium concentration from 5 mM to 10 mM hyperpolarized rat middle cerebral arterioles, and this hyperpolarization was prevented by barium ions (Edwards et al., 1988). An increase in $[K^+]_o$ in this range also dilated pressurized rat cerebral arteries (McCarron & Halpern, 1990). These dilations were prevented by 50 µM barium, but not by endothelium removal, inhibitors of other potassium channels, or by a number of receptor antagonists (McCarron & Halpern, 1990; Knot et al., 1994). Barium ions inhibit K_{IR} currents in rat cerebral arteries at a concentration of 50 µM (see below and Quayle et al., 1993), consistent with the hypothesis that potassium ions dilate cerebral arteries by activating the K_{IR} channel. A similar mechanism for K-induced dilation has been identified in rat coronary arteries (Knot et al., 1994). An increase in the extracellular potassium ion concentration in the 1–5 mM range causes a transient dilation of small cerebral arteries (McCarron & Halpern, 1990). This dilation is abolished by ouabain but not by barium ions, suggesting that over this concentration range potassium ions dilate arteries by activating the Na/K pump (McCarron & Halpern, 1990).

ATP-sensitive (K_{ATP}) potassium channels

ATP-sensitive potessium channels are inhibited by intracellular ATP and are also regulated by other cellular constituents such as nucleotide diphosphate levels. These channels are also modulated by both synthetic and endogenous vasodilators. Indeed, the arterial dilation to endogenous vasodilators such as adenosine and calcitonin gene-related peptide is sensitive to inhibition of K_{ATP} channels, and channel activation may therefore underlie dilation (von

Beckerath et al., 1991: Nelson et al., 1990a). The actions of several synthetic vasodilators are also sensitive to inhibition of K_{ATP} channels (Winquist et al., 1988; Standen et al., 1989).

K_{ATP} channel currents have been measured in single smooth muscle cells isolated from several vascular beds, including pulmonary arteries (Clapp & Gurney, 1992), coronary arteries (Dart & Standen, 1993), and mesenteric arteries (Standen et al., 1989; Russell et al., 1992). K_{ATP} channel currents have been also measured in cells from other types of smooth muscle, including portal vein (e.g. Beech et al., 1993a,b; Kajioka et al., 1991), urinary bladder (Bonev & Nelson, 1993a,b), and gallbladder (Zhang et al., 1994a,b). The reported properties show some variation, particularly at the single-channel level. However, channel activity appears to have either little or no dependence on the membrane potential, is inhibited by intracellular ATP and by sulphonylurea drugs like glibenclamide, and is enhanced by intracellular nucleotide diphosphates.

A number of synthetic compounds activate K_{ATP} channels. These potassium channel openers include minoxidil sulfate, diazoxide, pinacidil, nicorandil, lemakalim, and RP 49356. Vasodilation to all of these compounds is blocked by glibenclamide (Winquist et al., 1988; Standen et al., 1989). Several of these compounds have been shown to activate directly K_{ATP} channels in vascular smooth muscle cells (Standen et al., 1989; Kajioka et al., 1991; Russell et al., 1992; Beech et al., 1993a,b). Glibenclamide inhibits whole-cell K_{ATP} currents, with half inhibition at a concentration between 25 and 200 nM (Beech et al., 1993a,b). Arterial relaxation to K_{ATP} channel openers such as cromakalim and pinacidil are reversed by half by about 100 nM glibenclamide in rabbit mesenteric artery (Meisheri et al., 1993). Glibenclamide appears to be relatively selective for K_{ATP} channels, and has become an important tool in the investigation of the role of K_{ATP} channels in arterial physiology.

K_{ATP} channels have a number of physiological roles in arterial smooth muscle cells (Nelson & Quayle, 1995). The channel is activated by a number of vasodilators, and the associated membrane hyperpolarization causes part of the resulting vasodilation in many cases. The K_{ATP} channel may also be inhibited by vasoconstrictors, which would tend to cause membrane depolarization and constriction. The channel is involved in the metabolic regulation of blood flow: it is activated in conditions of increased blood demand, for example in hypoxia, either by release of vasodilators from the surrounding tissue or as a direct result of hypoxia on the vascular smooth muscle cells. Finally, the channel may be active in the resting state, as inhibition of K_{ATP} channels can lead to increased resistance to blood flow in some vascular beds. Studies addressing the physiological role of K_{ATP} channels have, in many cases, implicated K_{ATP} channels through the ability of glibenclamide to reverse a particular functional effect.

Hypoxia decreases resistance to blood flow in many vascular beds, presumably as a means of increasing blood flow to the hypoxic region. In several vascular beds, including the coronary, cerebral, and skeletal muscle circulations, this hypoxic vasodilation is partially blocked by glibenclamide, suggesting a role for K_{ATP} channels in the response (von Beckerath et al., 1991; Marshall et al., 1993: Reid et al., 1993). Activation of K_{ATP} channels in coronary artery cells mediates the hypoxic-induced dilation of coronary arteries, as glibenclamide completely blocks this response in isolated, intact hearts (von Beckerath et al., 1991). Hypoxia could activate K_{ATP} channels in smooth muscle cells of coronary arteries through a reduction in intracellular ATP, elevation in intracellular ADP, or through an oxygen sensor. Hypoxia also causes the release of adenosine from cardiac myocytes. Adenosine is a potent dilator of coronary arteries, and has been proposed as a metabolic vasodilator in the coronary circulation. Both adenosine and hypoxia activate K_{ATP} currents in single coronary artery smooth muscle cells (Dart & Standen, 1993; 1995).

Hyperpolarizations and part of the vasorelaxations to several endogenous vasodilators are blocked by inhibition of K_{ATP} channels (Standen et al., 1989; Nelson et al., 1990a; von Beckerath et al., 1991). Other endogenous vasodilators, such as adenosine diphosphate (ADP) and acetylcholine (ACh), act through releasing factors from the vascular endothelium. Some of these factors (endothelium-derived hyperpolarizing factor or EDHF) cause glibenclamide-sensitive membrane hyperpolarization of arterial smooth muscle (Brayden, 1991).

Calcitonin gene-related peptide (CGRP) and adenosine have been shown to activate K_{ATP} currents in smooth muscle cells isolated from rabbit mesenteric arteries and porcine coronary arteries, respectively (Nelson et al., 1990a; Dart & Standen, 1993). Several endogenous vasodilators, including CGRP, increase cAMP levels in smooth muscle cells through activation of adenylate cyclase, and the mechanism by which these adenylate cyclase coupled vasodilators activate K_{ATP} channels has been one focus of our recent work (see below and Quayle et al., 1994). CGRP is present in sensory nerve endings which innervate the mesenteric vasculature, and is a potent vasodilator. CGRP may have a protective role in this vascular bed, serving to increase blood flow in response to noxious stimuli, such as acid accumulation at the wall of the mesentery (Figure 1; see also review by Holzer, 1992).

METHODS

Cell preparation

Studies on the modulation of K_{ATP} current by CGRP were undertaken on the rabbit mesenteric artery. New Zealand white rabbits were killed by lethal injection of sodium pentobarbital and exsanguinated. A branch of the

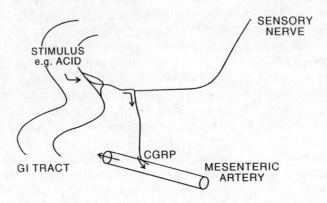

Figure 1 Role of calcitonin gene-related peptide (CGRP) in the mesenteric vasculature.

superior mesenteric artery (external diameter about 1 mM) was dissected in physiological saline solution (PSS) containing (in mM): 137 NaCl, 5.4 KCl, 0.44 NaH$_2$PO4, 0.42 Na$_2$HPO4, 4.17 NaHCO$_3$, 1 MgCl$_2$, 2.6 CaCl$_2$, 10 N-2-hydroxyethylpiperazine-N'-2-ethanesulfonic acid (HEPES), pH adjusted to 7.4 with NaOH. The artery was cut into approximately 5 mm long pieces and placed in PSS containing 0.1 mM CaCl$_2$. The tissue was incubated at 35°C in 0.1 Ca PSS containing 1.6 mg ml^{-1} papain and 1.0 mg ml^{-1} dithioerithritol for 30 mins, and then for a further 10 mins in solution containing 1.5 mg ml^{-1} collagenase and 1 mg ml^{-1} hyaluronidase. Single cells were released by trituration through a pasteur pipette, stored in 0.1 mM Ca PSS at 4°C, and used on the day of preparation. A similar cell isolation procedure was employed for the studies on the K$_{IR}$ current in the posterior cerebral artery of rat.

Data recording

The whole-cell configuration of the patch-clamp technique was used to record potassium currents through the ATP-sensitive potassium channels and inward rectifier potassium channels (Quayle *et al.*, 1993, 1994). Single cells were placed in a chamber through which experimental solutions were continuously perfused. Experiments were conducted at room temperature. Pipettes were fabricated from borosilicate glass (outer diameter 1.5 mm, internal diameter 1.17 mm; Sutter Instrument Co., Novato, CA, USA), and coated with wax to reduce capacitance. Whole-cell currents were amplified by an Axopatch 1C, filtered at 2 kHz, digitized, and stored on computer.

Currents were digitized and analysed using an Axon Instruments TL-1 interface and PCLAMP or AXOTAPE software (Axon Instruments, Burlingame, CA, USA).

Solutions

The pipette solution contained (in mM): 107 KCl, 33 KOH, 10 ethylene glycol-bis(*-aminoethyl ether)-N,N,N',N'-tetraacetic acid (EGTA), 1 $MgCl_2$, 1 $CaCl_2$, 10 HEPES, pH 7.2. ATP (0.1 or 3 mM) and ADP (0.1 mM) were added to the pipette solution on the day of the experiment, and the pH readjusted to 7.2 with NaOH. The extracellular solution contained (in mM): 60 KOH, 80 NaOH, 1 $MgCl_2$, 0.1 $CaCl_2$, 10 HEPES, pH adjusted to 7.4 with NaOH. The contribution of voltage-activated and calcium-activated potassium channels to measured inward potassium currents was minimized by the negative membrane potential and by buffering $[Ca^{2+}]i$ to less than 20 nM. Glibenclamide was made as a 10 mM stock solutions in DMSO on the day of the experiment. Drugs and channel inhibitors were added to the extracellular solution. Chemicals were obtained from Sigma Chemical Co., St. Louis, MO, USA.

RESULTS

Inward rectifier channels in cerebral arteries

Intact segments of arterioles from the rat cerebral circulation have K_{IR} currents (Edwards et al., 1988). To investigate further the basis of the K_{IR} current in arterial smooth muscle, and the mechanism by which potassium dilates arteries, we isolated single cells from the rat posterior cerebral artery (Quayle et al., 1993). Inward potassium currents were recorded negative to the potassium equilibrium potential (EK) in single cells in a solution containing 60 mM $[K^+]_o$ and with pipettes containing 140 mM $[K^+]_i$ (Figure 2).

Inward currents were identified as arising from K_{IR} channels using several criteria (see Quayle et al., 1993). Current reversed at a potential close to the potassium equilibrium potential when the extracellular potassium concentration ($[K^+]_o$) was altered. As $[K^+]_o$ changed, outward current remained small at membrane potentials positive to the potassium equilibrium potential. This dependence of channel activity on $[K^+]_o$ is a unique feature of the K_{IR} channel, and contrasts with the situation for other potassium channels, where activity may depend on the membrane potential (for the KV and KCa channels), or be relatively independent of membrane potential (for the K_{ATP} channel), but does not depend on $[K^+]_o$. As barium ions block K_{IR} currents in

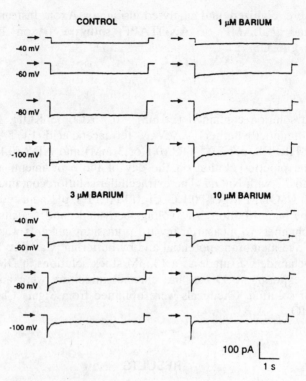

Figure 2 Inhibition of whole-cell currents through inward rectifier potassium channels in rat posterior cerebral artery by extracellular barium ions. The membrane potential was held at −20 mV and current recorded in response to a hyperpolarizing voltage pulse to −40, −60, −80, or −100 mV, as indicated. The extracellular solution contained no barium (CONTROL), or 1, 3 or 10 μM $[Ba^{2+}]_o$, as indicated. Reproduced from Quayle *et al.* (1993). *Am. J. Physiol.* **265** (Cell Physiol. 34), C1363–C1370.

other cells, and inhibit potassium induced dilations, we also investigated inhibition of inward currents by barium ions. Inward potassium currents activate rapidly in response to a hyperpolarizing voltage step in the absence of barium ions (Figure 2). In the presence of barium ions in the extracellular solution, currents recorded in response to a voltage step are smaller at the onset of the pulse and decay to a new steady-state level over the duration of the voltage step. These data suggest that barium ions block arterial K_{IR} channels, and that inhibition develops over the duration of the voltage pulse (several-hundred milliseconds). Inhibition increased with both membrane hyperpolarization and with barium concentration (Figure 2). The K_{IR} channel in arterial smooth muscle is very sensitive to inhibition by extracellular barium ions, with a dissociation constant in the micromolar range. Inhibition by barium ions is greater at more negative membrane potentials. The dissociation constant for barium block is an exponential function of membrane potential, decreasing e-fold for a 24 mV hyperpolarization, from 8 μM at −40 mV to 0.6 μM at −100 mV. Extracellular barium ions block other potassium channels, but at higher concentrations than required to the K_{IR} channel, and barium is therefore a useful tool for investigating the physiological role of this channel (Quayle et al., 1993).

Caesium also inhibited K_{IR} current in cerebral arteries, while these currents were relatively insensitive to blockers of the ATP-sensitive potassium channels (10 μM glibenclamide), Ca^{2+}-activated potassium channels (100 μM charybdotoxin, 1 mM tetraethyl ammonium), and voltage-dependent potassium channels (1 mM 4-aminopyridine: Quayle et al., 1993).

Modulation of K_{ATP} channels by calcitonin gene-related peptide (CGRP) in rabbit mesenteric artery

CGRP dilates rabbit mesenteric artery, in part through activation of K_{ATP} channels (Nelson et al., 1990b). We have studied the second-messenger pathways involved in CGRP activation of K_{ATP} channels in this artery using the whole-cell configuration of the patch-clamp technique (Quayle et al., 1994). CGRP activated whole-cell potassium selective currents and the magnitude of these currents was reduced by increasing the intracellular ATP concentration from 0.1 to 3 mM. CGRP induced currents were also suppressed by 10 μM glibenclamide, suggesting that CGRP activates K_{ATP} channels.

As CGRP is known to activate adenylate cyclase, we investigated whether the adenylate cyclase/cAMP/cAMP-dependent protein kinase system was involved in activation of K_{ATP} currents by CGRP. Forskolin, a membrane permeant activator of adenylate cyclase, increased K_{ATP} currents (Figure 3A). Adenylate cyclase catalyses the conversion of ATP to cAMP and the membrane permeant cAMP analogue, Sp-cAMPS, also activates K_{ATP} currents (Figure 3B). cAMP binds to the regulatory subunits of cAMP-dependent protein kinase, releasing the catalytic subunits, which can then phosphorylate membrane proteins. Inclusion of 100 U ml^{-1} of purified catalytic subunit of cAMP-dependent protein kinase into the pipette solution, which could therefore dialyse into the cell, activated K_{ATP} currents (Figure 3C). If CGRP increases K_{ATP} channel currents through activation of cAMP-dependent protein kinase, then inhibition of this kinase should abolish the response to CGRP. Inhibition with the nonspecific kinase inhibitor H-8, or with a specific inhibitor peptide which binds the catalytic site of cAMP-dependent protein kinase, both abolished activation of K_{ATP} currents by CGRP (Quayle et al., 1994).

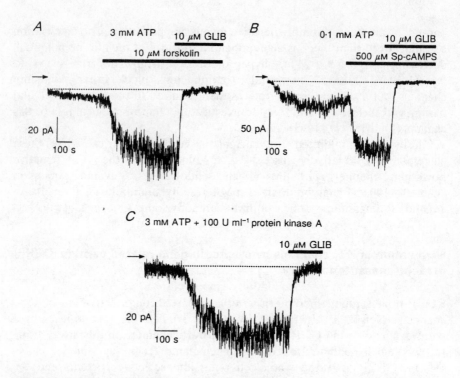

Figure 3 Activation of K_{ATP} currents by forskolin (A), Sp-cAMPS (B), and the catalytic subunit of cAMP-dependent protein kinase (C). $[K^+]_o = 60$ mM, $[K^+]_i = 140$ mM, membrane potential $= -70$ mV. Reproduced from Quayle *et al.* (1994). *J. Physiol.* **475**, 9–13.

CONCLUSIONS

Inward rectifier and ATP-sensitive potassium channels are present in the cell membrane of arterial smooth muscle cells and serve to regulate the cell membrane potential both in the resting state, and in response to vasodilators. The K_{ATP} channel is subject to complex regulation. Activation of the channel by both physiological and pharmacological vasodilators results in smooth muscle cell membrane hyperpolarization and vasorelaxation. Calcitonin gene-related peptide activates whole cell potassium currents through K_{ATP} channels in rabbit mesenteric arteries. Activation of K_{ATP} channels by CGRP underlies the membrane hyperpolarization, and part of the vasodilation, to CGRP in several vascular beds, including the mesenteric circulation. CGRP activates K_{ATP} channels through the adenylate cyclase/cAMP/cAMP-dependent protein kinase second messenger system. A similar mechanism of action for CGRP has recently been identified in guinea pig gall bladder (Zhang *et al.*, 1994a,b). Several other vasodilators which cause glibenclamide-sensitive vasodilations are coupled to adenylate cyclase, for example prostacyclin, adenosine acting at A2 receptors, and vasoactive intestinal peptide (Nelson & Quayle, 1995). Activation of K_{ATP} channels by this second messenger system may also be involved in these responses.

Small cerebral and coronary arteries contain K_{IR} channels. These channels may be involved in generating the resting membrane potential in these arteries. K_{IR} channels are also involved in the vasodilator response of small arteries to moderate elevations in the extracellular potassium concentration. It is possible that increasing $[K^+]_o$ can augment an outward, and therefore hyperpolarizing, membrane current through K_{IR} channels, as the activity of these channels is uniquely dependent on the extracellular potassium concentration. An increase in $[K^+]_o$ can act as a signal to cause an increase in local blood flow, and the vascular K_{IR} channel may therefore be involved in the metabolic regulation of blood flow.

ACKNOWLEDGEMENTS

This work was supported by the NIH. J.M.Q. is a British Heart Foundation Research Fellow.

REFERENCES

von Beckerath, N., Cyrys, S., Dischner, A. & Daut, J. (1991). Hypoxic vasodilatation in isolated, perfused guinea pig heart: an analysis of the underlying mechanisms. *J. Physiol.* **442**, 297–319.

Beech D.J., Zhang, H., Nakao, K. & Bolton, T.B. (1993a). K channel activation by nucleotide diphosphates and its inhibition by glibenclamide in vascular smooth muscle cells. *Br. J. Pharmacol.* **110**, 573–582.

Beech, D.J., Zhang, H., Nakao, K. & Bolton, T.B. (1993b). Single channel and whole-cell K-currents evoked by levcromakalim in smooth muscle cells from the rabbit portal vein. *Br. J. Pharmacol.* **110**, 583–590.

Bonev, A. & Nelson, M.T. (1993a). ATP-sensitive potassium channels in smooth muscle cells from guinea pig urinary bladder. *Am. J. Physiol.* **264**, C1190–C1200.

Bonev A.D. & Nelson, M.T. (1993b). Muscarinic inhibition of ATP-sensitive K^+ channels by protein kinase C in urinary bladder smooth muscle. *Am. J. Physiol.* **265**, C1723–C1728.

Bonev, A.D., Robertson, B.E. & Nelson, M.T. (1994). Inward rectifier K^+ currents from rat coronary artery smooth muscle cells. *Biophys. J.* **66**, A237. (Abstr.).

Brayden J.E. (1991). Hyperpolarization and relaxation of resistance arteries in response to adenosine diphosphate. *Circ. Res.* **69**, 1415–1420.

Clapp, L.H. & Gurney, A.M. (1992). ATP-sensitive K⁺ channels regulate resting
potential of pulmonary arterial smooth muscle cells. *Am. J. Physiol.* **262**,
H916–H920.

Dart C. & Standen, N.B. (1993). Adenosine-activated potassium current in smooth
muscle cells isolated from the pig coronary artery. *J. Physiol.* **471**, 767–786.

Dart C. & Standen, N.B. (1995). Activation of ATP-dependent K⁺ channels by
hypoxia in smooth muscle cells isolated from the pig coronary artery. *J. Physiol.*
483, 29–39.

Edwards, F.R. & Hirst, G.D.S. (1988). Inward rectification in submucosal arterioles of
guinea pig ileum. *J. Physiol.* **404**, 437–454.

Edwards, F.R., Hirst, G.D.S. & Silverberg, G.D. (1988). Inward rectification in rat
cerebral arterioles, involvement of potassium ions in autoregulation. *J. Physiol.* **404**,
455–466.

Hirst, G.D.S. & Edwards, F.R. (1989). Sympathetic neuroeffector transmission in
arteries and arterioles. *Physiolog. Rev.* **69**, 546–604.

Holzer, P. (1992). Peptidergic sensory neurones in the control of vascular functions,
mechanisms and significance in the cutaneous and splancnic vascular beds. *Rev.
Physiol. Biochem. Pharmacol.* **121**, 49–146.

Kajioka S., Kitamura, K. & Kuriyama, H. (1991). Guanosine diphosphate activates an
adenosine-5′-triphosphate-sensitive K⁺ channel in the rabbit portal vein. *J. Physiol.*
444, 397–418.

Kuchinsky, W., Wahl, M, Bosse, O. & Thurau, K. (1972). Perivascular potassium and
pH as determinants of local pial arterial diameter in cats. *Circ. Res.* **31**, 240–247.

Knot, H.J., Zimmermann, P.A. & Nelson, M.T. (1994). Activation of inward rectifier
K⁺ channels (K_{IR}) dilate small cerebral and coronary arteries in response to
elevated potassium. *Biophys. J.* **66**, A144. (Abstr.).

Maggi, C.A., Giuliani, S. & Santicioli, P. (1994). Multiple mechanisms in the smooth
muscle relaxant action of calcitonin gene-related peptide in the guinea pig ureter.
Naunyn-Schmiedebergs's Arch. Pharmacol. **350**, 537–547.

Marshall J.M., Thomas, T. & Turner, L. (1993). A link between adenosine, ATP-
sensitive K⁺ channels, potassium and muscle vasodilation in the rat in systemic
hypoxia. *J. Physiol.* **472**, 1–9.

McCarron, J.G. & Halpern, W. (1990). Potassium dilates rat cerebral arteries by two
independent mechanisms. *Am. J. Physiol.* **259**, H902–H908.

Meisheri, K.D., Kahn, S.A. & Martin, J.L. (1993). Vascular pharmacology of ATP-
sensitive K⁺ channels, Interactions between glyburide and K⁺ channel openers. *J.
Vasc. Res.* **30**, 2–12.

Nelson, M.T. & Quayle, J.M. (1995). Physiological roles and properties of potassium
channels in arterial smooth muscle. *Am. J. Physiol.* **268**, C1–C24.

Nelson, M.T., Huang, Y., Brayden, J.E., Hescheler, J. & Standen, N.B. (1990a).
Activation of K⁺ channels is involved in arterial dilations to calcitonin gene-related
peptide. *Nature* **344**, 770–773, 1990.

Nelson, M.T., Patlak, J.B., Worley, J.F. & Standen, N.B. (1990b). Calcium channels,
potassium channels, and the voltage-dependence of arterial smooth muscle tone.
Am. J. Physiol. **259**, C3–C18.

Newman, E.A. (1986). High potassium conductance in astrocyte endfeet. *Science* **233**,
453–454.

Quayle, J.M., McCarron, J.G., Brayden, J.E. & Nelson, M.T. (1993). Inward rectifier
K⁺ currents in smooth muscle cells from rat resistance-sized cerebral arteries. *Am.
J. Physiol.* **265**, C1363–C1370.

Quayle, J.M., Bonev, A.D., Brayden, J.E. & Nelson, M.T. (1994). Calcitonin gene related peptide activated ATP-sensitive K+ currents in rabbit arterial smooth muscle via protein kinase A. *J. Physiol.* **475**, 9–13.

Reid J.M., Paterson, D.J. Ashcroft, F.M. & Bergel, D.H. (1993). The effect of tolbutamide on cerebral blood flow during hypoxia and hypercapnia in the anaesthetized rat. *Pflügers Arch.* **425**, 362–364.

Russell, S.N., Smirnov, S.V. & Aaronson, P.I. (1992). Effects of BRL 38227 on potassium currents in smooth muscle cells isolated from rabbit portal vein. *Br. J. Pharmacol.* **105**, 549–556.

Standen, N.B., Quayle, J.M., Davies, N.W., Brayden, J.E., Huang, Y. & Nelson, M.T. (1989). Hyperpolarizing vasodilators activate ATP-sensitive K+ channels in arterial smooth muscle. *Science* **245**, 177–180.

Winquist, R.J., Heaney, L.A., Wallace, A.A., Baskin, E.P., Stein, R.B., Garcia, M.L. & Kaczorowski, G.J. (1988). Glyburide blocks the relaxation response to BRL 34915 (cromakalim), minoxidil sulfate and diazoxide in vascular smooth muscle. *J. Pharmacol. Exp. Therap.* **248**, 149–156.

Zhang, L., Bonev, A.D., Mawe, G.M. & Nelson, M.T. (1994a). Protein kinase A mediates activation of ATP-sensitive K+ currents by CGRP in gallbladder smooth muscle. *Am. J. Physiol.* **267**, G494–G499.

Zhang, L., Bonev, A.D., Nelson, M.T. & Mawe, G.M. (1994b). Activation of ATP-sensitive potassium currents in guinea pig gall-bladder smooth muscle by the neuropeptide CGRP. *J. Physiol.* **478**, 483–491.

9

ATP-sensitive Potassium Channels in Vascular Smooth Muscle Cells

Y. NAKAYA
H. MIYOSHI

*Department of Nutrition,
School of Medicine,
University of Tokushima,
Tokushima, Japan*

INTRODUCTION

Recent studies with patch clamp have shown that there are several different channels sensitive to glibenclamide (ATP-sensitive K channel; K_{ATP} channel) in different vascular smooth muscle cells. Standen *et al.* (1989) reported that the unitary conductance of this channel was 135 pS (K^+ concentration in pipette/bath solutions: 60 mM/140 mM). Their group later reported that in dispersed mesenteric artery smooth muscle cells the conductance of the K_{ATP} channel was 20 pS in cell-attached patches when the pipette contained 6 mM K^+ (Nelson *et al.*, 1990). Kajioka *et al.* (1990) reported that nicorandil opened K channels with a conductance of 20 pS (140 mM/140 mM) which were activated by intracellular Ca^{2+} and inhibited by intracellular ATP in portal vein of rabbits. Activation of the channel by intracellular Ca^{2+} was seen at a lower concentration of Ca^{2+} than that needed to activate Ca^{2+}-activated K channels with large conductance (K_{Ca} channel). We found, in cultured porcine coronary artery smooth muscle cells, that the K_{ATP} channel with a conductance of 30 pS (150 mM/150 mM) was activated not by intracellular Ca^{2+} but by extracellular Ca^{2+} (Inoue *et al.*, 1989). These differences might be due to differences in tissues or methods, such as cultured cells versus dispersed cells. Although there are differences in conductance and Ca^{2+} dependency among these reports, all of these studies agree that the K_{ATP} channel is suppressed by glibenclamide in addition to being blocked by intracellular ATP.

The membrane potential of vascular smooth muscle cell is determined by

SMOOTH MUSCLE EXCITATION
ISBN 0-12-112360-X

the relative membrane permeabilities to Na^+, Cl^- and K^+. The permeability to K^+ predominates, but other factors play a role as the resting membrane potential is displaced in a positive direction from the equibrium potential for K^+. Thus, the opening of this channel by potassium channel openers shifts the membrane potential closer to the K^+ equibrium potential, i.e. it hyperpolarizes the membrane and produces vasodilation. In physiological conditions, opening of K_{ATP} channels and membrane hyperpolarization also should be important mechanisms for a variety of endogenous vasodilators. In contrast to the pharmacological action of potassium channel openers, little is known about the regulation of this channel by endogenous substances. In the present review, we discuss the regulation of this channel by endogenous substances especially intracellular second messengers.

Effects of ATP and glibenclamide

In excised inside-out patches, K_{ATP} channels are present in various tissues, and are reversibly inhibited by the addition of ATP to the cytoplasmic surface of the membrane. Therefore, inhibition of channel activity by ATP in excised inside-out patches is through direct binding of the nucleotide to the channel and not through second-messenger regulation. The abundance, conductance and voltage independence of the K_{ATP} channels suggest that they play a major role in regulating membrane potential in pancreatic β-cells and vascular smooth muscle cells. It is, however, still unknown whether a change in intracellular concentration of ATP is the primary regulator of channel activity under physiological and pathological conditions or whether changes in the concentrations of other intracellular factors, such as ADP, or the action of vasoactive substances, are more important in keeping K_{ATP} channels open which would otherwise be held closed by a high concentration of ATP in the cell.

The K_{ATP} channels in the heart cell open only in extreme conditions, such as severe ischaemia in which ATP in the cell is depleted (Noma & Takano, 1991). In contrast, this channel is very active at the resting potential in pancreatic β-cells, and contributes to the generation of resting membrane potential. However, the concentration of ATP required to inhibit the K_{ATP} channel ($IC_{50} = 15$ mM; Cook & Hales, 1984) is much lower than the concentration of ATP present in the β-cell (3 to 6 mM).

The mechanism which allows continued K_{ATP} channel activity in smooth muscle cells in the presence of physiological concentration of ATP is not yet known and various hypotheses have been offered to explain why all the K_{ATP} channels are not closed at concentrations of ATP present in the cells. In cultured smooth muscle cells from porcine coronary artery, we (Miyoshi & Nakaya, 1991) have demonstrated that higher concentrations of ATP

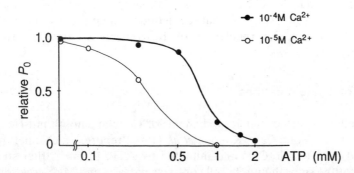

Figure 1 Inhibition of K_{ATP} channel by cytosolic ATP in an excised inside-out patch. ATP added to the cytosolic side blocked activity of K_{ATP} channel in a concentration-dependent manner between 0.1 to 2 mM in the presence of 10^{-5} to 10^{-4} M Ca^{2+} in the pipette solution. Reproduced with permission from Miyoshi & Nakaya (1991). *Biochem. Biophys. Res. Commun.* **181**, 700–706.

(1–5 mM) were required to block this channel substantially in inside-out patches when using a pipette solution containing 10^{-4} M Ca^{2+} (Figure 1). In vascular smooth muscle, the opening of this channel by K+ channel openers hyperpolarizes smooth muscle and this hyperpolarization is reversed by glibenclamide. These findings suggest that the K_{ATP} channel is active in vascular smooth muscle. Glibenclamide, however, causes only a small depolarization, which contradicts the finding that the K_{ATP} channel contributes significantly to the generation of the resting membrane potential. However, this finding does not rule out the possibility that the K_{ATP} channel contributes to the resting potential because depolarization by glibenclamide induces activation of other channels which counteract the depolarizing effect of glibenclamide.

Effect of nucleotide diphosphates

ADP partially reverses ATP-induced channel inhibition by competing with ATP for the same nucleotide-binding site. In support of this concept, changing the ATP:ADP ratio from 2.5:0.5 to 0.5:2.5 mM increased channel activity 20-fold in excised patches from rat β-cells (Misler *et al.*, 1986). K_{ATP} channels remain active when membrane patches are excised into solutions containing concentrations of ATP and ADP similar to those *in vivo*. These experiments demonstrate that the presence of ADP increases the concentration of ATP required for channel inhibition.

Recently, Kajioka *et al.*, (1991) found, in vascular smooth muscle cells, that GDP can open K_{ATP} channels in a concentration-dependent manner in the presence of pinacidil. Other nucleoside diphosphates are also effective as well. These results suggest that nucleotide diphosphates may play an important role in the regulation of K_{ATP} channels under physiological conditions.

Effects of divalent cations

Most studies reported that K_{ATP} channels of vascular smooth muscle are not sensitive to cytosolic Ca^{2+}. Kajioka *et al.* (1990) reported a channel that was activated by cytosolic Ca^{2+} and inhibited by ATP. In our earlier study, we found that the smooth muscle cell contracts in Ca^{2+}- and Mg^{2+}-free solutions. We referred to this phenomenon as 'Ca^{2+}-free contraction'. This contraction was considered to be due to block of the K_{ATP} channel which is activated by extracellular Ca^{2+} above $>10^{-6}$ M (Miyoshi & Nakaya, 1991). Thus, the K_{ATP} channel in smooth muscle cell is also active under resting conditions and this channel helps to control the membrane potential and maintain vascular tone. Mg^{2+} also activated K_{ATP} channels at higher concentrations (Inoue *et al.*, 1990). In vascular smooth muscle, we also found substates of K_{ATP} channels in the presence of Mg^{2+}.

Effect of endogenous vasoactive substances

Activation of K_{ATP} channel by vasodilators

Many K channels are known to be controlled by various peptides and intracellular second messengers. Endogenous vasoactive substances which are reported to activate K_{ATP} channels are prostacyclin, adenosine, calcitonin gene-related peptide (CGRP), endothelium-derived hyperpolarizing factor (EDHF) and endothelium-derived relaxing factor (EDRF).

Nelson *et al.* (1993) reported that arterial relaxation by CGRP involved activation of K_{ATP} channels. They also found that vasoactive intestinal peptide and EDHF act by opening K_{ATP} channels. In their studies, addition of CGRP (5 nM) to the bath solution activated K_{ATP} channels; however, CGRP, when added to the pipette solution, did not. We also tested the effect of Rp-cAMPS, a membrane permeable inhibitor of protein kinase A, on CGRP-induced activation of K_{ATP} channels. In the presence of RP-cAMPS, CGRP did not activate K_{ATP} channels (Miyoshi & Nakaya, 1995). From these results, we concluded that CGRP acts via an intracellular second messenger to increase channel activities and not by a direct G-protein gated mechanism. In cardiac muscle cells, various receptor-coupled activations of K_{ATP} channel have been reported through interaction with G proteins, but it is not yet known whether in vascular smooth muscle G-protein gating is responsible or not.

Adenosine is released as a consequence of cell metabolism in several tissues, such as the heart, brain, and skeletal muscle. Adenosine relaxes arterial smooth muscle and it has been proposed to serve as a link between tissue metabolic demand and local blood flow. Adenosine causes membrane hyperpolarization of bovine coronary artery and relaxation occurs through activation of A_1 and A_2 adenosine receptor subtypes. Glibenclamide inhibited only A_1 receptor-mediated relaxation.

Vascular endothelial cells produce endothelium-derived relaxing (EDRF) and hyperpolarizing factors (EDHF) in response to acetylcholine. EDRF has now been found to be a simple compound, nitric oxide (NO) (Ignarro et al., 1987; Palmer et al., 1987). Early studies showed that EDRF could not hyperpolarize the membrane, but recent studies revealed that NO derived from endothelium can hyperpolarize vascular smooth muscle (Tare et al., 1990). This hyperpolarization may involve activation of K_{ATP} channels. Nitrovasodilators, donors of NO, produce cGMP via activation of soluble guanylate cyclase and act on various ionic channels. Miyoshi et al. (1994) found that endogenous NO and also nitrovasodilators activated not only the K_{Ca} channel but also the K_{ATP} channel through production of cGMP. Recently, Bolotina et al., (1994) found that NO itself can activate K_{Ca} channels. However, contrary to their results, our study showed that endogenous NO could not activate K_{Ca} channels or K_{ATP} channels directly (Miyoshi et al., 1994).

Hyperpolarization by acetylcholine was almost blocked by methylene blue and specific nitric oxide synthase inhibitors, whereas hyperpolarization was unaffected (Chen et al., 1988). EDHF has yet to be identified and we do not know which channel is its target. Endothelium-dependent hyperpolarization of rabbit cerebral arteries was inhibited by glibenclamide, suggesting a role of K_{ATP} channels, whereas tetraethylammonium but not glibenclamide, inhibited acetylcholine-induced hyperpolarization, suggesting a role for KCa channels (Chen & Cheung, 1992).

Inhibition of K_{ATP} channel

Endothelin is a potent vasoconstrictor with an amino acid sequence similar to that of other peptide neurotoxins that bind directly to ionic channels. Endothelin caused a rapid but transient increase in the cytosolic Ca^{2+}, followed by a slower but sustained increase. The increase in cytosolic Ca^{2+} induced by endothelin was considered to be due, at least in part, to activation of the voltage dependent Ca^{2+} channels (Miyoshi et al., 1992). Figure 2 shows the effect of endothelin on K_{ATP} channels. In our studies, endothelin blocked this channel directly from outside of the cell membrane. This produced depolarization of the cells (Figure 3) and a sustained increase in vascular tension, in addition to Ca^{2+} mobilization owing to IP_3 production. Thus,

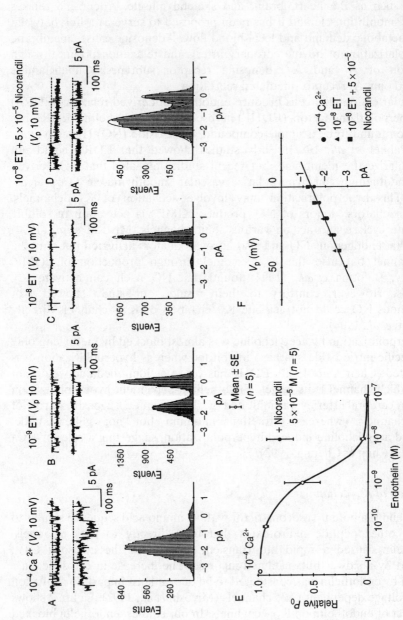

Figure 2 Effects of endothelin-1 (ET) on K_{ATP} channel activities. Recording from inside-out patch with 10^{-4} M Ca^{2+} in the pipette solution. Panels A–D, Channel recordings and amplitude histogram show that endothelin-1 inhibited K_{ATP} channel in a concentration-dependent manner. D, This block is reversed by nicorandil, a potassium channel opener. E, Graph shows fraction of open K_{ATP} channels at various endothelin concentrations. F, Current-voltage relation of channel. Reproduced with permission from Miyoshi et al. (1992). Circ. Res. **70**, 612–616.

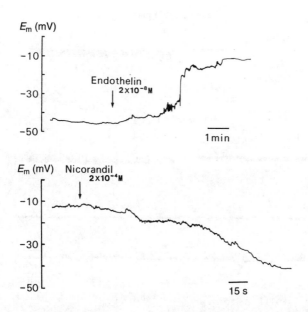

Figure 3 A whole-cell membrane potential (Em) recording showing depolarization induced by addition of endothelin-1. Panel B shows that depolarization by endothelin-1 is reversed by nicorandil. Reproduced with permission from Miyoshi et al. (1992). Circ. Res. 70, 612–616.

inhibition of K_{ATP} channels by vasoconstrictors might contribute membrane depolarization and contraction of smooth muscle. We have shown that angiotensin II (Miyoshi & Nakaya, 1991) and vasopressin (Wakatsuki et al., 1992) also blocked K_{ATP} channels.

These results suggest that the K_{ATP} channel of smooth muscle may be a common target for a number of vasorelaxing and vasoconstrictive agents and thus an important contributor to vascular tone.

Effect of intracellular second messengers

cAMP and cGMP are known to activate K_{Ca} channels in vascular smooth muscle cells. However, these effects on K_{ATP} channel are not well known. Figure 4 shows the effect of isoprenaline, a β-adrenoceptor agonist, and forskolin, an activator of adenylate cyclase. Both isoprenaline and forskolin activated K_{ATP} channels in cell-attached patches (Miyoshi & Nakaya, 1993) This effect can be mimicked by the catalytic subunit of protein kinase A. Figure 5 shows that in the presence of ATP and cAMP, protein kinase A activated K_{ATP} channels, suggesting that this activation was via cAMP-

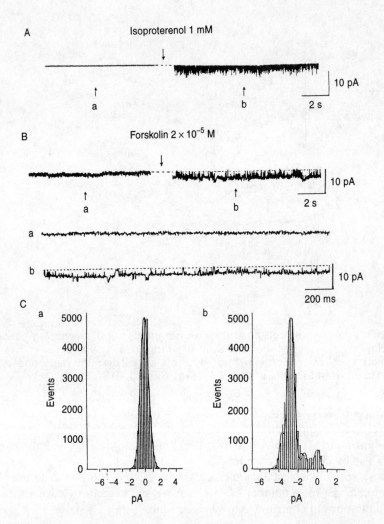

Figure 4 Effects of isoprenaline and forskolin on K_{ATP} channel activity. Reproduced with permission from Miyoshi & Nakaya (1993). *Biochem. Biophys. Res. Commun.* **193**, 240–247.

dependent protein kinase. Thus, many substances which activate adenylate cyclase and produce cAMP will open K_{ATP} channels in addition to their known effect on K_{Ca} channels.

Similar to cAMP, cGMP-protein kinase G pathway also activates both K_{Ca} and K_{ATP} channels. Activation of K_{ATP} channels by protein kinase G was not demonstrated directly, but dibutyryl-cGMP, a membrane permeable cGMP, can activate K_{ATP} channels in the rat aorta (Kubo *et al.*, 1994). In vascular

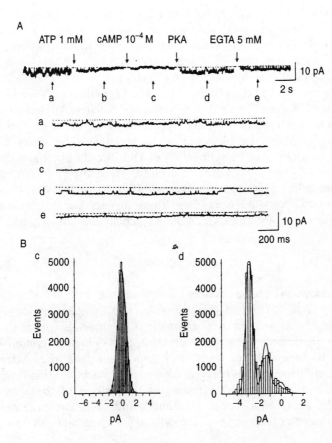

Figure 5   Effect of cAMP-dependent protein kinase (PKA) on K$_{ATP}$ channel activity in an inside-out patch. Pipette solution contained charybdotoxin (10^{-7} M) to block K$_{Ca}$ channel activity K$_{ATP}$ channel was activated by applying PKA (20 unit ml^{-1}) to the cytosolic side. Addition of 5 mM EGTA did not significantly suppress K$_{ATP}$ channel activity. Reproduced with permission from Miyoshi & Nakaya (1993). *Biochem. Biophys. Res. Commun.* **193**, 240–247.

smooth muscle, activation of these two types of K channels might produce relaxation of the artery. K$_{ATP}$ channels mainly contribute to the resting potential and also probably to the resting vascular tone. Conversely, K$_{Ca}$ channels counteract contraction by producing a large repolarizing current which is activated during increased intracellular Ca^{2+} and depolarization. Most of the vasoactive substances act on both channels at the same time and produce continuous vasodilation.

Protein kinase C is reported to produce a sustained contraction of smooth muscle cells and endothelin, angiotensin II and vasopressin, which activate protein kinase C through production of 1,2-diacylglycerol (DG), blocked K_{ATP} channels. We have reported that protein kinase C inhibited K_{Ca} channels (Minami *et al.*, 1993). Many vasoconstrictors are known to activate protein kinase C, and it has been reported that K_{ATP} channels were inhibited by muscarinic agonists through activation of protein kinase C in bladder smooth muscle. We also studied the effects of phorbol 12-myristate 13-acetate (PMA), an activator of protein kinase C in cell-attached patches. Application of PMA (10^{-6}M) to the bath solution did not significantly alter the open probability of K_{ATP} channels. Thus, the blockade of K_{ATP} channels by these vasoactive substances is not due to the production of DG. We do not know the precise mechanism of this blockade. Recently, Endothelin-1 inhibited the isoprenaline-induced increase in the cAMP content of ventricular slices measured by radioimmunoassay. Their study suggest that reduction of cAMP might be one reason for blockade of the K_{ATP} channel by endothelin.

CONCLUSION

In this review, we have mainly discussed the effects of endogenous substances on K_{ATP} channels, as there have been many studies of their pharmacological actions on these channels. K_{ATP} channels appear to operate at low to moderate open probability in physiological conditions, and contribute to generation of the resting membrane potential. Activation of K_{ATP} channels produces hyperpolarization and vasodilatation and closure plays a part in vasoconstrictor responses. Activation of these channels is regulated by many endogenous substances and plays an important role in controlling vascular tone in physiological and pathological conditions.

REFERENCES

Bolotina, V.M., Najibi, S., Palacino, J.J., Pagano, P.J. & Cohen, R.A. (1994) Nitric oxide directly activates calcium-dependent potassium channels in vascular smooth muscle. *Nature* **368**, 850–853.

Chen, G. & Cheung, D. W. (1992) Characterization of acetylcholine-induced membrane hyperpolarization in endothelial cells. *Circ. Res.* **70**, 257–263.

Chen, G., Suzuki, H. & Weston, A.H. (1988) Acetylcholine releases endothelium derived hyperpolarizing factor and EDRF from rat blood vessels. *Br. J. Pharmacol.* **95**, 1165–1174.

Cook, D.L. & Hales, C.H. (1984) Intracellular ATP directly blocks K channels in pancreatic β cells. *Nature* **311**, 271–273.

Ignarro, L.J., Buga, G.M., Wood, K.S., Byrns, R.E. & Chaudhuri, G. (1987) endothelium-derived relaxing factor produced and released from artery and vein is nitric oxide. *Proc. Natl Acad. Sci. USA* **84**, 9265–9269.

Inoue, I., Nakaya, Y., Nakaya, S. & Mori, H. (1989) Extracellular Ca^{2+}-activated K^+ channel in coronary artery smooth muscle cells and its role in vasodilation. *FEBS*

Lett. **255**, 281–284.

Inoue, I., Nakaya, S. & Nakaya, Y. (1990) An ATP-sensitive K+ channel activated by extracellular Ca^{2+} and Mg^{2+} in primary cultured arterial smooth muscle cells. *J. Physiol. (London)* **430**, 132P.

Kajioka, S., Oike, M. & Kitamura, K. (1990) Nicorandil opens a calcium dependent potassium channel in smooth muscle cells of the rat portal vein. *J. Pharmacol. Exp. Ther.* **254**, 905–913.

Kajioka, S., Kitamura, K. & Kuriyama, H. (1991) Guanosine diphosphate activates an adenosine 5'-triphosphate-sensitive K+ channel in the rabbit portal vein. *J. Physiol. (London)* **444**, 397–418.

Kubo, M., Nakaya, Y., Matuoka, S. & Kuroda, Y. (1994) Atrial natriuretic factor and isosorbide dinitrate modulate the gating of ATP-sensitive K+ channels in cultured vascular smooth muscle cells. *Circ. Res.* **74**, 471–476.

Minami, K., Fukuzawa, K. & Nakaya, Y. (1993) Protein kinase C inhibits the Ca(2+)-activated K+ channel of cultured porcine coronary artery smooth muscle cells. *Biochem. Biophys. Res. Commun.* **190**, 263–269.

Misler, S., Falke, L.C., Gillis, K. & McDaniel, M.L. (1986) A metabolite-regulated potassium channel in rat pancreatic β cells. *Proc. Natl Acad. Sci. USA* **83**, 7119–7123.

Miyoshi, Y. & Nakaya, Y. (1991) Angiotensin II blocks ATP-sensitive K+ channels in porcine coronary artery smooth muscle cells. *Biochem. Biophys. Res. Commun.* **181**, 700–706.

Miyoshi, H. & Nakaya, Y. (1993) Activation of ATP-sensitive K+ channels by cyclic AMP-dependent protein kinase in cultured smooth muscle cells of porcine coronary artery. *Biochem. Biophys. Res. Commun.* **193**, 240–247.

Miyoshi, H. & Nakaya, Y. (1994) Endotoxin-induced nonendothelial nitric oxide activates the Ca^{2+}-activated K+ channel in cultured vascular smooth muscle cells. *J. Mol. Cell. Cardiol.* **20**, 1487–1495.

Miyoshi, H. & Nakaya, Y. (1995) Calcitonin gene-related peptide activates K+ channels of vascular smooth muscle cells via adenylate cyclase. *Basic Res. Cardiol.* **90**, 332–336.

Miyoshi, Y., Nakaya, Y. , Wakatsuki, T., Fujino, K., Saito, K., Mori, H. & Inoue, I. (1992) Endothelin blocks ATP-sensitive K+ channels and depolarizes smooth muscle cells of porcine coronary artery. *Circ. Res.* **70**, 612–616.

Nelson, M. T., Huang,Y., Brayden, J.E., Hescheler, J. & Standen, N.B. (1990) Arterial dilations in response to calcitonin gene-related peptide involve activation of K+ channels. *Nature* **344**, 770–773.

Nelson, S. H., Suresh, M. S., Dehring, D.J. & Jonson, R.L. (1993). Relaxation by calcitonin gene-related peptide may involve activation of K+ channels in the human uterine artery. *Eur. J. Pharmacol.* **242**, 255–261.

Noma, A. & Takano, M. (1991) The ATP-sensitive K+ channel. *Jpn J. Physiol.* **41**, 177–187.

Palmer, R.M.J., Ferrige, A.G. & Moncada, S. (1987) Nitric oxide release accounts for the biological activity of endothelium-derived relaxing factor. *Nature* **327**, 524–526.

Standen, N. B., Quayle, J. M., Davies, N.W., Brayden, J.E., Huang, Y. & Nelson, M.T. (1989) Hyperpolarizing vasodilators activate ATP-sensitive K+ channels in arterial smooth muscle. *Science* **245**, 177–180.

Tare, M., Parkington, H.C., Coleman, H.A., Neild, T.O. & Dusting, G.J. (1990) Hyperpolarization and relaxation of arterial smooth muscle caused by nitric oxide derived from the endothelium. *Nature* **346**, 69–71.

Wakatsuki, T., Nakaya, Y. & Inoue, I. (1992) Vasopressin modulates K+-channel activities of cultured smooth muscle cells from porcine coronary artery. *Am. J. Physiol.* **32**, H491–H496.

10

Modulation of the Agonist-induced Ca²⁺ Mobilization by K⁺ Channel Openers in Arterial Smooth Muscle

TAKEO ITOH*
YOSHIMASA WATANABE*
HIKARU SUZUKI**

*Department of Pharmacology,
Nagoya City University Medical School,
Nagoya, Japan

**Department of Physiology,
Nagoya City University Medical School,
Nagoya, Japan

SUMMARY

1. The underlying mechanism of vaso-relaxation induced by K⁺ channel openers (KCOs) on agonist-induced contraction was investigated by measuring intracellular Ca²⁺ concentration ($[Ca^{2+}]_i$), isometric tension, membrane potential and production of inositol 1,4,5-trisphosphate (IP₃) in intact and chemically skinned smooth muscles of the rabbit mesenteric artery. Pinacidil, lemakalim and $(-)$-$(3S,4R)$-4-(N-Acetyl-N-hydroxy-amino)-6-cyano-3,4-dihydro-2,2-dimethyl-2H-1-benzopyran-3-ol (Y-26763) were used to open the K⁺ channel.

2. Pinacidil (0.1–10 μM), lemakalim (0.001–1 μM) and Y-26763 (0.01–1 μM) concentration-dependently hyperpolarized the smooth muscle membrane. Glibenclamide (10 μM) depolarized the membrane (4–7 mV) and inhibited the membrane hyperpolarization induced by these KCOs.

3. Noradrenaline (NA, 10 μM) depolarized the smooth muscle membrane with associated oscillations. Histamine (His, 3 μM) with ranitidine (3 μM, H₂-blocker) also depolarized the membrane to the same extent as NA (10 μM). KCOs inhibited the NA-induced membrane depolarization, and glibenclamide prevented the action of KCOs. In contrast, these KCOs did not modify the His-induced membrane depolarization.

SMOOTH MUSCLE EXCITATION
ISBN 0-12-112360-X

4. NA $(10\,\mu M)$ and His $(3\,\mu M)$ both produced a phasic, followed by a tonic increase in intracellular Ca^{2+} concentration $([Ca^{2+}]_i)$ and tension. Pinacidil, lemakalim and Y-26763 all inhibited the NA-induced phasic and tonic increase in $[Ca^{2+}]_i$ and tension. In contrast, these KCOs attenuated the His-induced phasic responses but had almost no effect on the tonic ones. Under these conditions, the inhibition of L-type Ca^{2+} channel by nicardipine attenuated the His-induced tonic increase in $[Ca^{2+}]_i$ and tension.

5. In ryanodine-treated smooth muscle cells, Y-26763 hyperpolarized the membrane and potently inhibited the membrane depolarization induced not only by NA but also by His. Thus, ryanodine-treatment of the muscle cells altered the potency of membrane hyperpolarizing activity of Y-26763 in the presence of His and thus enhances the vaso-relaxing activity of Y-26763 on His-induced tonic increase in $[Ca^{2+}]_i$ and tension.

6. In Ca^{2+}-free solution, NA $(10\,\mu M)$ and His $(3\,\mu M)$ both transiently increased $[Ca^{2+}]_i$, tension and synthesis of IP_3. KCOs inhibited the increases in $[Ca^{2+}]_i$ and tension induced by each NA and His in Ca^{2+}-free solution containing 5.9 mM K^+, but not in a similar solution containing 50 mM K^+. The inhibition of the NA-induced IP_3 synthesis was observed by an application of pinacidil or lemakalim in Ca^{2+}-free solution containing 5.9 mM K^+, but not in 40 mM K^+. Glibenclamide inhibited all these actions of KCOs. In β-escin treated-skinned strips, NA $(10\,\mu M)$ or IP_3 $(20\,\mu M)$ released Ca^{2+} from the storage sites. KCOs had no effect on Ca^{2+}-release induced by either NA or IP_3 in the skinned muscles. These results suggest that KCOs inhibit the agonist-induced Ca^{2+} release from storage sites through inhibition of IP_3 synthesis resulting from its membrane hyperpolarizing action.

7. In the presence of NA or His, Y-26763 and lemakalim had no measurable effect on $[Ca^{2+}]_i$-tension relationship in ryanodine-treated living and α-toxin-treated skinned smooth muscles.

8. It is concluded that in smooth muscle of the rabbit mesenteric artery, KCOs hyperpolarize the membrane and inhibit Ca^{2+} release activated by NA or His, possibly through an inhibition of these agonist-induced IP_3 production. It is also suggested that the membrane hyperpolarization induced by KCOs may not be enough to inhibit the His-activated Ca^{2+}-influx. Thus, the vaso-relaxing activity of KCOs differs between vaso-spasmogenic agonists.

INTRODUCTION

A variety of chemicals which hyperpolarize the membrane by opening glibenclamide-sensitive K^+ channels are called K^+ channel openers (KCOs) (see Quast, 1993 for a review). The KCOs by hyperpolarizing the membrane

(Standen et al., 1989) inhibit the activation of voltage-dependent L-type Ca^{2+} channels, which are sensitive to organic Ca^{2+}-channel blockers. In smooth muscle cells, Ca^{2+} influx can be increased by agonists through activation of both the L-type Ca^{2+} channel and the receptor-operated nonselective cation channel (Benham & Tsien, 1987; Nelson et al., 1988; Inoue & Isenberg, 1990a,b; Pacaud & Bolton, 1991). These channels are voltage sensitive, but the latter channel is insensitive to organic Ca^{2+}-channel blockers in longitudinal smooth muscle of the guinea pig ileum (Inoue & Isenberg, 1990a). In the rabbit mesenteric artery, noradrenaline (NA) enhances both organic Ca^{2+} channel blocker-sensitive and -insensitive Ca^{2+}-influxes (Kanmura et al., 1983; Itoh et al., 1994). Furthermore, it was also found that KCOs attenuate the NA-induced synthesis of inositol 1,4,5-trisphosphate (IP_3) and thus inhibit NA-induced Ca^{2+} release from intracellular storage sites in smooth muscle of the rabbit mesenteric artery (Ito et al., 1991; Itoh et al., 1992a). Therefore, an agent which hyperpolarizes the smooth muscle membrane would be likely to inhibit the NA-induced contraction more than an organic Ca^{2+}-channel blocker. However, it is not yet known whether KCOs inhibit the responses induced by other types of Ca^{2+}-mobilizing agonists in this tissue.

A newly synthesized drug, (+)-(3S,4R)-4-(N-acetyl-N-benzyloxyamino)-6-cyano-3,4-dihydro-2,2-dimethyl-2H-1-1-benzopyran-3-ol (Y-27152), has a long-lasting anti-hypertensive action and produces little tachycardia (Nakajima et al., 1992). The compound is pharmacologically inert but after oral administration it is converted to an active desbenzyl form (Y-26763) by cytochrome P_{450}. Y-26763 has also been supposed to be a KCO (Nakajima et al., 1992; Itoh et al., 1994). In preliminary experiments, we found that Y-26763, even at high concentrations ($10\,\mu M$), only marginally inhibited the maximum contraction induced by histamine (His) in smooth muscle of the rabbit mesenteric artery. This suggests that the vaso-relaxing actions of this agent in resistant vessels of the rabbit mesentery may differ against various vaso-spasmogenic agonists. However, the mechanisms underlying these differences remain unclear.

To investigate further the actions of KCOs their effects on membrane potential, $[Ca^{2+}]_i$ and tension were studied in the presence of His using smooth muscle tissues obtained from the third and fourth branches of the rabbit mesenteric artery (diameter 0.06–0.1 mm). The effects were compared with those in the presence of NA in the same muscle strips. To examine the effect of KCOs on the agonist-induced Ca^{2+} influx more precisely, the effects of KCOs were also studied in ryanodine-treated smooth muscles which functionally have lost the agonist-sensitive Ca^{2+} storage sites (Itoh et al., 1992b). The effects of KCOs on contractile proteins in the presence of His were assessed from a study of the $[Ca^{2+}]_i$-tension relationships in ryanodine-treated living and β-escin or α-toxin-treated skinned smooth muscles.

METHODS

Male albino rabbits, weighing 1.9–2.5 kg, were anaesthetized with
pentobarbitone sodium (40 mg kg^{-1}, i.v.) and then exsanguinated. A segment
from the third or fourth branch of the mesenteric artery distributing to the
ileum was excised, immediately immersed in Krebs solution and cleaned free
of connective tissue under a binocular microscope. All the experiments were
carried out at room temperature.

Electrophysiological experiments

A glass microelectrode filled with 3 M KCl was made from borosilicate glass
tube (o.d. 1.2 mm with a core inside, Hilgenberg, Germany). The tip
resistance of the electrodes was 40–80 MΩ. The artery was cut vertically and
the endothelial cells were removed by gentle rubbing the internal surface of
the vessels using small knives. NA (10 μM) or His (3 μM) was applied for
10–15 min by dissolving it in the superfusing Krebs solution and membrane
potentials were recorded from different cells by successive impalements with
the electrode. Ranitidine (3 μM) a histamine-H$_2$ receptor blocker was present
throughout the experiments. Microelectrodes which connected to a high
input impedance preamplifier (MEZ-7200, Nihon-Kohden, Tokyo, Japan)
were inserted into smooth muscle cells from the adventitial side, and the
responses were displayed on both a cathode-ray oscilloscope (SS-7602,
Iwatsu, Japan) and a pen recorder (Recticorder RJG-4024, Nihon-Kohden).

[Ca^{2+}]$_i$ and tension measurement

[Ca^{2+}]$_i$ and isometric tension were monitored simultaneously using
endothelium-denuded fine circularly-cut smooth muscle strips (0.3–0.5 mm
length, 0.04–0.05 mm width, 0.02–0.03 mm thickness) mounted horizontally
on an inverted-microscope (Diaphot TMD, Nikon, Tokyo, Japan), as
previously described (Itoh *et al.*, 1983, 1992 a,b). The preparation was moved
to the centre of the field and a mask (0.04 mm square) placed in an
intermediate image plane of the microscope. The resting tension was
adjusted to obtain a maximum contraction to 128 mM K$^+$.

Fura 2 was loaded into smooth muscle cells by application of 1 μM of the
acetoxy methyl ester of fura 2 (fura 2-AM) for 1 h in Krebs solution at room
temperature. After this period, the solution containing fura 2-AM was
washed with Krebs solution for 1 h to ensure sufficient esterification of fura
2-AM in the cells. The fura 2 fluorescence emission at 510 nm was passed
through the objective lens (20 × fluor, Nikon) through a band-pass
interference filter centred at 510 nm with half-transmission at ±20 nm and

collected with a photomultiplier tube (R928, side-on type, Hamamatsu Photonics, Japan) via a dichroic mirror which was substituted for the photochanger in a Nikon Diaphot TMD microscope. Two alternative excitation wavelengths, 340 nm and 380 nm (each slit 5 nm) were applied by a spectro-fluorimeter (Spex, NJ, USA or CA 200DP, Japan Spectroscopic Co. Ltd., Tokyo, Japan) and the data were analysed using customized software provided by Spex (DM-3000CM) or developed in our laboratory. The ratio of the fura 2 fluorescence intensities excited by 340 or 380 nm was calculated after subtraction of the background fluorescence and [Ca^{2+}]$_i$ were calculated using an *in vitro* calibration procedure (Poenie *et al.*, 1986).

NA (10 μM) or His (3 μM) was applied for 2 min at 20 min intervals in Krebs solution, so as to obtain reproducible responses. Pinacidil, lemakalim or Y-26763 was applied for 10 min before and during application of NA or His. Guanethidine (5 μM), propranolol (3 μM) and ranitidine (3 μM) were present throughout the experiments to prevent NA-outflow from sympathetic nerves, β-adrenoceptor stimulation by exogenously applied NA and H$_2$-receptor stimulation by His, respectively. Experiments were also carried out in Ca^{2+}-free solution containing 2 mM ethylene glycol-bis-(β-aminoethyl)-*N,N,N',N'*-tetraacetic acid (EGTA): after 2 min in Ca^{2+}-free solution, the strips were stimulated by NA or His for 2 min and then brought back to Ca^{2+}-containing Krebs solution ([Ca^{2+}] = 2.6 mM) for 20 min. Each KCO was applied for 5 min in Krebs solution and was present in the Ca^{2+}-free solution in the presence and absence of NA or His.

In some experiments, Ca^{2+} storage sites in smooth muscle cells were functionally removed by application of ryanodine (Fleischer *et al.*, 1985; Katsuyama *et al.*, 1991; Itoh *et al.*, 1992b). After recording the control responses induced by 10 μM NA or 3 μM His, ryanodine (50 μM) with 5 mM caffeine was applied for 5 min in Krebs solution followed by a 10-min application of a Krebs solution containing 10 μM ryanodine only, and either NA or His was again applied in the presence of ryanodine. The effect of KCOs on [Ca^{2+}]$_i$-tension relationships in the presence of NA or His was then studied in these ryanodine-treated smooth muscle strips in a Ca^{2+}-free solution containing 2 mM EGTA for 5 min with either 10 μM NA or 3 μM His applied for 30 s in the Ca^{2+}-free solution. Finally, Ca^{2+} (0.16–2.6 mM) was applied in an ascending concentration together with either NA or His in the presence or absence of Y-26763.

Measurement of IP$_3$

Endothelium-denuded muscle strips (10 mm length, 2.2–2.5 mm width, 0.1 mm thickness) were equilibrated for over 2 h at 32°C in Krebs solution. After the equilibration, the strips were transferred to Ca^{2+}-free Krebs solution containing 2 mM EGTA for 2 min, and then 10 μM NA was applied.

KCO or glibenclamide was given as pretreatment for 3 min in Krebs solution, for 2 min in Ca^{2+}-free solution and during application of NA. The reaction was stopped by addition of a large amount of ice-cold trichloroacetic acid and the strips were homogenized. The homogenate was centrifuged and the supernatant fraction was treated with ether three times and then assayed using a radioimmunoassay kit from Amersham International plc.

Experiments on chemically skinned smooth muscle

Chemically skinned smooth muscle strips were made using 400 units ml^{-1} α-toxin or $25\,\mu M$ β-escin for 25 min (Nishimura *et al.*, 1988; Kitazawa *et al.*, 1991; Itoh *et al.*, 1992a,b). The composition of the solutions have been described elsewhere (Itoh *et al.*, 1992a).

The Ca^{2+}-tension relationship was determined with 4 mM EGTA and $1\,\mu M$ ionomycin present to avoid spurious effects due to Ca^{2+} release from intracellular storage sites in the skinned muscle strips. Increasing concentrations of Ca^{2+} were applied cumulatively. The amplitude of contraction induced by Ca^{2+} was normalized with respect to that induced by $10\,\mu M$ Ca^{2+} in the same strip.

To enable measurement of NA-induced Ca^{2+} release from the storage sites, $0.3\,\mu M$ Ca^{2+} buffered with 4 mM EGTA was applied for 3 min (to load Ca^{2+} into the storage sites) and Ca^{2+} then removed from the solution by application of Ca^{2+}-free solution containing 4 mM EGTA for 0.5 min. Then, a solution containing $50\,\mu M$ EGTA, $10\,\mu M$ GTP and $2\,\mu M$ fura 2 was applied for 2 min. Finally, $10\,\mu M$ NA with $10\,\mu M$ GTP was applied for 2 min in a solution containing $50\,\mu M$ EGTA and $2\,\mu M$ fura 2.

Solutions

The ionic composition of the Krebs solution was as follows (mM): Na^+, 137.4; K^+, 5.9; Mg^{2+}, 1.2; Ca^{2+}, 2.6; HCO_3^-, 15.5; $H_2PO_4^-$, 1.2; Cl^-, 134; glucose, 11.5. The concentration of K^+ was modified by replacing NaCl with KCl, isosmotically. Ca^{2+}-free Krebs solution was made by substituting an equimolar concentration of $MgCl_2$ for $CaCl_2$ and adding 2 mM EGTA. The solutions were bubbled with 95% O_2 and 5% CO_2 and their pH maintained at 7.3–7.4.

The calibration solution for Ca^{2+} measurement contained 11 mM EGTA, 110 mM KCl, 1 mM $MgCl_2$, $2\,\mu M$ fura 2 and 20 mM N-2-hydroxyethyl-piperazine-N'-2-ethanesulphonic acid (HEPES) (pH 7.1) with or without 11 mM $CaCl_2$.

For experiments on skinned muscles, the composition of the relaxing solution was as follows: 87 mM potassium methanesulphonate (KMS), 20 mM piperazine-N,N'-bis-(2-ethanesulphonic acid) (PIPES), 5.1 mM Mg(MS)$_2$, 5.2 mM ATP, 5 mM phosphocreatine, 1 μM propranolol, 3 μM ranitidine and 4 mM EGTA. Various Ca^{2+} concentrations were prepared by adding appropriate amounts of Ca(MS)$_2$ to 4 mM EGTA, based on the calculations reported previously (Itoh et al., 1986). The pH of the solution was adjusted to 7.1 at 25°C with KOH and the ionic strength was standardized at 0.2 M by changing the amount of KMS added.

Drugs

Drugs used were fura 2, fura 2-AM, EGTA, PIPES and HEPES (Dojin, Japan), NA, GTP, nicardipine, ranitidine, β-escin and glibenclamide (Sigma), ryanodine (Agri-system), guanethidine (Tokyo Kasei, Japan), ATP (Na salt; Kohjin, Japan), histamine dihydrochloride (His) and propranolol (Nacalai, Japan), caffeine (Wako pure Chemical, Japan), α-toxin (Gibco BRL) and ionomycin (free acid; Calbiochem). Pinacidil, lemakalim and Y-26763 were provided by Yoshitomi Pharmaceutical Ind., Ltd. (Japan).

Statistics

The values recorded were expressed as mean ± standard deviation (sd) unless stated otherwise. Statistical significance was determined by a paired or unpaired Student's t-test. Probabilities less than 5% ($P < 0.05$) were considered significant.

RESULTS

KCOs hyperpolarize the smooth muscle cell membrane

In smooth muscle cells of the rabbit mesenteric artery, the resting membrane potential was −65 to −75 mV (mean −70.2 ± 1.8 mV, $n = 26$). Application of lemakalim (>1 nM), pinacidil (>0.1 μM) and Y-26763 (>10 nM) hyperpolarized the membrane, in a concentration-dependent manner (Figure 1). The sustained hyperpolarization produced by these KCOs lasted for up to 15 min. On removal of KCOs from the superfusate, the membrane potential returned to the resting level with a very slow time course: complete recovery required 25–30 min.

Glibenclamide (1 and 10 μM) depolarized the membrane by 4–7 mV. In the presence of 10 μM glibenclamide, Y-26763 (1 μM), lemakalim (1 μM) or pinacidil (1 μM) produced only a small hyperpolarization after a very long delay: (1) the time to the start of the hyperpolarization and that for the

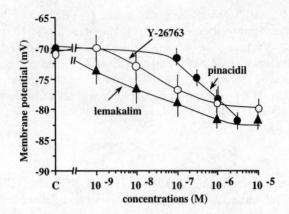

Figure 1 Concentration-dependent effects of lemakalim, pinacidil and Y-26763 on membrane potential in smooth muscle cells of the rabbit mesenteric artery. The membrane potential was measured 10 min after application of these KCOs. Results shown are each as the mean of 5–12 observations with ± SD shown by vertical bars. (▲), lemakalim; (○), Y-26763; (●), pinacidil.

hyperpolarization to reach peak amplitude were both greatly prolonged, (2) the amplitude of the hyperpolarization was greatly reduced and (3) the time required for recovery from the hyperpolarization was shortened to 7–10 min.

KCOs have very weak effect on the His-induced tonic increase in $[Ca^{2+}]_i$ and tension

In the presence of $3\,\mu M$ ranitidine, His (over $0.3\,\mu M$) produced contraction (ED_{50} values $= 0.8 \pm 0.2\,\mu M$, $n = 4$) with a just submaximal response obtained at $3\,\mu M$. The contractions induced by $10\,\mu M$ NA and $3\,\mu M$ His were blocked by $3\,\mu M$ prazosin and $3\,\mu M$ mepyramine, respectively.

The resting $[Ca^{2+}]_i$ was $116 \pm 12\,nM$ for smooth muscle strips of the rabbit mesenteric artery set to a resting tension of $0.3 \pm 0.1\,mg$ ($n = 4$). NA ($10\,\mu M$) and His ($3\,\mu M$) produced a phasic, followed by a tonic increase in both $[Ca^{2+}]_i$ and tension (Figure 2). The maximum increases in $[Ca^{2+}]_i$ induced by NA and His were $552 \pm 137\,nM$ and $534 \pm 102\,nM$ respectively ($n = 4$). Y-26763 (0.1–$10\,\mu M$) lowered the resting $[Ca^{2+}]_i$ and strongly inhibited both the phasic and a tonic increases in $[Ca^{2+}]_i$ and tension induced by NA, in a concentration-dependent manner. In contrast, Y-26763 (0.1–$10\,\mu M$) attenuated the His-induced phasic response to some extent, but had no significant effect on the His-induced tonic increase in $[Ca^{2+}]_i$ and tension. Similar effects were also observed by an application of $1\,\mu M$ lemakalim or $1\,\mu M$ pinacidil. Glibenclamide ($10\,\mu M$) prevented all the inhibitory actions of Y-26763 and of lemakalim on increases in $[Ca^{2+}]_i$ and tension induced by NA or His.

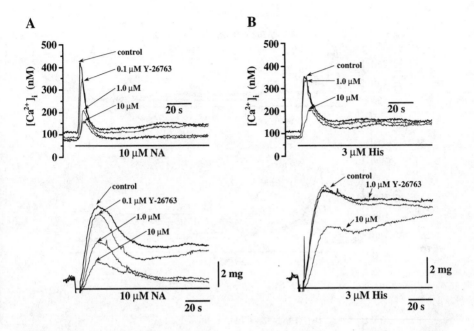

Figure 2 Effects of Y-26763 on the increase in $[Ca^{2+}]_i$ and tension induced by noradrenaline (NA, A) or histamine (His, B) in smooth muscle of rabbit mesenteric artery. $[Ca^{2+}]_i$, upper panel; tension, lower panel. NA (10 μM) or His (3 μM) was applied for 2 min at 20-min intervals in the presence or absence of Y-26763. Y-26763 was applied for 10 min before and during application of NA or His.

KCOs inhibit the agonist-induced $[Ca^{2+}]i$ increase in Ca^{2+}-free solution

To study the effect of KCOs on Ca^{2+} release induced by NA or His, the effect of Y-26763 was examined on the agonist-induced $[Ca^{2+}]_i$ increase in Ca^{2+}-free solution containing 2 mM EGTA with 5.9 mM K^+. Changeover of the Krebs solution to the Ca^{2+}-free solution was rapid with no increase in $[Ca^{2+}]_i$ induced by 128 mM K^+ after 15 s application. Following application of the Ca^{2+}-free solution, the resting $[Ca^{2+}]_i$ rapidly decreased from 116 ± 18 nM to 65 ± 12 nM ($n = 4$) within 1 min and then remained at this new steady level. Under these conditions, NA (10 μM) or His (3 μM) transiently increased $[Ca^{2+}]_i$. In Ca^{2+}-free solution, Y-26763 (10 μM) lowered the resting $[Ca^{2+}]_i$ to 46 ± 12 nM ($n = 4$) and attenuated both the NA- and His-induced increases in $[Ca^{2+}]_i$ (Figure 3). Similar effects on NA- and His-induced $[Ca^{2+}]_i$ increase in

A

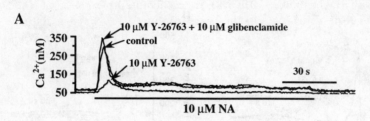

B

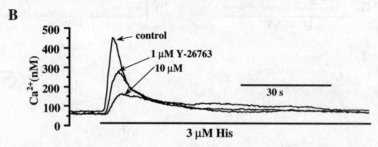

C

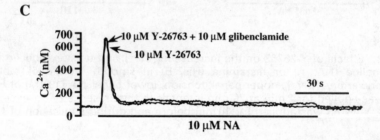

D

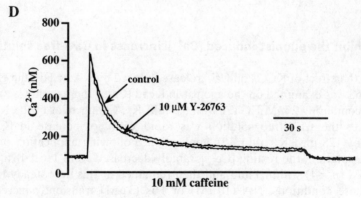

Ca^{2+}-free solution were also observed by an application of lemakalim or pinacidil. Glibenclamide (10 μM) blocked the inhibitory action of Y-26763 on both the resting [Ca^{2+}]$_i$ and the agonist-induced response in the Ca^{2+}-free solution. In contrast, Y-26763 had no effect on the increase in [Ca^{2+}]$_i$ and tension induced by 10 mM caffeine in Ca^{2+}-free solution containing 5.9 mM K$^+$ (Figure 3D).

Figure 3C shows the effects of Y-26763 on the increases in [Ca^{2+}]$_i$ induced by NA in Ca^{2+}-free solution containing 50 mM K$^+$. Following an application of Ca^{2+}-free solution containing 5.9 mM K$^+$ for 1 min, the solution containing 50 mM K$^+$ failed to increase [Ca^{2+}]$_i$ but enhanced the increase in [Ca^{2+}]$_i$ and tension induced by subsequently applied NA. In Ca^{2+}-free solution containing 50 mM K$^+$, Y-26763 had no effect on either the resting [Ca^{2+}]$_i$ or the NA-induced increases in [Ca^{2+}]$_i$ and force. Similarly, lemakalim (1 μM) had no effect on the NA-induced increase in [Ca^{2+}]$_i$ in Ca^{2+}-free solution containing 50 mM K$^+$.

Effects of KCOs on inositol 1,4,5-trisphosphate (IP$_3$) production induced by NA

In Ca^{2+}-free solution containing 2 mM EGTA, NA (10 μM) transiently increased IP$_3$ within 10 s and the effect gradually decayed (Figure 4). Pinacidil (1 μM) slightly lowered the concentration of IP$_3$ at the resting level and inhibited maximum increase in the synthesis of IP$_3$ measured at 10 s after application of NA. Similarly, lemakalim (1 μM) also attenuated the NA-induced IP$_3$ production. Glibenclamide (1 μM) did not significantly modify the IP$_3$ production induced by 10 μM NA but did block the inhibitory actions of 1 μM pinacidil or 1 μM lemakalim on the NA-induced IP$_3$ synthesis. When the extracellular concentration of K$^+$ was over 40 mM K$^+$, the inhibitory action of pinacidil or lemakalim on NA-induced synthesis of IP$_3$ was abolished.

Figure 3 Effects of 10 μM Y-26763 on increase in [Ca^{2+}]$_i$ induced by 10 μM NA (A, C), 3 μM His (B) or 10 mM caffeine (D) in Ca^{2+}-free solution containing 2 mM EGTA with 5.9 mM K$^+$ (A, B and D) or 50 mM K$^+$ (C). Each stimulant was applied for 2 min after a 2-min period of Ca^{2+} removal, then Ca^{2+}-free solution was applied for 3 min to wash out the stimulant. This protocol was repeated at 30-min intervals with the strips being kept in Krebs solution (containing 2.6 mM Ca^{2+}) for the 25-min period between tests. When used, Y-26763 was applied for 10 min before and was present throughout the experiment. In C, Ca^{2+}-free solution containing 50 mM K$^+$ was applied for 1 min after a 1-min removal of Ca^{2+} by Ca^{2+}-free solution containing 5.9 mM K$^+$. NA (10 μM) was then applied for 2 min in Ca^{2+}-free solution containing 50 mM K$^+$.

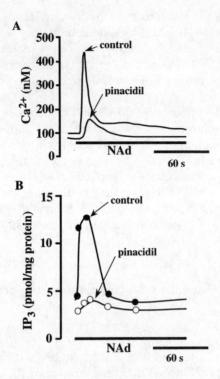

Figure 4 Effects of pinacidil on increase in $[Ca^{2+}]_i$ (A) and IP_3-synthesis (B) induced by 10 μM NA in Ca^{2+}-free solution in smooth muscles of the rabbit mesenteric artery. NA (10 μM) was applied in Ca^{2+}-free solution containing 2 mM EGTA after 2 min removal of Ca^{2+}. Pinacidil (1 μM) was applied for 5 min before, and throughout application of NA. B, time-dependent changes in the synthesis of IP_3 following application of 10 μM NA in the presence (o) or absence (●) of 1 μM pinacidil. NA (10 μM) was applied at time 0.

Actions of KCOs on NA-induced Ca^{2+} release in β-escin-skinned smooth muscle

The direct effects of Y-26763 on NA-induced Ca^{2+} release were observed in β-escin-treated skinned smooth muscle strips which cannot generate a membrane potential. NA (10 μM) increased $[Ca^{2+}]_i$ in Ca^{2+}-free solution after brief application of Ca^{2+} (Figure 5). Y-26763 (10 μM) had no significant effect on this NA-induced Ca^{2+} release. Similarly, lemakalim (1 μM) or pinacidil (1 μM) had no effect on the NA-induced Ca^{2+} release in β-escin skinned smooth muscle.

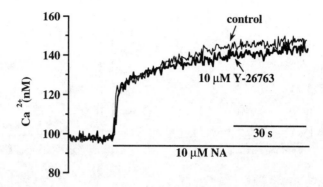

Figure 5   Effects of Y-26763 on increase in Ca^{2+} induced by 10 μM NA in a β-escin-skinned smooth muscle. After the strip was skinned by β-escin, 0.3 μM Ca^{2+} buffered with 4 mM EGTA was applied for 3 min and Ca^{2+}-free solution containing 4 mM EGTA then applied for 0.5 min to remove Ca^{2+} from the solution. Subsequently, 10 μM NA was applied for 2 min in Ca^{2+}-free solution containing 50 μM EGTA, 10 μM GTP and 2 μM fura 2 following a 2-min application of Ca^{2+}-free solution containing 50 μM EGTA, 10 μM GTP and 2 μM fura 2. Y-26763 (10 μM) was applied for 10 min prior to and was present throughout application of NA. The figure was reproduced from Itoh *et al.*, 1994. (Thinner line, in the absence of Y-26763; thicker line, in the presence of Y-26763).

Actions of nicardipine on agonist-induced increase in [Ca^{2+}]$_i$

Effects of nicardipine (0.3 μM) on the increase in [Ca^{2+}]$_i$ and tension induced by 10 μM NA or 3 μM His were examined. At this concentration, nicardipine completely inhibited the contraction induced by 128 mM K$^+$. Nicardipine did not affect either the resting [Ca^{2+}]$_i$ or the phasic increase in [Ca^{2+}]$_i$ and tension induced by NA (10 μM) or His (3 μM), but attenuated the tonic increase in [Ca^{2+}]$_i$ and tension induced by these agonists (Figure 6). In the presence of 0.3 μM nicardipine, neither Y-26763 (10 μM) nor lemakalim (1 μM) had any effect on the His-induced tonic increase in [Ca^{2+}]$_i$ and tension (data not shown). These results indicate that nicardipine inhibits the His-induced tonic increase in [Ca^{2+}]$_i$ and tension more potently than KCOs.

Effect of Y-26763 on membrane potential in the presence of NA or His

In endothelium-denuded muscle strips, the resting membrane potential was -53.5 ± 1.7 mV ($n = 6$). Y-26763 (> 30 nM) hyperpolarized the membrane in a concentration-dependent manner, and the maximum hyperpolarization

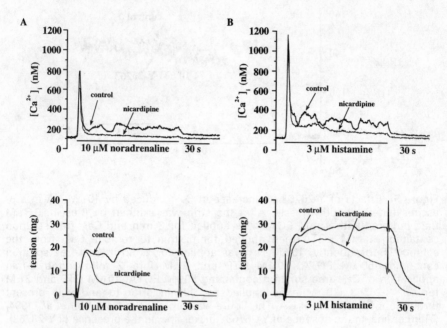

Figure 6 Effects of 0.3 μM nicardipine on increase in [Ca²⁺]ᵢ and tension induced by 10 μM NA (A) or 3 μM His (B). Nicardipine (0.3 μM) was given as pretreatment for 5 min, and NA or His was then applied in the presence of nicardipine.

obtained by $10 \mu M$ Y-26763 was to $-71.6 \pm 1.0 \, mV$ ($n = 5$). NA ($10 \mu M$) depolarized the membrane and generated spike potentials (Figure 7A). The mean amplitude of the NA-induced membrane depolarization was $10.6 \pm 2.7 \, mV$. In the presence of $10 \mu M$ NA, Y-26763 ($10 \mu M$) hyperpolarized the membrane and greatly attenuated the NA-induced membrane depolarization ($1.6 \pm 1.2 \, mV$). In the presence of $3 \mu M$ His together with $3 \mu M$ ranitidine, Y-26763 ($10 \mu M$) hyperpolarized the membrane. The extent of membrane hyperpolarization induced by Y-26763 was less in the presence of His than in that of NA (Figure 7B).

Following application of ryanodine, agonist-sensitive Ca^{2+} storage sites are functionally lost in smooth muscle of the rabbit mesenteric artery (Itoh *et al.*, 1992b). To examine the role of Ca^{2+} released from the storage sites on the membrane hyperpolarization induced by Y-26763 in the presence of His, the effect of Y-26763 on membrane potential was studied in the presence of His in ryanodine-treated muscle cells. The effects of Y-26763 on membrane

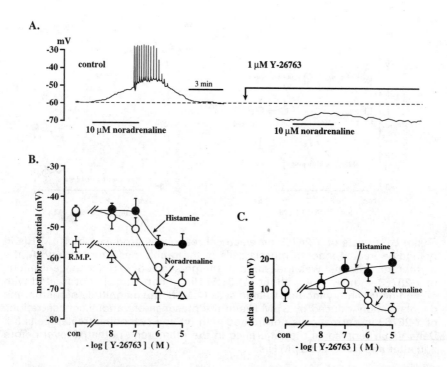

Figure 7   Effects of Y-26763 on electrical responses produced by 10 μM NA or 3 μM His in smooth muscle cells of rabbit mesenteric artery. A, Y-26763 (1 μM) was applied before and during application of 10 μM NA. B, concentration-dependent effect of Y-26763 in the absence (Δ) and presence of 10 μM NA (○) or 3 μM His (●). C, the magnitude of membrane depolarization induced by 10 μM NA or 3 μM His in the presence of various concentrations of Y-26763. Delta value represents the difference in the membrane potential level before and after application of 10 μM NA or 3 μM His.

potential in the presence and absence of 3 μM His in ryanodine-treated cells are presented in Figure 8. Ryanodine treatment did not affect either the resting membrane potential or the membrane depolarization induced by 3 μM His. In the absence of His, the magnitude of the membrane hyperpolarization induced by Y-26763 was not modified by the ryanodine treatment. However, Y-26763 (10 μM) potently hyperpolarized the membrane in the presence of 3 μM His in ryanodine-treated cells (from -40.2 ± 2.6 mV, $n = 6$, to -66.1 ± 4.7 mV, $n = 5$) and thus strongly attenuated the His-induced membrane depolarization.

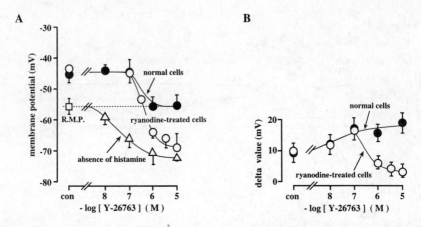

Figure 8 Effects of Y-26763 on electrical responses produced by 3 μM His in ryanodine-treated smooth muscle cells of the rabbit mesenteric artery. A, the membrane potential was measured in the presence of various concentrations of Y-26763 with (●,○) or without (Δ) 3 μM His in normal cells not treated with ryanodine (●) and ryanodine-treated cells (○,Δ). B, the magnitude of membrane depolarization induced by 3 μM His in the presence of various concentrations of Y-26763 in normal cells not treated with (●) and ryanodine-treated cells (○). Delta value represents the difference in the membrane potential level before and after application of 3 μM His.

Y-26763 attenuates the increase in $[Ca^{2+}]_i$ and tension induced by His in ryanodine-treated strips

To study the effect of KCOs on His-induced Ca^{2+}-influx more precisely, the effect of Y-26763 on the changes in $[Ca^{2+}]_i$ and tension induced by 3 μM His was studied in ryanodine-treated muscle strips and the effects were compared with those induced by 10 μM NA.

Following the application of ryanodine, the resting $[Ca^{2+}]_i$ was slightly increased (from 119 ± 10 nM to 158 ± 18 nM, $n = 4$) and additional application of NA failed to induce either the phasic or the subsequent oscillatory increases in $[Ca^{2+}]_i$ and force. In ryanodine-treated strips, $[Ca^{2+}]_i$ and tension were induced to increase slowly by NA and the time to peak was delayed (Figure 9A). Y-26763 (10 μM) lowered the resting $[Ca^{2+}]_i$ to 117 ± 10 nM, ($n = 4$) and almost completely inhibited the increases in $[Ca^{2+}]_i$ and tension induced by 10 μM NA. Figure 9B shows the effects of Y-26763 on the increase in $[Ca^{2+}]_i$ and tension induced by His in ryanodine-treated muscle strips. His (3 μM) failed to induce the phasic increase in $[Ca^{2+}]_i$ and tension.

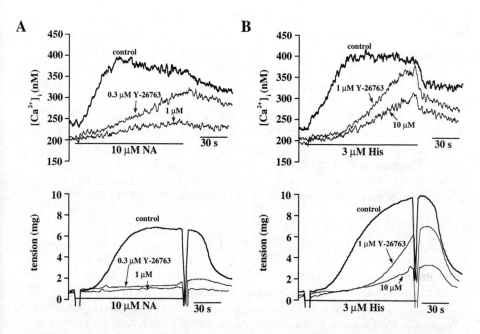

Figure 9 Concentration-dependent effects of Y-26763 on increases in $[Ca^{2+}]_i$ and tension induced by 10 µM NA (A) and 3 µM His (B) in ryanodine-treated smooth muscle strips. Upper panel, $[Ca^{2+}]_i$; lower panel, tension. After muscle strips were treated with ryanodine, NA or His was applied for 2 min at 20-min intervals in Krebs solution. Y-26763 was given as pretreatment for 10 min and was present during application of the agonist.

Under these conditions, the $[Ca^{2+}]_i$ and tension induced by His increased slowly and the time to peak was delayed. Y-26763 (1 and 10 µM) lowered the resting $[Ca^{2+}]_i$ and inhibited the maximum increase in $[Ca^{2+}]_i$ and tension induced by His.

Y-26763 has no effect on the $[Ca^{2+}]_i$-tension relationships in both ryanodine-treated intact and skinned smooth muscles

The $[Ca^{2+}]_i$-tension relationship was obtained by cumulative applications of solutions with various concentrations of Ca^{2+} (from 0 to 2.6 mM) in solutions containing either NA (10 µM) or His (3 µM) in ryanodine-treated muscle strips. In the absence of Y-26763, the sensitivity of the contraction at a given Ca^{2+} concentration seemed to be higher in the presence of 3 µM His than in 10 µM NA. Y-26763 (0.1–1 µM) did not shift the relationship between $[Ca^{2+}]_i$ and tension in the presence of either NA or His.

The direct actions of Y-26763 on contractile proteins were also estimated from the effects of this drug on Ca^{2+}-tension relationships in the presence and absence of $3 \mu M$ His or $10 \mu M$ NA together with $30 \mu M$ GTP in β-escin- or α-toxin-treated skinned muscle strips. In the skinned muscles, the minimum concentration of Ca^{2+} that produced contraction was $0.1 \mu M$ and the maximum contraction was obtained at $10 \mu M$. The concentration of Ca^{2+} required for half-maximal contraction (ED_{50}) was $0.49 \pm 0.05 \mu M$. NA shifted the Ca^{2+}-tension relationship to the left with a slight increase in the amplitude of the maximum Ca^{2+}-induced contraction ($ED_{50} = 0.31 \pm 0.03 \mu M$ Ca^{2+}). His also shifted the Ca^{2+}-tension relationship to the left ($ED_{50} = 0.28 \pm 0.03 \mu M$ Ca^{2+}). In the skinned muscles, Y-26763 ($10 \mu M$) did not modify the Ca^{2+}-tension relationship in the presence and absence of His or NA.

DISCUSSION

In various types of vascular smooth muscle, agents that activate the ATP-sensitive K^+ channel, such as pinacidil, cromakalim, lemakalim and Y-26763 induce membrane hyperpolarization and muscle relaxation (Hamilton & Weston, 1989; Quast & Cook, 1989; Standen et al., 1989; Kajioka et al., 1991; Itoh et al., 1992a, 1994; Nakajima et al., 1992). The hyperpolarization can be selectively inhibited by a sulphonylurea, glibenclamide (Standen et al., 1989; Kajioka et al., 1991; Itoh et al., 1992a). These results suggest that KCOs hyperpolarizes the vascular smooth muscle cell membrane by activating the glibenclamide-sensitive (probably ATP-sensitive) K^+ channel.

In the rabbit mesenteric artery, NA ($10 \mu M$) depolarizes the membrane and produces a contraction with two phases: the transient phasic increase in both $[Ca^{2+}]_i$ and tension is possibly induced by release of Ca^{2+} from its storage sites, while the subsequent tonic phase and the associated oscillations may be due to activation of Ca^{2+}-influx (Itoh et al., 1983; Kanmura et al., 1983). KCOs inhibited all of these NA-induced responses. The tonic increases in $[Ca^{2+}]_i$ and tension induced by NA were abolished by high concentration of KCOs, while they were inhibited only partly by nicardipine. Glibenclamide attenuated the inhibitory actions of KCOs on the membrane depolarization and the increases in $[Ca^{2+}]_i$ and tension induced by NA. These results suggest that the membrane hyperpolarization induced by KCOs inhibits the NA-induced increases in $[Ca^{2+}]_i$ and tension through mechanisms in addition to simple inhibition of L-type Ca^{2+} channels.

In the rabbit mesenteric artery, His also produced a phasic, followed by a tonic increase in $[Ca^{2+}]_i$ and tension. The former response is possibly due to the His-induced Ca^{2+} release from intracellular storage sites, as the response was maintained in Ca^{2+}-free solution and abolished in ryanodine-treated smooth muscle, while the latter response may be caused by His-activated

Ca^{2+} influx since the response was greatly inhibited by nicardipine and abolished in Ca^{2+}-free solution. Pinacidil, Y-26763 and lemakalim had little effect on the His-induced tonic increase in [Ca^{2+}]$_i$ and tension, although these agents inhibited the phasic responses. In contrast, Y-26763 (10 μM) strongly attenuated both the NA-induced phasic and tonic responses. The level of membrane depolarization attained by an application of 3 μM His was similar to that by 10 μM NA, but the effect of the KCOs on membrane potential was different in the presence of NA and His; in the presence of 10 μM NA, Y-26763 (10 μM) hyperpolarized the membrane close to the level in the absence of NA (−70 mV) and thus, the NA-induced delta membrane potential change (difference in the membrane potential before and after application of 10 μM NA) was strongly reduced by application of 10 μM Y-26763 (about 2 mV). In the presence of 3 μM His, Y-26763 hyperpolarized the membrane close to the resting potential (−50 mV) and thus, the His-induced delta membrane potential change was not reduced by 10 μM Y-26763. Under these conditions, His might activate voltage-dependent L-type Ca^{2+} channels even at the resting membrane potential level because Ca^{2+} mobilizing agonists shift the voltage-dependency of the L-type Ca^{2+} channels to a more negative potential in smooth muscle of the rabbit mesenteric artery (Nelson et al., 1988). This might explain our observation that nicardipine further attenuated the His-induced tonic increases in [Ca^{2+}]$_i$ and tension in the presence of Y-26763. Thus, these results suggest that in the presence of His, the level of the membrane potential achieved by Y-26763 may not be enough to inhibit the His-induced Ca^{2+} influx.

In smooth muscles of the rabbit mesenteric artery, ryanodine causes the functional loss of NA-sensitive Ca^{2+} store sites (Itoh et al., 1992b). In the present experiments, following application of ryanodine, both NA and His failed to produce the phasic increase in [Ca^{2+}]$_i$ and produced only a mono-tonic response, suggesting that ryanodine causes the loss of function to both NA and His in this arterial muscle. Thus, it is likely that both NA and His increase [Ca^{2+}]$_i$ and tension through agonist-activated Ca^{2+}-influx in ryanodine-treated muscles. In ryanodine-treated smooth muscles, Y-26763 (10 μM) completely abolished the His-induced increase in [Ca^{2+}]$_i$ and tension. Moreover, after ryanodine treatment, the membrane potential levels obtained by Y-26763 in the presence and absence of His were the same (−72 mV and −70 mV respectively), indicating that the membrane depolarization induced by His was completely blocked by 10 μM Y-26763. These results indicate that in the presence of His, ryanodine enhances the membrane hyperpolarizing activity of Y-26763 and thus greatly potentiates the KCO-induced inhibition of Ca^{2+}-influx activated by His. Alternatively, His may inhibit the membrane hyperpolarization induced by Y-26763 through activation of ryanodine-sensitive intracellular Ca^{2+} storage sites. It has recently been reported that in bladder smooth muscle cells of the guinea pig, carbachol activates protein kinase C which then inhibits the ATP-sensitive K^+ channel (Bonev and Nelson, 1993). It is also known that Ca^{2+} released from the storage sites activates receptor-operated nonselective cation channels in longitudinal smooth muscle cells of the guinea pig ileum (Inoue and Isenberg, 1990b). These mechanisms may be activated by His and then attenuate the membrane hyperpolarization induced by Y-26763. The underlying mechanisms for this have not been clarified.

Ca^{2+} mobilizing agonists bind to their own receptor and synthesize IP_3 which releases Ca^{2+} from the intracellular storage sites in vascular smooth muscle cells (Hashimoto et al., 1986; Itoh et al., 1992α). In living smooth muscles, pinacidil, lemakalim and Y-26763 inhibited the increase in $[Ca^{2+}]_i$ induced by NA and His, but not that induced by caffeine in Ca^{2+}-free solution containing 5.9 mM K^+. This inhibitory action of KCOs was prevented by glibenclamide and was not seen in Ca^{2+}-free solution containing 50 mM K^+. In skinned smooth muscle strips made using β-escin, NA increased Ca^{2+}. Such NA-induced increases in Ca^{2+} are inhibited by prazosin (an α-receptor blocker) or heparin (a blocker of IP_3 receptors) (Kobayashi et al., 1989; Itoh et al., 1992b), suggesting that in the skinned smooth muscle, NA releases Ca^{2+} from intracellular storage sites through the action of synthesized IP_3 via α-receptor–phospholipase C coupling. In the skinned smooth muscles, pinacidil, lemakalim and Y-26763 did not modify this NA-induced Ca^{2+} release, indicating that these KCOs has no direct effect on either IP_3-production through α-receptor-phospholipase C coupling or the IP_3-induced Ca^{2+} release mechanism. These results suggest that the membrane hyperpolarization may be the essential factor for the inhibitory action of KCO on agonist-induced Ca^{2+} release. Pinacidil and lemakalim did not modify the resting concentrations of IP_3 but inhibited the synthesis of IP_3 induced by NA and, these actions were inhibited by glibenclamide (Ito et al., 1991; Itoh et al., 1992a). These results suggest that KCOs inhibit the NA-induced Ca^{2+} release through an inhibition of the NA-induced IP_3 synthesis. Thus, the membrane hyperpolarization induced by KCO negatively controls the hydrolysis of phosphatidylinositol 4,5-bisphosphate (PIP_2) induced by agonist and inhibit agonist-induced Ca^{2+} release from the intracellular storage sites in smooth muscle cells of the rabbit mesenteric artery.

In the present experiments, Y-26763 had no effect on the $[Ca^{2+}]_i$ -tension relationship when activated by either 10 μM NA or 3 μM His under conditions where the membrane was polarized. Moreover, in α-toxin and β-escin skinned smooth muscle strips, Y-26763 had no direct effect on the Ca^{2+}-tension relationship in the presence and absence of His with GTP. These results suggest that neither KCOs nor the membrane hyperpolarization induced by KCOs modify the myofilament Ca^{2+} sensitivity when activated by His, although it has been demonstrated that some of KCOs, such as pinacidil at high concentration ($>3 \mu$M), posses a direct inhibitory action on the contractile proteins (Itoh et al., 1991).

In conclusion, in smooth muscle of the rabbit mesenteric artery, KCOs hyperpolarize the membrane and inhibit Ca^{2+} release activated by NA and His, possibly through inhibition of the agonist-induced production of IP$_3$. The magnitude of the membrane hyperpolarization induced by KCOs may be different in the presence of NA and His. Thus, the vaso-relaxing actions of K channel openers may not be the same in the presence of different types of vaso-spasmogenic agonists.

ACKNOWLEDGEMENTS

This work was partly supported by a Grant-In-Aid from the Ministry of Education of Japan. Y-26763, lemakalim and pinacidil were a gift from Yoshitomi Pharmaceutical Ind., Ltd. (Japan).

REFERENCES

Benham, C.D. & Tsien, R.W. (1987). A novel receptor-operated Ca^{2+}-permeable channel activated by ATP in smooth muscle. *Nature* **328**, 275–278.

Bonev, A.D., & Nelson, M.T. (1993). Muscarinic inhibition of ATP-sensitive K$^+$ channels by protein kinase C in urinary bladder smooth muscle. *Am. J. Physiol.* **265**, C1723–C1728.

Fleischer, S., Ogunbunmi, E.M., Dixon, M.C. & Fleer, E.A.M. (1985). Localization of Ca^{2+} release channels with ryanodine in junctional terminal cisternae of sarcoplasmic reticulum of fast skeletal muscle. *Proc. Natl Acad. Sci. USA* **82**, 7256–7259.

Hamilton, T.C. & Weston, A.H. (1989). Cromakalim, nicorandil and pinacidil: novel drugs which open potassium channels in smooth muscle. *Gen. Pharmacol.* **20**, 1–9.

Hashimoto, T., Hirata, M., Itoh, T., Kanmura, Y. & Kuriyama, H. (1986). Inositol 1,4,5-trisphosphate activates pharmacomechanical coupling in smooth muscle of the rabbit mesenteric artery. *J. Physiol.* **370**, 605–618.

Inoue, R. & Isenberg, G. (1990a). Effect of membrane potential on acetylcholine-induced inward current in guinea pig ileum. *J. Physiol.* **424**, 57–71.

Inoue, R. & Isenberg, G. (1990b). Intracellular calcium ions modulate acetylcholine-induced inward current in guinea pig ileum. *J. Physiol.* **424**, 73–92.

Ito, S., Kajikuri, J., Itoh, T. & Kuriyama, H. (1991). Effects of lemakalim on changes in Ca^{2+} concentration and mechanical activity induced by noradrenaline in the rabbit mesenteric artery. *Br. J. Pharmacol.* **104**, 227–233.

Itoh, T., Kuriyama, H. & Suzuki, H. (1983). Differences and similarities in the noradrenaline- and caffeine-induced mechanical responses in the rabbit mesenteric artery. *J. Physiol.* **337**, 609–629.

Itoh, T., Kanmura, Y. & Kuriyama, H. (1986). Inorganic phosphate regulates the contraction-relaxation cycle in skinned muscles of the rabbit mesenteric artery. *J. Physiol.* **376**, 231–252.

Itoh, T., Suzuki, S. & Kuriyama, H. (1991). Effects of pinacidil on contractile proteins in high K$^+$-treated intact, and in β-escin-treated skinned smooth muscle of the rabbit mesenteric artery. *Br. J. Pharmacol.* **103**, 1697–1702.

Itoh, T., Seki, N., Suzuki, S., Ito, S., Kajikuri, J. & Kuriyama, H. (1992a). Membrane hyperpolarization inhibits agonist-induced synthesis of inositol 1,4,5-trisphosphate in rabbit mesenteric artery. *J. Physiol.* **451**, 307–328.

Itoh, T., Kajikuri, J. & Kuriyama, H. (1992b). Characteristic features of noradrenaline-induced Ca^{2+} mobilization and tension in arterial smooth muscle of the rabbit. *J. Physiol.* **457**, 297–314.

Itoh, T., Ito, S., Shafiq, J. & Suzuki, H. (1994). Effects of a newly synthesized K$^+$ channel opener, Y-26763, on noradrenaline-induced Ca^{2+} mobilization in smooth muscle of the rabbit mesenteric artery. *Br. J. Pharmacol.* **111**, 165–172.

Kajioka, S., Kitamura, K. & Kuriyama, H. (1991). Guanosine diphosphate activates an adenosine 5′-triphosphate-sensitive K$^+$ channel in the rabbit portal vein. *J. Physiol.* 397–418.

Kanmura, Y., Itoh, T., Suzuki, H., Ito, Y. & Kuriyama, H. (1983). Effects of nifedipine on smooth muscle cells of the rabbit mesenteric artery. *J. Pharmacol. Exp. Ther.* **226**, 238–248.

Katsuyama, H., Ito, S., Itoh, T. & Kuriyama, H. (1991). Effects of ryanodine on acetylcholine-induced Ca^{2+} mobilization in single smooth muscle cells of the porcine coronary artery. *Pflügers Archiv.* **419**, 460–466.

Kitazawa, T., Gaylinn, B.D., Denny, G.H. & Somlyo, A.P. (1991). G-protein-mediated Ca^{2+} sensitization of smooth muscle contraction through myosin light chain phosphorylation. *J. Biol. Chem.* **266**, 1708–1715.

Kobayashi, S., Kitazawa, T., Somlyo, A.V. & Somlyo, A.P. (1989). Cytosolic heparin inhibits muscarinic and α-adrenergic Ca^{2+} release in smooth muscle. *J. Biol. Chem.* **264**, 17997–18004.

Nakajima, T., Shinohara, T., Yaoka, O., Fukunari, A., Shinagawa, K., Aoki, K., Katoh, A., Yamanaka, T., Setoguchi, M. & Tahara, T. (1992). Y-27152, a long-acting K$^+$ channel opener with less tachycardia: antihypertensive effects in hypertensive rats and dogs in conscious state. *J. Pharmacol. Exp. Ther.* **261**, 730–736.

Nelson, M.T., Standen, N.B., Brayden, J.E. & Worley III, J.F. (1988). Noradrenaline contracts arteries by activating voltage-dependent calcium channels. *Nature* **336**, 382–385.

Nishimura, J., Kolber, M & Van Breemen, C. (1988). Norepinephrine and GTP-γ-S increase myofilament Ca^{2+} sensitivity in α-toxin permeabilized arterial smooth muscle. *Biochem. Biophys. Res. Commun.* **157**, 677–683.

Pacaud, P. & Bolton, T.B. (1991). Relation between muscarinic cationic current and internal calcium in guinea pig jejunal smooth muscle cells. *J. Physiol.* **441**, 477–499.

Poenie, M., Alderton, J., Steinhardt, R. & Tsien, R. (1986). Calcium rises abruptly and briefly throughout the cell at the onset of anaphase. *Science* **233**, 886–889.

Quast, U. (1993). Do the K$^+$ channel openers relax smooth muscle by opening K$^+$ channels? *Trends Pharmacol. Sci.* **14**, 332–337.

Quast, U. & Cook, N.S. (1989). Moving together: K$^+$ channel openers and ATP-sensitive K$^+$ channels. *Trends Pharmacol. Sci.* **10**, 431–435.

Standen, N.B., Quayle, J.M., Davies, N.W., Brayden, J.E., Huang, Y. & Nelson, M.T. (1989). Hyperpolarizing vasodilators activate ATP-sensitive K$^+$ channels in arterial smooth muscle. *Science* **245**, 177–180.

11

Molecular Cloning, Expression and Characterization of Smooth Muscle K+ Channels

BURTON HOROWITZ

Department of Physiology,
University of Nevada School of Medicine,
Reno, Nevada, USA

ABSTRACT

Smooth muscles display a heterogeneous collection of K+ conductances which contribute to phasic or tonic contraction through excitation–contraction coupling. Electrophysiological studies in dispersed smooth muscle cells have generated a considerable body of information concerning the properties of these currents, however, molecular characterization of the K+ channel genes responsible for these currents has been slow. We have been investigating the molecular basis for the electrical activity in smooth muscles and have cloned, characterized and expressed cDNAs representing smooth muscle K+ channels. While this work focuses on canine colonic smooth muscle, the molecular distribution of these K+ channels has been determined for other canine vascular and visceral smooth muscles.

SMOOTH MUSCLE ELECTRICAL ACTIVITY

The contractile behaviour of smooth muscles depends to a considerable extent upon the electrical activities of these muscles. Electrical activity can vary from a tonic membrane potential that changes slowly in response to regulatory substances to fast Ca^{2+} action potentials that occur in response to excitatory agonists. Gastrointestinal (GI) smooth muscles exhibit the complete range of electrical events, and the cause of this diversity has been a central point of investigation for at least 50 years.

Prevalent in the electrical repertoire of GI muscles is the activity known as electrical slow waves (Prosser & Mangel, 1982). The major ionic currents that appear to be responsible for these events have recently been reviewed (Sanders, 1992), and among these currents, voltage-dependent (non-Ca^{2+}-dependent) K^+ currents appear to play a critical role. For example, in circular muscle cells at physiological temperatures these currents activate rapidly and tend to limit the amplitude of the upstroke of the depolarization phase of slow waves (Thornbury et al., 1992b). They may also balance inward Ca^{2+} currents at certain potentials allowing development of the plateau phase of slow waves that is critical for excitation-contraction coupling in some regions of the GI tract (Thornbury et al., 1992b). Voltage-dependent K^+ currents with different properties appear to be expressed in muscles that exhibit fast Ca^{2+} action potentials, such as the longitudinal muscles of the colon (Thornbury et al., 1992a). These studies have suggested that the diversity in electrical activity in GI muscles may be related to the expression of different species of voltage-dependent K^+ channels, but definitive descriptions of the properties of these currents have been difficult to obtain because of inadequate means of dissecting specific components of K^+ currents from whole-cell currents.

MOLECULAR CLONING OF K⁺ CHANNEL GENES

Molecular biological studies have been extremely useful in isolating specific ionic currents. This approach has identified and allowed rigorous description of the properties of several classes of voltage-dependent K^+ channels, such as the A-type and delayed rectifier gene family (Stuhmer et al., 1989), Ca^{2+}-activated K^+ channels encoded by the slo gene in Drosophila and its homologues in mammalian tissues (Atkinson et al., 1991; Tseng-Crank et al., 1994), eag (Warmke et al., 1991) whose function has yet to be firmly established, and inwardly rectifying (Morishige et al., 1994) as well as ATP-sensitive K^+ channels (Ho et al., 1993). Studies of smooth muscle K^+ channels have lagged far behind other excitable cells. The functional diversity of K^+ channels is exemplified by the different types and number of these ion channels expressed in excitable cells. Distinctions between channel types have classically been made on the basis of electrophysiological and pharmacological properties. As more of the cDNAs encoding K^+ channel proteins are cloned and their primary structure becomes known, it is becoming clear that their functional diversity is based on molecular and genetic heterogeneity. While there appears to be a great deal of homology between the families of K^+ channel proteins, small variations in amino acid sequence leads to diverse functional properties (Stuhmer et al., 1989). Further diversity occurs because K^+ channel properties are modulated in a cell- and tissue-specific manner by the action of neurotransmitter- and hormone receptor-activated second messenger systems (Vogalis & Sanders, 1989). In addition, the possibility of heterotetramer formation between K+ channel subunits from the same family exists, further leading to channels with diverse functional characteristics (Hopkins *et al.*, 1994; Russell *et al.*, 1994b). We have cloned and characterized $cK_v1.2$ (Hart *et al.*, 1993) and $cK_v1.5$ (Overturf *et al.*, 1994) from canine colonic smooth muscle and recently cloned a $K_v1.1$ from human colonic smooth muscle (data not shown).

HETEROLOGOUS EXPRESSION OF K+ CHANNELS

By expressing channel proteins in *Xenopus* oocytes, it has been possible to characterize the properties of individual channels and analyze regulatory mechanisms related to molecular structure (Sigel, 1990). Heterologous expression systems have revolutionized the manner in which we examine the structure–function relationships of ion channels. K+ channels have been especially accessible to this approach because of their relatively simple subunit structure and small size when compared to other cation, anion and non selective channels. Detailed information concerning the voltage sensor (Papazian *et al.*, 1991), ion permeation pathway (Kirsch *et al.*, 1991), inactivation mechanisms (Hoshi *et al.*, 1990), pharmacological interactions (Snyders *et al.*, 1992), membrane topology and subunit association (MacKinnon, 1991) have been obtained employing heterologous expression systems. While these studies have determined many common features of K+ channel structure, they have also shown the tremendous diversity of K+ channels from different gene families and even within the same gene family with respect to conductance, voltage dependence, and gating kinetics (Jan & Jan, 1990). Indeed, we have demonstrated that significant pharmacological differences exist between K+ channels of the $K_v1.2$ gene class which may lead to the structural identification of the region and/or amino acids involved in 4-AP binding (Russell *et al.*, 1994a) and we have determined mechanism of 4-AP block on the smooth muscle $cK_v1.2$ channel (Russell *et al.*, 1994c).

REGULATION OF K+ CHANNELS IN SMOOTH MUSCLES

Although release of acetylcholine from parasympathetic nerve endings is a principal mechanism for the neural control of smooth muscle tone and rhythmicity, few details about the specific ionic processes associated with muscarinic stimulation of smooth muscle are known.

Several different mechanisms account for modulation of K+ channels by second   messenger   systems.   The   most   common   pathways   involve phosphorylation–dephosphorylation events of either the ion channel or some modulatory intermediate (Catterall *et al.*, 1991). Most often protein kinase C (Akerman *et al.*, 1988), protein kinase A or other cyclic nucleotide kinases (Sieglebaum *et al.*, 1982), mediates these events. K^+ channels are also modulated by other mechanisms, including direct interaction with a G protein (Yatani *et al.*, 1987), actions of phospholipase A_2 products (Piomelli *et al.*, 1987), or direct interaction with Ca^{2+} (Dubinsky & Oxford, 1985).

Much of the work concerning K^+ channel regulation in smooth muscles has focused on the K_{Ca} current (Kume & Kotlikoff, 1991). Cole & Sanders (1989) implicated a G-protein linked second messenger system in this regulation. However, in atrial myocytes, investigators have identified K_{ACh} currents which are inwardly rectifying in nature and linked directly to G-protein activation (Brown *et al.*, 1990). There have been no studies examining the effects of muscarinic stimulation on Ca^{2+}-independent voltage gated K^+ channels in smooth muscle. However, in neuronal tissue, the fast transient outward K^+ current (Baraban *et al.*, 1985) and also a delayed rectifier K^+ current (Hoger *et al.*, 1991) have been demonstrated to be modulated by G-protein linked second messenger systems. An important question in smooth muscle relates to whether these K^+ conductances are modulated by signal transduction. In the colon, inhibition of the delayed rectifier K^+ current by 4-aminopyridine increases the amplitude and rate of rise of the upstroke potential and increases the amplitude and prolongs the plateau phase of the electrical slow wave (Thornbury *et al.*, 1991). It is not known whether these effects are mimicked by muscarinic stimulation. One strategy to explore the effects of signal transduction mechanisms on these Ca^{2+}-independent voltage-gated K^+ channels is the expression of these channels in heterologous systems. Expression in oocytes would effectively remove the K_{ca} conductance and allow the unobstructed regulatory examination of the expressed K^+ channel. Exogenous ion channels expressed in oocytes undergo modulation, as demonstrated by Dascal *et al* (1986) who showed in that heart mRNA-encoded Ca^{2+} channel currents were increased by isoproterenol or cAMP injections. We have determined that phorbol 12,13-dibutyrate (PDBu, 3×10^{-9}–10^{-7} M) decreased K^+ current (I_{Kv}) in oocytes injected with cRNA encoding $cK_v1.2$, $cK_v1.5$ (Figure 1) and those coinjected with both clones. Overnight pretreatment of expressing oocytes with the specific PKC inhibitor staurosporine (500 nM) decreased the PDBu-mediated inhibition of I_{Kv} from 90% to 60 %. Calphostin C (10^{-7}M), however, another putative PKC-inhibitor alone inhibited I_{Kv} and failed to antagonize the PDBu-mediated suppression of I_{Kv}. The inactive phorbol ester, 4-phorbol 12,13-didecanoate (10^{-8}M) caused a 20% reduction in I_{Kv} suggesting that the action of PDBu is specific and mediated by activation of PKC (Vogalis *et al.*, 1995).

Studies have shown that the contraction of smooth muscle is temperature dependent (Nasu, 1990), and while this effect can be partly explained by

A. **B.**

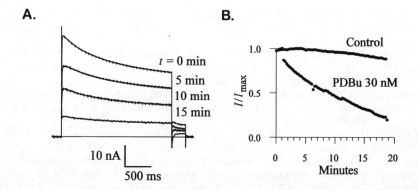

Figure 1 Regulation of $cK_v1.5$ by protein kinase C. Panel A: Oocytes expressing $cK_v1.5$ were stepped from a holding potential of −80mV to a test potential of 0mV. Phorbol 12, 13-dibutyrate (PDBu, 3×10^{-9}–10^{-7} M) was applied and oocytes were stepped after the time points indicated. Panel B: Time course of the effects of PDBu on currents elicited by expressed $cK_v1.5$.

effects on energy metabolism it has been postulated that other proccesses may be involved. For example, in guinea pig taenia coli cooling results in an increase in the smooth muscle membrane resistance (Brading *et al.*, 1969) suggesting the inhibition of membrane conductance with a decrease in temperature. Indeed, raising the temperature from 17°C to 37°C in chick sensory neurones caused an increase in open probability of Ca^{2+} channels and a drastic acceleration in their activation and inactivation characteristics (Nobile *et al.*, 1990). Thornbury *et al.* (1992b) have shown that the delayed rectifier K⁺ current in single cells isolated from the circular muscle of the canine proximal colon is similarly enhanced at physiological temperatures. It is now apparent that the delayed rectifier K⁺ current in these cells is a heterologous current made up of at least two different components (Thornbury *et al.*, 1992b). We have identified the characteristics of $cK_v1.2$ component in isolation at room temperature and at physiological temperature. At 34°C the *I–V* relationship and inactivation curve shifted to more negative potentials. Increasing the temperature to 34°C did not alter the degree of block by 4-AP, although the rate of onset of block was greatly enhanced (Russell *et al.*, 1994c).

REFERENCES

Akerman, K.E.O., Envist, M.G.K. & Halpainen, I. (1988). Activators of protein kinase C and phenylephrine depolarize the astrocyte membrane by reducing the potassium permeability. *Neurosci.Lett.* **92**, 265–269.

Atkinson, N.S., Robertson, G.A. & Ganetzky, B. (1991). A component of calcium-activated potassium channels encoded by the Drosophila slo locus. *Science* **253**, 551–555.

Baraban, J.M., Gould, R.J., Peroutka, S.J. & Snyder, S.H. (1985). Phorbol ester effects on neurotransmission: Interaction with neurotransmitters and calcium in smooth muscle. *Proc. Natl Acad. Sci.* **82**, 604–607.

Brading, A., Bulbring, E. & Tomita, T. (1969). The effect of temperature on the membrane conductance of the smooth muscle of the guinea pig taenia coli. *J. Physiol.* **200**, 621–635.

Brown, A.M., Yatani, A., Codina, J. & Birnbaumer, L. (1990). Gating of atrial muscarinic K$^+$ channels by G proteins. *Prog. Clin. Biol. Res.* **334**, 303–312.

Catterall, W.A., Scheuer, T., Thomsen, W. & Rossie, S. (1991). Structure and modulation of voltage-gated ion channels. *Ann. NY Acad. Sci.* **625**, 174–180.

Cole, W.C. & Sanders, K.M. (1989). G proteins mediate suppression of Ca^{2+}-activated K current by acetylcholine in smooth muscle cells. *Am. J. Physiol.* **257**, C596–C600.

Dascal, N., Snutch, T.P., Lubbert, H., Davidson, N. & Lester, H. A. (1986). Expression and modulation of voltage gated calcium channels after RNA injection in Xenopus oocytes. *Science* **231**, 1147–1150.

Dubinsky, J.M. & Oxford, G.S. (1985). Dual modulation of potassium channels by thyrotropin-releasing hormone in clonal pituitary cells. *Proc. Natl Acad. Sci.* **82**, 4282–4286.

Hart, P.J., Overturf, K.E., Russell, S.N., Carl, A., Hume, J.R., Sanders, K.M. & Horowitz, B. (1993). Cloning and expression of a $K_v1.2$ class delayed rectifier K$^+$ channel from canine colonic smooth muscle. *Proc. Natl Acad. Sci. USA* **90**, 9659–9663.

Ho, K., Nichols, C.G., Lederer, W.J., Lytton, J., Vassilev, P.M., Kanazirska, M.V. & Hebert, S.C. (1993). Cloning and expression of an inwardly rectifying ATP-regulated potassium channel. *Nature* **362**, 31–38.

Hoger, J.H., Walter, A.E., Vance, D., Yu, L., Lester, H.A. & Davidson, N. (1991). Modulation of a cloned mouse brain potassium channel. *Neuron* **6**, 227–236.

Hopkins, W.F., Demas, V. & Tempel, B.L. (1994). Both *N*- and *C*-terminal regions contribute to the assembly and functional expression of homo- and heteromultimeric voltage-gated K$^+$ channels. *J. Neurosci.* **14**, 1385–1393.

Hoshi, T., Zagotta, W.N. & Aldrich, R.W. (1990). Biophysical and molecular mechanisms of Shaker potassium channel inactivation. *Science* **250**, 533–538.

Jan, L.Y. & Jan, Y.N. (1990). A superfamily of ion channels. *Nature* **345**, 672.

Kirsch, G.E., Taglialatela, M. & Brown, A.M. (1991). Internal and external TEA block in single cloned K$^+$ channels. *Am. J. Physiol. Cell Physiol.* **261**, C583–C590.

Kume, H. & Kotlikoff, M.I. (1991). Muscarinic inhibition of single K_{Ca} channels in smooth muscle cells by a pertussis-sensitive G protein. *Am. J. Physiol. Cell Physiol.* **261**, C1204–C1209.

MacKinnon, R. (1991). Determination of the subunit stoichiometry of a voltage-activated potassium channel. *Nature* **350**, 232–235.

Morishige, K.-I., Takahashi, N., Jahangir, A., Yamada, M., Koyama, H., Zanelli, J.S. & Kurachi, Y. (1994). Molecular cloning and functional expression of a novel brain-specific inward rectifier potassium channel. *FEBS Lett.* **346**, 251–256.

Nasu, T. (1990). Effects of cooling on smooth muscle contraction. *Comp. Biochem. Physiol.* [*A*] **95A**, 201–207.

Nobile, M., Carbonne, E., Lux, H.D. & Zucker, H. (1990). Temperature sensitivity of Ca currents in chick sensory neurones. *Pflügers Arch.* **415**, 658–663.

Overturf, K.E., Russell, S.N., Carl, A., Vogalis, F., Hart, P.J., Hume, J.R., Sanders, K.M. & Horowitz, B. (1994). Cloning and characterization of a $K_v1.5$ delayed rectifier K^+ channel from vascular and visceral smooth muscles. *Am. J. Physiol. Cell Physiol.* **267**, C1231–C1238.

Papazian, D.M., Timpe, L.C., Jan, Y.N. & Jan, L.Y. (1991). Alteration of voltage-dependence of Shaker potassium channel by mutations in the S4 sequence. *Nature* **349**, 305–310.

Piomelli, O., Volterra, A., Dale, N., Sieglebaum, S.A., Kandel, E.R., Schwartz, J.H. & Belandetti, F. (1987). Lipoxygenase metabolites or arachidonic acid as second messengers for presynaptic inhibition of Aplysia cells. *Nature* **328**, 38–43.

Prosser, C.L. & Mangel, A.W. (1982). Mechanisms of spike and slow wave pacemaker activity in smooth muscle cells. In *Cellular Pacemakers, Vol. 1: Mechanisms of Pacemaker Generation* (Carpenter, D.O., ed.), pp. 273-301. John Wiley & Sons, New York.

Russell, S.N., Overturf, K.E., Hart, P.J. & Horowitz, B. (1994a). Localization of the 4-aminopyridine binding site on a $K_v1.2$ K^+ channel through chimera construction and site-directed mutagenesis. *Biophys. J.* **66**, A208(Abstr.).

Russell, S.N., Overturf, K.E. & Horowitz, B. (1994b). Heterotetramer formation and charybdotoxin sensitivity of two K^+ channels cloned from smooth muscle. *Am. J. Physiol. Cell Physiol.* **267**, C1729–C1733.

Russell, S.N., Publicover, N.G., Hart, P.J., Carl, A., Hume, J.R., Sanders, K.M. & Horowitz, B. (1994c). Block by 4-aminopyridine of a $K_v1.2$ delayed rectifier K^+ current expressed in Xenopus oocytes. *J. Physiol. (London)* **481**, 571–584.

Sanders, K.M. (1992). Ionic mechanisms of electrical rhythmicity in gastrointestinal smooth muscles. *Annu. Rev. Physiol.* **54**, 439–453.

Sieglebaum, S.A., Camardo, J.S. & Kandel, E.R. (1982). Serotonin and cAMP close single potassium channels in Aplysia sensory neurons. *Nature* **299**, 413–417.

Sigel, E. (1990). Use of Xenopus oocytes for the functional expression of plasma membrane proteins. *J. Membr. Biol.* **117**, 201–221.

Snyders, D.J., Knoth, K.M., Roberds, S.L. & Tamkun, M.M. (1992). Time-, voltage-, and state-dependent block by quinidine of a cloned human cardiac potassium channel. *Mol. Pharmacol.* **41**, 322–330.

Stuhmer, W., Ruppersberg, J.P., Schroter, K.H., Sakmann, B., Stocker, M., Giese, K.P., Perschke, A., Baumann, A. & Pongs, O. (1989). Molecular basis of functional diversity of voltage-gated potassium channels in mammalian brain. *EMBO J.* **8**, 3235-3244.

Thornbury, K.D., Ward, S.M. & Sanders, K.M. (1991). Characteristics of fast outward current in canine colonic circular muscles. *Biophys. J.* **59**, 234a (Abstr.).

Thornbury, K.D., Ward, S.M. & Sanders, K.M. (1992a). Outward currents in longitudinal colonic muscle cells contribute to spiking electrical behavior. *Am. J. Physiol. Cell Physiol.* **263**, C237–C245.

Thornbury, K.D., Ward, S.M. & Sanders, K.M. (1992b). Participation of fast-activating, voltage-dependent K currents in electrical slow waves of colonic circular muscle. *Am. J. Physiol. Cell Physiol.* **263**, C226–C236.

Tseng-Crank, J., Foster, C.D., Krause, J.D., Mertz, R., Godinot, N., Dichiara, T.J. & Reinhart, P.H. (1994). Cloning, expression, and distribution of functionally distinct Ca^{2+}-activated K^+ channel isoforms from human brain. *Neuron* **13**, 1315–1330.

Vogalis, F. & Sanders, K.M. (1989). Excitatory and inhibitory neural regulation of canine pyloric smooth muscles. *Am. J. Physiol.* **259**, G125–G133.

Vogalis, F., Ward, M.W. & Horowitz, B. (1995). Regulation of cloned smooth muscle K^+ channels $cK_v1.2$ and $cK_v1.5$ by protein kinase C. *Biophys. J.* **68**, A47(Abstr.).

Warmke, J., Drysdale, R. & Ganetzky, B. (1991). A distinct potassium channel polypeptide encoded by the Drosophila eag locus. *Science* **252**, 1560–1562.

Yatani, A., Codina, J., Brown, A.M. & Birnbaumer, L. (1987). Direct activation of mammalian atrial muscarinic potassium channels by GTP regulatory protein Gk. *Science* **235**, 207–211.

12

ATP-sensitive Potassium Channels and their Modulation by Nucleotides and Potassium Channel Openers in Vascular Smooth Muscle Cells

H-L. ZHANG
T. B. BOLTON

*Department of Pharmacology and Clinical Pharmacology,
St George's Hospital Medical School,
London, UK*

INTRODUCTION

In 1983 Noma reported the presence of a K-selective ion channel in guinea pig and rabbit ventricular cells that was inhibited by intracellular ATP ($[ATP]_i$). This channel was rarely seen under normal conditions but was activated by cyanide in cell-attached patches and by forming inside-out patches into ATP-free solution (Noma *et al.*, 1983). Almost at the same time, similar results were reported by Trube and Hescheler (1983, 1984). Since then, the ATP-sensitive K (K_{ATP}) channel has been described in the membrane of cardiac muscle (Kakei & Noma, 1984; Kakei *et al.*, 1985), skeletal muscle (Spruce, *et al.*, 1985, 1987), pancreatic β-cells (Cook & Hales, 1984; Findlay *et al.*, 1985; Rorsman & Trube, 1985), neurone (Ashford *et al.*, 1988) and smooth muscle (Standen, *et al.*, 1989). Among these, the K_{ATP} channels in cardiac muscle and pancreatic β-cells have been most intensively investigated (reviewed by Ashcroft & Ashcroft, 1990; Nichols & Lederer, 1991; Dunne 1992; Takano & Noma, 1993).

The data available concerning the K_{ATP} channel in smooth muscle present a confusing and complex picture. In many studies, the presence of K_{ATP} channels has been claimed on the basis of activation of channel activity by potassium channel openers (KCOs) and inhibition by the sulphonylurea glibenclamide. However, the Ca-activated large-conductance K channel (BK channel) in smooth muscle was also found to be activated by cromakalim and

SMOOTH MUSCLE EXCITATION
ISBN 0-12-112360-X

inhibited by glibenclamide (Carl et al., 1992). In cardiac muscle and β-cells, creation from cell-attached patches of isolated inside-out patches into ATP-free solution results in a high level of K_{ATP} channel activity as the inhibitory effect of ATP is lost. However, this property of K_{ATP} channels has seldom been seen in smooth muscle and most experiments on smooth muscle have failed to identify K_{ATP} channel activity in inside-out patches simply in the absence of ATP (Kajioka et al., 1991; Nakao & Bolton, 1991; Robertson et al., 1992; Beech et al., 1993a,b; Bonev & Nelson, 1993; Kamouchi et al., 1993; Zhang & Bolton, 1995) unless GDP and levcromakalim ((−)Ckm) or pinacidil were present (Kajioka et al., 1991; Beech et. al, 1993a, b; Kamouchi et al., 1993, Zhang & Bolton, 1995). Thus, in smooth muscle the term 'K_{ATP} channel,' has been used by authors either to refer to the single K channels shown to be inhibited by ATP or glibenclamide, or activated by GDP and KCOs (but not BK channels), or to refer to the target channels underlying whole-cell currents which have been shown to be inhibited by intracellular ATP and glibenclamide and stimulated by extracellular KCOs.

RESPONSE TO ATP

One of the characteristics of the K_{ATP} channels in cardiac myocytes and pancreatic β-cells is the dual effect of ATP on the channels. K_{ATP} channel activity ceases a short period after patch isolation i.e., the channel activity exhibits 'run-down'. ATP in the presence, but not in the absence of Mg^{2+} could prevent or reverse the channel rundown (Findlay & Dunne, 1986; Misler et al., 1986; Ohno-Shosaku et al., 1987; Takano et al., 1990). When K_{ATP} channels are active, ATP inhibits channel activity with half-maximal inhibition (K_i) at about 20–30 μM in cardiac cells (Findlay, 1988; Lederer & Nichols, 1989), and 10–20 μM in pancreatic β-cells (Cook & Hales, 1984; Kakei et al., 1986; Ashcroft & Kakei, 1989; Ohno-Shosaku et al., 1987). There have been no reports that the K_{ATP} channel in smooth muscle can be reactivated by Mg-ATP in inside-out patches. Only a few studies have quantitatively investigated the inhibitory effects of ATP on the K_{ATP} channel. Kajioka et al. (1991) observed single K channel activity in the presence of GDP 1 mM and pinacidil 100 μM together in rabbit portal vein smooth muscle cells. ATP, in the absence of Mg, inhibited this channel with a K_i of 28 μM. Mg or MgATP interacted with the inhibitory actions of ATP. The slope of the inhibitory curve was well fitted by a value of 2, suggesting two binding sites for ATP. However, more recently the same group reported a much higher K_i (about 200 μM without Mg and about 1 mM with Mg) for ATP inhibiting the channel activity activated by UDP 1 mM and pinacidil 100 μM together (Kamouchi & Kitamura, 1994). Kovacs & Nelson (1991) reported a large conductance K channel incorporated into bilayers from aortic smooth muscle cells which was inhibited by ATP with a K_i of 41 μM and a Hill coefficient of 1. Another large conductance K channel from rat tail artery smooth muscle was found to be inhibited by ATP with a K_i of 125 μM (Furspan & Webb, 1993). In other studies, a single high concentration of ATP (1–5 mM) has generally been used to show substantial channel inhibition or complete inhibition of K_{ATP} channel activity (Standen et al., 1989; Kajioka et al., 1990).

The K_{ATP} channels would be expected to open under conditions where intracellular ATP falls. Attempts have been made to identify the K_{ATP} channel in smooth muscle by depleting $[ATP]_i$ in single cells. Glibenclamide is normally used to identify the current presumed to result from K_{ATP} channel opening in these kinds of studies, and so the studies rely quite heavily on the specificity of this agent at the concentrations used. In rabbit pulmonary artery smooth muscle cells, whole-cell holding currents were larger when ATP was omitted from the intracellular solution; such currents could be inhibited by glibenclamide or by release of ATP intracellularly by flash photolysis of caged ATP (Clapp & Gurney, 1992). Similarly, in rabbit mesenteric artery, Quayle et al., (1994) found the glibenclamide-sensitive whole-cell K current to be three times larger when ATP was included in the pipette at 0.1 mM (free ATP was 10 μM) than when the pipette ATP was 3 mM (free ATP was 371 μM). However, in the above studies either GDP and ADP (Quayle et al., 1994) or GTP (Clapp & Gurney, 1992) was present in the pipette solution which makes it difficult to argue that these currents were induced simply by the low concentration of $[ATP]_i$. In rat portal vein smooth muscle, Noack et al., (1992a) observed a glibenclamide-sensitive whole-cell current which was induced by removing glucose and carboxylic acids from the pipette solution and also removing extracellular glucose, a combination of procedures designed to lead to ATP depletion. Using the 'perforated patch' method (nystatin was included in the pipette) Silberberg and van Breemen (1992) reported that metabolic inhibition could induce a glibenclamide-sensitive current in rabbit mesenteric artery cells. More recently, Xu & Lee (1994) reported a glibenclamide-sensitive sustained K current in dog coronary artery smooth muscle cells which was induced by depletion of $[ATP]_i$. This current could be inhibited by $[ATP]_i$ concentration-dependently with a K_i for ATP of 350 μM in the presence of 1 mM Mg.

CHANNEL CONDUCTANCE AND OTHER PROPERTIES

The unitary conductance of the K_{ATP} channel is about 50–80 pS in cardiac muscle and pancreatic β-cells when the internal K concentration is 140 mM and external K concentration is about 100–140 mM (Noma, 1983; Cook & Hales, 1984; Trube & Hescheler, 1984; Kakei et al., 1985; Rorsman & Trube,

1985; Trube *et al.*, 1986). The unitary conductance of the K_{ATP} channel became smaller when the external K concentration was reduced and was around 20–25 pS when physiological K gradients (external K 5 mM) were used (Noma, 1983; Trube & Hescheler, 1984; Findlay *et al.*, 1985; Kakei *et al.*, 1985; Trube *et al.*, 1986; Nichols & Lederer, 1990).

K_{ATP} channels in smooth muscle have widely varying properties, including channel conductance and channel sensitivity to Ca and voltage. Large conductance (130-260 pS) K_{ATP} channels have been observed in rabbit and rat mesenteric artery (Standen *et al.*, 1989) in lipid bilayers from aorta (Kovacs & Nelson, 1991) in rabbit afferent arteriole of kidney (Lorenz *et al.*, 1992) and in rat tail artery (Furspan & Webb, 1993). The conductance reported by Standen *et al.*, (1989) was 135 pS in inside-out patches when the K gradient was 60 mM:120 mM. These channels were clearly inhibited by ATP with an K_i of 50–300 μM and were Ca- and voltage-insensitive. Cromakalim reactived the channels after they had been inhibited by ATP and the effects of cromakalim were blocked by glibenclamide. Similar K channels were observed in lipid bilayers (Kovacs & Nelson, 1991). The conductance reported by Lorenz *et al.*, (1992) was 258 pS in inside-out patches with symmetrical K concentrations of 150 mM. These channels were voltage-dependent and were inhibited by ATP and glibenclamide.

Small conductance (10–30 pS) K_{ATP} channels were reported in rat and rabbit portal vein (Kajioka *et al.*, 1990, 1991; Beech *et al.*, 1993a,b; Kamouchi *et al.*, 1993; Kamouchi & Kitamura, 1994), rat mesenteric artery (Zhang & Bolton, 1995), urinary bladder (Bonev & Nelson, 1993) and pig coronary artery (Inoue *et al.*, 1989; Miyoshi & Nakaya, 1991, 1993; Miyoshi *et al.*, 1992; Wakatsuki *et al.*, 1992). Kajioka *et al.*, (1990) observed 10 pS K channel activity (6 mM:138 mM K-gradient) in outside-out and inside-out patches from rat portal vein smooth muscle cells. These channels were Ca dependent and were inhibited by 5 mM NaATP but not MgATP. Similar K channels have been observed in patches from cultured coronary artery smooth muscle cells, which had a conductance of 30 pS under symmetrical K concentrations of 150 mM, and these were inhibited by glibenclamide and ATP (Wakatsuki *et al.*, 1992). K channels with 15 pS conductance that require GDP and KCO for activation have been observed by Kajioka *et al.* (1991) and Kamouchi *et al.* (1993) in cell-attached and inside-out patches from rabbit portal vein (6 mM:140 mM K gradient). The channel conductance was increased to 50 pS when symmetrical K concentrations of 140 mM were used. These channels opened only when pinacidil (or LP-805, a potassium channel opener) and GDP were present together. The channels were not Ca-dependent and showed little voltage-dependence and were inhibited completely by 100 μM glibenclamide. Similar channels (K_{NDP} channels as they were called) were reported by Beech *et al.* (1993a,b) and Zhang & Bolton (1995); conductance of K_{NDP} channels was 20–24 pS when K-gradient was 60 mM:130 mM.

The conductance of the target channel underlying the whole-cell current which is induced by depletion of [ATP]$_i$ or by KCOs can be estimated by means of noise analysis; the unitary current is calculated from the relationship between the variance of the whole-cell currents and its mean level. Noise analysis studies of the whole-cell currents activated by $(-)$Ckm in rat portal vein smooth muscle cells suggested an underlying unitary conductance of 17 pS in physiological extracellular K (6 mM) concentration (Noack *et al.*, 1992b), while the current induced by metabolic inhibition gave a value of 10-20 pS (Noack *et al.*, 1992a). In rabbit pulmonary artery smooth muscle cells, the conductance of the channel underlying the whole-cell current induced by $(-)$Ckm was estimated to be 16 pS with symmetrical 143 mM K (Langton *et al.*, 1992). Thus, although both large and small channel conductances have been reported in single channel studies, the K_{ATP} channel primarily activated by either ATP deletion or KCO in whole-cell recordings is of small rather than large conductance.

BK channels in smooth muscle could also be inhibited by intracellular ATP (Silberberg & van Breemen, 1990; Groschner *et al.*, 1991). However, this effect of ATP was ascribed to the chelation of intracellular Ca^{2+} (Klöckner & Isenberg, 1992).

PHARMACOLOGY OF K_{ATP} CHANNELS

Almost all K_{ATP} channels reported in smooth muscle are sensitive to glibenclamide, a suggested specific K_{ATP} channel blocker in cardiac myocytes and pancreatic β-cells (Sturgess *et al.*, 1985; Ashcroft & Ashcroft, 1990; Nichols & Lederer, 1991). However, quantitative data concerning inhibition of K_{ATP} channels by glibenclamide in smooth muscle cells are very limited. Beech *et al.*, (1993a) reported that the whole-cell current induced by intracellular GDP was inhibited by glibenclamide with a K_i of 25 nM. A similar K_i for glibenclamide (20 nM) was obtained for the inhibition of whole-cell current induced by depletion of intracellular ATP in canine coronary smooth muscle cells (Xu & Lee, 1994).

KCOs are particularly potent relaxants of smooth muscle and are of promise for the treatment of diseases such as asthma, essential hypertension and urinary incontinence (reviewed by Robertson & Steinberg, 1990). An important difference between vascular smooth muscle and β-cells or cardiac myocytes is the much greater sensitivity of smooth muscle to KCOs (Quast & Cook, 1989). Cromakalim, pinacidil, RP 49356 and nicorandil in hypotensive doses do not affect the control of blood sugar, and in isolated patches from β-cells they have little effect on channel opening below 100 μM when the concentration of [ATP]$_i$ is in the millimolar range (Dunne & Petersen, 1991). A major mechanism underlying the relaxant effects of KCO appears to be the opening of K channels in the cell membrane which leads to membrane hyperpolarization (Edwards *et al.*, 1992).

It is quite clear that KCOs open the K_{ATP} channels in cardiac myocytes and pancreatic β-cells (Nichols & Lederer, 1991; Dunne, 1992). The target K channel for the effect of KCOs on smooth muscle has not been determined. Both large and small conductance ATP-sensitive K channels (Standen *et al.* 1989; Kajioka *et al.*, 1990, 1991), BK channels (Carl *et al.*, 1992; Gelband & McCullough, 1993) and delayed rectifier K channels (K_{DR}) (Beech & Bolton, 1989; Edwards *et al.*, 1993) have been suggested as targets for the actions of KCOs. It is surprising that there is so much inconsistency in the literature regarding the target K channel of KCOs in smooth muscle. In a series of detailed studies (Gelband *et al.*, 1989, 1990; Gelband & McCullough, 1993) obtained evidence that BK channels are involved in the actions of cromakalim and pinacidil; in experiments using either cultured aortic smooth muscle or following the incorporation of BK into planar lipid bilayers, the channel opened by cromakalim was extremely similar to charybdotoxin-sensitive BK channels and the effects of cromakalim and pinacidil were inhibited by glibenclamide. However, although KCOs appear to open several types of K channel in isolated patches of membrane, there are numerous studies that show that the hyperpolarization and relaxation of intact smooth muscle by KCOs are blocked by glibenclamide and are unaffected by blockers of BK channels (charybdotoxin or 1–5 mM tetraethyl ammonium (TEA) (reviewed by Edwards & Weston, 1993). In addition, data from noise analysis suggested that the channels underlying the whole-cell current induced by KCOs are of small conductance (Langton *et al.*, 1992; Noack *et al.*, 1992b; Criddle *et al.*, 1994) implying that large conductance channels do not open in response to KCOs in the intact cell or tissue and that K_{ATP} channels are most likely the target channel of KCOs.

Table 1 summarizes some of the properties of the K_{ATP} channels described in smooth muscle cells. It is clear that not only is there great variety among these channels but also that the available data reveal only a limited similarity to the K_{ATP} channels in tissues other than smooth muscle.

METHODS

Single cells were enzymatically isolated from rat portal vein and experiments were performed at room temperature (22°C). Cell-attached and isolated inside-out patch recordings (Hamill *et al.*, 1981) were used in the experiments. Bathing solution (mM): NaCl 9, KCl 120, HEPES 18, EDTA 5, pH 7.4 with KOH. For Mg-containing bathing solution, MgCl$_2$ 0.1, 1, 2 or 3 mM was added and EDTA was replaced by EGTA. Pipette solution (mM): NaCl 80, KCl 60, MgCl$_2$ 1.2, HEPES 10, glucose 10, pH 7.4 with NaOH.

Table 1 Characteristics of K-channels sensitive to ATP in smooth muscles

Conductance (pS)	Tissue	Ki:Ko (mM)	Active in nucleotide-free solution	Inhibition of ATP	NDPs	KCOs (in the presence of)	Glibenclamide
260*	Rabbit preglomerular artery (Lorenz et al., 1992)	145:145	Yes	1 mM (82%)	–	↑(ATP)	↓1 µM
230	Rat tail artery (Furspan, 1992; Furspan & Webb, 1993)	150:150	Yes	1 mM (95%) K$_i$ 125 µM	–	↑(ATP)	↓10 µM K$_i$ 0.43 nM
135	Rabbit mesenteric artery (Standen et al., 1989)	60:120	Yes	1 mM (95%)	–	↑(ATP)	↓20 µM
50	Dog aorta (Kovacs & Nelson, 1991)	5:120	Yes	K$_i$ 41 µM	–	↑(ATP)	↓50 µM
40	Rabbit mesenteric artery (Nelson et al., 1990)	6:120	Yes	–	–	–	↓30 µM
30†	Pig coronary artery (Inoue et al., 1989; Miyoshi & Nakaya, 1991; 1993; Miyoshi et al., 1992; Wakatsuki et al., 1992)	150:150	Yes	1 mM K$_i$ 0.3–0.5 mM	–	↑	↓20 µM
10†	Rat portal vein (Kajioka et al., 1990)	6:140	Yes	5 mM	–	↑ (Outside)	–
7.5	Guinea pig urinary bladder (Bonev & Nelson, 1993)	6:140	No	–	No	↑ (Outside)	↓10 µM
24	Rabbit portal vein (Beech et al., 1993a, 1993b)	60:130	No	1 mM	Activation	↑(NDP)	↓10 µM
20	Rat mesenteric artery (Zhang & Bolton, 1995)	60:130	No	–	Activation	↑(NDP)	↓10 µM
15	Rabbit portal vein (Kajioka et al., 1991; Kamouchi et al., 1993; Kamouchi & Kitamura, 1994)	6:140	No	K$_i$ 29–200 µM	Activation	↑(NDP or ATP)	↓100 µM
10–20‡	Rat mesenteric artery and portal vein (Noack et al., 1992a; Criddle et al., 1994)	6:120	–	–	–	↑	↓10 µM

* Voltage-dependent.
† Ca^{2+} dependent.
‡ From noise analysis of whole-cell current.
– No data available.

RESULTS

There were two types of ATP-sensitive K channels in rat portal vein smooth muscle cells. When inside-out patches from rat portal vein smooth muscle cells were created in nucleotide-free solution, a K channel was activated in about 80 patches. This channel, which showed very similar characteristics to the K_{ATP} channel described in cardiac myocytes and pancreatic-β cells, will be called here the LK channel. The LK channel showed a high probability of open state immediately after inside-out patches were isolated. In most of the patches, 3–5 channels opened simultaneously while in other patches up to 10 channels could be seen opening simultaneously. The channel conductance was about 50 pS (60:130 K gradient) in the linear region (−20 to −100 mV) of the current-voltage relationship which showed some inwardly rectification even in the absence of Mg (Figure 1c). Channel activity declined (channel run-down) after the initial dramatic openings and gradually decreased over a period ranging from 40 s to a few minutes; in a few patches no run-down of channel activity was observed even after up to 20 or 30 min. ATP in the presence of Mg could reactivated the LK channel after its partial or total run-down. In some patches,

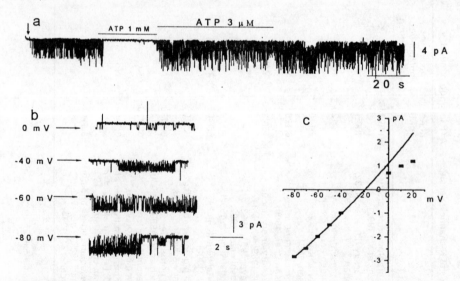

Figure 1 a, Inhibition of the LK channel by ATP in an inside-out patch. The patch was held at −60 mV. 130 mM K was in the bathing solution and 60 mM K was in the pipette. An inside-out patch was created at the time indicated by arrow. ATP (1 mM and 3 μM) was applied to the inner side of the patch via bathing solution. b, Unitary current amplitude of the LK channel at different holding potentials. c, Current–voltage relationship of the LK channel. The data was fitted with Goldman–Hodgkin–Katz current equation (solid line).

LK channel activity was greater after ATP treatment than before run-down of channel activity. NDPs could also reactivate the LK channel after it had run-down. ATP, either in the absence or presence of Mg, inhibited the LK channel potently (Figure 1a); K_i of ATP was 11 and 23 μM in the absence and presence of 1 mM Mg, respectively. The LK channel was also inhibited by glibenclamide with a K_i of 3 μM. In some patches LK channel activity was also observed in the cell-attached mode. If LK channels were active in the cell-attached mode, channel activity generally declined upon creating an inside-out patch. (−)Ckm or pinacidil 10 μM had little effect on LK channel activity either in the absence or presence of ATP or NDPs in inside-out patches. In the cell-attached patches, these KCOs did not activate the LK channel although the channel was proved to be present after the creation of isolated inside-out patches.

A second type of K channel with a smaller channel conductance was also observed in rat portal vein smooth muscle cells. This channel, which was very similar to the K_{NDP} channels described in rabbit portal vein and rat mesenteric artery (Beech et al., 1993a; Zhang & Bolton, 1995) will here be called the MK channel. The MK channel seemed more active than the LK channel in cell-attached patches (Figure 2a). However, it was rare to see the

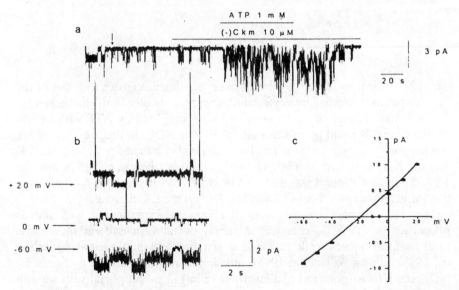

Figure 2 a, Activation of the MK channel by ATP and (−)Ckm in an inside-out patch. The patch was held at −60 mV. 130 mM K was in the bathing solution and 60 mM K was in the pipette. An inside-out patch was created at the time (indicated by arrow). ATP (1 mM) and (−)Ckm (10 μM) were applied to the inner side of the patch via the bathing solution. b, Unitary current amplitude of the MK channel at different holding potentials (brief openings of BK channels are apparent at +20 mV). c, Current–voltage relationship of the MK channel. The data was fitted with Goldman–Hodgkin–Katz current equation (solid line).

MK channel activity in isolated inside-out patches in the absence of nucleotides. If MK channels were active in the cell-attached patch mode, activity eventually declined on creating an inside-out patch into nucleotide-free solution. ATP or UDP 1 mM alone could stimulate MK channel activity in inside-out patches either in patches where the MK channel had been active before application of ATP or in patches where no channel activity had been observed prior to application of ATP. After washing out ATP, MK channel activity disappeared almost immediately without a transient increase. Lower concentrations of ATP (10 µM) had no effect on MK channel activity while increasing the concentration of ATP from 1 mM to 3 or 5 mM inhibited channel activity compared with that in 1 mM ATP. KCOs alone could not activate MK channels unless ATP (Figure 2a) or NDPs were present. In other patches, ATP alone could not activate MK channels unless $(-)$Ckm 10 µM or pinacidil 10 µM were also added. KCOs could also increase activity of the MK channels activated by ATP or UDP alone. The current–voltage relationship of the MK channel showed only slight inward rectification in the region of -70 to $+30$ mV (in the presence of 1 or 2 mM Mg) and the channel conductance was 22 pS (Figure 2c).

DISCUSSION

The LK channel we describe here has very similar properties to those of the K_{ATP} channels in cardiac myocytes and pancreatic β-cells; both channels were active in the absence of nucleotides and were inhibited by ATP with similar K_i; the channels could be reactivated by ATP or NDPs in the presence of Mg after channel activity had run down; the channel conductance of both the LK and the K_{ATP} were very similar. The only difference between the LK and the K_{ATP} channels we found was that KCOs which activate in the K_{ATP} channel in cardiac myocytes and β-cells had little effect on the LK channel.

The MK channel described in the present experiments had similar properties to the K_{NDP} channels in rabbit portal vein and rat mesenteric artery smooth muscle cells reported in our previous publications (Beech et al., 1993a; Zhang & Bolton, 1995) and similar to the channels activated by NDP and KCOs (pinacidil and levcromakalim) in rabbit portal vein smooth muscles (Kajioka et al., 1991; Kamouchi & Kitamura, 1994). These channels have the following common characteristics: (1) they were activated by NDPs or KCOs in the presence of ATP or NDPs; (2) they were not active in the absence of nucleotide; (3) they have a smaller channel conductance of 20–24 pS when external K was 60 mM (Figure 2b; Beech et al., 1993a; Zhang & Bolton, 1995) or 140 mM (Kamouchi & Kitamura, 1994). However, the K_{NDP} channel was not activated by ATP (Beech et al., 1993a; Zhang &

Bolton, 1995). In our previous experiments (Beech *et al.*, 1993a; Zhang & Bolton, 1995), we did not test at the single-channel level the effect of ATP on the K_{NDP} channels after they were activated by NDPs. However, ATP 1 mM in the presence of 2 mM Mg inhibited about 63% of the whole-cell currents induced by 1 mM GDP (Beech *et al.*, 1993a). Kamouchi & Kitamura (1994) reported that K_i for ATP inhibiting the channel activity induced by 1 mM UDP and 100 μM pinacidil was about 200 μM to 1 mM in the absence and presence of Mg. In the present studies, channel activity of the MK channel induced by 1 mM ATP in the presence of 3 mM Mg could be inhibited by a higher concentration (3–5 mM) ATP. Thus, the MK channel and similar channels were not very sensitive to the inhibitory action of ATP, at least in the presence of Mg.

The LK and MK channels could be observed in the same patches, either in cell-attached patches or in isolated inside-out patches. In some inside-out patches ATP (1 mM) inhibited LK channel activity and activated the MK channel at the same time; after washing out of ATP, the LK channel was reactivated and MK channel activity disappeared. The MK channel could also be activated when KCOs in the presence of ATP or NDPs were applied to the patches where LK channels had been active.

The relationship of the LK and the MK channels (K_{NDP} in other tissues) is not yet clear from the present experiments. It is possible that the LK and the MK channels were two different modes of the same population channel as they had some common properties (Table 2); perhaps the LK channel can be transformed into the MK channel in the presence of ATP, NDPs or the nucleotides and KCOs together.

Table 2 Summary of properties of K-channels described in this chapter

	Rabbit portal vein K_{NDP}	Rat mesenteric artery K_{NDP}	Rat portal vein K_{NDP} (MK)	Rat portal vein K_{ATP} (LK)
Conductance	24 pS $60K_i:130K_o$	20 pS $60K_i:130K_o$	22 pS $60K_i:130K_o$	50 pS $60K_i:130K_o$
NDPs	↑ Needs Mg^{2+}	↑ Needs Mg^{2+}	↑ Needs Mg^{2+}	↑ After run-down needs Mg^{2+}
ATP	↑ If Mg^{2+} and KCO present; if NDP present then inhibits; high concentration inhibits	–	↑ If Mg^{2+} present; high concentration inhibits	↓ K_i 11 μM–23 μM
KCO	↑ If NDP or ATP present	↑ If NDP present	↑ If NDP or ATP present	No effect
Glibenclamide	$I_{K(GDP)}$ ↓ K_i 25 nM $I_{K(CKm)}$ ↓ K_i 200 nM	Inhibits (10 μM)	Inhibits (10 μM)	Inhibits K_i 3 μM (no Mg^{2+})

However, it is more likely that the LK and the MK were two different channels but related to each other in some way (probably, genetically both belong to the family of inward rectifier K channels, K_{IR}; Ho et al., 1993; Krapivinsky et al., 1995). The following facts support the latter suggestion: (1), KCOs activated the K_{ATP} channels in cardiac myocytes and in pancreatic β-cells but the MK channel has not been reported in these tissues (K_{IR} in cardiac cells had a similar conductance to that of the MK channel and could also be activated by ATP (Trube & Hescheler, 1984; Takano et al., 1990). (2) No LK channel was observed in rabbit portal vein (Kajioka et al., 1991; Beech et al., 1993a,b; Kamouchi & Kitamura, 1994) and rat mesenteric artery (Zhang & Bolton, 1995) smooth muscle cells where the MK (or K_{NDP}) channels were present. For the same reasons mentioned above it may not be too surprising that KCOs could activate MK but not LK channels.

ACKNOWLEDGEMENT

Work described in this chapter was supported by the British Heart Foundation.

REFERENCES

Ashcroft, S.J.H. & Ashcroft, F.M. (1990). Properties and functions of ATP-sensitive K-channels. Cell. Signal. 2, 197–214.

Ashcroft, F.M. & Kakei, M. (1989) ATP-sensitive K channels in rat pancreatic β-cells, modulation by ATP and Mg ions. J. Physiol. 416, 349–367.

Ashford, M.L.J., Sturgess, N.C., Trout, N.J., Gardner, N.J. & Hales, C.H. (1988) Adenosine-5'-triphosphate-sensitive ion channels in neonatal rat culture neurones. Pflügers Arch. 412, 297–304.

Beech, D.J. & Bolton, T.B. (1989) Properties of the cromakalim-induced potassium conductance in smooth muscle cells isolated from the rabbit portal vein. Br. J. Pharmacol. 98, 851–864 .

Beech, D.J., Zhang, H., Nakao, K. & Bolton, T.B. (1993a). K channel activation by nucleotide diphosphates and its inhibition by glibenclamide in vascular smooth muscle cells. Br. J. Pharmacol. 110, 573–582.

Beech, D.J., Zhang, H., Nakao, K. & Bolton, T.B. (1993b). Single channel and whole-cell K-currents evoked by levcromakalim in smooth muscle cells from the rabbit portal vein. Br. J. Pharmacol. 110, 583–590.

Bonev, A.D. and Nelson, M.T. (1993) ATP-sensitive potassium channels in smooth muscle cells from guinea pig urinary bladder. Am. J. Physiol. 264, C1190–C1200.

Carl, A., Bowen, S.M., Gelband, K.M., Sanders, K.M. & Hume, J.R. (1992) Cromakalim and lemakalim activates Ca^{2+}-dependent K^+ channels in canine colon. Pflügers Arch. 421, 67–76.

Clapp, L.H. and Gurney, A.M. (1992) ATP-sensitive K^+ channels regulate resting potential of pulmonary arterial smooth muscle cells. Am. J. Physiol. 262, H916–H920.

Cook, D.L. & Hales, C.N. (1984) Intracellular ATP directly blocks K⁺ channels in pancreatic β-cells. *Nature* **311**, 271–273.

Criddle, D.N, Greenwood, I.A. & Weston, A.H. (1994) Levcromakalim-induced modulation of membrane potassium currents, intracellular calcium and mechanical activity in rat mesenteric artery. *Naunyn-Schmiedebergs Arch. Pharmacol.* **349**, 422–430.

Dunne, M. J. (1992) Physiology and pharmacology of ATP-regulated potassium channels in insulin-secreting cells. In *Potassium Channel Modulators, Pharmacological. Molecular and Clinical Aspects*, (Weston, A.H. & Hamilton, T.C. eds), pp. 110–143. Blackwell Scientific Publications, Oxford.

Dunne, M.J & Petersen, O.H. (1991) Potassium selective ion channels in insulin-secreting cells, Physiology, pharmacology and their role in stimulus-secretion coupling. *Biochem. Biophys. Acta.* **1071**, 67–82.

Edwards, G. & Weston, A.H. (1993). The pharmacology of ATP-sensitive potassium channels. *Ann. Rev. Pharmacol. Toxicol.* **33**, 597–637.

Edwards, G., Duty, S., Trezise, D.J. & Weston, A.H. (1992). Effects of potassium channel modulators on the cardiovascular system. In *Potassium Channel Modulators, Pharmacological. Molecular and Clinical Aspects*, (Weston, A.H. & Hamilton, T.C. eds), pp. 110–143. Blackwell Scientific Publications, Oxford.

Edwards, G., Ibbotson, T., Weston, A.H. (1993) Levcromakalim may induce a voltage-independent K-current in rat portal veins by modifying the gating properties of the delayed rectifier. *Br. J. Pharmacol.* **110**, 1037–1048.

Findlay, I. (1988) ATP⁴⁺ and ATP-Mg inhibit the ATP-sensitive K channel of rat ventricular myocyte. *Pflügers Arch.* **412**, 37–41.

Findlay, I. & Dunne. M.J. (1986) ATP maintains ATP-inhibited K channel in an operational state. *Pflügers Arch.* **407**, 238–240.

Findlay, I, Dunne, M.J. & Petersen, O.H. (1985) ATP-sensitive inward rectifier and voltage- and calcium activated K⁺ channels in cultured insulin secreting cells. *J. Membrane Biol.* **88**, 165–172.

Furspan, P. B. (1992) WAY 120,491 activates ATP-sensitive potassium channels in rat tail artery. *Eur. J. Pharmacol.* **223**, 201–203.

Furspan, P.B. & Webb, R.C. (1993) Decreased ATP sensitivity of a K⁺ channel and enhanced vascular smooth muscle relaxation in genetically hypertensive rats. *J. Hypertension* **11**, 1067–1072.

Gelband, C.H. and McCullough, J.R. (1993) Modulation of rabbit aortic Ca²⁺-activated K⁺ channel by pinacidil, cromakalim, and glibenclamide. *Am. J. Physiol.* **264**, C1119–C1127.

Gelband, C.H., Lodge N.J. & van Breemen, C. (1989) A Ca²⁺-activated K⁺ channel from rabbit aorta, modulation by cromakalim. *Eur. J. Pharmacol.* **167**, 201–210.

Gelband, C.H., Silberberg, S.D., Groschner, K., & van Breemen, C. (1990) ATP inhibits smooth muscle Ca²⁺-activated K⁺ channels. *Proc. Roy. Soc. London*, Ser. B, Biolog. Sci. **242**, 23–28.

Groschner, K, Silberberg S.D., Gelband, C. H. & van Breemen, C. (1991) Ca²⁺-activated K⁺ channels in airway smooth muscle were inhibited by cytoplasmic adenosine triphosphate. *Pflügers Arch.* **417**, 517–522.

Hamill, O.P., Marty, E., Neher, B., Sakmann, B. & Sigworth, F.J. (1981). Improved patch-clamp techniques for high-resolution current recording from cells and cell-free membrane patches. *Pflügers Arch.* **391**, 85–100.

Ho, K., Nichols, C.G., Lederer, W.J., Lytton J., Vassilev, P.M., Kanazriska, M.V. & Hebert, S.C. (1993). Cloning and expression of an inwardly rectifying ATP-regulated potassium channel. *Nature* **362**, 31–38.

Inoue, I., Nakaya, Y., Mori, H. (1989) Extracellular Ca^{2+}-activated K-channel in coronary artery smooth muscle cells and its role in vasodilation. *FEBS Lett.* **255**, 282–284.

Kajioka, S., Oike, M. & Kitamura, K. (1990) Nicorandil opens a calcium-dependent potassium channel in smooth muscle cells of the rat portal vein. *J. Pharmacol. Exper. Ther.* **254**, 905–913.

Kajioka, S., Kitamura, K., & Kuriyama, H. (1991) Guanosine diphosphate activates an adenosine $5'$-triphosphate-sensitive K^+ channel in the rabbit portal vein. *J. Physiol.* **444**, 397–418.

Kakei, M., Noma, A. (1984) Adenosine $5'$-triphosphate-sensitive single potassium channels in the atrioventricular node cell of the rabbit heart. *J. Physiol.* **352**, 265–84.

Kakei, M., Noma, A. & Shibasaki, T. (1985) Properties of adenosine-triphosphate-regulated potassium channels in guinea pig ventricular cells. *J. Physiol.* **363**, 441–462.

Kakei, M., Kelly, R.P., Ashcroft, F.M. & Ashcroft. S.H. (1986) The ATP-sensitivity of K^+ channel in rat pancreatic β-cells. *FEBS Lett.* **208**, 63–66.

Kamouchi, M & Kitamura, K. (1994). Regulation of ATP-sensitive K^+ channels by ATP and nucleotide diphosphate in rabbit portal vein. *Am. J. Physiol.* **266**, H1687–1698.

Kamouchi, M., Kajioka, S., Sakai, T., Kitamura, K., & Kuriyama, H. (1993) A target K^+ channel for the LP-805-induced hyperpolarization in smooth muscle cells of the rabbit portal vein. *Naunyn-Schmiedebergs Arch. Pharmacol.* **347**, 329–335.

Klöckner, U. & Isenberg, G. (1992). ATP suppresses activity of Ca^{2+}-activated K^+ channels by Ca^{2+} chelation. *Pflügers Arch.* **420**, 101–105.

Kovacs, R.J. & Nelson, M.T. (1991) ATP-sensitive K^+ channels from aortic smooth muscle incorporated into planar lipid bilayers. *Am. J. Physiol.* **261**, H604–H609..

Koyano, T., Kakei, M., Nakashima, H., Yoshinaga, M., Matsuoka, T. & Tanaka, H. (1993) ATP-regulated K^+ channels are modulated by intracellular H^+ in guinea pig ventricular cells. *J. Physiol.* **463**, 747–766.

Krapivinsky, G., Gordon, E.A., Wickman, K., Vellmirovic, B., Krapivinsky, L. & Clapham, D.E. (1995) The G-protein-gated atrial K^+ channel I_{KACh} is a heteromultimer of two inwardly rectifying K^+-channel proteins. *Nature* **374**, 135–141.

Langton, P.D., Clapp, L.H., Dart, C., Gurney, A.M. & Standen, N.B. (1992) Whole cell K^+ current activated by lemakalim in isolated myocytes from rabbit pulmonary artery: estimate of unitary conductance and density by noise analysis. *J. Physiol.* **459**, 254.

Lederer, W.J. & Nichols. C.G. (1989) Nucleotide modulation of the activity of rat heart K_{ATP} channels in membrane patches. *J. Physiol.* **419**, 193–211.

Lorenz, J.N., Schnermann, J., Brosius, F.C., Briggs, J.P. & Furspan, P.B. (1992) Intracellular ATP can regulate afferent arteriolar tone via ATP-sensitive K^+ channels in the rabbit. *J. Clin. Invest.* **90**, 733–740..

Misler, S., Falke, L.C., Gillis, K. & McDaniel. M.L. (1986) A metabolite regulated potassium channel in rat pancreatic β-cells. *Proc. Natl Acad. Sci. USA* **83**, 7119–7123.

Miyoshi, H. & Nakaya, Y. (1991) Angiotensin II blocks ATP-sensitive K^+ channels in porcine coronary artery smooth muscle cells. *Biochem. Biophys. Res. Commun.* **181**, 700–706.

Miyoshi, H. & Nakaya, Y. (1993) Activation of ATP-sensitive K^+ channels by cyclic AMP-dependent protein kinase in cultured smooth muscle cells of porcine coronary artery. *Biochem. Biophys. Res. Commun.* **193**, 240–247.

Miyoshi, Y., Nakaya, Y., Wakatsuki, T., Nakaya, S., Fujino, K., Saito, K. & Inoue, I. (1992) Endothelin blocks ATP-sensitive K⁺ channels and depolarizes smooth muscle cells of porcine coronary artery. *Cir. Res.* **70**, 612–616.

Nakao, K. & Bolton. (1991) Cromakalim-induced potassium currents in single dispersed smooth muscle cells of rabbit artery and vein. *Br. J. Pharmacol.* **102**, 155p.

Nelson, M.T., Huang, Y., Brayden, J.E., Hescheler, J. & Standen, N.B. (1990) Arterial dilations in response to calcitonin gene-related peptide involve activation of K⁺ channels. *Nature* **344**, 770–773.

Nichols, C.G. & Lederer, W.J. (1990) The regulation of ATP-sensitive K channel activity in intact and permeabilized rat ventricular myocytes. *J. Physiol.* **423**, 91–110.

Nichols, C.G. & Lederer, W.J. (1991) Adenosine triphosphate-sensitive potassium channels in the cardiovascular system. *Am. J. Physiol.* **261**, H1675–1686.

Noack, T., Edwards, G., Deitmer, P. & Weston, A.H. (1992a) Potassium channel modulation in rat portal vein by ATP depletion, a comparison with the effects of levcromakalim (BRL 38227). *Br. J. Pharmacol.* **107**, 945–955.

Noack, T., Deitmer, P, Edwards, G. & Weston, A.H. (1992b) Characterization of potassium currents modulated by BRL 38227 in rat portal vein. *Br. J. Pharmacol.* **106**, 717–726..

Noma, A. (1983) ATP-regulated single K channels in cardiac muscle. *Nature* **305**, 147–148.

Ohno-Shosaku, T., Zunckler, B. & Trube. G. (1987) Dual effects of ATP on K currents of mouse pancreatic β-cells. *Pflügers Arch.* **408**, 133–138 .

Quast, U. & Cook, N.S. (1989) Moving together, K⁺ channel openers and ATP-sensitive K⁺ channels. *TIPS.* **10**, 431–434.

Quayle, J.M., Bonev, A.D., Brayden, J.E. & Nelson, M.T. (1994) Calcitonin gene related peptide activates ATP-sensitive K⁺ currents in rabbit arterial smooth muscle via protein kinase. *Am. J. Physiol.* **475**, 9–13.

Robertson, B.E., Corry, P.R., Nye, P.C. & Kozlowski, R.Z. (1992) Ca²⁺ and Mg-ATP activated potassium channels from rat pulmonary artery. [corrected and republished article originally printed in Pflügers Arch. 1992 May; 421(1), 97–9]. *Pflügers Arch.* **421**, 94–96.

Robertson, D.W. & Steinberg, M.I. (1990) Potassium channel modulators, scientific applications and therapeutic promise. *J. Med. Chem.* **33**, 1529–1541.

Rorsman, P. & Trube. G. (1985) Glucose-dependent K channels in pancreatic β-cells are regulated by intracellular ATP. *Pflügers Arch.* **405**, 305–309..

Silberberg, S.D. & van Breemen, C. (1990) An ATP, calcium and voltage sensitive potassium channel in porcine coronary artery smooth muscle cells. *Biochem. Biophys. Res. Commun.* **172**, 517–522.

Silberberg, S.D. & van Breemen, C. (1992) A potassium current activated by lemakalim and metabolic inhibition in rabbit mesenteric artery. *Pflügers Arch.* **420**, 118–120 .

Spruce, A.E., Standen, N.B. & Stanfield, P.R. (1985) Voltage-dependent ATP-sensitive potassium channels of skeletal muscle membrane. *Nature* **316**, 736–738 .

Spruce, A.E., Standen, N.B. & Stanfield, P.R. (1987) Studies of the unitary properties of adenosine-5'-triphosphate-regulated potassium channels of frog skeletal muscle. *J. Physiol.* **382**, 213–237.

Standen, N.B., Quayle, J.M, Davies, N.W., Brayden, J.E., Huang, Y. & Nelson. M.T. (1989) Hyperpolarizing vasodilators activate ATP-sensitive channels in arterial smooth muscle. *Science* **245**, 177–180 .

Sturgess, N.C., Ashford, M.L.J., Cook, D.L. & Hales. C.N. (1985). The sulphonylurea receptor may be an ATP-sensitive potassium channel. *Lancet* **ii**, 474–475.

Takano, M. and Noma, A. (1993) The ATP-sensitive K⁺ channel. *Prog. Neurobiol.* **41**, 21–30.

Takano, M., Qin, D. & Noma, A. (1990) ATP-dependent decay and recovery of K channels in guinea pig cardiac myocytes. *Am. J. Physiol.* **258** (Heart Circ. Physiol), H45–H50.

Trube, G. & Hescheler, J. (1983). Potassium channels in isolated patches of cardiac cell membrane. *Naunyn-Schmiedebergs Arch. Pharmacol.* **322**, R64.

Trube, G. & Hescheler, J. (1984) Inward-rectifying channel in isolated patches of the heart cell membrane, ATP-dependence and comparison with cell-attached patches. *Pflügers Arch.* **401**, 178–184.

Trube, G., Rorsman, P. & Ohno-Shoshaku, T. (1986) Opposite effects of tolbutamide and diazoxide on the ATP-dependent K channel in mouse pancreatic β-cells. *Pflügers Arch.* **407**, 493–499.

Wakatsuki, T., Nakaya, Y. & Inoue, I. (1992) Vasopressin modulates K⁺-channel activities of cultured smooth muscle cells from porcine coronary artery. *Am. J. Physiol.* **263**, H491–H496.

Xu, X-P. & Lee, K.S. (1994). Characterization of the ATP-inhibited K⁺ current in canine coronary smooth muscle cells. *Pflügers Arch.* **427**, 110–120.

Zhang, H-L. & Bolton, T.B. (1995). Intracellular GDP, metabolic inhibition and pinacidil activate a glibenclamide-sensitive K-channel in smooth muscle cells of rat mesenteric artery. *Br. J. Pharmacol.* **114**, 662–672 .

13

Properties of the Muscarinic Cationic Channel in Longitudinal Smooth Muscle of Guinea Pig Small Intestine

A. V. ZHOLOS
T. B. BOLTON

*Department of Pharmacology & Clinical Pharmacology,
St. George's Hospital Medical School,
London, UK*

It has been known for 40 years that acetylcholine depolarizes visceral and other smooth muscles. Associated with the depolarization is an increase in the frequency of action potential discharge and a decline in size and increase in duration of action potentials; in addition there is an increased efflux of potassium which can be detected by radioactive tracers. Such observations led to the idea, by analogy with the nicotinic receptor at the neuromuscular junction, that there was a 'non-specific' increase in ionic permeability following muscarinic receptor activation (Bülbring, 1954, 1955; Lembeck & Strobach 1955; Born & Bülbring, 1956; Burnstock, 1958; Durbin & Jenkinson, 1961; Bülbring & Burnstock 1960; Bülbring & Kuriyama, 1963). In 1963, Bülbring & Kuriyama concluded that the acetylcholine depolarization was mainly due to an increase in sodium permeability but that it arose because of a 'non-selective' increase in permeability. Their doubt about whether the increase in permeability involved only cations probably arose because Durbin & Jenkinson (1961) had showed increased flux of chloride and of cations, in depolarized smooth muscle of taenia caeci; the reason for the increased movement of chloride which occurs in that tissue is still unclear.

It is now generally accepted that channels passing only cations, and not anions, are commonly present in a variety of smooth muscle cells. Cation channels are sometimes referred to as 'non-selective' cation channels although they are highly selective for cations over anions. While several monovalent cation species are permeant through them (including Cs^+) the relative permeabilities to K^+, Na^+ and sometimes Ca^{2+} are normally

SMOOTH MUSCLE EXCITATION
ISBN 0-12-112360-X

important under physiological conditions; adenosine triphosphate (ATP) receptor-operated cation channels allow divalent cations (Ba^{2+}, Ca^{2+}) to pass readily (Benham et al., 1987b; Benham & Tsien, 1987; Benham, 1989) whereas muscarinic receptor-operated channels seem relatively less permeable to Ca^{2+} ions (Pacaud & Bolton, 1991).

GATING OF CATION CHANNELS IN SMOOTH MUSCLE

In the absence of the gating stimulus cation channels generally remain closed, or their probability of occupying the open state is so low that no detectable cation current is observed. Gating, leading to opening of the channels, occurs in response to several different events, namely receptor activation, voltage change at the plasma membrane, stretch, or rise in internal ionized calcium concentration above some level. In the case of receptor gating, G-proteins appear to be involved, in several cases, in the increase in probability of the channel open state occuring.

Gating of cationic channels, a cationic inward current, and depolarization occur in response to the application of a muscarinic agonist, acetylcholine or carbachol, to longitudinal smooth muscle of guinea pig and rabbit small intestine (Bolton, 1972, 1975; Benham et al., 1985). In guinea pig there is good evidence that opening of cationic channels involves a pertussis-toxin sensitive link between the receptor and channel (Inoue & Isenberg, 1990c; Komori et al., 1992). In rabbit the evidence for a G-protein link is less compelling, perhaps suggesting that other mechanisms may be involved (Komori & Bolton, 1990). Cationic currents are evoked in several smooth muscles by activation of receptors for various other hormones or transmitters – noradrenaline (Amédée et al., 1990; Wang & Large, 1991; Wang et al., 1993; Inoue & Kuriyama, 1993) vasopressin (van Renterghem et al., 1988; Chen & Wagoner, 1991) endothelin (Chen & Wagoner, 1991) oxytocin (Arnaudeau et al., 1994; Shimamura et al., 1994) and ATP (Benham et al., 1987b; Nakazawa & Matsuki, 1987). In these instances, binding of agonist to the receptor is necessary for a detectable probability of the open state, and observable cationic current, to occur. However, in some cases it has been suggested that the gating stimulus is the rise in internal ionized calcium concentration which occurs (Janssen & Sims, 1992), in others the gating stimulus is not known but may involve a G-protein. Activation of a protein kinase C can also open cationic channels (Oike et al., 1993).

Potential change can also gate cationic channel opening in smooth muscle. A current passing sodium and potassium ions was discovered to be activated by hyperpolarization in single cells of longitudinal smooth muscle of rabbit small intestine (Benham et al., 1987a). It is sensitive to block by caesium

(1 mM). It seems likely that this current is a cationic current similar to i_f in sino-atrial node cells (DiFrancesco, 1985) and i_h in mouse spinal sensory ganglion neurones (Mayer & Westbrook, 1983) and elsewhere. Significant contribution of chloride ions to i_f and i_h is unlikely (Mayer & Westbrook, 1983; van Bogaert & Carmeliet, 1985) and it seems that this is probably also true for the smooth muscle current. Single cation channels activated by hyperpolarization have been found in smooth muscle of toad stomach (Hisada et al., 1991, 1993a,b) and uterus (Cole & Parkington, 1990). Other smooth muscle cation currents, such as that gated by muscarinic receptor activation, are affected by potential (Benham et al., 1985; Inoue & Isenberg, 1990a). This current is absent if muscarinic receptors are not stimulated; however, during their activation the cation conductance elicited increases in size upon depolarization from about $-50\,mV$ (Benham et al., 1985).

Cationic currents in smooth muscle can also be gated by a rise in internal ionized calcium concentration. A 25 pS cation channel, poorly permeable to calcium, was activated by a rise in internal ionized calcium concentration in rabbit ear artery smooth muscle cells (Wang et al., 1993). A much larger conductance channel (200 pS) was activated by internal calcium in rat portal vein smooth muscle cells (Loirand et al., 1991). Caffeine also elicited an inward current, presumably owing to a rise in internal ionized calcium concentration, in single cells of circular muscle from dog gastric corpus (Sims, 1992) although it is uncertain whether a rise in internal ionized calcium is necessary because Guerrero et al. (1994) showed that caffeine activated a cationic current in single smooth muscle cells of toad stomach even when the cells were dialysed with 10 mM 1,2-bis(2-aminophenoxy)ethane N,N,N',N'-tetraacetic acid (BAPTA) which would be expected to prevent much rise in internal ionized calcium.

Stretching the membrane also causes cationic channels to open in several smooth muscles. In toad stomach muscle stretch-activated channels which pass Na^+, K^+ and Ca^{2+} ions were observed (Kirber et al., 1988). These were not significantly permeable to Cl^- ions, had a conductance of about 60 pS, and some of them were activated by hyperpolarization alone (Kirber et al., 1988; Hisada et al., 1991) an effect potentiated by aluminofluoride (Hisada et al., 1993b). An 8pS cation channel inactivated by membrane stretch has also been seen in toad stomach muscle (Hisada et al., 1993a). Stretch-activated cation channels in guinea pig bladder had a conductance of about 35 pS and were permeable to both monovalent and divalent cations; hyperpolarization predisposed to opening. Whole-cell stretch-activated currents could be observed which were increased by cAMP (Wellner & Isenberg, 1993, 1995). Stretch-activated cation channels were also found in pig coronary artery (Davis et al., 1992a,b) where a nifedipine-resistant increase in internal ionized calcium occurred when whole-cells were stretched (Davis et al., 1992a).

ATP-RECEPTOR CATION CURRENT

Application of ATP to smooth muscle of rabbit ear artery (Benham *et al.*, 1987b) rat vas deferens (Nakazawa & Matsuki, 1987; Friel, 1988) rat uterus (Honoré *et al.*, 1989) guinea pig bladder (Marchenko *et al.*, 1987; Schneider *et al.*, 1991) cultured rat aortic cells (von der Weid *et al.*, 1993) and rabbit portal vein (Xiong *et al.*, 1991) evokes a cationic current; in some other smooth muscles calcium store release and an inward calcium-activated chloride current are seen which may be associated with calcium-activated potassium current (Droogmans *et al.*, 1991; Hoiting *et al.*, 1990; Molleman *et al.*, 1989; von der Weid *et al.*, 1993).

The current evoked by ATP-receptor activation in rabbit ear artery is transient owing to rapid desensitization. The relation between peak current evoked and potential is linear between about $+50\,mV$ and $-50\,mV$, but negative to this inward rectification is seen (Benham & Tsien, 1987; Benham *et al.*, 1987b). Calcium ions carry a substantial component of the current through these channels, which have a conductance of about $20\,pS$ (Benham & Tsien, 1987; Benham 1989). In two fairly systematic studies K^+, Na^+, Cs^+, Ba^{2+} and Ca^{2+} ions were found to pass relatively freely through the channels; Mg^{2+} is permeable but to a lesser extent (Benham & Tsien, 1987; Benham *et al.*, 1987b). The cationic conductance is not calcium activated and it was suggested (Benham & Tsien, 1987) that no diffusible messenger was involved between activated receptor and channel opening.

In rabbit portal vein (Xiong *et al.*, 1991) and in rat uterus (Honoré *et al* 1989) the ATP-evoked cationic current is more long-lasting than in ear artery cells. Current–voltage relations are linear over the physiological range. However, during single-cell recording the cationic current was potentiated when GTP-γS was present in the pipette and inhibited by GDP-βS in the pipette or by treatment of the cells with Pertussis toxin (Xiong *et al.*, 1991). The mRNA from rat vas deferens when injected into oocytes gave rise to a cationic current and its cDNA was cloned and sequenced (Valera *et al.*, 1994). The ATP cationic channel in rat vas deferens and that in rabbit portal vein may be very different; it appears that there are several types of cation channel linked to various ATP receptors in different smooth muscles.

MUSCARINIC RECEPTOR CATIONIC CURRENT

The cation current which is evoked by activating the muscarinic receptor in smooth muscle of guinea pig or rabbit small intestine is not evoked simply by a rise in internal ionized calcium concentration, such as that produced by caffeine application, and so it is a receptor-evoked rather than a calcium-gated cation channel (Benham & Bolton, 1986; Komori & Bolton, 1990). It is opened apparently by a G-protein mechanism in guinea pig (Inoue & Isenberg 1990c; Komori *et al.*, 1992). It shows conspicuous voltage-dependence, and cation current almost disappears in some cells upon hyperpolarization to about -100 mV (Bolton 1975; Benham *et al.*, 1985; Inoue & Isenberg, 1990a). In these experiments the ionized calcium in the cell was weakly buffered and it is known that changes in internal ionized calcium concentration have a strong effect on the size of this cationic current (Inoue & Isenberg, 1990b; Pacaud & Bolton, 1991). This property and the strong voltage-dependence are unusual properties for receptor-gated currents. The sensitivity of the channels to internal ionized calcium explains the large slow (seconds) oscillations of the cationic current that occur in these cells when similar oscillations occur in the internal ionized calcium probably owing to periodic calcium store release (Komori *et al.*, 1993). Earlier work suggested that the single channel conductance was about 25 pS (Inoue *et al.*, 1987). Despite the permeability of this cation channel to Na^+, K^+, Li^+, Cs^+, Ba^{2+} and Ca^{2+} ions (Inoue & Isenberg, 1990a) in solutions with high Na^+ to Ca^{2+} ion ratio, in contrast to the situation in ATP cationic channels (Benham, 1989), no detectable increase in internal ionized calcium concentration occurs upon cationic current flow (Pacaud & Bolton, 1991). Thus, unlike ATP-cationic channels, muscarinic receptor cation channels do not appear to be an important portal of calcium entry, and their effects on internal ionized calcium are mediated mainly indirectly via changes in calcium entry through voltage-dependent calcium channels. The cationic channel is affected by protons (Inoue *et al.*, 1995) and is blocked by a number of divalent cations in the external solution (Cd^{2+}, Ni^{2+}, Co^{2+}, Mn^{2+} and Mg^{2+}) (Inoue, 1991) and by tetraethylammonium, 4-aminopyridine, procaine, quinine, diphenylamine-2-carboxylate (DPC, a chloride-channel blocker) flufenamic acid or caffeine (Chen *et al.*, 1993). Tyrosine kinases have been implicated in the regulation of this cationic channel (Inoue *et al.*, 1994; Minami *et al.*, 1994). The cation channel activated by muscarinic receptors in dog stomach (Sims, 1992) and colon smooth muscle (Lee *et al.*, 1993) have a similar voltage-dependence to that in guinea pig or rabbit small intestine. However, in dog stomach, caffeine also elicits an inward current which may indicate that the muscarinic current is evoked via a rise in internal ionized calcium and not via a G-protein or other mechanism (Sims, 1992). In dog pyloric smooth muscle the muscarinic cationic current is also voltage-dependent in some cells and single-channel conductance was 30 pS. Frequency of single channel opening was decreased negative to -65 mV (Vogalis & Sanders, 1990). It appears likely that gastro-intestinal muscle of several species possesses a muscarinic cation channel resembling that studied in most detail in guinea pig longitudinal muscle of small intestine.

METHODS

Male adult guinea pigs were killed by decapitation after dislocation of the neck. Experiments were performed at room temperature on single ileal smooth muscle cells obtained after collagenase treatment (1 mg ml^{-1}, type 1A from Sigma Chemical Co., Poole, Dorset, UK) at 36°C for 25–30 min. Membrane current recordings were made from the whole cell using borosilicate patch pipettes (1 to 3 MΩ) and a List EPC-7 (List-electronic, Darmstadt, Germany) or an Axopatch 200A (Axon Instruments Inc., Foster City, CA, USA) patch-clamp amplifier. Pipettes were filled with the following solution (in mM): CsCl 80, MgATP 1, creatine 5, glucose 20, HEPES 10, BAPTA 10, CaCl$_2$ 4.6 ([Ca^{2+}]$_i$=100 nM); pH was adjusted to 7.4 with CsOH. In experiments with caged compounds caged GTP or GDP-S (obtained from Calbiochem or Molecular Probes) were added to the pipette solution at 2.5 mM. The external solution consisted of (in mM): CsCl 120, glucose 12, HEPES 10; pH was adjusted to 7.4 with CsOH. Data were analysed and plotted using MicroCal Origin software. Values are given as the means±SEM.

RESULTS

When cationic current (I_{CAT}) was activated in an isolated intestinal or gastric smooth muscle cell by applying acetylcholine at the same concentration but at different holding potentials it showed a U-shaped dependence on membrane potential (Benham *et al.*, 1985; Sims, 1992). Thus, the current became smaller closer to its reversal potential, which was about 0 mV, but it also decreased with hyperpolarization despite an increased driving force. We studied further this interesting phenomenon of an apparent loss of sensitivity at negative potentials by applying the stable muscarinic agonist carbachol (CCh) at different concentrations while I_{CAT} was monitored at two different membrane potentials using the voltage protocol shown in Figure 1A (top trace). At low CCh concentrations (such as 5 μM), I_{CAT} during a negative step demonstrated considerable relaxation towards a new (quasi)steady-state level by the end of the pulse which was significantly smaller than at −40 mV (Figure 1A) in keeping with its U-shaped steady-state current–voltage (I–V) relationship. To avoid possible complications from interactions of divalent cations with this process, we performed experiments in Ca^{2+}- and Mg^{2+}-free conditions in symmetrical 125 mM–125 mM Cs$^+$ solutions with an intracellular Ca^{2+} concentration strongly buffered to 100 nM using 10 mM BAPTA. A new and important observation was that if the agonist was applied to the same cell again but this time at a saturating concentration (Figure 1A, 300 μM) both the extent and the rate of relaxation at −120 mV

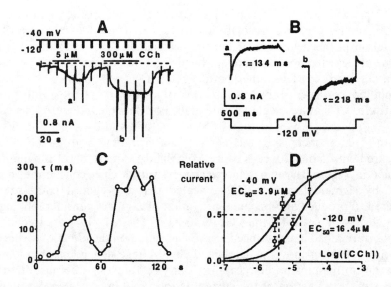

Figure 1 Agonist concentration affects voltage-dependent properties of I_{CAT} in single ileal smooth muscle cell. A, Membrane current responses evoked by different CCh concentrations as indicated while membrane potential was stepped every 8 s from -40 to -120 mV as shown at the top. B, I_{CAT} during steps indicated in A is shown expanded after appropriate correction for any CCh-independent current. Note that I_{CAT} decay was fitted with a single exponential function. C, The time constant of I_{CAT} relaxation at -120 mV is plotted versus time on the same scale as in A. D, Concentration-effect curves for the relative steady-state I_{CAT} at -40 mV (squares) and -120 mV (circles). Maximal current was -867 ± 88 pA ($n = 20$) at -40 mV and -1208 ± 214 pA ($n = 20$) at -120 mV.

were strongly affected. This can be better seen in Figure 1B where currents obtained at times indicated in panel A are plotted on an extended time scale and after CCh-independent currents were subtracted. The steady-state I_{CAT} amplitude at -120 mV in the presence of high CCh concentration became larger than that at -40 mV, indicating considerable linearization of the I–V relationship. In fact in a few cells a linear I–V relationship in the range from 0 to -120 mV was observed with strong receptor stimulation proving, first, that the unusual U-shape of the I–V relationship is determined by an unknown process linked somehow with fractional receptor occupancy and, second, another hypothetical mechanism such as ion block of the channel can be excluded from consideration; because no divalent cations are present.

The relaxation of I_{CAT} at -120 mV could be well fitted by a single exponential function as shown in Figure 1B. The mean time constant was

94 ± 12 ms with $3\,\mu M$ CCh and it increased to a mean value of 178 ± 14 ms ($n = 20$) at the peak response to 300 μM CCh. There was also a striking parallelism in the behaviour of the time constant of I_{CAT} relaxation (τ) and the current size (compare Figures 1 A and C plotted on the same time scale), as if a single process determined both.

Another consistent observation was that I_{CAT} was apparently more sensitive to CCh at less negative potentials. For example in Figure 1B steady-state I_{CAT} increased by a factor of 1.86 at $-40\,mV$ and by a factor of 6.28 at $-120\,mV$ upon increasing the agonist concentration from 3 to $300\,\mu M$. Measurements from 20 cells were combined, plotted in a conventional manner in Figure 1D as a relative current versus CCh concentration and fitted by sigmoidal curves. This revealed that the agonist concentration required to produce half-maximal activation of I_{CAT} was considerably higher at $-120\,mV$ ($16.4\,\mu M$) than at $-40\,mV$ ($3.9\,\mu M$). It appeared as if depolarization had a pronounced sensitising action on the effect of carbachol. However, this cannot be explained by voltage-dependent binding of carbachol to the muscarinic receptor (Marty & Tan, 1989) because both the decline and reactivation of the current is too rapid upon a step in potential with time constants in the order of several hundred milliseconds. For comparison, activation and deactivation of the cationic current when carbachol was applied or removed from the bathing solution was 10–100 times slower. These metabotropic receptor responses also have a minimum latency of at least 100 ms, generally much more (Bolton, 1976) presumably due to the G-protein link between receptor and channel.

The loss of cellular sensitivity following or during an application of an agonist is a global phenomenon known for a wide variety of cells and receptors and described generally as desensitization regardless of the quite diverse cellular processes involved. Therefore we aimed to see next whether at high CCh concentration, but after desensitization had developed (maintained application), the I_{CAT} properties would, or would not be any different from those at a low CCh concentration. To test this CCh was applied and maintained at $50\,\mu M$ whereas the membrane potential was stepped repeatedly between $+40$, -40 and $-120\,mV$ (Figure 2A). Traces in Figure 2B show fragments of this protocol (bottom) and also current traces at the peak response (left) and after desensitization had fully developed (right). The I_{CAT} relaxation during a negative step accelerated with desensitization as expected if it was equivalent to a lower CCh concentration (fitted exponentials in panel B) as did the steady-state current amplitude. Very little change was seen at $+40\,mV$ whereas the current decreased by 27% at $-40\,mV$ and by 47% at $-120\,mV$ over the same time interval. Relative I_{CAT} at three different membrane potentials is plotted in Figure 2C. As in the experiment shown in Figure 1 A and C we found a good correlation between τ and I_{CAT} size, as shown in Figure 2D.

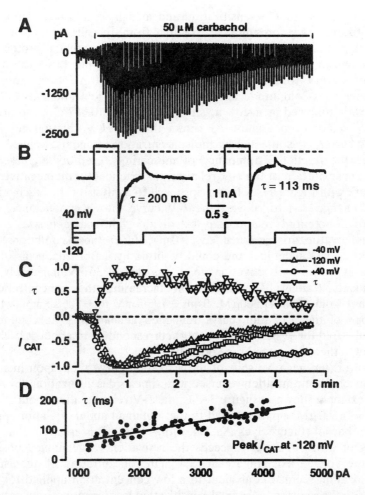

Figure 2 Desensitization affects I_{CAT} properties. A, A representative example where CCh was applied for several minutes while membrane potential was stepped repeatedly between +40, −40 and −120 mV. B, Examples at maximal response to CCh (left) and at the end of CCh application of current traces obtained and voltage protocol used. C, Relative steady-state I_{CAT} at three different membrane potentials (peak normalized as −1.0) and its time constant of relaxation at −120 mV plotted during receptor desensitization on the same scale as in A. D, The time constant correlated strongly with the peak I_{CAT} at −120 mV ($r = 0.85$; $P < 0.0001$).

In the next series of experiments CCh was applied at low concentration (usually 3 μM) and then at high concentration (300 μM) and for a long period to evoke desensitization and to make possible direct comparison on the same cell between the peak effect of a low CCh concentration, a high CCh concentration without desensitization and a high CCh concentration after desensitization. A representative example from 16 cells studied with this protocol is illustrated in Figure 3A; a more complex voltage protocol was used, as shown in the inset. Voltage steps were first applied to $-120\,$mV and then to $+80\,$mV from the holding potential of $-40\,$mV to monitor both steady-state I_{CAT} amplitude and the kinetics of its relaxation at $-120\,$mV. These were followed by a slow negative-going ramp ($0.067\,$V$\,$s^{-1}) to measure the I–V relationship. Figure 3B shows that the I–V relationship of the cationic current was affected by the concentration of agonist applied to the cell. As the fractional occupancy of muscarinic receptors increased, the nearly linear portion of the I–V relation was extended in the negative range (compare with Figure 1). A better approach to analysis of the mechanism of such a change was to convert the I–V curve into a conductance versus membrane potential relationship by dividing the current size at each potential by the driving force ($E_{Cs} = 0\,$mV under these conditions). This relationship was sigmoidal and could be fitted by a Boltzmann distribution (Figure 3C). The half-activation point was shifted $36\,$mV negatively in 16 experiments (range 17–$89\,$mV) upon increasing the concentration of carbachol from 3μM to 300μM, from $-70\pm5\,$mV to $-106\pm5\,$mV, whereas the slope of the activation curve remained unchanged. The conductance changed e-fold for $19.3\pm0.9\,$mV ($n = 14$) corresponding to about 1.25 charges exposed to the whole membrane potential.

However, the negative shift of the activation curve seen upon increasing the carbachol concentration reversed with time as desensitization developed. In the example shown in Figure 3A–C, the I–V relation after about 3 min in carbachol ($300\,\mu$M) approximated to that obtained about $20\,$s after applying $3\,\mu$M carbachol (Figure 3; cf. Aa, Ba, with Ac, Bc). It is apparent that as the process of desensitization proceeds the activation range moved positively along the voltage axis (Figure 3C). A high concentration of agonist after desensitization seemed equivalent to a low concentration applied for a few seconds to the same cell. Again, desensitization was less at positive potentials than at negative ones and was often negligible over $2\,$min or more if cells were held at $+30$ to $+80\,$mV.

Desensitization may be explained by some internal process (e.g. a decline in the production of activated G-protein subunits) which reduces the effectiveness of activated muscarinic receptors in maintaining channels in their open state at negative potentials; this same process might also explain the different I–V relations obtained with low, and with high concentrations of carbachol, without invoking any voltage dependence of CCh binding to the receptor.

We speculated that the activating portion of the G-protein may be an α-subunit in the GTP bound form or the dissociated $\beta\gamma$ subunit, and that the availability of these α-GTP subunits declines during desensitization both due

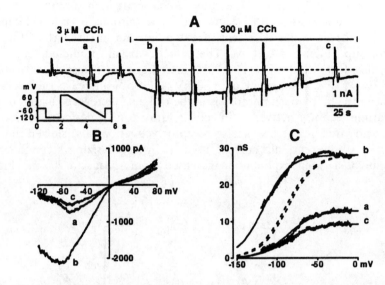

Figure 3 Comparison between a low CCh concentration and a high CCh concentration before and after desensitization had developed. A, Voltage-dependent properties of the cationic current were evaluated repeatedly at 30 s intervals using the voltage protocol shown in the inset. B, I–V relationships for the cationic current evaluated with the slow ramp pulses from +80 to −120 mV (3 s) at times indicated in A (a, CCh at 3 μM; b and c, 20 s and 170 s after application of 300 μM CCh, respectively). Dotted lines were fitted to linear portions of the I–V curves between −25 and −5 mV to obtain maximal slope conductance in each case. C, Activation curves obtained by dividing current amplitudes in B by the driving forces. Data were fitted by a Boltzmann distribution:

$$G = \frac{G_{max}}{1 + \exp((V - V_{0.5})/k)}$$

with the following best fit parameters for conditions of a, b and c, respectively: the maximal chord conductance, G_{max}, was 13, 28 and 9 nS; the potential of half-maximal activation, $V_{0.5}$, was −86, −116 and −89 mV; the slope factor, k, was −17, −16 and −17 mV. The dashed lines show the activation curves a and c after scaling; notice they have the same slope but different $V_{0.5}$ to b.

to G-protein and GTP depletion; in support of this, when 1 mM GTP was added to the pipette solution, desensitization and all related phenomena such as the positive shift of the activation curve were strongly retarded ($n = 5$, data not illustrated). In contrast, desensitization was considerably faster with the addition of 50 μM of GDP-βS to the pipette solution.

To investigate the mechanism of desensitization further we filled pipettes with a solution without GTP but which contained its inert 'caged' precursor. Photolysis of the precursor to release around 0.4 mM GTP inside the cell had the expected effect of extending the linear part of the I–V relationship (Figure 4A, top). The effect was, as predicted, especially pronounced at -120 mV ($111 \pm 23\%$ increase, $n = 9$), less so at -40 mV ($37 \pm 7\%$), and very small at $+80$ mV ($11 \pm 5\%$ increase on average). Release of GTP by flash photolysis in the cell also increased current during muscarinic receptor activation in cells held for longer periods at -120 mV (it had no effect in the absence of receptor activation) and slowed the rate of decay of the cationic current upon a hyperpolarizing step: the time constant of a fitted exponential increased from 158 ms to 205 ms (Figure

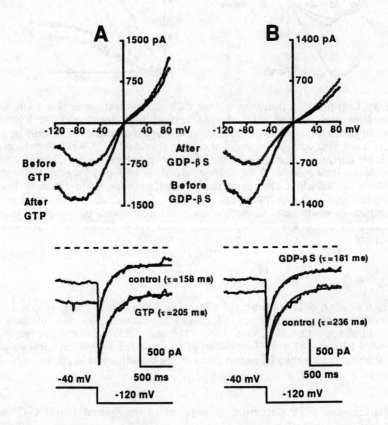

Figure 4 Effects of flash-released GTP and GDP-βS. A, I–V curves (top) and I_{CAT} relaxation during a step to -120 mV, at the peak of the response to 50 μM CCh before and a few seconds after light flash application (300–380 nm) to release GTP. The pipette solution contained 2.5 mM caged GTP. B, Similar experiment but with 2.5 mM caged GDP-βS added to the pipette solution.

4A, bottom). Flash release of GDP-βS from a 'caged' precursor had the opposite effect to release of GTP: cationic current was reduced especially at negative potentials and the decay of current upon a negative step accelerated (Figure 4B).

DISCUSSION

The shifts of the cationic conductance activation curve negatively during increased receptor occupancy and positively during desensitization provide sufficient grounds to explain both the 'sensitizing' action of depolarization (Figure 1) and the apparent voltage-dependence of desensitization as disproportional changes in I_{CAT} sizes at different potentials are expected from a purely parallel shift in the activation curve (more pronounced the more negative the potential). Moreover, as we observed in our experiments when the activation range changes, steps from -40 to -120 mV would not be expected to produce similar rates of I_{CAT} relaxation. Thus, a single process within the cell which affects the position of the activation curve on the voltage axis can explain all details of I_{CAT} behaviour. The molecular basis of this control remains unclear but it is evident that the activation range for the cationic channel gating depends critically upon the concentration of activated G-protein generated at any time in the cell. It should be emphasized, however, that the voltage-dependent gating of the channel (the slope of the activation curve) is an inherent property and can be explained in the same way as for other voltage-dependent channels by the existence of charges on the channel protein which are subject to part or all of the membrane field. This conclusion is based on the remarkably constant slope of the voltage dependence seen in the same cell under different conditions (Figure 3C).

One possible explanation for the shift in the position of the activation curve would be binding of two (or more) α-GTP (or βγ) subunits to the same channel having the effect of increasing channel lifetime at any potential as the slower relaxation of I_{CAT} suggests (Figures 1B and 4A). Such an effect would be increasingly larger with hyperpolarization. However, because of the intrinsic voltage dependence, the channel already has high open probability at positive potentials with one activated G-protein bound (at least one subunit is prerequisite for its opening). The predictions of such a model can be tested. Following agonist application, activated G-protein concentration increases from a very low (if non-zero) background to a higher level. Therefore, a more rapid onset of I_{CAT} would be expected at positive potentials. To test this, CCh was applied to the same cell at two different holding potentials such as $+80$ and -80 mV.

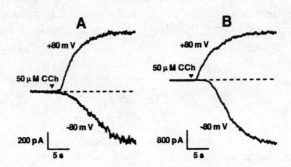

Figure 5   Onset of I_{CAT} activation at two different holding potentials. A and B show traces obtained from two different cells.

Figure 5A and B shows examples obtained from two different cells. Despite some variations between the cells, the latency was always shorter and the rate of current development greater the more positive the holding potential. It is interesting to note here that voltage-dependent latency and the characteristic S-shaped time course of activation are in a good agreement with the idea that several activated α-subunits may gate the channel. This situation was well presented in the Hodgkin–Huxley model which suggested that K channel opening was controlled by several independent membrane-bound 'particles' to explain the S-shaped delayed increase of G_K on depolarization (n^4 kinetics).

All experiments described were done with a strongly buffered intracellular ionized calcium concentration. However, under more physiological conditions, internal ionized calcium rises as a result of both the calcium-releasing action of acetylcholine and calcium influx during depolarization. Calcium is known to modulate cationic channels (Inoue & Isenberg, 1990b; Pacaud & Bolton, 1991) but the mechanism of its action is not clear. Therefore, it was important to compare the I–V relationships obtained in the same cell with low and high intracellular calcium concentrations. When intracellular calcium is weakly buffered, I_{CAT} size correlated well with the calcium concentration and large oscillations of internal ionized calcium and I_{CAT} occur in phase (Komori et al., 1993). Using 50 μM EGTA in the pipette solution, the I–V relationship was obtained at the peak of I_{CAT} in response to 10 μM CCh corresponding to maximal calcium release and later when I_{CAT} had decayed (Figure 6A; a and b, respectively). It seems that, when Ca^{2+} acts as a ligand, a very similar mechanism may be involved resulting in a considerable linearization of the I–V curve (compare Figure 6B and Figure 3B).

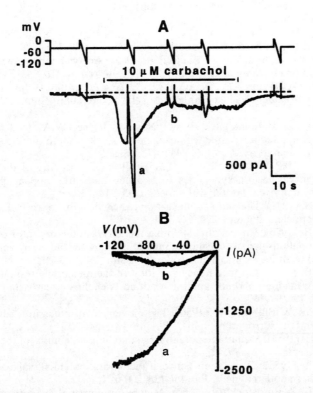

Figure 6 Effect of intracellular ionized calcium on I_{CAT} voltage dependence. A, I_{CAT} was activated by 10 μM CCh when intracellular calcium was weakly buffered (50 μM EGTA in the pipette solution). When I_{CAT} is large, and ionized calcium in the cell is high, the I–V relationship is nearly linear to −80 mV; however, when I_{CAT} is small, and ionized calcium in the cell is low, the linear portion of the I–V relationship is reduced (B).

REFERENCES

Amédée, T., Benham, C.D., Bolton, T.B., Byrne, N.G. & Large, W.A. (1990). Potassium, chloride and non-selective cation conductances opened by noradrenaline in rabbit ear artery cells. *J. Physiol.* **423**, 551–568.

Arnaudeau, S., Leprêtre N. & Mironneau, J. (1994). Chloride and monovalent ion-selective cation currents activated by oxytocin in pregnant rat myometrial cells. *Am. J. Obst. Gynaecol.* **171**, 491–501.

Benham, C.D. (1989). ATP-activated channels gate calcium entry in single smooth muscle cells dissociated from rabbit ear artery. *J. Physiol.* **419**, 689–701.

Benham, C.D. & Bolton, T.B. (1986). Spontaneous transient outward currents in single visceral and vascular smooth muscle cells of the rabbit. *J. Physiol.* **381**, 385–406.

Benham, C.D. & Tsien, R.W. (1987). A novel receptor-operated Ca^{2+}-permeable channel activated by ATP in smooth muscle. *Nature* **328**, 275–278.

Benham, C.D., Bolton, T.B. & Lang, R.J. (1985). Acetylcholine activates an inward current in single mammalian smooth muscle cells. *Nature* **316**, 345–346.

Benham, C.D., Bolton, T.B., Denbigh, J.S. & Lang, R.J. (1987a). Inward rectification in freshly isolated single smooth muscle cells of the rabbit jejunum. *J. Physiol.* **383**, 461–476.

Benham, C.D., Bolton, T.B., Byrne, N.G. & Large, W.A. (1987b). Action of externally applied adenosine triphosphate on single smooth muscle cells dispersed from rabbit ear artery. *J. Physiol.* **387**, 473–488.

van Bogaert, P.P. & Carmeliet, E. (1985). Chloride sensitivity of the I_f pacemaker current in cardiac Purkyne fibes from sheep and atrial appendage fibres from human hearts. *Arch. Int. Physiol. Biochim.* **93**, P14–15.

Bolton, T.B. (1972). The depolarizing action of acetylcholine or carbachol in intestinal smooth muscle. *J. Physiol.* **220**, 647–671.

Bolton, T.B. (1975). Effects of stimulating the acetylcholine receptor on the current-voltage relationships of the smooth muscle membrane studied by voltage clamp of potential recorded by micro-electrode. *J. Physiol.* **250**, 175–202.

Bolton, T.B. (1976). On the latency and form of the membrane responses of smooth muscle to the iontophoretic application of acetylcholine or carbachol. *Proc. R. Soc. Lond. B.* **194**, 99–119.

Born, G.V.R. & Bülbring, E. (1956). The movement of potassium between smooth muscle and the surrounding fluid. *J. Physiol.* **131**, 690–703.

Bülbring, E. (1954). Membrane potential of smooth muscle fibres of the taenia coli of the guinea pig. *J. Physiol.* **125**, 302–315.

Bülbring, E. (1955). Correlation between membrane potential, spike discharge and tension in smooth muscle. *J. Physiol.* **128**, 200–221.

Bülbring, E. & Burnstock, G. (1960). Membrane potential changes associated with tachyphylaxis and potentiation of the response to stimulating drugs in smooth muscle. *Br. J. Pharmacol. Chemother.* **15**, 611–624.

Bülbring, E. & Kuriyama, H. (1963). Effect of changes in ionic environment on the action of acetylcholine and adrenaline on the smooth muscle cells of guinea pig taenia coli. *J. Physiol.* **166**, 59–74.

Burnstock, G. (1958). The effect of acetylcholine on membrane potential, spike frequency, conduction velocity and excitability in the taenia coli of the guinea pig. *J. Physiol.* **143**, 165–182.

Chen, S., Inoue, R. & Ito, Y. (1993). Pharmacological characterization of muscarinic receptor-activated cation current in guinea pig ileum. *Br. J. Pharmacol.* **109**, 793–801.

Chen, C. & Wagoner, P.K. (1991). Endothelin induces a nonselective cation current in vascular smooth muscle cells. *Circu. Res.* **69**, 447–454.

Cole, H.A. and Parkington, H.C. (1990). Hyperpolarization-activated channels in myometrium: a patch clamp study. In *'Frontiers in Smooth Muscle Research'* (Sperelakis, N. and Wood, J.D., eds) Wiley, New York. *Prog. Clin. Biol. Res.* **327**, 665–672.

Davis, M.J., Meininger, G.A. & Zawieja, D.C. (1992a). Stretch-induced increases in intracellular calcium of isolated vascular smooth muscle cells. *Am. J. Physiol.* **263**, H1292–H1299.

Davis, M.J., Donovitz, J.A. & Hood, J.D. (1992b). Stretch-activated single-channel and whole cell currents in vascular smooth muscle cells. *Am. J. Physiol.* **263**, C1083–C1088.

DiFrancesco, D. (1985). The cardiac hyperpolarizing-activated current, I_f, origins and developments. *Progr. Biophys. Mol. Biol.* **46**, 163–183.

Droogmans, G., Callewaert, G., Declerck, I. & Casteels, R. (1991). ATP-induced Ca^{2+} release and Cl^- current in cultured smooth muscle cells from pig aorta. *J. Physiol.* **440**, 623–634.

Durbin, R.P. & Jenkinson, D.H. (1961). The effect of carbachol on the permeability of depolarized smooth muscle to inorganic ions. *J. Physiol.* **157**, 74–89.

Friel, D.D. (1988). An ATP-sensitive conductance in single smooth muscle cells from the rat vas deferens. *J. Physiol.* **401**, 361–380.

Guerrero, A., Fay, F.S. & Singer, J.J. (1994). Caffeine activates a Ca^{2+}-permeable, nonselective cation channel in smooth muscle cells. *J. Gen. Physiol.* **104**, 375–394.

Hisada, T., Ordway, R.W., Kirber, M.T., Singer, J.J. & Walsh, J.V. (1991). Hyperpolarization-activated cationic channels in smooth muscle cells are stretch sensitive. *Pflügers Arch.* **417**, 493–499.

Hisada, T., Walsh, J.V. & Singer, J.J. (1993a). Stretch-inactivated cationic channels in single smooth muscle cells. *Pflügers Arch.* **422**, 393–396.

Hisada, T., Singer, J.J. & Walsh, J.V (1993b). Aluminofluoride activates hyperpolarization- and stretch-activated cation channels in single smooth muscle cells. *Pflügers Arch.* **422**, 397–400.

Hoiting, B., Molleman, A., Nelemans, A. & Den Hertog, A. (1990). P_2-purinoceptor-activated membrane currents and inositol tetrakisphosphate formation are blocked by suramin. *Eur. J. Pharmacol.* **181**, 127–131.

Honoré, E., Martin, C., Mironneau, C. & Mironneau, J. (1989). An ATP-sensitive conductance in cultured smooth muscle cells from pregnant rat myometrium. *Am. J. Physiol.* **257**, C297–C305.

Inoue, R. (1991). Effect of external Cd^{2+} and other divalent cations on carbachol-activated non-selective cation channels in guinea pig ileum. *J. Physiol.* **442**, 447–463.

Inoue, R. & Isenberg, G. (1990a). Effect of membrane potential on acetylcholine-induced inward current in guinea pig ileum. *J. Physiol.* **424**, 53–71.

Inoue, R. & Isenberg, G. (1990b). Intracellular calcium ions modulate acetylcholine-induced inward current in guinea pig ileum. *J. Physiol.* **424**, 73–92.

Inoue, R. & Isenberg, G. (1990c). Acetylcholine activates nonselective cation channels in guinea pig ileum through a G protein. *Am. J. Physiol.* **258**, C1173–C1178.

Inoue, R. & Kuriyama, H. (1993). Dual regulation of cation-selective channels by muscarinic and α_1-adrenergic receptors in the rabbit portal vein. *J. Physiol.* **465**, 427–448.

Inoue, R., Kitamura, K. & Kuriyama, H. (1987). Acetylcholine activates single sodium channels in smooth muscle cells. *Pflügers Arch.* **410**, 69–74.

Inoue, R., Waniishi, Y., Yamada, K. & Ito, Y. (1994). A possible role of tyrosine kinases in the regulation of muscarinic receptor-activated cation channels in guinea pig ileum. *Biochem. Biophys. Res. Comm.* **203**, 1392–1397.

Inoue, R., Waniishi, Y. & Ito, Y. (1995). Extracellular H^+ modulates acetylcholine-activated nonselective cation channels in guinea pig ileum. *Am. J. Physiol.* **37**, C162–C170.

Janssen, L.J. & Sims, S.M. (1992). Acetylcholine activates non-selective cation and chloride conductances in canine and guinea pig tracheal myocytes. *J. Physiol.* **453**, 197–218.

Kirber, M.T., Walsh, J.V. & Singer, J.J. (1988). Stretch-activated ion channels in smooth muscle: a mechanism for the initiation of stretch-induced contraction. *Pflügers Arch.* **412**, 339–345.

Komori, S. & Bolton, T.B. (1990). Role of G-protein in muscarinic receptor inward and outward currents in rabbit jejunal smooth muscle. *J. Physiol.* **427**, 395–419.

Komori, S., Kawai, M., Takewaki, T. & Ohashi, H. (1992). GTP-binding protein involvement in membrane currents evoked by carbachol and histamine in guinea pig ileal muscle. *J. Physiol.* **450**, 105–126.

Komori, S., Kawai, M., Pacaud, P., Ohashi, H. & Bolton, T.B. (1993). Oscillations of receptor-operated cationic current and internal calcium in single guinea pig ileal smooth muscle cells. *Pflügers Arch.* **424**, 431–438.

Lee, H.K., Bayguinov, O. & Sanders, K.M. (1993). Role of nonselective cation current in muscarinic responses of canine colonic muscle. *Am. J. Physiol.* **265**, C1463–C1471.

Lembeck, F. & Strobach, R. (1955). Kaliumabgabe aus glatter muskulatur. *Arch. Exp. Pathol. Pharmacol.* **228**, 130–131.

Loirand, G., Pacaud, P., Baron, A., Mironneau, C. & Mironneau, J. (1991). Large conductance calcium-activated non-selective cation channel in smooth muscle cells isolated from rat portal vein. *J. Physiol.* **437**, 461–475.

Marchenko, S.M., Volkova, T.M. & Fedorov, O.I. (1987). ATP-activated ionic permeability in smooth muscle cells isolated from the guinea pig urinary bladder. *Neuropharmacology* **19**, 82–86.

Marty, A. and Tan, Y.P. (1989). The initiation of calcium release following muscarinic stimulation in rat lacrimal glands. *J. Physiol.* **419**, 665–687.

Mayer, M. & Westbrook, G.L. (1983). A voltage-clamp analysis of inward (anomalous) rectification in mouse spinal sensory ganglion neurones. *J. Physiol.* **366**, 365–368.

Minami, K., Fukuzawa, K. & Inoue, I. (1994). Regulation of a non-selective cation channel of cultured porcine coronary artery smooth muscle by tyrosine kinase. *Pflügers Arch.* **426**, 254–257.

Molleman, A., Nelemans, A. & Den Hertog, A. (1989). P_2-purinoceptor-mediated membrane currents in DDT_1 MF-2 smooth muscle cells. *Eur. J. Pharmacol.* **169**, 167–174.

Nakazawa, K. & Matsuki, N. (1987). Adenosine trisphosphate-activated inward current in isolated smooth muscle cells from rat vas deferens. *Pflügers Arch.* **409**, 644–646.

Oike, M., Kitamura, K. & Kuriyama, H. (1993). Protein kinase C activates the non-selective cation channel in the rabbit portal vein. *Pflügers Arch.* **424**, 159–164.

Pacaud, P. & Bolton, T.B. (1991). Relation between muscarinic receptor cationic current and internal calcium in guinea pig jejunal smooth muscle cells. *J. Physiol.* **441**, 477–499.

van Renterghem, C., Romey, G. & Lazdunski, M. (1988). Vasopressin modulates the spontaneous electrical activity in aortic cells (line A7r5) by acting on three different types of ionic channels. *Proc. Natl Acad. Sci. USA* **85**, 9365–9369.

Schneider, P., Hopp, H.H. & Isenberg, G. (1991). Ca^{2+} influx through ATP-gated channels increments $[Ca^{2+}]_i$ and inactivates I_{Ca} in myocytes from guinea pig urinary bladder. *J. Physiol.* **440**, 479–496.

Shimamura, K., Kusaka, M. & Sperelakis, N. (1994). Oxytocin induces an inward current in pregnant rat myometrial cells. *Can. J. Physiol. Pharmacol.* **72**, 759–763.

Sims, S.M. (1992). Cholinergic activation of a non-selective cation current in canine gastric smooth muscle is associated with contraction. *J. Physiol.* **449**, 377–398.

Valera, S., Hussy, N., Evans, R.J., Adami, N., North, R.A., Surprenant, A. & Buell, G.

(1994). A new class of ligand-gated ion channel defined by P_{2x} receptor for extracellular ATP. *Nature* **371**, 516–519.

Vogalis, F. & Sanders, K.M. (1990). Cholinergic stimulation activates a non-selective cation current in canine pyloric circular muscle cells. *J. Physiol.* **429**, 223–236.

Wang, Q. & Large, W.A. (1991). Noradrenaline-evoked cationic conductance recorded with the nystatin whole-cell method in rabbit portal vein cells. *J. Physiol.* **435**, 21–39.

Wang, Q., Hogg, R.C. & Large, W.A. (1993). A monovalent ion-selective cation current activated by noradrenaline in smooth muscle cells of rabbit ear artery. *Pflügers Arch.* **423**, 28–33.

von der Weid, P.-Y., Serebryakov, V.N., Orallo, F., Bergmann, C., Snetkov, V.A. & Takeda, K. (1993). Effects of ATP on cultured smooth muscle cells from rat aorta. *Br. J. Pharmacol.* **108**, 638–645.

Wellner, M-C & Isenberg, G. (1993). Properties of stretch-activated channels in myocytes from the guinea pig urinary bladder. *J. Physiol.* **466**, 213–227.

Wellner, M-C & Isenberg, G. (1995). cAMP accelerates the decay of stretch-activated inward currents in guinea pig urinary bladder myocytes. *J. Physiol.* **482**, 141–156.

Xiong, Z., Kitamura, K. & Kuriyama, K. (1991). ATP activates cationic currents and modulates the calcium currents through GTP binding protein in rabbit portal vein. *J. Physiol.* **440**, 143–165.

14

Muscarinic Activation of Cation Channels in Airway Smooth Muscle Cells

MICHAEL I. KOTLIKOFF
BERND K. FLEISCHMANN

Department of Animal Biology,
School of Veterinary Medicine,
University of Pennsylvania, Philadelphia, USA

INTRODUCTION

Exposure of airway myocytes to muscarinic agonists elicits characteristic electrical responses. The general features of these responses have been demonstrated using microelectrode and double sucrose gap methods (Kirkpatrick, 1975; Suzuki *et al.*, 1976; Farley & Miles, 1977; Coburn, 1977; Small, 1982). These data demonstrated that a graded, sustained depolarization occurs following exposure to contractile agonists. In recent years the characterization of specific calcium transport proteins has been greatly facilitated by technical advances in the measurement of ion channel currents and the noninvasive measurement of calcium concentration in cells (Neher & Sakmann, 1976; Hamill *et al.*, 1981; Tsien *et al.*, 1985; Korn & Horn, 1989). The combination of these techniques yields substantial experimental power in the dissection of specific transport processes that contribute to rises in cytosolic calcium. In smooth muscle, the relationship between tension and calcium has long been appreciated, and a rise in cytosolic calcium and activation of myosin light chain kinase has been shown to be a necessary and sufficient event for contraction (Itoh *et al.*, 1989). While calcium-independent regulatory processes may exist in smooth muscle (Kitazawa *et al.*, 1989), full activation of contractile proteins does not occur in the absence of a rise in $[Ca^{2+}]_i$, and following force development, decreases in $[Ca^{2+}]_i$ result in muscle relaxation (Somlyo & Himpens, 1989).

Whereas intracellular calcium release plays an important role in the initiation of contraction (Baron *et al.*, 1984; Somlyo & Himpens, 1989) of smooth muscle and calcium falls following initial peak transients (Morgan &

SMOOTH MUSCLE EXCITATION
ISBN 0-12-112360-X

Morgan, 1982), sustained contractile responses require a sustained elevation of $[Ca^{2+}]_i$, which is dependent on extracellular calcium (Himpens et $al.$, 1988; Murray & Kotlikoff, 1991). The study of membrane calcium channels has focused on two classes of channel proteins. Voltage-dependent calcium channels have been extensively characterized at the molecular and biophysical level, and good antagonists of their function acting in the submicromolar range are available. Although these channels have been shown to play a dominant role in excitation-contraction coupling in some smooth muscle tissues (Nelson et $al.$, 1988), they are by no means the only calcium-permeant channel proteins. An extensive literature on smooth muscle (Benham et $al.$, 1986; Benham & Tsien, 1987; Rüegg et $al.$, 1989; Inoue & Isenberg, 1990a,b; Loirand et $al.$, 1991; Murray & Kotlikoff, 1991; Pacaud & Bolton, 1991; Sims, 1992; Inoue & Kuriyama, 1993; Guerrero et $al.$, 1994) has documented the existence of cation channels and agonist-activated calcium permeation through these channels. Recent reports indicate that in addition to a calcium-activated chloride current, a cation conductance is activated during E–C coupling in airway smooth muscle (Janssen & Sims, 1992). Experiments in this laboratory have focused on the characterization of the cation conductance, and its correlation with agonist-stimulated increases in $[Ca^{2+}]_i$. This manuscript will briefly summarize our recent findings with respect to the activation of cation channels by muscarinic agonists in airway smooth muscle.

METHODS

Single equine tracheal myocytes were dissociated by previously described methods and loaded with fura 2AM. As described previously (Fleischmann et $al.$, 1994), cells were loaded by incubation in $2\,\mu M$ fura 2AM for 10 min and then voltage clamped using the nystatin whole-cell method. All recordings were performed at 35°C. Application of agonists and rapid solution changes were accomplished by means of one or more puffer pipettes. Unless otherwise stated, the intracellular solution was (mM): CsCl (130), $MgCl_2$ (5), $CaCl_2$ (1), EGTA (3), HEPES (10), pH 7.3 (CsOH). The standard extracellular solution was composed of (mM): NaCl (125), KCl (5), $MgSO_4$ (1), $CaCl_2$ (1.8), HEPES (10), pH 7.4 (NaOH).

RESULTS

Application of the muscarinic agonist methacholine $(50–200\,\mu M)$ to voltage-clamped myocytes resulted in a transient rise in cytosolic calcium followed by a sustained elevation over basal levels that persisted as long as the agonist

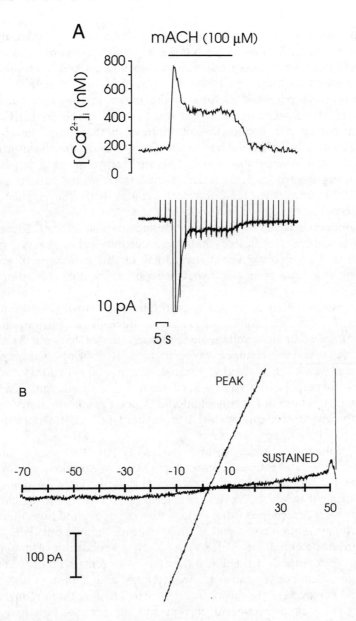

Figure 1 Methacholine activates transient and sustained currents. $[Ca^{2+}]_i$ and current measurements from a nystatin voltage-clamped equine tracheal myocyte. A, Application of 100 μM methacholine triggered a transient and sustained increase in $[Ca^{2+}]_i$ and current. B, Currents obtained from 150 ms voltage ramps indicate that both currents reversed at approximately 0 mV. The calculated chloride and cation reversal potentials for this experiment were 1.6 and 0 mV (assuming no calcium permeability), respectively.

was applied. Like previous findings (Byrne & Large, 1987; 1988; Pacaud *et al.*, 1989; Janssen & Sims, 1992), a large, rapidly inactivating inward current was associated with the initial calcium transient evoked by application of the muscarinic agonist. Following the decay of this current, a sustained inward current persisted as long as the muscarinic agonist was applied. Figure 1a shows an example of the simultaneous recording of $[Ca^{2+}]_i$ and current during the application of 100 μM methacholine to an equine tracheal myocyte voltage-clamped at −50 mV using the nystatin method. Application of the agonist resulted in the activation of a large, rapidly inactivating inward current. A small, sustained inward current persisted, and this current was temporally correlated with the agonist-induced increase in $[Ca^{2+}]_i$.

Instantaneous current/voltage relationships obtained from 150 ms voltage ramps (Figure 1b) indicated that large current had a reversal potential consistent with chloride selectivity (0 mV in this experiment), similar to cholinergic currents in airway myocytes reported by others (Janssen & Sims, 1992).

The sustained increase in $[Ca^{2+}]_i$ associated with muscarinic stimulation is consistent with the influx of calcium through a calcium permeant conductance other than voltage dependence calcium channels. As shown in Figure 2, a voltage clamped myocyte held at −40 mV was exposed to methacholine and then stepped alternatively to −80 or +20 mV. When the cell was hyperpolarized, the inward current increased, and $[Ca^{2+}]_i$, was increased (the normal fall was blunted). Depolarization to 20 mV evoked a net outward current and resulted in a sharp fall in $[Ca^{2+}]_i$, which then increased following repolarization.

The voltage dependence and selectivity of the small amplitude, noninactivating current was examined in a series of experiments in which the chloride and cation reversal potentials were shifted. Figure 3A demonstrates an experiment in which the time course of the selectivity of the cholinergic currents were determined using voltage ramps, under conditions in which the extracellular solution contained 38.6 mM chloride and the calculated chloride equilibrium potential was 34.5 mV. As shown, application of methacholine evoked typical rapidly activating and sustained currents, with distinct reversal potentials. Sequential ramps at 1-s intervals and a plot of the reversal potential versus time are shown in Figure 3B. The first three ramps occur at the beginning of the transient current and the reversal potential reached 28 mV. Subsequent ramps occur during the decay of the transient current, and the reversal potential became progressively more negative until it reached the cation equilibrium potential of 0 mV. Similarly, experiments in which the cation gradient was shifted, while the chloride concentrations were symmetrical, demonstrated a zero reversal potential for the transient current and a negatively shifted reversal potential for the sustained current. These

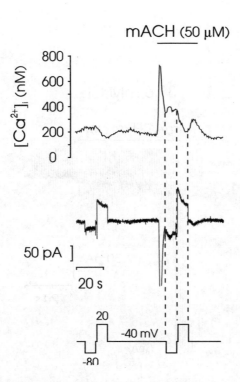

Figure 2 Voltage-dependence of $[Ca^{2+}]_i$ and current during cholinergic stimulation. Following application of methacholine (50 µM), hyperpolarizing voltage-clamp steps increased, and depolarizing steps decreased, $[Ca^{2+}]_i$ and current.

experiments are consistent with the sustained current being a nonselective cation current.

The sustained current is calcium permeant, as shown in Figure 4. In this experiment, a cell that was pre-exposed to 5 mM nisoldipine to block the voltage-dependent calcium current was exposed to 110 mM $CaCl_2$, (calcium was the only external cation) and then to the cholinergic agonist and 110 mM $CaCl_2$. One second steady-state voltage steps were imposed before and after exposure to the agonist. The reversal potential determined from this voltage protocol was 14 mV under conditions of 130 mM internal Cs^+ and 110 mM $CaCl_2$; the calculated Ca^{2+}/Cs^+ permeability ratio was 4.1, which compares well to previous determinations (Benham & Tsien, 1987). This experiment also demonstrates a prominent feature of the voltage dependence of the cation current. As shown in the I–V curve, the nonselective cation conductance departs substantially from ohmic behaviour at negative

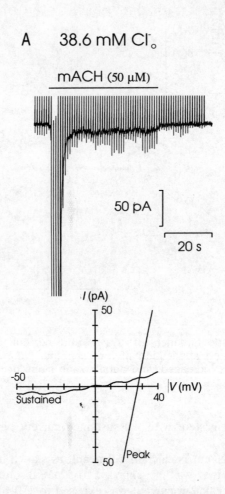

Figure 3 Dissection of selectivity of transient and sustained cholinergic currents. Extracellular chloride was decreased to 38.6 mM by substitution with Cs Acetate. A, The transient and sustained currents had distinct reversal potentials, with the transient current being shifted positively by chloride substitution by 28 mV. B, The time-course of the shift in current selectivity during agonist exposure is shown. The transient current is mainly chloride selective, but becomes progressively more cation selective as the transient current decays.

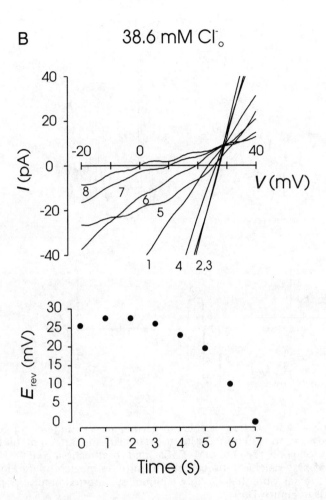

potentials. At potentials negative to −40 or −50 mV, the current rectifies strongly, with little additional inward current observed negative to −50 mV.

As previously reported in airway myocytes and other cells (Byrne & Large, 1987, 1988; Pacaud *et al.*, 1989), the chloride current is calcium activated. However, a rise in $[Ca^{2+}]_i$ is not sufficient to activate the cation current. Experiments in which the same cell was sequentially exposed to caffeine and methacholine resulted in activation of the large transient chloride current, but not the sustained current, and no sustained elevation of calcium was observed. Subsequent application of methacholine (50 μM) resulted in activation of the chloride current followed by the cation current.

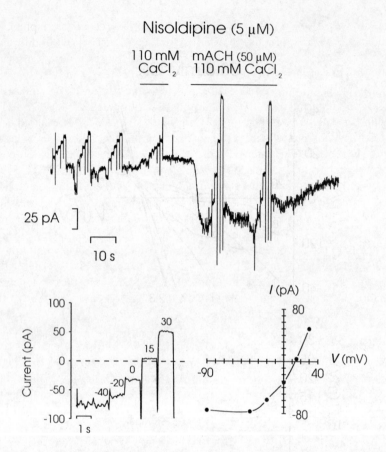

Figure 4 The cation current is calcium permeant. A voltage-clamped myocyte is exposed first to 110 mM $CaCl_2$, to establish the effect of high calcium exposure, followed by 110 mM $CaCl_2$ and methacholine (50 μM). In the presence of high calcium, the cation current is larger (compare Figures 1–3), and the reversal potential is right shifted by approximately 14 mV (same solutions as in Figure 1).

DISCUSSION

Simultaneous recordings of $[Ca^{2+}]_i$ and current in equine tracheal myocytes indicate that cholinergic agonists activate a large, rapidly inactivating chloride current and a sustained cation current that is calcium permeant. The chloride current is activated by calcium, and inactivates completely within seconds of exposure to the agonist. The nonselective current is not activated simply by a rise in $[Ca^{2+}]_i$, but requires agonist–receptor coupling. This conductance is generally less than 30 pA under physiological conditions, but appears to underlie a substantial component of calcium flux during muscarinic stimulation of airway myocytes. The cation currents reported bear substantial similarity to those reported in gastrointestinal smooth muscle (Benham et al., 1986; Inoue & Isenberg, 1990a; Pacaud & Bolton, 1991; Sims, 1992) and vascular smooth muscle (Wang & Large, 1991; Inoue & Kuriyama, 1993). Interestingly, current activation mechanisms appear to differ somewhat from previously reported currents. That is, whereas caffeine evokes cation current in several preparations (Sims, 1992; Wang et al., 1993; Guerrero et al., 1994), it did not activate the current in airway myocytes. The acetylcholine-activated cation current in equine tracheal myocytes appears to bear substantial similarity to the noradrenaline- and acetylcholine-activated current in rabbit portal vein cells (Wang & Large, 1991, Inoue & Kuriyama, 1993) and the acetylcholine or carbachol-activated current in guinea pig small intestine myocytes (Inoue & Isenberg, 1990a; Pacaud & Bolton, 1991). In these studies of noradrenaline or acetylcholine-activated chloride and cation conductances, the chloride conductance was activated by an increase in $[Ca^{2+}]_i$ alone, whereas the cation conductance was not activated by caffeine-induced calcium rises (Wang & Large, 1991), and was still activated when intracellular calcium was strongly buffered (Inoue & Kuriyama, 1993). Further studies of the coupling mechanisms interposed between muscarinic receptor binding and channel activation may provide important information with respect to the mechanisms of excitation–contraction coupling in airway smooth muscle.

REFERENCES

Baron, C.B., Cunningham, M., Strauss, J.F. III & Coburn, R.F. (1984). Pharmacomechanical coupling in smooth muscle may involve phosphatidylinositol metabolism. Proc. Natl Acad. Sci. USA **81**, 6899–6903.

Benham, C.D. & Tsien, R.W. (1987). A novel receptor-operated Ca2+-permeable channel activated by ATP in smooth muscle. Nature **328**, 275–278.

Benham, C.D., Bolton, T.B. & Lang, R.J. (1986). Acetylcholine activates an inward current in single mammalian smooth muscle cells. Nature **316**, 345–347.

Byrne, N.G. & Large, W.A. (1987). Action of noradrenaline on single smooth muscle cells freshly dispersed from the rat anococcygeus muscle. J. Physiol. **389**, 513–525.

Byrne, N.G. & Large, W.A. (1988). Membrane ionic mechanisms activated by noradrenaline in cells isolated from the rabbit portal vein. J. Physiol. (London) **404**, 557–573.

Coburn, R.F. (1977). The airway smooth muscle cell. Federation Proc. **36**, 2692–2697.

Farley, J.M. & Miles, P.R. (1977). Role of depolarization in acetylcholine-induced contractions of dog trachealis muscle. J. Pharmacol. Exp. Ther. **201**, 199–205.

Fleischmann, B.K., Murray, R.K. & Kotlikoff, M.I. (1994). A voltage window for sustained elevation of cytosolic calcium in smooth muscle cells. Proc. Natl Acad. Sci. USA **91**, 11914–11918.

Guerrero, A., Fay, F.S. & Singer, J.J. (1994). Caffeine activates a Ca^{2+} permeable, non-selective cation channel in smooth muscle cells. *J. Gen. Physiol.* **104**, 375–394.

Hamill, O.P., Marty, A., Neher, E., Sakmann, B. & Sigworth, F.J. (1981). Improved patch-clamp techniques for high-resolution current recording from cells and cell-free membrane patches. *Pflügers Archiv.* **391**, 85–100.

Himpens, B., Matthijs, G., Somlyo, A.V., Butler, T.M. & Somlyo, A.P. (1988). Cytoplasmic free calcium, myosin light chain phosphorylation, and force in phasic and tonic smooth muscle. *J. Gen. Physiol.* **92**, 713–729.

Inoue, R. & Isenberg, G. (1990a). Intracellular calcium ions modulate acetylcholine-induced inward current in guinea pig ileum. *J. Physiol. (London)* **424**, 73–92.

Inoue, R. & Isenberg, G. (1990b). Effect of membrane potential on acetylcholine-induced inward current in guinea pig ileum. *J. Physiol. (London)* **424**, 57–71.

Inoue, R. & Kuriyama, H. (1993). Dual regulation of cation-selective channels by muscarinic and α_1-adrenergic receptors in the rabbit portal vein. *J. Physiol. (London)* **465**, 427–448.

Itoh, T., Ikebe, M., Kargacin, G.J., Hartshorne, D.J., Kemp, B.E. & Fay, F.S. (1989). Effects of modulators of myosin light-chain kinase activity in single smooth muscle cells. *Nature* **338**, 164–167.

Janssen, L.J. & Sims, S.M. (1992). Acetylcholine activates non-selective cation and chloride conductances in canine and guinea pig tracheal smooth muscle cells. *J. Physiol.* **453**, 197–218.

Kirkpatrick, C.T. (1975). Excitation and contraction in bovine tracheal smooth muscle. *J. Physiol. (London)* **244**, 263–281.

Kitazawa, T., Kobayashi, S., Horiuti, K., Somlyo, A.V. & Somlyo, A.P. (1989). Receptor coupled, permeabilized smooth muscle: role of the phosphatidylinositol cascade, G-proteins and modulation of the contractile response to Ca^{2+}. *J. Biol. Chem.* **264**, 5339–5342.

Korn, S.J. & Horn, R. (1989). Influence of sodium-calcium exchange on calcium current rundown and the duration of calcium-dependent chloride currents in pituitary cells, studied with whole cell and perforated patch recording. *J. Gen. Physiol.* **94**, 789–812.

Loirand, G., Pacaud, P., Baron, A., Mironneau, C. & Mironneau, J. (1991). Large conductance calcium-activated non-selective cation channel in smooth muscle cells isolated from rat portal vein. *J. Physiol. (London)* **437**, 461–475.

Morgan, J.P. & Morgan, K.G. (1982). Vascular smooth muscle: the first recorded Ca2+ transients. *Pflügers Arch.* **395**, 75–77.

Murray, R.K. & Kotlikoff, M.I. (1991). Receptor-activated calcium influx in human airway smooth muscle cells. *J. Physiol. (London)* **435**, 123–144.

Neher, E. & Sakmann, B. (1976). Single channel currents recorded from membrane of denervated frog muscle fibres. *Nature* **260**, 799–802.

Nelson, M.T., Standen, N.B., Brayden, J.E. & Worley, J.F. (1988). Noradrenaline contracts arteries by activating voltage-dependent calcium channels. *Nature* **336**, 382–385.

Pacaud, P. & Bolton, T.B. (1991). Relation between muscarinic receptor cationic current and internal calcium in guinea pig jejunal smooth muscle cells. *J. Physiol. (London)* **441**, 477–499.

Pacaud, P., Loirand, G., Lavie, J.L., Mironneau, C. & Mironneau, J. (1989). Calcium-activated chloride current in rat vascular smooth muscle cells in short-term primary culture. *Pflügers Arch.* **413**, 629–636.

Rüegg, U.T., Wallnöfer, A., Weir, S. & Cauvin, C. (1989). Receptor-operated calcium-permeable channels in vascular smooth muscle. *J. Cardiovasc. Pharmacol.*

14, S49–S58.

Sims, S.M. (1992). Cholinergic activation of a non-selective cation current in canine gastric smooth muscle is associated with contraction. *J. Physiol. (London)* **449**, 377–398.

Small, R.C. (1982). Electrical slow waves and tone of guinea pig isolated trachealis muscle: effects of drugs and temperature changes. *Br. J. Pharmacol.* **77**, 45–54.

Somlyo, A.P. & Himpens, B. (1989). Cell calcium and its regulation in smooth muscle. *FASEB J.* **3**, 2266–2276.

Suzuki, H., Morita, K. & Kuriyama, H. (1976). Innervation and properties of the smooth muscle of the dog trachea. *Japan. J. Physiol.* **26**, 303–320.

Tsien, R.Y., Rink, T.J. & Poenie, M. (1985). Measurement of cytosolic free Ca2+ in individual small cells using fluorescence microscopy with dual excitation wavelengths. *Cell Calcium* **6**, 145–157.

Wang, Q. & Large, W.A. (1991). Noradrenaline-evoked cation conductance recorded with the nystatin whole-cell method in rabbit portal vein cells. *J. Physiol. (London)* **435**, 21–39.

Wang, Q., Hogg, R.C. & Large, W.A. (1993). A monovalent ion-selective cation current activated by noradrenaline in smooth muscle cells of rabbit ear artery. *Pflügers Arch.* **423**, 28–33.

15

Characteristics of Carbachol- and Caffeine-induced Inward Currents in Rat Intestinal Smooth Muscle Cells

SHIGEO ITO
TOSHIO OHTA
YOSHIKAZU NAKAZATO

Laboratory of Pharmacology,
Graduate School of Veterinary Medicine,
Hokkaido University, Sapporo, Japan

INTRODUCTION

Acetylcholine acts on muscarinic receptors on the smooth muscle membrane to cause depolarization and contraction. A number of conductance mechanisms are involved in the current response to acetylcholine. In intestinal smooth muscle cells, muscarinic receptor stimulation is proposed to activate nonselective cation channels (Benham *et al.*, 1985). In tracheal smooth muscle cells, however, acetylcholine activates chloride channels in addition to nonselective cation channels (Janssen & Sims 1992). Chloride channels activated by noradrenaline are proposed to be activated by increasing the intracellular Ca^{2+} concentration in vascular smooth muscles (Pacaud *et al.*, 1989). The purpose of the present study was to examine the characteristics of current responses to carbachol and caffeine in the smooth muscle cells of the rat intestine.

METHODS

Male Wistar rats were killed by stunning and bleeding and smooth muscle cells were enzymatically isolated from the longitudinal smooth muscle layer of the rat intestine with collagenase and papain as described previously (Ohta *et al.*, 1993). Membrane currents were measured with standard whole-cell

SMOOTH MUSCLE EXCITATION
ISBN 0-12-112360-X

patch-clamp technique. In some experiments, nystatin-perforated patch clamp technique was used to prevent run-down of the carbachol-induced response. Intracellular Ca^{2+} was measured using fura-2 in two ways; fura-2 was introduced into the cell through a patch pipette and when the nystatin-perforated-patch technique was used, cells were pretreated with fura-2AM. In most of the conventional patch-clamp experiments, the patch pipette solution contained 0.1 mM fura-2.

RESULTS AND DISCUSSION

Using a pipette solution containing 132 mM potassium chloride, carbachol was applied at various holding potentials. As shown in Figure 1, at a holding potential of -60 mV, carbachol evoked an inward current and at -20 mV it produced an outward current. At -40 mV, both inward and outward currents were observed in most of the cells. Very similar results were obtained when caffeine was used instead of carbachol. The outward currents were identified as potassium currents. Inward currents at these potentials were not due to inward movement of potassium ion because the equilibrium potential of potassium ion was calculated to be -75 mV. To remove the outward potassium currents, potassium chloride in the pipette and external solutions was replaced by sodium chloride in the following experiments. The reversal

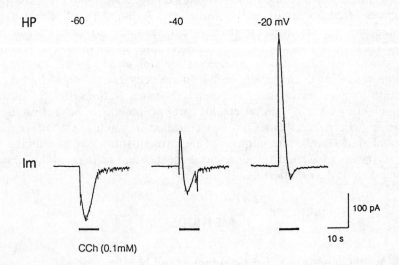

Figure 1 Membrane current responses to carbachol (CCh) at various holding potentials (HP) in K^+-containing pipette solution. Reproduced from Ito *et al.* (1993) with permission.

Table 1 Reversal potentials of the current responses to carbachol (CCh) and caffeine in various external solutions (132 mM). Reproduced from Ito *et al.* (1993) with permission.

Cation	Anion	n	CCh (0.1 mM)	Caffeine (10 mM)
Na^+	SCN^-	5	-27.0 ± 4.8	-60.6 ± 3.2
	I^-	5	-21.2 ± 2.2	-37.7 ± 0.7
	Cl^-	8	-0.9 ± 0.9	-3.0 ± 0.7
	Glutamate$^-$	6	$+18.3 \pm 3.0$	$+30.0 \pm 3.2$

potentials of the current response to carbachol and caffeine were about 0 mV in the sodium-containing, potassium-free environment. To examine the ionic mechanisms underlying the inward current, the reversal potentials of current responses to carbachol and caffeine were investigated in the presence of various external anions such as thiocyanate, iodine, glutamate and chloride. These are summarized in Table 1. In the presence of external chloride, reversal potentials of current responses to both drugs were close to 0 mV. Substitution of sodium iodide or sodium thiocyanate for sodium chloride produced a shift of reversal potential to more negative values and substitution of sodium glutamate to more positive values. These values of the reversal potentials of caffeine-induced currents in the presence of foreign anions were similar to those of noradrenaline-induced chloride currents in rabbit ear artery (Amédée *et al.*, 1990). However, reversal potentials of carbachol-induced currents in the presence of foreign anions were closer to 0 mV than those of caffeine-induced currents. If caffeine activated only chloride channels, other conductance mechanisms in addition to chloride conductance would appear to be involved in the current response to carbachol. Therefore, we examined the effect of external sodium ions on current responses to carbachol and caffeine. The amplitude and reversal potential of the caffeine-induced current were changed little by replacement of external sodium chloride with Tris chloride or choline chloride. However, when sodium chloride was replaced by Tris chloride, the carbachol-induced current decreased in amplitude and recovered after restoration of sodium chloride. It appears likely that an increase in sodium conductance is involved in the inward current response to carbachol, probably resulting from activation of cation channels as in guinea pig and rabbit intestinal smooth muscle cells. These results suggest that caffeine activates chloride channels, and carbachol activates both chloride and cation channels in rat intestinal smooth muscle cells.

In vascular smooth muscle cells, noradrenaline has been shown to activate Ca^{2+}-dependent chloride channels (Pacaud *et al.*, 1989). Thus, we examined the Ca^{2+}-transient and membrane current in response to caffeine and

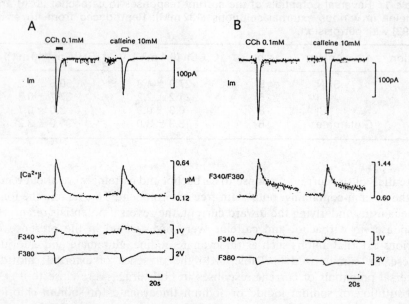

Figure 2 Simultaneous measurements of [Ca²⁺]ᵢ and membrane current in response to carbachol (CCh) and caffeine at a holding potential of −60 mV using standard whole-cell recording (A) and nystatin-perforated whole-cell recording (B). Reproduced from Ito *et al.* (1993) with permission.

carbachol using standard and nystatin-perforated patch clamp methods (Figure 2). Changes in both excitation wavelength signals (340 nm and 380 nm) were symmetrical, indicating changes in the Ca^{2+} concentration in the cell. Caffeine and carbachol evoked simultaneous increases in intracellular Ca^{2+} concentration ($[Ca^{2+}]_i$) and inward current at a holding potential of −60 mV and there was no significant difference in the peak currents between conventional and nystatin methods. In the whole-cell patch-clamp recording, increases in the EGTA concentration in the pipette solution blocked current responses to both drugs. Therefore, an increase in $[Ca^{2+}]_i$ appeared to play an important role in producing inward current. Next, we examined the effect of removal of extracellular Ca^{2+} on the current and Ca^{2+}-transient in response to caffeine. One minute after the removal of Ca^{2+}, caffeine was still effective in producing both responses. Five minutes after Ca^{2+} removal, however, responses to caffeine were greatly decreased. It was noted that more than 20% of the Ca^{2+} transient still remained but there was no current response 5 min after Ca^{2+} removal (Figure 3A). Similar results were obtained with the responses to carbachol. The peak inward current was plotted against the increment of $[Ca^{2+}]_i$ in each cell in the presence and

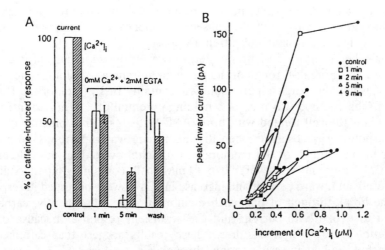

Figure 3 Effect of removal of external Ca^{2+} on the inward current and Ca^{2+}-transient in response to caffeine. Reproduced from Ohta *et al.* (1993) with permission.

absence of Ca^{2+} to obtain the threshold Ca^{2+} concentration producing inward current (Figure 3B). A more than 100 nM increase in $[Ca^{2+}]_i$ seemed to be required to activate the chloride current.

Ryanodine has been reported to inhibit Ca^{2+}-induced Ca^{2+} release (Fleischer *et al.*, 1985). We investigated the effect of ryanodine on the current and Ca^{2+}-transient in response to caffeine at a holding potential of -60 mV. After a control response to caffeine was obtained, cells were treated with caffeine, together with ryanodine. This treatment produced an initial rise and then a sustained increase in $[Ca^{2+}]_i$ and a transient inward current. Caffeine subsequently applied evoked negligible or no effect on the current and $[Ca^{2+}]_i$. In contrast to caffeine, activation of muscarinic receptors has been proposed to cause the release of Ca^{2+} from intracellular Ca^{2+} stores through the production of inositol-1,4,5-trisphosphate ($InsP_3$) (Komori & Bolton, 1990, 1991). As $InsP_3$-induced Ca^{2+} release is reported to be inhibited by heparin (Kobayashi *et al.*, 1989); the effect of heparin on the current and Ca^{2+}-transient in response to carbachol was examined. At a holding potential of -60 mV, carbachol was continuously applied for 1 min and then caffeine was applied for 20 s to cells dialysed with fura-2 in the presence and absence of heparin in the pipette solution. In the absence of heparin, continuous application of carbachol produced a transient increase in $[Ca^{2+}]_i$ and inward current. Caffeine applied subsequently produced only a minute increase in $[Ca^{2+}]_i$ and a small current response, probably because stored Ca^{2+} had been depleted by the pretreatment with carbachol. Conversely, in the presence of heparin, carbachol failed to produce any response, but the subsequent application of caffeine evoked a substantial Ca^{2+}-transient and current response.

It has been reported that a marked outward potassium current is evoked just following break-through of the patch membrane at a holding potential of 0 mV when the patch pipette solution contains $InsP_3$ (Komori & Bolton, 1991). This method was used at a holding potential of $-60\,mV$ to introduce $InsP_3$ into the cell treated with fura-2AM. With $InsP_3$-free pipette solution, no response was observed when the membrane was ruptured. One minute after break-through of the membrane, carbachol evoked an inward current and Ca^{2+} transient. However, when 0.1 mM $InsP_3$-containing pipette solution was used, an inward current and increase in $[Ca^{2+}]_i$ were observed in response to the break-through of the patch membrane and, subsequently, carbachol failed to evoke both current and Ca^{2+}-transient responses because of the depletion of Ca^{2+} in the stores. These results suggest that caffeine and carbachol evoked inward currents through Ca^{2+}-induced Ca^{2+} release and $InsP_3$-induced Ca^{2+} release, respectively.

Recently, it has been reported that $InsP_3$-induced Ca^{2+} release is potentiated in the presence of submicromolar concentrations of Ca^{2+} but inactivated by increasing Ca^{2+} (Iino, 1990) and that $InsP_3$-induced Ca^{2+} release occurs in a regenerative manner (Iino *et al.*, 1993). We studied, therefore, the effects of various concentrations of carbachol on increases in $[Ca^{2+}]_i$ and current. Figure 4A shows Ca^{2+}-transient responses to carbachol in two cells treated with fura-2AM without voltage clamping. In the cell shown in the upper traces, no change in $[Ca^{2+}]_i$ occurred in response to $0.2\,\mu M$ carbachol, but $0.5\,\mu M$ carbachol was effective in increasing $[Ca^{2+}]_i$. The amplitude of the rise in $[Ca^{2+}]_i$ was not significantly different at concentrations over $0.2\,\mu M$. Qualitatively, the same results were obtained in another cell shown in the lower traces, although a higher concentration of carbachol was needed to cause the increase in $[Ca^{2+}]_i$. The Ca^{2+}-transient elicited by $1\,\mu M$ carbachol was little affected by removal of extracellular Ca^{2+}, or application of $1\,\mu M$ nifedipine or 1 mM lanthanum, but was inhibited by thapsigargin, suggesting that the Ca^{2+}-transient was attributable to Ca^{2+} released from intracellular Ca^{2+} stores but not to Ca^{2+} influx. The amplitude of the Ca^{2+}-transient was plotted against the concentration of carbachol (Figure 4B). The amplitude was not significantly different for concentrations of carbachol over $0.2\,\mu M$ when a Ca^{2+}-transient occurred. The Ca^{2+}-transient response to carbachol appeared to be all or nothing in these cells. It was therefore determined whether this was also true for the carbachol-induced inward current at a holding potential of $-60\,mV$ using sodium-containing, potassium-free pipette solution. In the cell shown in the upper traces of Figure 5A, carbachol failed to evoke any current responses at $0.2\,\mu M$, but did evoke a large inward current at $0.5\,\mu M$. However, in some cells, a current

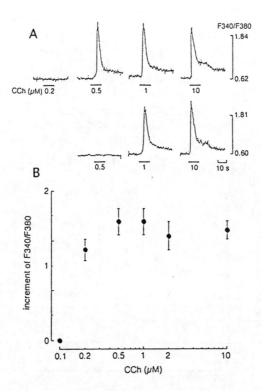

Figure 4 Ca^{2+}-transient responses to various concentrations of carbachol (CCh) in the cells pretreated with fura-2AM. Reproduced from Ohta *et al.* (1994) with permission.

response started to occur at 1 μM, as indicated in the lower traces. There was no significant difference between the amplitude of the inward current with concentrations over 0.2 μM (Figure 5B). Similar experiments were carried out in cells held at −30 mV using a potassium-containing pipette solution. As with the inward current responses, an outward current of almost full magnitude was elicited by a threshold concentration of carbachol, which differed slightly among cells.

The threshold dose for carbachol varied from cell to cell, although there was no concentration-dependent increase in the amplitude of the Ca^{2+}-transient and membrane current in the same cell. The number of cells responding to various concentrations of carbachol was counted and expressed as a percentage of the total number of cells responding to the highest concentration of carbachol used (10 μM). In addition, the number of cells contracted by carbachol was also counted by microscopic observation and the percentages of responding cells were also plotted against the log

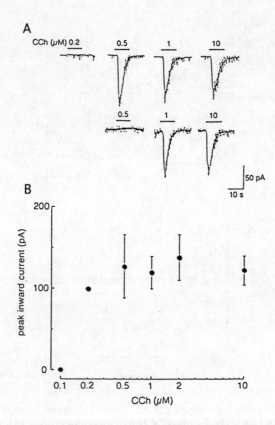

Figure 5 Inward current responses to various concentrations of carbachol (CCh) at a holding potential of −60 mV. If no response occurred at a particular concentration then it was ignored when calculating average responses; i.e. at any concentration only responding cells were included. Reproduced from Ohta *et al.* (1994) with permission.

concentration of carbachol (Figure 6). The curves for all responses (Ca^{2+} transient, current and contractile responses) appeared to be sigmoidal and to overlap each other. These results may provide further evidence that carbachol-induced inward currents are dependent on the increase in Ca^{2+} released from internal Ca^{2+} stores.

Finally, we constructed the concentration-response curve for carbachol-induced contraction, which was dependent on Ca^{2+} released from Ca^{2+} stores, using muscle strips isolated from longitudinal smooth muscle of the rat intestine. The muscle strips were prepared as small as possible in order to facilitate penetration of carbachol to cells deeper in the strip. After the muscle bundles were placed in a Ca^{2+}-containing solution, they were exposed

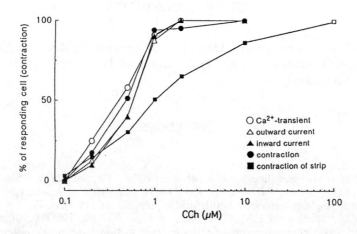

Figure 6 Concentration-dependent increases in the number of cells responding (Ca^{2+} transient, inward current, outward current and contraction) to given concentrations of carbachol (CCh). Filled black squares indicate a dose-response curve for the carbachol-induced contraction dependent on Ca^{2+} released from Ca^{2+} stores in thin bundle of the longitudinal smooth muscle. Reproduced from Ohta *et al.* (1994) with permission.

to a Ca^{2+}-free solution containing 2 mM EGTA and then stimulated by various concentrations of carbachol. Carbachol over 0.2 μM evoked a transient contraction, the amplitude of which increased with increasing concentrations (Figure 6). The threshold concentration of carbachol evoking contraction was similar to those obtained in single cells. The concentration–response curve in the muscle bundle extended to higher concentrations of carbachol than those obtained from single cells. This may be explained by the diffusion rate of carbachol being slower in muscle bundles than in single cells.

CONCLUSION

Carbachol-induced inward current results from an increase in chloride and cation conductance and caffeine-induced inward current from an increase in chloride conductance in the smooth muscle cells of the rat intestine. The increase in chloride conductance appears to depend on Ca^{2+} released from the Ca^{2+} stores. Muscarinic receptor activation elicits a Ca^{2+}-transient and inward current in an all-or-nothing manner. This may be explained by the characteristics of $InsP_3$-induced Ca^{2+} release mechanisms.

ACKNOWLEDGEMENTS

This work was supported by a Grant-in-Aid for Scientific Research from the Ministry of Education, Science and Culture of Japan, and by The Naito Foundation (Japan).

REFERENCES

Amédée, T., Large, W.A. & Wang, Q. (1990). Characteristics of chloride currents activated by noradrenaline in rabbit ear artery cells. *J. Physiol.* **428**, 501–516.

Benham, C.D., Bolton, T.B. & Lang, R.J. (1985). Acetylcholine activates an inward current in single mammalian smooth muscle cells. *Nature* **316**, 345–347.

Fleischer, S., Ogunbunmi, E.M., Dixon, M.C. & Fleer, E.A.M. (1985). Localization of Ca^{2+} release channels with ryanodine in junctional terminal cisternae of sarcoplasmic reticulum of fast skeletal muscle. *Proc. Natl Acad. Sci. USA* **82**, 7256–7259.

Iino, M. (1990). Biphasic Ca^{2+} dependence of inositol 1,4,5-trisphosphate-induced Ca release in smooth muscle cells of the guinea pig taenia caeci. *J. Gen. Physiol.* **95**, 1103–1122.

Iino, M., Yamazawa, T., Miyashita, Y., Endo, M. & Kasai, H. (1993). Critical intracellular Ca^{2+} concentration for all-or-none Ca^{2+} spiking in single smooth muscle cells. *EMBO J.* **12**, 5287–5291.

Ito, S., Ohta, T. & Nakazato, Y. (1993). Inward current activated by carbachol in rat intestinal smooth muscle cells. *J. Physiol.* **470**, 395–409.

Janssen, L.J. & Sims, S.M. (1992). Acetylcholine activates non-selective cation and chloride conductances in canine and guinea pig tracheal myocytes. *J. Physiol.* **453**, 197–218.

Kobayashi, S., Kitazawa, T., Somlyo, A.V. & Somlyo, A.P. (1989). Cytosolic heparin inhibits muscarinic and α-adrenergic Ca^{2+} release in smooth muscle: Physiological role of inositol 1,4,5-trisphosphate in pharmacomechanical coupling. *J. Biol. Chem.* **264**, 17997–18004.

Komori, S. & Bolton, T.B. (1990). Role of G-proteins in muscarinic receptor inward and outward currents in rabbit jejunal smooth muscle. *J. Physiol.* **427**, 395–419.

Komori, S. & Bolton, T.B. (1991). Calcium release induced by inositol 1,4,5-trisphosphate in single rabbit intestinal smooth muscle cells. *J. Physiol.* **433**, 495–517.

Ohta, T., Ito, S. & Nakazato, Y. (1993). Chloride currents activated by caffeine in rat intestinal smooth muscle cells. *J. Physiol.* **465**, 149–162.

Ohta, T., Ito, S. & Nakazato, Y. (1994). All-or-nothing responses to carbachol in single intestinal smooth muscle cells of rat. *Br. J. Pharmacol.* **112**, 972–976.

Pacaud., Loirand, G., Mironneau, C. & Mironneau, J. (1989). Noradrenaline activates a calcium-activated chloride conductance and increases the voltage-dependent calcium current in cultured single cells of rat portal vein. *Br. J. Pharmacol.* **97**, 139–146.

16

Multiplicity of Regulatory Mechanisms for Receptor-operated Cation-permeable Channels in Guinea Pig Ileum – A Possible Contribution of Mechanical Forces

RYUJI INOUE
YOSHIKI WANIISHI
YUSHI ITO

Department of Pharmacology,
Faculty of Medicine,
Kyushu University,
Fukuoka, Japan

MULTIPLICITY OF REGULATIONS FOR RECEPTOR-OPERATED CATION CHANNELS

Many receptors capable of mobilizing internally stored calcium in smooth muscle are also known to activate cation-permeable channels (CCs). Because these channels often show higher selectivity for divalent cations than monovalent ones (based on the biionic reversal potential measurements; Benham & Tsien, 1987; Byrne & Large, 1988; Inoue and Isenberg, 1990a), they have been implicated in Ca entry into the cell during receptor stimulation (Bolton, 1979). It is now believed that CCs can elevate the intracellular free Ca concentration ($[Ca^{2+}]_i$) in two different ways, i.e., direct permeation of external Ca through CCs *per se* and secondary activation of voltage-dependent Ca channels by membrane depolarization owing to increased Na and Ca permeability. However, a recent $[Ca^{2+}]_i$ study using the fluorescent dye indo-1 in single cells of mammalian gut muscle suggested that the $[Ca^{2+}]_i$ rise due to Ca entry via CCs is only of the order of 10 nanomolar (Pacaud & Bolton, 1991). However, because this measurement represents the overall $[Ca^{2+}]_i$ change rather than the change localized to the subsarcolemmal space, the physiological importance of direct Ca entry through CCs in agonist-mediated Ca mobilization cannot be entirely excluded.

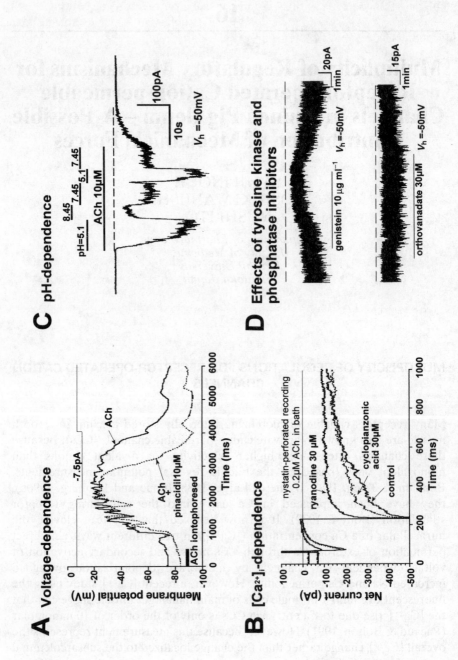

A Voltage-dependence

B [Ca²⁺]ᵢ-dependence

C pH-dependence

D Effects of tyrosine kinase and phosphatase inhibitors

In agreement with this argument, recent investigations attempting to characterize CCs have revealed other unexpected aspects. For instance, muscarinic receptor CCs in guinea pig ileal smooth muscle are found to be regulated in a variety of ways such as by membrane potential, $[Ca^{2+}]_i$, by external pH and possibly by tyrosine phosphorylation (Figure 1; Benham et al., 1985; Inoue & Isenberg, 1990a; Inoue & Isenberg, 1990b; Pacaud & Bolton, 1991; Inoue et al., 1994, 1995). The effective ranges of these regulations appear to correspond to their dynamic ranges under physiological conditions, therefore providing an idea that there may be close a functional collaboration between CCs and other cellular effectors associated with Ca^{2+} homeostasis such as voltage-dependent Ca and K channels, the Na/K pump, and Na/Ca exchange during receptor stimulation (Figure 2; Inoue & Chen, 1993; Inoue, 1995). For this reason, further exploration of as yet unknown regulatory mechanisms which are convergent on, or divergent from, CCs may be essential to understand the precise role of CCs in agonist-mediated Ca mobilization.

In the following part of this paper, we briefly describe a novel regulatory mechanism, the effects of mechanical stimulus on CCs of muscarinic receptors in guinea pig ileal smooth muscle. The potency and importance of this regulation appears to be comparable to those described above as regulating CCs in this muscle.

Figure 1 Factors which affect the activity of muscarinic receptor-operated nonselective cation channels in guinea pig ileum. A, Acetylcholine (ACh)-induced depolarization recorded with nystatin perforated-patch recording under current clamp conditions in the absence or presence of 10 μM pinacidil. Pinacidil (10 μM) hyperpolarized the membrane close to the K equilibrium potential, and significantly retarded and shortened the ACh-induced depolarization. B, Potentiating effect of voltage-dependent Ca influx (I_{Ca}) on ACh-induced inward current. Following I_{Ca}, the amplitude of ACh-induced inward current was greatly increased, which was attenuated in the presence of ryanodine or cyclopiazonic acid. Nystatin perforated patch recording. The pipette and bath contained physiological saline (2 mM Ca) and caesium aspartate, respectively. Holding potential was −70 mV. I_{Ca} was activated by a voltage step pulse to 0 mV. Ryanodine or cyclopiazonic acid was added into the bath about 2 min before administration of 0.2 μM ACh. C, Effects of external proton activity on ACh-induced inward current, where acidosis increased and alkalosis reduced the current. Conventional whole-cell recording with the internal solution containing Cs aspartate and 10 mM EGTA and 4.5 mM Ca. External pH was switched rapidly by shifting a voltage-clamped cell between the orifices of four tandem-arranged small tubes. D, Effects of genistein and orthovanadate on GTP-$_\gamma$S-induced inward current. Cells were dialysed with a pipette solution of the same ionic composition as in C which was supplemented with 50 μM GTP-$_\gamma$S. A, C and D are reproduced from Inoue (1995), Inoue & Chen (1993), and Inoue et al. (1994), respectively.

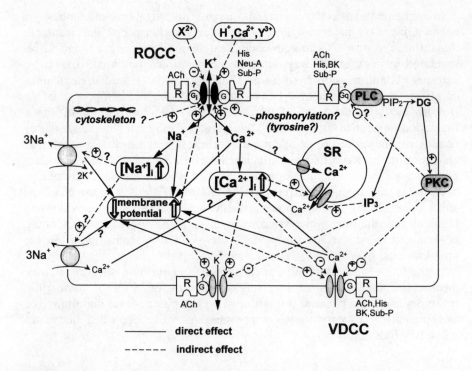

direct effect

- - - - indirect effect

Figure 2 Conceptual network of feedforward and feedback regulations for receptor-operated cation channels in gut smooth muscle. Abbreviations: ROCC, receptor-operated cation-permeable channel; VDCC, voltage-dependent Ca channel; G, GTP-binding protein; R; Ca-mobilizing receptors; PLC, phospholipase C; PKC, protein kinase C ; DG, diacylglycerol; IP$_3$, inositol 1,4,5-trisphosphate; PIP$_2$, phosphatidylinositol 4,5-bisphosphate; ACh, acetylcholine; BK, bradykinin; His, histamine; Neu-A, neurokinin A; Sub-P, substance P; X^{2+}; divalent cations; Y^{3+}, trivalent cations. (Inoue & Isenberg, 1990a,b,c; Komori et al., 1992; Pacaud & Bolton, 1992; Beech, 1993; Lee et al., 1993, Inoue et al., 1995, 1994). Question marks indicate that this route is in question. Reproduced from Inoue (1995) with minor modifications.

ALTERED OSMOLARITY CHANGES CELL VOLUME AND ACh-INDUCED CATIONIC CURRENTS

Exposing single ileal cells to hypotonic solutions (from 308 mOsm to 258 or 208 mOsm, keeping the ionic composition constant) resulted in a varying amount of swelling of cells. This was characterized by increased cell width which was sometimes accompanied by rounding of the cell ends. In contrast with this, cells started to shrink when they were exposed to hypertonic solutions (358 or 408 mOsm). These changes were usually progressive and when cells were persistently exposed to anisosmotic solutions, they were sometimes irreversibly deformed if the extent of change in osmolarity was severe (e.g., progressive expansion and eventual rupture upon hypotonic challenge). It was therefore necessary to limit the time of exposure to a short period (usually 2 min).

With nystatin-perforated patch recording (KCl electrode) and in the absence of acetylcholine (ACh), membrane currents activated by depolarizing step pulses were hardly affected by mild changes in the osmolarity of external solution (258 mOsm or 358 mOsm), despite the fact that cells had changed shape. In contrast, the amplitude of inward cationic currents evoked by iontophoretic application of ACh (I_{ACh}) was significantly increased in hypotonic solutions, while reduced in hypertonic ones. With ±100 mOsm change, the amplitude of I_{ACh} became 42 ± 7 and 211 ± 32% of the control (308 mOsm), respectively. The current–voltage relationship evaluated by voltage step pulses applied during iontophoresis revealed that the current component sensitive to osmotic change reverses more positively than −30 mV, thus suggesting that this component is cationic.

The effects of osmotic change on I_{ACh} was still observed under the conditions where $[Ca^{2+}]_i$ was strongly buffered. Even when the cell was dialysed with 10 mM EGTA or BAPTA/4~5 mM Ca mixtures, the amplitude of I_{ACh} was increased under hypotonic conditions, while reduced under hypertonic ones (Figure 3). These results were quantitatively unchanged when I_{ACh} was activated via a G-protein by adding 50 μM GTP-γS to the pipette solution (Inoue & Isenberg, 1990c; Komori et al., 1992; hereafter referred to as $I_{GTP-γS}$). Thus, the amplitude of I_{ACh} and $I_{GTP-γS}$ (normalized to that at 308 mOsm) can be expressed as a decremental function of external osmolarity with no obvious mininum or maximum in the tested range (208 to

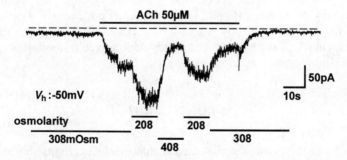

Figure 3 Effects of osmotic change on ACh-induced inward current. The pipette contained the internal solution of the same composition as in Figure 1C except that EGTA was replaced by BAPTA. External solutions with different osmolarity were applied using four tandem-arranged small tubes.

around 408 mOsm) and mutually superimposable. These results suggest that neither $[Ca^{2+}]_i$ nor the muscarinic receptor plays a major role in the effects of osmotic change on I_{ACh} .

PROPERTIES OF THE EFFECTS OF HYPOTONIC SWELLING ON I$_{GTP-\gamma S}$

Desensitization of $I_{GTP-\gamma S}$ proceeded more slowly than that of I_{ACh} . This enabled us to investigate further details of the effects of hypotonic swelling on the cationic currents.

Simultaneous measurements of cell size and $I_{GTP-\gamma S}$ revealed a good temporal and quantitative relationship between cell width change and $I_{GTP-\gamma S}$ amplitude, that is, the increasing and decreasing phases of $I_{GTP-\gamma S}$, respectively, closely matched those of cell size change. This coincidence could be dissociated by potent inhibitors of CCs in this muscle such as 10 mM procaine and 400 µM zinc (Chen *et al.*, 1993; Inoue *et al.*, 1995). These compounds almost completely inhibited the increased inward cationic curents during hypotonic challenge, while having little effect on hypotonicity-induced cell swelling. These results support the idea that the component sensitive to osmotic change reflects the modified activity of CCs *per se* rather than another membrane conductance which is induced by hypotonic swelling such as a volume-sensitive Cl current (Oike *et al.*, 1994).

The effect of altered osmolarity on $I_{GTP-\gamma S}$ was still observed when external cations were substituted with a single species of monovalent (Na+, Li+, or Cs+) or divalent (Ba^{2+}, Mn^{2+}) cations but their reversal potentials were affected differently. For example, the rightward shift (shift toward more positive potentials) was more pronounced for Na+ than for Cs+. These results imply that mechanical stimuli such as hypotonic swelling might affect the structure of the channel pore and significantly alter its permeability preferentially to some cations. The voltage-dependence of $I_{GTP-\gamma S}$ do not appear to change much by varying the osmolarity, but the maximam conductance, which is observed at strongly depolarized potentials, was clearly increased in hypotonic solutions.

CONCLUSION

The results of the present study suggest that mechanical stimuli imposed on the cell membrane such as membrane stretch could be an efficient regulator of receptor-operated CC activity in gut smooth muscle, providing a novel powerful mechanism for the control of agonist-induced Ca mobilization in the organs whose mechanical activity is dynamically changing.

REFERENCES

Beech, D.J. (1993). Inhibitory effects of histamine and bradykinin on calcium current in smooth muscle cells isolated from guinea pig ileum. *J. Physiol. (London)* **463**, 565–583.

Benham, C.D. & Tsien, R.W. (1987). A novel receptor-operated Ca^{2+}-permeable channel activated by ATP in smooth muscle. *Nature* **328**, 275–278.

Benham, C.D., Bolton, T.B. & Lang, R.J. (1985). Acetylcholine activates an inward current in single mammalian smooth muscle cells. *Nature* **316**, 345–347.

Bolton, T.B. (1979). Mechanisms of action of transmitters and other substances on smooth muscle. *Physiol. Rev.* **59**, 606–718.

Byrne, N.G. & Large, W.A. (1988). Membrane ionic mechanisms activated by noradrenaline in cells isolated from the rabbit portal vein. *J. Physiol. (London)* **404**, 557–573.

Chen, S., Inoue, R. & Ito, Y. (1993). Pharmacological characterization of muscarinic receptor-activated cation channels in guinea pig ileum. *Br. J. Pharmacol.* **109**, 793–801.

Inoue, R. (1995). Biophysical and pharmacological characterization of receptor-operated nonselective cation channels (ROCC) and their regulatory mechanisms in smooth muscle. *Folia Pharmacolog. Japon.* **105**, 11–22.

Inoue, R. & Chen, S. (1993). Physiology of muscarinic receptor-operated nonselective cation channels in guinea pig ileal smooth muscle. In *Nonselective Cation Channels – Pharmacology, Physiology and Biophysics.* (Siemen, D. & Hescheler, J. eds), pp. 261–268. Birkhäuser Verlag, Basel, Switzerland.

Inoue, R. & Isenberg, G. (1990a). Effect of membrane potential on acetylcholine-induced inward current in guinea pig ileum. *J. Physiol. (London)* **424**, 57–71.

Inoue, R. & Isenberg, G. (1990b). Intracellular calcium ions modulate acetylcholine-induced inward current in guinea pig ileum. *J. Physiol. (London)* **424**, 73–92.

Inoue, R. & Isenberg, G. (1990c). ACh activates non-selective cation channels in guinea pig ileum through a G-protein. *Am. J. Physiol.* **258**, C1173–C1178.

Inoue, R., Waniishi, Y., Yamada, K. & Ito,Y. (1994). A possible role of tyrosine kinases in the regulation of muscarinic receptor-activated cation channels in guinea pig ileum. *Biochem. Biophys. Res. Comm.* **203**, 1392–1397.

Inoue, R, Waniishi,Y. & Ito, Y. (1995). Extracellular protons modulate acetylcholine-activated cation channels in guinea pig ileum. *Am. J. Physiol.* **268**, C162–C170.

Komori, S., Kawai, M., Takewaki, T. & Ohashi, H. (1992). GTP-binding protein involvement in membrane currents evoked by carbachol and histamine in guinea pig ileal muscle. *J. Physiol. (London)* **450**, 105–126.

Lee, H.K, Shuttleworth C.W. & Sanders, K.M. (1993). Nonselective cation current in canine colonic myocytes is activated by cholinergic and peptide neurotransmitters. In *Abstr. 32nd Congr. Int. Union of Physiological Sciences,* 140.47P.

Oike, M., Droogmans,G. & Nilius,B. (1994). The volume-activated chloride current in human endothelial cells depends on intracellular ATP. *Pflügers Arch., Eur. J. Physiol.* **427**, 184–186.

Pacaud, P. & Bolton, T.B. (1991). Relation between muscarinic receptor cationic current and intestinal calcium in guinea pig jejunal smooth muscle cells. *J. Physiol. (London)* **441**, 447–499.

17

Mechanisms of Cytosolic Ca²⁺ Oscillations Following Muscarinic Receptor Activation in Single Smooth Muscle Cells

S. KOMORI
H. OHASHI

Laboratory of Pharmacology,
Department of Veterinary Science,
Faculty of Agriculture,
Gifu University,
Gifu, Japan

The cytosolic concentration of free Ca^{2+}, ($[Ca^{2+}]_i$), is a critically important factor for the control of cellular function. $[Ca^{2+}]_i$ is increased in response to receptor agonists including hormones and neurotransmitters. In many different cell types, the increase in $[Ca^{2+}]_i$ has been shown to be an oscillatory one which occurs as a result of periodic Ca^{2+} release from the intracellular stores. The underlying process of the $[Ca^{2+}]_i$ oscillations is that agonists activate a G protein-coupled phosphoinositide pathway leading to an accelerated formation of D-myo-inositol 1,4,5-trisphosphate ($InsP_3$) and $InsP_3$ in turn acts on intracellular Ca^{2+} stores to release Ca^{2+}. To date, several models of the phenomenon have been proposed; these differ in respects such as whether the $InsP_3$ concentration itself oscillates, the relative contributions of $InsP_3$-gated channels ($InsP_3$ receptor) and Ca^{2+}-gated channels (ryanodine receptor) responsible for Ca^{2+} release from the stores, and the sites of positive and/or negative feedback required for oscillatory behavior (for reviews, see Tsien & Tsien, 1990; Meyer & Stryer, 1991; Fewtrell, 1993).

The changes in $[Ca^{2+}]_i$ have been detected directly using fluorescent Ca^{2+}-sensitive dyes introduced into the cell or inferred from measurement of ionic currents flowing through membrane channels which are controlled by intracellular Ca^{2+}. In visceral and vascular smooth muscle cells held under whole-cell voltage clamp, repetitive discharge of spontaneous transient outward currents (STOCs) or inward currents (STICs) occurs as a result of openings of Ca^{2+}-sensitive K^+ channels and Ca^{2+}-sensitive Cl^- channels,

SMOOTH MUSCLE EXCITATION
ISBN 0-12-112360-X

respectively. STOCs and STICs are considered to result from sporadic release of Ca^{2+} from the intracellular stores, representing Ca^{2+}-store-dependent $[Ca^{2+}]_i$ oscillations. However, these currents are of short duration (50–100 ms) and are rarely detected using the fluorescent dye method. STOCs and STICs seem likely to reflect Ca^{2+} oscillations which are localized phenomena in the vicinity of these ionic channels. Further, the Ca^{2+} release does not require $InsP_3$ as an indispensable factor, since the discharge of STOCs is not blocked by heparin, a putative $InsP_3$ antagonist, even at concentrations sufficient to block a massive release of Ca^{2+} induced by endogenous $InsP_3$ produced by muscarinic receptor stimulation and by $InsP_3$ liberated by flash-photolysis from its inert precursor (caged $InsP_3$) loaded within the cell (Komori & Bolton, 1990, 1991). Observations of $InsP_3$-controlled $[Ca^{2+}]_i$ oscillations in visceral and vascular smooth muscle cells have been limited.

Recently, we demonstrated in single intestinal smooth muscle cells, using the whole-cell patch-clamp technique, that stimulation of muscarinic receptors can elicit current oscillations which are closely correlated with changes in $[Ca^{2+}]_i$ (Komori et al., 1992, 1993; Zholos et al., 1994). In this article, we will describe some properties and underlying mechanisms of the muscarinic receptor-mediated oscillations in $[Ca^{2+}]_i$.

MUSCARINIC $[Ca^{2+}]_i$ OSCILLATIONS

Single cells were prepared by enzymic dispersion of the longitudinal muscle layer of guinea pig ileum. To monitor changes in $[Ca^{2+}]_i$, membrane currents which are potentiated or activated by intracellular Ca^{2+} were recorded using the patch-clamp technique in the whole-cell recording mode. Muscarinic receptors have been shown to relay the information via two different G-proteins in the cells, one is a pertussis toxin (PTX)-sensitive G-protein (G_i or G_o) linking to activation of cationic channels, and the other is a PTX-insensitive G-protein (G_q) linking to phospholipase C activation, which ultimately leads to $InsP_3$-induced Ca^{2+} release from intracellular stores (Komori et al., 1992). In cells under voltage clamp at a holding potential (V_h) of -40 to -60 mV, a muscarinic agonist carbachol (CCh) evoked an inward current (I_{cat}) due to activation of the muscarinic receptor-coupled cationic channels. Micromolar concentrations of CCh usually elicited I_{cat} with an oscillatory component (Figure 1A, B). The oscillation had a more or less regular frequency, appeared for the entire or early period during the drug application and was usually superimposed on a sustained component of I_{cat} which slowly developed to a maximum. The muscarinic-receptor-coupled cation channels are not activated by a rise in $[Ca^{2+}]_i$ itself, but their activation

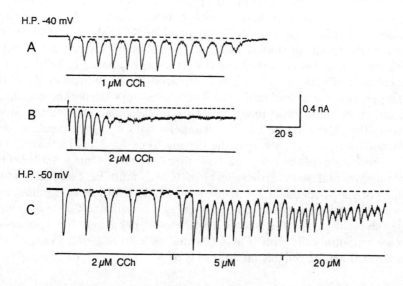

Figure 1 Oscillations in the inward cationic current evoked by carbachol (CCh) in single smooth muscle cells from guinea pig ileum. The cells in A and B were dialysed with a potassium-rich solution and voltage-clamped at −40 mV. The concentration of CCh in the bathing solution is marked. A, Current oscillations persisting for the entire period of the drug application, which were superimposed on a slowly developing, sustained inward current. B, Current oscillations waning with time to end in a sustained inward current in the presence of CCh. C, The oscillation frequency increased with increasing CCh concentration in a cell held at −50 mV with a CsCl-filled pipette. (From Komori *et al.*, 1993).

during stimulation of muscarinic receptors is strongly potentiated by intracellular Ca^{2+} (Inoue & Isenberg, 1990; Pacaud & Bolton, 1991). Therefore, I_{cat} can be changed in strength if $[Ca^{2+}]_i$ is altered by an internal process that is operated also through stimulation of muscarinic receptors. The $[Ca^{2+}]_i$ oscillations were blocked by introduction of a chelating substance, EGTA, into the cell and, under these circumstances, CCh evoked a small sustained I_{cat} without an oscillatory component. The current oscillations were associated with similar changes in the Indo-1 (Ca^{2+}-sensitive fluorescent dye)-signal. Thus, it is highly probable that the oscillations in I_{cat} are brought about by fluctuations of Ca^{2+} level in the cytosol of the smooth muscle cell. The frequency of oscillations in I_{cat} varied from 0.08 to 0.9 Hz in different cells and increased with increasing CCh concentration in one cell, as shown in Figure 1C. However, when used at higher concentrations (> 50 μM), CCh usually elicited a biphasic I_{cat} without any oscillatory component (an initial, fast phase followed by a late, slow phase).

In K^+-filled cells voltage-clamped at a V_h of 0 mV, close to the reversal potential for I_{cat}, CCh evoked a brief outward current (I_{CCh-o}) which is considered to reflect opening of Ca^{2+}-dependent K^+ channels. As expected, in view of the results of studies on I_{cat}, I_{CCh-o} was repeatedly generated with a frequency ranging between 0.02 and 0.3 Hz in cells exposed to 1–2 μM CCh. The repeated discharge of I_{CCh-o} was replaced by an oscillatory I_{cat} if the holding potential was displaced from 0 mV to −40 mV during the continued stimulation of muscarinic receptors. This replacement presumably arises because the Ca^{2+}-dependent K^+ channels are voltage-dependent and deactivated at −40 mV, whereas the driving force for I_{cat} is increased. The main difference between I_{CCh-o} and I_{cat} is that I_{CCh-o} arose from a flat baseline. This suggests that some critical level of $[Ca^{2+}]_i$ must be exceeded before opening of Ca^{2+}-dependent K^+ channels occurs. In contrast, I_{cat} continuously changed because the cationic channel opening is sensitive to Ca^{2+} over a wide range, and unlike I_{CCh-o}, it shows no threshold behaviour but appears to increase monotonically with $[Ca^{2+}]_i$ (Pacaud & Bolton, 1991). Thus, I_{cat} can be utilized as a more reliable monitor of $[Ca^{2+}]_i$.

THE MUSCARINIC $[Ca^{2+}]_i$ OSCILLATIONS INVOLVE A G-PROTEIN-DEPENDENT SIGNALLING PATHWAY

A reliable way for judging involvement of a G-protein in signal transduction is to see whether or not GTP-γS, a nonhydrolysable analogue of GTP, can mimic the receptor-mediated effect. Inclusion of GTP-γS (0.1–0.2 mM) in the pipette solution generated an oscillatory inward current in cells held under the same conditions as used for CCh application. The oscillation frequency ranged between 0.08 and 0.2 Hz and the time-dependent changes in the oscillation amplitude were very similar to those induced in I_{cat} by 1–2 μM CCh, suggesting that a G-protein participates in transmitting the muscarinic signal (muscarinic $[Ca^{2+}]_i$ oscillations).

THE ROLE OF InsP$_3$ IN THE MUSCARINIC $[Ca^{2+}]_i$ OSCILLATIONS

Pretreatment with ryanodine (0.05–0.1 mM) to cause depletion of intracellular Ca^{2+} stores by locking the Ca^{2+}-gated Ca^{2+} release channels in an open state, prevented CCh from evoking any oscillatory component but a sustained component of I_{cat} persisted under these conditions. Similar results were obtained with thapsigargin (1–5 μM), an inhibitor of Ca^{2+}-transporting ATPase in Ca^{2+} store membrane. The thapsigargin treatment does not allow the Ca^{2+} stores to be refilled with Ca^{2+} and ultimately results in their depletion. Therefore, a functional intracellular Ca^{2+} store may be required for the generation of the muscarinic [Ca^{2+}]$_i$ oscillations.

Intracellular application of heparin (2–5 mg ml^{-1}), which inhibits binding of InsP$_3$ to the purified receptor (Supattapone et al., 1988) and also the release of Ca^{2+} from intracellular stores (Ghosh et al., 1988; Kobayashi et al., 1988), prevent the generation of oscillations in I_{cat}. The inhibition is attributable to the action of heparin on the InsP$_3$ receptor, but does not arise through depletion of Ca^{2+} stores or a decrease in Ca^{2+} sensitivity of I_{cat}, since caffeine (5–10 mM), which acts as a potentiator of Ca^{2+}-induced Ca^{2+} release mechanism to cause a massive release of Ca^{2+} from intracellular stores, produced a brief increase in the sustained I_{cat} in the continued presence of heparin. These results suggest a critical role of InsP$_3$ in mediating the muscarinic [Ca^{2+}]$_i$ oscillations.

REQUIREMENT OF Ca^{2+} INFLUX FOR PERSISTENCE OF THE MUSCARINIC [Ca^{2+}]$_i$ OSCILLATIONS

CCh still elicited an oscillatory I_{cat} in cells treated with nifedipine (1–3 μM) or D 600 (5 μM) to block Ca^{2+} entry across the plasma membrane through voltage-dependent Ca^{2+} channels. However, removal of the extracellular Ca^{2+} during CCh-induced [Ca^{2+}]$_i$ oscillations resulted in an immediate arrest of the oscillations in I_{cat}. Lowering Ca^{2+} concentration in the extracellular fluid to 0.2 or 0.05 mM decreased gradually the oscillation frequency and amplitude over a period during which the amplitude was somewhat increased and finally caused the oscillations to cease. Oscillations in I_{cat} reappeared on returning to the normal Ca^{2+} level (2 mM) and were restored in their frequency and amplitude. After elevation of the extracellular Ca^{2+} concentration to 5–8 mM, the oscillations remained unchanged or increased their frequency in some cells exhibiting the oscillations with a relatively low frequency. In addition, by changing V$_h$ within a range between −60 and 40 mV stepwise and in a random order in the presence of nifedipine, it was found that the more positive was V$_h$, the lower was the oscillation frequency, suggesting that the oscillation generator is accelerated by increasing the driving force for Ca^{2+}. Thus, during muscarinic receptor activation, Ca^{2+} influx across the plasma membrane may occur through nifedipine- and D 600-insensitive Ca^{2+} pathways (unidentified Ca^{2+} channels) and contribute to refilling of intracellular Ca^{2+} stores in such a manner that the Ca^{2+} store-dependent Ca^{2+} oscillations can be sustained. In the same cell type, Pacaud & Bolton (1991) suggested the existence of D 600-insensitive Ca^{2+} channels that open if the intracellular Ca^{2+} stores are depleted with caffeine or CCh. In many other cell types, agonist-induced depletion of Ca^{2+} stores is known to trigger Ca^{2+} influx through an unusual type of pathway in the plasma membrane which plays an important role for sustained oscillations in $[Ca^{2+}]_i$ (Putney, 1986).

MECHANISMS OF OSCILLATORY Ca^{2+} STORE RELEASE

One of the models of $[Ca^{2+}]_i$ oscillation in which $InsP_3$ plays a primary role involves an oscillatory change in cytosolic $InsP_3$ level, and the other a steady level of $InsP_3$. A variety of feedback loops have been assumed to regulate $InsP_3$ formation in the former but to regulate Ca^{2+} release from the stores in the latter. In many cell types, two classes of intracellular Ca^{2+}-release channels, the Ca^{2+}-gated channel (ryanodine receptor) and $InsP_3$-gated channel, are essential for spatiotemporal Ca^{2+} signalling. In ileal smooth muscle cells, $InsP_3$- and caffeine-releasable Ca^{2+} stores are indistinguishable from each other (Komori et al., 1992, 1995; Fukami et al., 1993), and this implies coexistence of both types of Ca^{2+}-release channels in the same stores. It is, therefore, possible that Ca^{2+} release via the Ca^{2+}-gated channels (CICR) acts as a positive feedback mechanism in muscarinic Ca^{2+} signalling. We tested this possibility using caffeine, an agonist, and ruthenium red, a blocker, for CICR. When K^+-filled cells were held at -10 or $0\,mV$ and then caffeine $(0.5-2\,mM)$ was applied, periodic outward currents (Ca^{2+}-activated K^+ currents) reminiscent of those evoked by CCh appeared only rarely in cells. Potentiation of CICR could trigger an oscillation of $[Ca^{2+}]_i$ only if for some reason resting $InsP_3$ levels are higher than usual (Prestwich & Bolton, 1991). In Cs^+-filled cells held at $-50\,mV$, application of caffeine $(0.5-2\,mM)$ during the oscillations of I_{cat} evoked by CCh resulted in a decrease in their frequency and amplitude or their immediate arrest. In addition, in cells that responded to CCh with a sustained I_{cat} alone, caffeine did not evoke current oscillation but instead produced a transient increase of I_{cat}. In cells treated with ruthenium red $(30-50\,\mu M)$, CCh $(2\,\mu M)$ evoked an oscillatory I_{cat}, as observed in normal cells. The concentrations of ruthenium red have been shown to be high enough to block CICR induced by Ca^{2+} entry brought about by membrane depolarization (Zholos et al., 1991) and strongly reduce caffeine-induced outward current, a K^+ current arising from activation of Ca^{2+}-dependent K^+ channels owing to a massive release of Ca^{2+} through CICR.

The CICR mechanism does not appear to be directly involved in the oscillation of $[Ca^{2+}]_i$ produced by muscarinic receptor activation in ileal smooth muscle cells. This view is supported by our recent finding in β-escin permeabilized muscle strips that Ca^{2+} released by CCh from the intracellular stores cannot activate Ca^{2+}-gated Ca^{2+}-release channel (Komori et al., 1995).

Feedback loops, necessary to explain $[Ca^{2+}]_i$ oscillations at a steady $InsP_3$

level, could be attributed to fluctuations in InsP$_3$-induced Ca^{2+} release (IICR). It has been reported that Ca^{2+} decreases the binding of InsP$_3$ to its receptor (Supattapone et al., 1988), and inhibits IICR in Xenopus oocytes (Parker & Ivorra, 1990), permeabilized smooth muscle cells (Iino, 1990) and brain microsomes (Finch et al., 1991). These results led us to test the sensitivity of the Ca^{2+} stores to InsP$_3$ at different phases of [Ca^{2+}]$_i$ oscillations by flash release of InsP$_3$ from caged InsP$_3$ within the cell.

In Cs$^+$-filled cells loaded with caged InsP$_3$ (30 μM) and held at -50 mV, CCh elicited I_{cat} oscillations. If a flash to liberate an additional amount of InsP$_3$ was applied close to the peak of an I_{cat} oscillation or its descending phase the response was small or absent, but if a flash was applied during the trough between two peaks this resulted in a large Ca^{2+} release, as judged from the change in I_{cat}. The Ca^{2+} stores remained undepleted even at the peak, as they responded to caffeine with an appreciable Ca^{2+} release (Zholos et al., 1994). One possible explanation for this is that IICR became inactive, or desensitized, for a while owing to an increase in [Ca^{2+}]$_i$ or a decrease in the amount of stored Ca^{2+}. In K$^+$-filled, caged InsP$_3$-loaded cells, a depolarizing pulse (a potential step from -50 to 10 mV) with a 15-s duration elicited transient outward current as a result of activation of Ca^{2+}-dependent K$^+$ channels during regenerative CICR following voltage-activated Ca^{2+} entry (Zholos et al., 1991; Zholos, 1992). The K$^+$ current developed to reach a peak and then decayed to a small current. If flash release of InsP$_3$ or caffeine was applied before the K$^+$ current attained its peak, large, full-sized responses to both agents were obtained. However, after the peak of the K$^+$ current had been reached, responses to a flash or to caffeine were severely depressed. Full recovery of the responses to both occurred within 30 s, but the caffeine response recovered considerably more quickly than the flash response. The difference in recovery time implies the existence of a period during which Ca^{2+} stores are refilled with Ca^{2+} and are able to be discharged by caffeine, but they are refractory to release by InsP$_3$. If caffeine was applied briefly and repeatedly by means of pressure ejection from a micropipette (10 mM caffeine, 0.1–0.5 s pressure pulses), reproducible current responses could be obtained at intervals of 20 s or longer, suggesting complete reuptake of released Ca^{2+} during the interval. The results of the experiments in which caffeine and flashes to release InsP$_3$ from caged InsP$_3$ were applied at an interval of 25 s in all possible combinations showed that InsP$_3$- or caffeine-induced Ca^{2+} release did not prevent subsequent caffeine-induced Ca^{2+} release, whereas InsP$_3$-induced Ca^{2+} release was inhibited by previous caffeine- or InsP$_3$-induced Ca^{2+} release (Zholos et al., 1994).

Elevation of [Ca^{2+}]$_i$ through any mechanism of caffeine-, InsP$_3$- or Ca^{2+}-induced Ca^{2+} release inactivates the InsP$_3$-gated Ca^{2+} release channel (InsP$_3$ receptor) probably in a concentration-dependent manner and the inhibitory effect is sustained for a period that is long enough to allow Ca^{2+} stores to be refilled. This mechanism may account for the generation of $[Ca^{2+}]_i$ oscillations. In addition, IICR has been shown to display a bell-shaped dependence on $[Ca^{2+}]_i$ (Iino, 1990; Iino & Endo, 1992), and Ca^{2+} also appears to be involved as a positive feedback loop in the $[Ca^{2+}]_i$ oscillations.

CONCLUDING REMARKS

Stimulation of muscarinic receptors elicits membrane current brought about by opening of cationic channels in smooth muscle cells of guinea pig ileum. The cationic current was found to change its intensity in a manner closely correlated with the cytosolic Ca^{2+} level because of the high sensitivity to Ca^{2+} in the cytoplasm. Thus, recording the cationic current was utilized as a probe to characterize $[Ca^{2+}]_i$ oscillations evoked by stimulation of muscarinic receptors. As in many other cell types, the muscarinic $[Ca^{2+}]_i$ oscillations involve activation of a phosphoinositide pathway through a pertussis toxin-insensitive G-protein and $InsP_3$ plays a primary role in the $[Ca^{2+}]_i$ oscillations in intestinal smooth muscle cells. Negative feedback of Ca^{2+} on $InsP_3$-mediated Ca^{2+} release from the intracellular stores may, at least in part, account for oscillations in $[Ca^{2+}]_i$ evoked by muscarinic receptor activation. Ca^{2+} influx across the plasma membrane, which occurs through nifedipine- and D 600-insensitive Ca^{2+} pathways, appears to contribute to refilling of the Ca^{2+} stores so that the Ca^{2+} store-dependent oscillations in $[Ca^{2+}]_i$ can be sustained.

REFERENCES

Fewtrell, C. (1993). Ca^{2+} oscillations in non-excitable cells. *Annu. Rev. Physiol.* **55**, 427–454.

Finch, E.A., Turner, T.J. & Goldin, S.M. (1991). Calcium as a coagonist of inositol 1,4,5-trisphosphate-induced calcium release. *Science* **252**, 443–446.

Fukami, K., Itagaki, M., Komori, S. & Ohashi, H. (1993). Contractile responses to histamine and GTPγS in β-escin-treated skinned smooth muscle of guinea pig ileum. *Jpn. J. Pharmacol.* **63**, 171–179.

Ghosh, T.K., Eis, P.S., Mullaney, J.M., Ebert, C.L. & Gill, D.L. (1988). Competitive, reversible and potent antagonism of inositol 1,4,5-trisphosphate-activated calcium release by heparin. *J. Biol. Chem.* **263**, 11075–11079.

Iino, M. (1990). Biphasic Ca^{2+}-dependence of inositol 1,4,5-trisphosphate-induced Ca^{2+}-release in smooth muscle cells of the guinea pig taenia caeci. *J. Gen. Physiol.* **95**, 1103–1122.

Iino, M. & Endo, M. (1992). Calcium-dependent immediate feedback control of inositol 1,4,5-trisphosphate-induced Ca^{2+}-release. *Nature* **360**, 76–78.

Inoue, R. & Isenberg, G. (1990). Intracellular calcium ions modulate acetylcholine-induced inward current in guinea pig ileum. *J. Physiol.* **424**, 73–92.

Kobayashi, S., Somlyo, A.V. & Somlyo, A.P. (1988). Heparin inhibits the inositol 1,4,5-trisphosphate-dependent, but not the independent, calcium release induced by guanine nucleotide in vascular smooth muscle. *Biochem. Biophys. Res. Comm.* **153**, 625–631.

Komori, S. & Bolton, T.B. (1990). Role of G-proteins in muscarinic receptor inward and outward currents in rabbit jejunal smooth muscle. *J. Physiol.* **427**, 393–419.

Komori, S. & Bolton, T.B. (1991). Calcium release induced by inositol 1,4,5-trisphosphate in single intestinal smooth muscle cells. *J. Physiol.* **433**, 495–517.

Komori, S., Kawai, M., Takewaki, T. & Ohashi, H. (1992). GTP-binding protein involvement in membrane currents evoked by carbachol and histamine in guinea pig ileal muscle. *J. Physiol.* **450**, 105–126.

Komori, S., Kawai, M., Pacaud, P., Ohashi, H. & Bolton, T.B. (1993). Oscillations of receptor-operated cationic current and internal calcium in single guinea pig ileal smooth muscle cells. *Pflügers Arch.* **424**, 431–438.

Komori, S., Itagaki, M., Unno, T. & Ohashi, H. (1995). Caffeine and carbachol act on common Ca^{2+}-stores to release Ca^{2+} in guinea pig ileal smooth muscle. *Eur. J. Pharmacol.* **277**, 173–180.

Mayer, T. & Stryer, L. (1991). Calcium spiking. *Annu. Rev. Biophys. Chem.* **20**, 153–174.

Pacaud, P. & Bolton, T. B. (1991). Relation between muscarinic receptor cationic current and internal calcium in guinea pig jejunal smooth muscle cells. *J. Physiol.* **441**, 477–499.

Parker, I. & Ivorro, I. (1990). Inhibition by Ca^{2+} of inositol trisphosphate-mediated Ca^{2+} liberation: a possible mechanism for oscillating release of Ca^{2+}. *Proc. Natl Acad. Sci. USA* **87**, 260–264.

Prestwich, S. A. & Bolton, T. B. (1991). Measurement of picomole amounts of any inositol phosphate isomer separable by h.p.l.c. by means of a bioluminescence assay. *Biochem. J.* **274**, 663–672.

Putney, J.W. Jr. (1986). A model for receptor-regulated calcium entry. *Cell Calcium* **7**, 1–12.

Supattapone, S., Worley, P.F., Barahan, J.M. & Snyder, S.H. (1988). Solubilization, purification, and characterization of an inositol trisphosphate receptor. *J. Biol. Chem.* **263**, 1530–1534.

Tsien, R.W. & Tsien, R.Y. (1990). Calcium channels, stores, and oscillations. *Annu. Rev. Cell Biol.* **6**, 715–760.

Zholos, A. V., Baidan, L. V. & Shuba, M. F. (1991). Properties of the late transient outward current in isolated intestinal smooth muscle cells of the guinea pig. *J. Physiol.* **443**, 555–574.

Zholos, A. V., Baidan, L. V. & Shuba, M. F. (1992). Some properties of Ca^{2+}-induced Ca^{2+} release mechanism in single visceral smooth muscle cell of the guinea pig. *J. Physiol.* **457**, 1–25.

Zholos, A.V., Komori, S., Ohashi, H. & Bolton, T.B. (1994). Ca^{2+} inhibition of inositol trisphosphate-induced Ca^{2+} release in single smooth muscle cells of guinea pig small intestine. *J. Physiol.* **481**, 97–109.

18

Muscarinic Action on Smooth Muscle Membrane of Guinea Pig Urinary Bladder

M. YOSHINO*
K. TSUTAI
H. YABU

Department of Physiology, School of Medicine,
Sapporo Medical University,
Sapporo, Japan

**Department of Biology,*
Tokyo Gakugei University,
Koganei, Tokyo, Japan

INTRODUCTION

Muscarinic receptor activation induces membrane depolarization, action potential generation, and ultimately contraction in a variety of smooth muscles (Bolton, 1981). Membrane depolarization so far described in visceral smooth muscles is brought about by the opening of cation channels (CCs) (Benham *et al.*, 1985; Komori & Bolton, 1990; Inoue & Isenberg, 1990a,b,c; Vogalis & Sanders, 1990; Sims, 1992) and Ca^{2+}-activated Cl^- channels (Janssen & Sims, 1992; Ito *et al.*, 1993). Muscarinic receptor activation also modifies voltage-dependent currents such as inward calcium current (Clapp *et al.*, 1987; Beech, 1993; Nakayama, 1993), outward potassium current (Cole *et al.*, 1989) or M-current (Sims *et al.*, 1985).

In guinea pig detrusor smooth muscle, adenosine 5'-triphosphate (ATP) and acetylcholine (ACh) have been proposed by many researchers as excitatory neurotransmitters. The membrane depolarization response to these neurotransmitters, however, differs; ATP produces a large depolarization, whereas ACh and carbachol (CCh) produce only a small depolarization (Fujii, 1988; Brading & Mostwin, 1989). In experiments on single cells from guinea pig detrusor, it has been revealed that ATP binds to the P_{2X}-purinoceptor and induces a large inward current through ATP-gated nonselective cation channels (Inoue & Brading, 1990; Schneider *et al.*, 1991). However, little attention has been paid to understanding the cholinergic excitatory actions and the ACh-induced conductance. This may partly be due to the minor role of cholinergic nerves in causing membrane depolarization.

SMOOTH MUSCLE EXCITATION
ISBN 0-12-112360-X

In this paper, we describe the properties of the inward current elicited by CCh and the modulatory mechanism of voltage-dependent Ca channels by CCh in smooth muscle cells of the guinea pig urinary bladder.

RESULTS AND DISCUSSION

The effect of CCh on the action potential

In guinea pig detrusor cells, the rising phase of action potential (AP) is generated by an inward Ca current (I_{Ca}), whereas the repolarization phase is primarily generated by an outward K current that is Ca^{2+}-dependent (I_{K-Ca}) (Klöckner & Isenberg, 1985; Kura *et al.*, 1992). The effect of the muscarinic agonist, CCh, on the action potential (AP) has been examined (Figure 1). APs were elicited by current injections of the minimum strength required to cause an AP. Under control conditions, only two distinct APs were elicited during the period of current injection. After application of CCh (1 µM), the number of AP which were induced increased, but many of these APs were of a lower amplitude and longer duration. In these cells, 25 s after CCh application, the membrane potential (MP) was depolarized by about 20 mV to −36 mV from the resting potential of −56 mV. This depolarization by itself did not trigger an AP since it did not reach the voltage threshold required for activation of Ca channels.

A detectable membrane depolarization by CCh was observed in about 50% of the cells tested. However, even in the cells where no membrane depolarization was not observed on application of CCh, a reduction of AP amplitude and a prolongation in AP duration were observed. This result suggests that the changes in AP shape and the membrane depolarization are mediated by separate mechanisms. The observed change in AP shape implies that both I_{Ca} and I_{K-Ca} are suppressed by CCh. The membrane depolarization which occurs upon CCh addition, however, implies that there is a change in membrane conductance near the resting potential. In order to investigate the underlying mechanisms, we have carried out voltage-clamp experiments in guinea pig detrusor cells.

The effect of CCh on the membrane currents

The membrane current in smooth muscle cells of the guinea pig urinary bladder was recorded using the whole-cell patch-clamp technique at a holding potential of −60 mV (140 mM KCl in the patch pipette). Application of CCh (1–10 µM) to the cell produced an inward current which increased much more slowly and to a much less extent than the inward current elicited

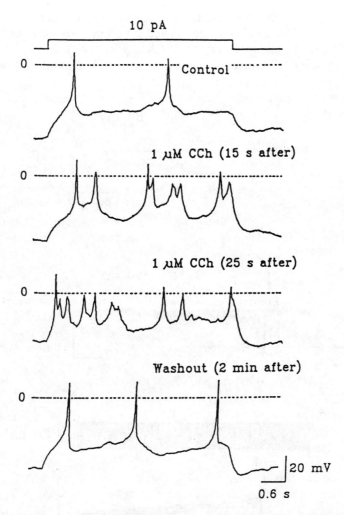

Figure 1 Effect of carbachol (CCh) on action potentials in guinea pig detrusor cells. The action potentials were elicited by applying a constant current at a minimum strength (10 pA). The action potentials were recorded 15 s, 25 s after application of 1 μM CCh and 2 min after wash-out of CCh. The resting membrane potential (−56 mV, control) depolarized to −50 mV (15 s after) and −36 mV (25 s after). After wash-out of CCh, it returned to −54 mV.

by 10 μM ATP (Figure 2A, B). However, CCh evoked a response that was far more sustained than the ATP-evoked response. Unfortunately, this sustained inward current was not always detected; in about 50% of the cells tested, CCh elicited a detectable inward current while in the remaining cells, CCh induced only an increase in baseline noise or a very small inward current.

However, in those cells where a detectable current was not seen, a detectable inward current could sometimes be elicited by applying a series of voltage command pulses to induce I_{Ca} prior to CCh application. This effect was not observed when the Ca antagonist, nifedipine, was present in the bath solution

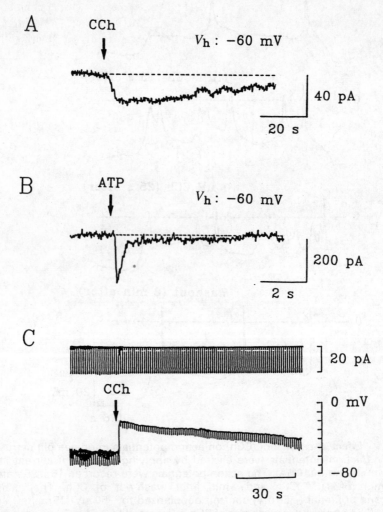

Figure 2 Effect of excitatory agonists on membrane current and membrane potential in guinea pig detrusor cells. Inward current elicited by 1 μM carbachol (CCh) (A) and 10 μM ATP (B). The holding potential was set to −60 mV. The patch pipette contained mainly 140 mM KCl with 0.05 mM EGTA. C, Effect of CCh (10 μM) on membrane potential and conductance. Constant hyperpolarizing pulses (top trace) were applied every 1 s. Application of CCh (10 μM) depolarized the cell and decreased the membrane resistance as indicated by a decrease in the amplitude of the electrotonic potentials.

or when external Ca^{2+} was replaced with equimolar Ba^{2+}. This suggests that Ca^{2+} influx through L-type Ca channels refills the internal Ca^{2+} store and so contributes to the inward current (Yoshino *et al.*, 1995b).

The reversal potential of the inward current evaluated by ramp voltage-clamp command was close to 0 mV (Figure 3) and was not significantly affected by replacing KCl with CsCl in the pipette solution. Replacing CsCl with caesium aspartate in the pipette solution or replacing NaCl with sodium glutamate in the bath solution also did not affect the reversal potential. Therefore, we conclude that the inward current is mediated by CCs. When

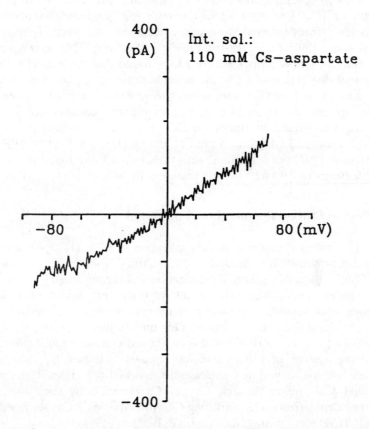

Figure 3 Current–voltage relationship for carbachol (CCh)-induced inward current obtained with ramp clamp. A ramp from −90 mV to +70 mV was performed within 1.5 s. CCh-induced current was obtained by subtracting the membrane current measured in the absence of CCh from the membrane current measured in the presence of CCh. The patch pipette contained mainly 110 mM Cs aspartate with 0.05 mM EGTA. The predicted reversal potential of Cl^- current (E_{Cl}) was −50.4 mV. Note the reversal potential of the CCh-induced current was 0 mV.

we included heparin ($3\,mg\,ml^{-1}$) in the patch pipette, application of CCh failed to induce a sustained inward current (Yoshino & Yabu, 1995), suggesting that this current is activated by Ca^{2+} release from an inositol 1,4,5-triphosphate ($InsP_3$)-sensitive internal store.

In guinea pig ileum and jejunal smooth muscles, it has been shown that an elevation of $[Ca^{2+}]_i$ enhances a cation current (Inoue & Isenberg, 1990c; Pacaud & Bolton, 1991). In this case, agonist is required for channel activation even if $[Ca^{2+}]_i$ is high. Thus, Ca^{2+} enhances the cation current but cannot activate channels in itself. This effect is therefore called facilitatory action. CCs in several smooth muscles, however, are activated directly by elevation of $[Ca^{2+}]_i$ without agonist stimulation. Caffeine, an agent that releases Ca^{2+} from internal store can elicit a cation current (portal vein, Loirand *et al.*, 1991; canine gastric muscle cells, Sims, 1992; airway smooth muscle cell, Janssen & Sims, 1992). We have found that, caffeine (10–20 mM) could mimic the action of CCh; the caffeine-induced current was similar to the current elicited by CCh with respect to reversal potential, a linear I–V relationship and its association with a membrane conductance increase. Therefore, CCs found in smooth muscle cells of the guinea pig urinary bladder are more like to those found in airway (Janssen & Sims, 1992) and gastric (Sims, 1992) smooth muscle cells rather than those found in intestinal (Inoue & Isenberg, 1990a,b) smooth muscle cells.

The effect of CCh on the membrane potential

Under the current clamp condition, application of CCh (1–10 μM) caused a sustained depolarization to around -30 to $-20\,mV$ from the resting potential near $-50\,mV$ (Figure 2C). This depolarization was accompanied by an increase in membrane conductance. The result suggests that under physiological conditions, the sustained inward current can mediate the CCh-induced depolarization of the cell membrane. Our unpublished experiments suggest that sustained inward current can also be elicited without agonist stimulation by applying a series of voltage command pulses to induce I_{Ca}. Addition of nifedipine, a dihydropyridine Ca antagonist, blocked this effect. These results imply that Ca^{2+} influx through L-types Ca channels by itself can cause membrane depolarization by activating CCs probably via a Ca^{2+}-induced Ca^{2+} release (CICR) mechanism (Ganitkevich & Isenberg, 1991, 1992).

The effect of CCh on the voltage-activated Ca channels

Muscarinic receptor activation has been reported to increase I_{Ca} in amphibian smooth muscles (Clapp *et al.*, 1987). Contrary to this, I_{Ca} has been shown to be suppressed by muscarinic agonist in several types of mammalian visceral smooth muscles. The underlying mechanism is thought to be via a Ca^{2+}-mediated inactivation of Ca channels caused by Ca^{2+} release from $InsP_3$ sensitive internal stores, although Ca^{2+} mobilization from the internal store does not always appear to be essential for Ca^{2+}-mediated inactivation of Ca channels to occur (Yoshino *et al.*, 1995a). Beech (1993) proposed a mechanism other than this to be responsible for I_{Ca} suppression when excitatory agonists are applied. This is a G-protein mediated mechanism which does not require Ca^{2+} release from $InsP_3$ sensitive internal store but does require internal $[Ca^{2+}]_i$ at resting state. In guinea pig detrusor cells, we found that application of CCh causes a sustained suppression of I_{Ca} (Yoshino & Yabu, 1995) (Figure 4). Approximately half of the total I_{Ca} suppression induced by CCh is due to Ca^{2+}-release from $InsP_3$ sensitive internal store. The other portion of I_{Ca} suppression is caused by a G-protein mediated mechanism which requires internal $[Ca^{2+}]_i$ at resting state but does not require the activation of protein kinase C (Yoshino & Yabu, 1995).

The suppresion of I_{Ca} induced by muscarinic receptor activation would at first glance appear to be contrary to the excitatory role of muscarinic agonist. A reduction of I_{Ca}, however, would tend to suppress Ca^{2+}-activated K^+ channels. This would allow depolarization rather than after-hyperpolarization following an AP as Ca^{2+}-activated K^+ channels are responsible

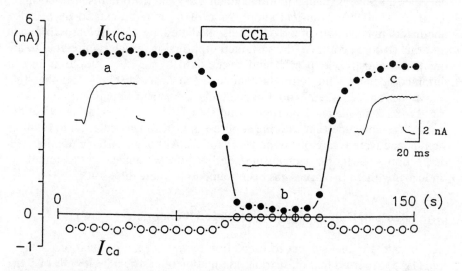

Figure 4 Effect of CCh on net membrane currents. The cell was depolarized from −60 mV to 10 mV (100 ms duration) every 5 s. The patch pipette contained mainly 140 mM KCl with 0.05 mM EGTA. The time course of changes in the peak inward current (mainly I_{Ca}) (open circles) and the peak outward current (mainly I_{K-Ca}) (closed circles) by 10 μM CCh. The bar indicates the perfusion time of CCh.

for AP repolarization in this cell. Suppression of Ca^{2+}-activated K^+ channel would prolong the AP duration and also lead to an increase in AP frequency. Our unpublished experiments show that there is a significant positive correlation (correlation coefficient, $r = 0.96$) between the amplitude of I_{Ca} and $I_{K\text{-}Ca}$ measured from the net membrane currents in guinea pig detrusor cells. This positive correlation was disrupted by applying cyclopiazonic acid ($r = 0.16$) or caffeine ($r = 0.59$) to the bath solution, which suggests that the activation of Ca^{2+}-activated K^+ channels involves a CICR mechanism which is triggered by Ca^{2+} influx through Ca channels. Therefore, it appears that the inhibition of Ca channels causes reduction of Ca^{2+}-activated K^+ channel current by reducing CICR.

The effect of caffeine on the voltage-activated Ca channels

The use of caffeine has become one of the standard tools used to indicate an involvement of internal Ca^{2+} store in cellular function. Recent studies have shown that caffeine suppresses voltage-activated Ca channels not only through its Ca^{2+} releasing action (Zholos *et al.*, 1991) but also by possible direct actions on the channel (Martin *et al.*, 1989; Hughes *et al.*, 1990; Zholos *et al.*, 1991). We have shown that caffeine suppresses I_{Ca} via two different mechanisms; one is related to intracellular Ca^{2+} and the other is not (Yoshino *et al.*, 1993, 1996). Transient suppression of I_{Ca} may be caused by a Ca^{2+}-mediated inactivation of Ca channels mediated by Ca^{2+} release from an internal store. In contrast, the sustained suppression, which is unrelated to an increase in cytosolic $[Ca^{2+}]_i$ and cyclic AMP, may be due to a direct interaction of caffeine with Ca channels. We have further found that the direct action of caffeine on Ca channels is voltage dependent; the drug producing a significant hyperpolarizing shift in the steady-state inactivation curve. We conclude that caffeine suppresses I_{Ca} through preferential binding to the inactivated state of L-type Ca channels. Although caffeine mimics well the action of CCh, the mechanism underlying the sustained suppression of I_{Ca} induced by these two drugs has been found to be quite different.

The effects of CCh on the Ca^{2+}-activated K channels

K currents are also subject to regulation by muscarinic stimulation. Sims *et al.*, (1985) reported that muscarinic stimulation of gastric muscle cells of *Bufo marinus* suppresses a K current (designated M-current) which was first described while investigating sympathetic neurones. In mammalian smooth muscle cells, there is no evidence for a M current; instead, Ca^{2+} activated K^+ channels may be the primary site of regulation. It has been reported that $I_{K\text{-}Ca}$ is suppressed by muscarinic receptor activation in several mammalian visceral smooth muscle cells. This is also the case in guinea pig detrusor cells (Figure 4). The mechanisms underlying I_{K-Ca} suppression appear to differ from tissue to tissue. Suzuki *et al.*, (1992) have shown that depletion of Ca^{2+} in the internal store may be responsible for the suppresion of I_{K-Ca} in guinea pig detrusor cells. It seems that the suppression of I_{K-Ca} together with the suppression of I_{Ca} is an essential mechanism of cholinergic excitatory neurotransmission in mammalian visceral smooth muscles.

CONCLUSION

In smooth muscle cells isolated from guinea pig urinary bladder, muscarinic stimulation induces a membrane depolarization accompanied by a membrane conductance increase. This depolarization has been found to be mediated by an opening of cation conductance which is elicited by Ca^{2+} release from the $InsP_3$ sensitive internal store. The depolarization may, in turn, cause activation of voltage-dependent Ca channels. The resultant Ca^{2+} entry through Ca channels may contribute to the refilling of internal Ca^{2+} store and to the activation of CCs through CICR. Suppression of I_{Ca} induced by muscarinic receptor activation is mediated by a dual mechanism: Ca^{2+}-mediated suppression via Ca^{2+} release from the $InsP_3$-sensitive internal store and G-protein-mediated suppression which requires internal Ca^{2+} at the resting level. The suppression of I_{Ca} may lead to a reduction in the CICR mechanism and therefore lower activation of Ca^{2+}-activated K^+ channels. As a result, we believe that the after-hyperpolarization of the AP is reduced, thus allowing more rapid Ca channel reactivation which would lead to an increase in AP frequency. Suppression of I_{K-Ca} induced by muscarinic receptor activation may further reduce the size of the AP after-hyperpolarization. It appears that the suppression of both I_{Ca} and I_{K-Ca} may participate in the regulatory mechanisms brought into play by cholinergic excitatory nerves and which are responsible for the increased frequency of action potential discharge and ultimately contraction of the muscle.

REFERENCES

Beech, D.J. (1993) Inhibitory effects of histamine and bradykinin on calcium current in smooth muscle cells isolated from guinea pig ileum. *J. Physiol.* **463**, 565–583.

Benham, C.D., Bolton, T.B. & Lang, R.J. (1985) Acetylcholine activates an inward current in single mammalian smooth muscle cells. *Nature* **316**, 345–347.

Bolton, T.B. (1981) Action of acetylcholine on the smooth muscle membrane. In *Smooth Muscle: An Assessment of Current Knowledge*, (Bulbring, E., Brading, A.F., Jones, A.W. & Tomita, T., eds), pp.199–217. Arnold, London.

Brading, A.F. & Mostwin, J.L. (1989) Electrical and mechanical responses of guinea pig bladder muscle to nerve stimulation. *Br. J. Pharmacol.* **98**, 1083–1090.

Clapp, L.H., Vivaudou, M.B., Walsh, J.V.Jr. & Singer, J.J. (1987). Acetylcholine increases voltage-activated Ca^{2+} current in freshly dissociated smooth muscle cells. *Proc. Natl Acad. Sci. USA* **84**, 2092–2096.

Cole, W.C., Carl, A. & Sanders, K.M. (1989) Muscarinic suppression of Ca^{2+}-dependent K current in colonic smooth muscle. *Am. J. Physiol.* **257** (*Cell Physiol.* 26), C481–C487.

Fujii, K. (1988) Evidence for adenosine triphosphate as an excitatory transmitter in guinea pig, rabbit and pig urinary bladder. *J. Physiol.* **404**, 39–52.

Ganitkevich, V.Y.A. & Isenberg, G. (1991) Depolarization-mediated intracellular calcium transients in isolated smooth muscle cells of guinea pig urinary bladder. *J. Physiol. (London)* **435**, 187–205.

Ganitkevich, V.Y.A & Isenberg, G. (1992) Contribution of Ca^{2+}-induced Ca^{2+} release to the $[Ca^{2+}]_i$ transients in myocytes from guinea pig urinary bladder. *J. Physiol. (London)* **458**, 119–147.

Hughes, A.D., Hering, S. & Bolton, T.B. (1990) The action of caffeine on inward barium current throgh voltage-dependent calcium channels in single rabbit ear artery cells. *Pflügers Arch.* **416**, 462–466.

Inoue, R. & Brading, A.F. (1990) The properties of the ATP-induced depolarization and current in single cells isolated from guinea pig urinary bladder. *Br. J. Pharmacol.* **100**, 619–625.

Inoue, R. & Isenberg, G. (1990a) Acetylcholine activates non-selective cation channels in guinea pig ileum through G protein. *Am. J. Physiol.* **258** (*Cell Physiology* 27), C1173–C1178.

Inoue, R. & Isenberg, G. (1990b) Effect of membrane potential on acetylcholine-induced inward current in guinea pig ileum. *J. Physiol. (London)* **424**, 57–71.

Inoue, R. & Isenberg, G. (1990c) Intracellular calcium ions modulate acetylcholine-induced inward current in guinea pig ileum. *J. Physiol. (London)* **424**, 73–92.

Ito, S., Ohta, T. & Nakazato, Y. (1993) Inward current activated by carbachol in intestinal smooth muscle cells. *J. Physiol. (London)* **470**, 395–409.

Janssen, L.J. & Sims, S.M. (1992) Acetylcholine activates non-selective cation and chloride conductances in canine and guinea pig tracheal smooth muscle cells. *J. Physiol. (London)* **453**, 197–218.

Klöckner, U. & Isenberg, G. (1985) Action potentials and net membrane currents of isolated smooth muscle cells (urinary bladder of the guinea pig). *Pflügers Arch.* **405**, 329–339.

Komori, S. & Bolton, T.B. (1990) Role of G-proteins in muscarinic receptor inward and outward currents in rabbit jejunal smooth muscle. *J. Physiol.* **427**, 395–419.

Kura, H., Yoshino, M. & Yabu, H. (1992) Blocking action of terodiline on calcium channels in single smooth muscle cells of the guinea pig urinary bladder. *J. Pharmacol. Exp. Ther.* **261**, 724–729.

Loirand, G.P., Pacaud, A., Baron, C. Mironneau, C & Mironneau, J. (1991) Large conductance calcium-activated non-selective cation channel in smooth muscle cells isolated from rat portal vein. *J. Physiol. (London)* **437**, 461–475.

Martin, C., Dacquet, C., Mironneau, C. & Mironneau, J. (1989) Caffeine-induced inhibition of calcium channel current in cultured smooth muscle cells from pregnant rat myometrium. *Br. J. Pharmacol.* **98**, 493–498.

Nakayama, S. (1993) Effects of excitatory neurotransmitters on Ca channel current in smooth muscle cells isolated from guinea pig urinary bladder. *Br. J. Pharmacol.* **110**, 317–325.

Pacaud, P. & Bolton, T.B. (1991) Relationship between muscarinic receptor cationinc current and internal calcium in guinea pig jejunal smooth muscle. *J. Physiol. (London)* **441**, 477–499.

Schneider, P. Hopp, H.H. & Isenberg, G. (1991) Ca^{2+} influx through ATP-gated channels increments $[Ca^{2+}]_i$ and inactivates Ica in myocytes from guinea pig urinary bladder. *J. Physiol. (London)* **440**, 479–496.

Sims, S.M. (1992) Cholinergic activation of non-selective cation current in canine gastric smooth muscle is associated with contraction. *J. Physiol. (London)* **449**, 377–398.

Sims, S.M., Singer, J.J. & Walsh, J.V. Jr. (1985) cholinergic agonists suppress a potasium current in freshly dissociated smooth muscle cells of the toad. *J. Physiol. (London)* **367**, 503–529.

Suzuki, M. Muraki, K. Imaizumi, Y. & Watanabe, M. (1992) Cyclopiazinic acid, an inhibitor of the sarcoplasmic reticulum Ca^{2+}-pump, reduces Ca^{2+}-dependent K^+ currents in guinea pig smooth muscle cells. *Br. J. Pharmacol.* **107**, 134–140.

Vogalis, F. & Sanders, K.M. (1990) Cholinergic stimulation activates a non-selective cation current in canine pyloric circular muscle cells. *J. Physiol.* **429**, 223–236.

Yoshino, M. & Yabu, H. (1995) Muscarinic suppression of Ca current in smooth muscle cells of the guinea pig urinary bladder. *Exp. Physiol.* **80**, 575–587.

Yoshino, M., Matsufuji, Y. & Yabu, H. (1993) Voltage-dependent block of L-type Ca channels by caffeine in smooth myocytes of the guinea pig urinary bladder. *Ann. Acad. Sci.* **707**, 362–364.

Yoshino, M., Matsufuji, Y. & Yabu, H.(1995a) Properties of Ca^{2+}-mediated inactivation of Ca current in smooth muslce cells of the guinea pig urinary bladder. *Can. J. Physiol. Pharmacol.* **73**, 27–35.

Yoshino, M., Matsufuji, Y. & Yabu, H. (1996) Voltage-dependent suppression of calcium current by caffeine in smooth muscle cells of the guinea pig urinary bladder. *Naunyn-Schmiedeberg's Arch. Pharmacol.* **353**, 334–341.

Yoshino M, Tsutai K & Yabu H (1995b) Non-selective cation channels in smooth muscle cells of the guinea pig urinary bladder. *J. Muscle Res. Cell Motility.* **16**(3), 347.

Zholos, A.V., Baidan, L.V. & Shuba, M.F. (1991) The inhibitory action of caffeine on calcium currents in isolated intestinal smooth muscle cells. *Pflügers Arch.* **419**, 267–273.

19

Transduction Pathways Activated by α-Adrenoceptors in Vascular Myocytes: Effects on Release of Stored Ca²⁺ and Voltage-dependent Ca²⁺ Channels

JEAN MIRONNEAU
NATHALIE MACREZ-LEPRÊTRE
CHANTAL MIRONNEAU

*Laboratoire de Physiologie Cellulaire et Pharmacologie Moléculaire,
CNRS URA 1489, Université de Bordeaux II,
Bordeaux, France*

SUMMARY

1. The effects of noradrenaline, methoxamine, phenylephrine, clonidine and oxymetazoline were studied on release of intracellular Ca^{2+}, inositol phosphate accumulation and voltage-dependent Ca^{2+} channel stimulation in rat portal vein smooth muscle.
2. The free cytoplasmic Ca^{2+} concentration ($[Ca^{2+}]_i$) was estimated using emission from fura-2 or Indo-1 dyes in single myocytes. Using subtype-selective adrenoceptor agonists and antagonists we showed that only α_{1A}-adrenoceptors mediated intracellular Ca^{2+} release and inositol phosphate accumulation (measured with a biochemical assay in intact strips). The α_{1A}-adrenoceptor-induced responses were insensitive to pertussis toxin-pretreatment, but were blocked in a concentration-dependent manner by intracellular dialysis with a pipette solution containing anti-$G\alpha_q/\alpha_{11}$ or anti-phosphatidylinositol antibodies (whole-cell recording mode of the patch-clamp technique).
3. The Ca^{2+} channel current was enhanced by both α_1- and α_2-adrenoceptor agonists. Using subtype-selective antagonists we showed that both α_{1A}- and α_{2A}-adrenoceptors modulate Ca^{2+} channels. However, internal applications of anti-phosphatidylinositol and anti-$G\alpha_q/\alpha_{11}$ antibodies had no effect on the α_{2A}-adrenoceptor-induced enhancement of Ca^{2+} channel

SMOOTH MUSCLE EXCITATION
ISBN 0-12-112360-X

current. In contrast, the α_{2A}-adrenoceptor-induced enhancement of Ca^{2+} channel current was blocked by pertussis toxin-pretreatment and internal applications of anti-$G\alpha_{i1,2}$ antibody.

4. Modulation of Ca^{2+} channels by α_{1A}- and α_{2A}-adrenoceptors was inhibited by external application of a protein kinase C inhibitor (GF109203X) and a long-term (24 h) treatment with 0.1 μM phorbol dibutyrate to decrease the activity of protein kinase C.

5. The effect on voltage-dependent Ca^{2+} channels of α_{2A}-adrenoceptor activation alone produces a slow, small and sustained increase in $[Ca^{2+}]_i$ without Ca^{2+} release from intracellular stores. These effects result in an increase of spontaneous contractile activity but no tetanus occurs. Activation of α_{1A}-adrenoceptors induces a large release of stored Ca^{2+} which activates chloride- and cation channels leading to membrane depolarization and opening of Ca^{2+} channels. In addition, Ca^{2+} channels are stimulated via the DAG-activated protein kinase C coupling. The contractile response corresponds to a tetanus.

INTRODUCTION

Molecular cloning studies have identified the existence of three or four subtypes of α_1- and α_2-adrenoceptors (for reviews, see: Ford *et al.*, 1994; McKinnon *et al.*, 1994). The subdivision of α-adrenoceptors is derived principally from binding and functional studies and the pharmacological profile of each subtype is determined by using selective agonists and antagonists.

In vascular smooth muscle, noradrenaline evokes contractions which are dependent on both Ca^{2+} influx through voltage-dependent Ca^{2+} channels and Ca^{2+} release from intracellular stores (Mironneau & Gargouil, 1979). However, the multiplicity of adrenoceptor subtypes and ion channels leads us to reinvestigate the effects of noradrenaline in rat portal vein myocytes in order to identify: (1) the subtypes of α_1- and α_2-adrenoceptors involved in the noradrenaline action; (2) the Ca^{2+} sources activated by the different α-adrenoceptor subtypes, and (3) the transduction pathways which couple α-adrenoceptors to Ca^{2+} channels and Ca^{2+} release from intracellular stores.

METHODS

The enzymatic dispersion procedure for isolating single myocytes from rat portal vein was identical to that previously described (Leprêtre *et al.*, 1994b). Voltage-clamp and membrane current recordings were made with a standard patch-clamp technique. Whole-cell membrane currents were measured with either the perforated-patch method or the classical whole-cell mode. In order to obtain a perforated patch, nystatin (80–100 μg ml^{-1}) was present in the patch pipette solution (Leprêtre *et al.*, 1994c). Simultaneous measurements of intracellular Ca^{2+} concentration were carried out in some experiments. Briefly, $100 \mu M$ fura-2 or $50 \mu M$ Indo-1 were added to the pipette solution and entered cells following establishment of the whole-cell recording mode. $[Ca^{2+}]_i$ was estimated from fluorescence ratio using a calibration determined within cells.

[^{3}H]inositol phosphate measurements were performed, as previously described (Leprêtre *et al.*, 1994b). Rat portal vein strips (20–25 mg wet weight) were cleaned free of endothelium and incubated with 407 kBq of myo-[2-^{3}H]-inositol (0.6 μM) in 1 ml of fresh buffer for 3.5 h. After washing the tissues, 10 mM LiCl were added for 10 min before applications of adrenoceptor antagonists. Antagonists were added 5 min before addition of adrenoceptor agonists. Separation of inositol phosphates was made on anion exchange resin columns (Marc *et al.*, 1986).

Purification and specificity of the antibodies directed against phosphatidylinositol and the α-subunits of G_o, G_i, G_q and G_{11} proteins have been previously reported (Leprêtre *et al.*, 1994b,c ; Leprêtre & Mironneau, 1994). Antibodies were added to the pipette solution to allow dialysis of the cell after a breakthrough in whole-cell recording mode.

Isometric contractions of longitudinal strips from rat portal vein were recorded as previously described (Mironneau *et al.*, 1980).

The normal physiological solution contained (in mM) : 130 NaCl, 5.6 KCl, 1 $MgCl_2$, 2 $CaCl_2$, 11 glucose, 10 HEPES, pH 7.3 with NaOH. The basic pipette solution contained (in mM): 130 CsCl, 10 HEPES, pH 7.3 with CsOH. Ca^{2+}-free external solution was prepared by omitting $CaCl_2$ and by adding 0.5 mM EGTA. For the recordings of Ca^{2+} channel current, 5 mM $BaCl_2$ was substituted for $CaCl_2$ in the physiological solution and 5 mM EGTA, 5 mM Na_2ATP and 1 mM $MgCl_2$ were added to the basic pipette solution. Adrenoceptor agonists were applied to the recorded cell by pressure ejection from a glass pipette for the period indicated on the records. Before each experiment a fast application of physiological solution was tested, and cells with movement artefacts were excluded.

The results are expressed as means ± SE Significance was tested by means of Student's t-test. P values of <0.05 were considered as significant. Inhibition and concentration-dependent curves were analysed by a nonlinear least-square fitting program, according to models involving one or two binding sites.

RESULTS

Effects of α-adrenoceptor agonists on cytoplasmic Ca^{2+} concentration and inositol phosphate accumulation

In single myocytes isolated from rat portal vein, ejection of 10 μM noradrenaline (a non-specific α-adrenoceptor agonist) or phenylephrine (an

α_1-adrenoceptor agonist) caused a biphasic Ca^{2+} response (Figure 1). The rapid, initial increase in $[Ca^{2+}]_i$ was still present in Ca^{2+}-free solution whereas the sustained phase was absent. In the presence of $1\,\mu M$ oxodipine or elgodipine (light-stable dihydropyridines; Baron et al., 1994 ; Leprêtre et al., 1994a), the transient Ca^{2+} response and the sustained phase were reduced by about 20% and 50%, respectively. In contrast, clonidine (an α_2-adrenoceptor agonist) was unable to induce a Ca^{2+} response in the presence of oxodipine (Figure 1). These results support the idea that the release of Ca^{2+} from the intracellular store is mediated through activation of α_1-adrenoceptors alone.

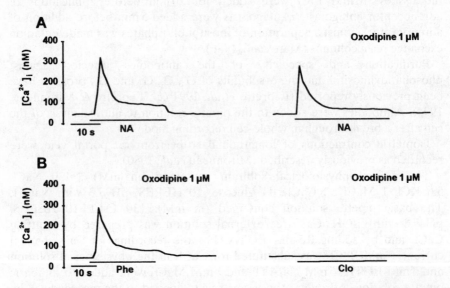

Figure 1 Effects of applications of $10\,\mu M$ noradrenaline (NA), phenylephrine (Phe) and clonidine (Clo) on $[Ca^{2+}]_i$ in single myocytes of rat portal vein. The cells were loaded with fura-2AM and not patch-clamped. A, Ejections of NA for 30s induced a transient increase in $[Ca^{2+}]_i$ followed by a sustained phase. Addition of $1\,\mu M$ oxodipine for 4 min decreased both Ca^{2+} phases. B, In the presence of $1\,\mu M$ oxodipine, $10\,\mu M$ Phe evoked a biphasic Ca^{2+} response whereas Clo was ineffective. Similar results were obtained in 12–25 cells.

The pharmacological profile of the α_1-adrenoceptor-induced Ca^{2+} release was studied with compounds selective for the different α_1-adrenoceptor subtypes. Preincubation with $50\,\mu M$ chloroethylclonidine (an agent which alkylated irreversibly the α_{1B}-adrenoceptor subtype) for 3 min had no effect on the transient Ca^{2+} responses evoked by noradrenaline, phenylephrine or methoxamine (an α_{1A}-adrenoceptor agonist). Prazosin, WB4101 and HV723 antagonized the Ca^{2+} response with the following concentrations producing half-maximal inhibition (IC_{50}): 0.04 nM for prazosin, 0.12 nM for WB4101 and 0.18 nM for HV723. The Hill coefficient was close to unity for each antagonist. The rank order of potency was, therefore, prazosin >WB4101 >HV723.

Noradrenaline and methoxamine stimulated, in a concentration-dependent manner, the generation of inositol phosphates. Prazosin, WB4101 and HV723 inhibited inositol phosphate accumulation with IC_{50} values somewhat higher than those obtained on the Ca^{2+} responses but with the same order of potency (Leprêtre et al., 1994b).

Effects on chloride channels

Ejection of 10 μM noradrenaline or phenylephrine on single myocytes held at -50 mV evoked a large and transient depolarizing current (Mironneau, 1991; Mironneau, 1995). In contrast, 10 μM clonidine evoked a slow, sustained and small inward current. Using various chloride concentrations in the bathing and pipette solutions we showed that only $α_1$-adrenoceptor agonists activated a chloride current when the transient increase in $[Ca^{2+}]_i$ was larger than 180 nM. In addition, the gating of the chloride channels was mainly controlled by the $[Ca^{2+}]_i$ level, independently of the rate of increase in cytoplasmic Ca^{2+}.

Effects on voltage-dependent Ca^{2+} channels

The maximal Ca^{2+} channel current, evoked by a depolarization to 0 mV from a holding potential of -60 mV, was increased by 43% by 10 μM noradrenaline, and 30% by 10 μM phenylephrine or clonidine. The phenylephrine-induced stimulation of the Ca^{2+} channel current was selectively inhibited by prazosin with an IC_{50} of 0.25 nM. The clonidine-induced stimulation was inhibited by rauwolscine with an IC_{50} of 0.70 nM. The Hill coefficients were close to unity, suggesting homogenous receptor populations. In contrast, prazosin produced a biphasic inhibition of the noradrenaline-induced stimulation of the Ca^{2+} channel current. If prazosin bound to two different sites, the estimated IC_{50} could be 5 nM and 7 μM, respectively. In addition, the stimulatory effect of noradrenaline on Ca^{2+} channel current was inhibited by rauwolscine with an IC_{50} of 1.6 nM, suggesting that noradrenaline activated both $α_1$- and $α_2$-adrenoceptors (Leprêtre et al., 1994c).

The phenylephrine-induced stimulation of the Ca^{2+} channel current was insensitive to chloroethylclonidine pretreatment (50 μM; 30 min), but inhibited by WB4101 with a high potency (0.2 nM) similar to that of prazosin. These results suggest that activation of $α_{1A}$-adrenoceptors is involved in both

Ca^{2+} release from intracellular stores and stimulation of voltage-dependent Ca^{2+} channels.

The clonidine-induced stimulation of the Ca^{2+} channel current was selectively inhibited by oxymetazoline, RX821002 and rauwolscine with the following IC_{50} values: 0.19 nM for oxymetazoline, 0.39 nM for RX821002 and 0.70 nM for rauwolscine. As expected from its partial agonist properties, ejections of 10 μM oxymetazoline produced an increase of Ca^{2+} channel current that reached about 25%. Therefore, in venous myocytes, the $α_2$-adrenoceptor-induced stimulation of Ca^{2+} channels corresponds to the $α_{2A}$-adrenoceptors (Leprêtre *et al.*, 1994c).

Transduction pathways

Antibodies directed against phosphatidylinositols have been used to identify the membrane phospholipids involved in the $α_1$- and $α_2$-adrenoceptor-activated transduction pathways. Intracellular applications of 15 μg ml^{-1} anti-phosphatidylinositol antibody specifically inhibited phenylephrine-induced Ca^{2+} release and stimulation of Ca^{2+} channels. In contrast, the clonidine-induced enhancement of Ca^{2+} channel current was insensitive to internal applications of 15–20 μg ml^{-1} anti-PtdIns antibody.

Similarly, incubation of the myocytes with 0.4 μg ml^{-1} pertussis toxin (PTX) for 24 h at 37°C had no effect on the phenylephrine-induced Ca^{2+} release and stimulation of Ca^{2+} channels, but completely abolished the clonidine-induced enhancement of Ca^{2+} channel current. The noradrenaline-induced enhancement of the Ca^{2+} channel current was reduced by about 65%. Moreover, internal applications of antibodies directed against the α-subunits of G_{o1}, G_{o2}, $G_{i1,2}$, G_{i3} and G_q/G_{11} proteins showed that the anti-$α_q/α_{11}$ antibodies selectively suppressed the stimulatory effects of phenylephrine on Ca^{2+} channels, whereas anti-$α_{i1,2}$ antibodies selectively suppressed the stimulatory effects of clonidine (Leprêtre *et al.*, 1994c; Macrez-Leprêtre *et al.*, 1995.

Involvement of protein kinase C in the α-adrenoceptors-induced stimulation of Ca^{2+} channels was examined by testing the effects of a protein kinase C inhibitor (GF109203X; Toullec *et al.*, 1991) and prolonged (24 h) pretreatment with phorbol dibutyrate. Both application of 1 μM GF109203X and 24 h pretreatment with 0.1 μM phorbol dibutyrate suppressed the enhancement of the Ca^{2+} channel current evoked by 10 μM noradrenaline, phenylephrine and clonidine or 0.1 μM phorbol dibutyrate.

Ca^{2+} influx induced by $α_2$-adrenoceptor agonists

In the presence of 0.1 μM prazosin, 10 μM noradrenaline evoked a slow, sustained and maintained increase in $[Ca^{2+}]_i$ (Figure 2A) which was selectively inhibited by 0.1 μM rauwolscine. This Ca^{2+} response was similar to

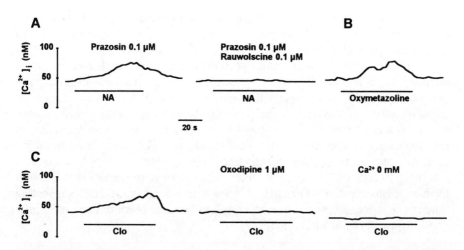

Figure 2 Effect of α-adrenoceptor agonists and antagonists on $[Ca^{2+}]_i$. The cells were loaded with fura-2AM and not patch-clamped. A, Long ejections of $10\,\mu M$ NA, in the presence of 0.1 mM prazosin, evoked a slow and sustained increase in $[Ca^{2+}]_i$ which was blocked by $0.1\,\mu M$ rauwolscine. B, Ejection of $10\,\mu M$ oxymetazoline induced a Ca^{2+} response similar to that shown with NA (in the presence of prazosin). C, The clonidine (Clo)-induced increase in $[Ca^{2+}]_i$ was completely blocked after addition of $1\,\mu M$ oxodipine or after incubation in Ca^{2+}-free solution for 3 min. External solution contained $1\,\mu M$ propranolol.

those evoked by $10\,\mu M$ clonidine (Figure 2C) and oxymetazoline (a selective α_{2A}-adrenoceptor agonist, Figure 2B). The mean increase in $[Ca^{2+}]_i$ reached about 30–35 nM. The clonidine-induced Ca^{2+} response was suppressed in Ca^{2+}-free external solution for 30 s and in the presence of $1\,\mu M$ oxodipine for 5 min (Figure 2C). These results suggest that the α_2-adrenoceptor-activated Ca^{2+} response results from Ca^{2+} influx through voltage-dependent L-type Ca^{2+} channels.

After pertussis toxin treatment $(0.4\,\mu g\,ml^{-1}$ for 24 h) the clonidine-activated Ca^{2+} response was reduced by 50% but not completely removed. In addition, application of $1\,\mu M$ GF109203X depressed the clonidine-induced Ca^{2+} response by 70%. These results indicate that the Ca^{2+} influx is mediated by activation of protein kinase C via a coupling involving, presumably, a G_i protein (Leprêtre & Mironneau, 1994; Macrez-Leprêtre et al., 1995).

Contractions induced by α-adrenoceptor agonists

In Ca^{2+}-containing solution, noradrenaline produced large and complex contractions which depended on the concentrations used. Low concentrations of noradrenaline (100 nM) augmented the frequency of spontaneous contractions with a small increase in the basal tone (Figure 3A). After removal of noradrenaline, the frequency of contractions returned to control, but the amplitude was strongly increased subsequently for 5–6 min. This response was similar to that induced by a high concentration (10 μM) of clonidine (Figure 3C), suggesting that the α_2-adrenoceptor-activated coupling was primarily involved with low concentrations of noradrenaline. In contrast, high concentrations (10 μM) of noradrenaline produced a large increase in the basal tone and a corresponding reduction of the spontaneous contraction amplitude (Figure 3B). After noradrenaline removal, the spontaneous contractions had a larger amplitude before returning to control. This type of contractile response resembles that induced by high concentrations (10 μM) of phenylephrine (Figure 3D), suggesting that the α_1-adrenoceptor-activated coupling became predominant with high concentrations of noradrenaline.

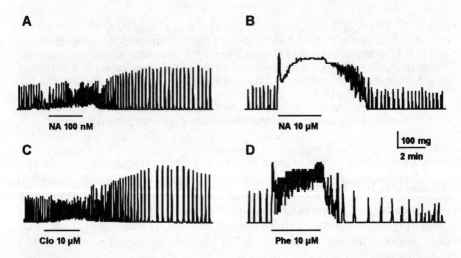

Figure 3 Typical contractions of intact rat portal vein strips induced by 100 nM (A) and 10 μM noadreline (NA) (B), by 10 μM clonidine (Clo) (C) and 10 μM phenylephrine (Phe) (D).

DISCUSSION

In this study, we show that stimulation of voltage-dependent Ca^{2+} channels in myocytes of rat portal vein is promoted by activation of both α_{1A}- and α_{2A}-adrenoceptors through two distinct transduction pathways involving different G-proteins and membrane phospholipids, both leading to activation of protein kinase C.

We demonstrated that, in native venous myocytes, activation of α_{1A}-adrenoceptors alone leads to phosphatidylinositol hydrolysis and release of Ca^{2+} from intracellular stores through a coupling process involving a G_q/G_{11} protein, insensitive to pertussis toxin, which activates a phospholipase C isoform and the subsequent generation of inositol 1,4,5-trisphosphate. This conclusion is in good agreement with data obtained in transfected cells which show that all three of the α_1-adrenoceptors can activate phosphatidylinositol-specific phospholipase Cβ by coupling to G_q-protein (Wu et al., 1992). Whether this or other transduction pathways may have a role in regulating voltage-dependent Ca^{2+} channels has not been previously established in vascular myocytes. We showed that both α_{1A}- and α_{2A}-adrenoceptors led to stimulation of Ca^{2+} channels through two distinct transduction pathways. Our finding that pertussis toxin partially inhibited the noradrenaline-induced enhancement of Ca^{2+} channel current disagrees with a previous study showing insensitivity of this noradrenaline-induced effect to pertussis toxin (Loirand et al., 1992). Possible explanations for this discrepancy are the too- limited number of cells tested and the use of nonselective α-adrenoceptor agonists and antagonists in the experiments of Loirand et al. (1992), and the application of the less intrusive method of perforated-patch recording in the present study. This interpretation is supported by the observation that treatment with pertussis toxin abolishes the clonidine-induced stimulation of Ca^{2+} channels but has no effect on the phenylephrine-induced response. The pertussis toxin-insensitive G-protein involved in the coupling mechanism activated by α_{1A}-adrenoceptors belongs to the G_q family, as demonstrated by addition of anti-α_q/α_{11} antibody in the pipette solution. In contrast, the pertussis toxin-sensitive G-protein involved in the coupling mechanism activated by α_{2A}-adrenoceptors is a G_{i1} or G_{i2} protein. Furthermore, our results show that the anti-phosphatidylinositol antibody is effective only in blocking the transduction pathway evoked by α_{1A}-adrenoceptor activation; it has no effect on the stimulation of Ca^{2+} channels induced by α_{2A}-adrenoceptors.

A common step in α_{1A}- and α_{2A}-adrenoceptor-induced stimulation of Ca^{2+} channels results from activation of protein kinase C because the down-regulation of protein kinase C by a long-term (24 h) pretreatment with phorbol dibutyrate and application of GF109203X blocks the enhancement of Ca^{2+} channel current evoked by the α_1- and α_2-adrenoceptor agonists and phorbol dibutyrate. As the α_2-adrenoceptor response does not involve hydrolysis of phosphatidylinositols, the production of diacylglycerol may depend on hydrolysis of phosphatidylcholine mediated by phospholipases C or D. The protein kinase C-induced stimulation of Ca^{2+} channel current is supported by previous data showing that both noradrenaline and phorbol dibutyrate increase isradipine affinity for its specific binding sites on Ca^{2+} channels, an effect that has been attributed to protein kinase C-induced phosphorylation of Ca^{2+} channels (Mironneau et al., 1991).

From whole-cell patch-clamp experiments and $[Ca^{2+}]_i$ measurements, it has been established that α_{1A}-adrenoceptor-induced Ca^{2+} release activates chloride channels and promotes a 25–30 mV depolarization. This depolarization activates, in turn, the voltage-dependent Ca^{2+} channels producing Ca^{2+} entry. In addition, Ca^{2+} channel activity is enhanced by diacylglycerol-induced activation of protein kinase C, when high (10 μM) noradrenaline concentrations are used. In contrast, α_{2A}-adrenoceptor activation of Ca^{2+} channels acts without a prior major depolarization and release of intracellular stored Ca^{2+} and is explained only by an increased activity of protein kinase C. It is proposed that protein kinase C-induced phosphorylation of Ca^{2+} channels is sufficient to increase their open probability at potentials close to the resting potential. This possibility is supported by contraction experiments which show a strong similarity between clonidine-induced contractions and contractions evoked by low (100 nM) concentrations of noradrenaline. Similarly, the phenylephrine-induced contractions resembles those evoked by high (10 μM) concentrations of noradrenaline. Taken together, these observations suggest that the modulation of Ca^{2+} channel activity and spontaneous contractions is mainly mediated by α_{2A}-adrenoceptor activation, whereas both release of intracellular Ca^{2+} and depolarization-dependent activation of Ca^{2+} channels, responsible for the tetanus contractions, are mainly mediated by α_{1A}-adrenoceptor activation.

REFERENCES

Baron, A., Rakotoarisoa, L., Leprêtre, N. & Mironneau, J. (1994). Inhibition of L-type Ca^{2+} channels in portal vein myocytes by the enantiomers of oxodipine. *Eur. J. Pharmacol. Mol. Pharmacol. Sect.* **269**, 105–113.

Ford, A.P.D.W., Williams, T.J., Blue, D.R. & Clarke, D.E. (1994). α_1-adrenoceptor classification: sharpening Occam's razor. *Trends Pharmacol. Sci.* **15**, 167–170.

Leprêtre, N. & Mironneau, J. (1994). α_{2A}-adrenoceptors activate dihydropyridine-sensitive calcium channels via G_i-proteins and protein kinase C in rat portal vein myocytes. *Pflügers Arch.* **429**, 253–261.

Leprêtre, N., Arnaudeau, S., Mironneau, J., Rakotoarisoa, L., Mironneau, C. & Galiano, A. (1994a). Electrophysiological and radioligand binding studies of elgodipine and derivatives in portal vein myocytes. *J. Pharmacol. Exp. Ther.* **271**, 1209–1215.

Leprêtre, N., Mironneau, J., Arnaudeau, S., Tanfin, Z., Harbon, S., Guillon, G. & Ibarrondo, J. (1994b). Activation of α_{1A}-adrenoceptors mobilizes calcium from the intracellular stores in myocytes from rat portal vein. *J. Pharmacol. Exp. Ther.* **268**, 167–174.

Leprêtre, N., Mironneau, J. & Morel, J.L. (1994c). Both α_{1A}- and α_{2A}-adrenoreceptor subtypes stimulate voltage-operated L-type calcium channels in rat portal vein myocytes: evidence for two distinct transduction pathways. *J. Biol. Chem.* **269**, 29546–29552.

Loirand, G., Faiderbe, S., Baron, A., Geffard, M. & Mironneau, J. (1992). Autoanti-phosphatidylinositol antibodies specifically inhibit noradrenaline effects on Ca^{2+} and Cl^- channels in rat portal vein myocytes. *J. Biol. Chem.* **267**, 4312–4316.

Macrez-Leprêtre, N., Ibarrondo, J., Arnaudeau, S., Morel, J.L., Guillon, G. & Mironneau, J. (1995). A G_{i1-2}-protein is required for α_{2A}-adrenoceptor-induced stimulation of voltage-dependent Ca^{2+} channels in rat portal vein myocytes. *Pflügers Arch.* **430**, 590–592.

Marc, S., Leiber, D. & Harbon, S. (1986). Carbachol and oxytocin stimulate the generation of inositol phosphates in the guinea pig myometrium. *FEBS Lett.* **201**, 9–14.

McKinnon, A.C., Spedding, M. & Brown, C.M. (1994) α_2-adrenoceptors: more subtypes but fewer functional differences. *Trends Pharmacol. Sci.* **15**, 119–123.

Mironneau J. (1991). Noradrenaline modulation of ionic channels in vascular smooth muscle cells. In *Ion channels of Vascular Smooth Muscle Cells and Endothelial Cells* (Sperelakis, N. & Kuriyama, H., eds), pp. 47–54. Elsevier, Amsterdam.

Mironneau, J. (1995). Regulation of calcium and chloride channels in vascular smooth muscle cells by norepinephrine. In *Physiology and Pathophysiology of the Heart* (Sperelakis, N., ed.), pp. 909–918. Kluwer, Dordrecht.

Mironneau, J. & Gargouil, Y.M. (1979). Action of indapamide on excitation-contraction coupling in vascular smooth muscle. *Eur. J. Pharmacol.* **57**, 57–67.

Mironneau, J., Mironneau, C., Grosset, A., Hamon, G. & Savineau, J.P. (1980). Action of angiotensin II on the electrical and mechanical activity of rat uterine smooth muscle. *Eur. J. Pharmacol.* 1980, **68**, 275–285.

Mironneau, C., Rakotoarisoa, L., Sayet, I. & Mironneau, J. (1991). Modulation of [^{3}H]dihydropyridine binding by activation of protein kinase C in rat vascular smooth muscle. *Eur. J. Pharmacol. Mol. Pharmacol. Sect.* **208**, 223–230.

Toullec, D., Pianetti, P., Coste, H., Bellevergue, P., Grand-Perret, T., Ajakane, M., Baudet, V., Boissin, P., Boursier, E., Loriolle, F., Duhamel, L., Charon, D. & Kirilovsky, J. (1991). The bisindolyleimide GF109203X is a potent and selective inhibitor of protein kinase C. *J. Biol. Chem.* **266**, 15771–15781.

Wu, D., Katz, A., Lee, C.H. & Simon, M.I. (1992). Activation of phospholipase C by α_1-adrenergic receptors is mediated by the α subunits of G_q family. *J. Biol. Chem.* **267**, 25798–27802.

20

Ca^{2+} Release Mechanisms in Smooth Muscle

MASAMITSU IINO

Department of Pharmacology,
Faculty of Medicine,
University of Tokyo,
Tokyo, Japan

It has long been recognized that smooth muscle cells have intracellular Ca^{2+} stores that are capable of inducing maximum contractions even in the absence of Ca^{2+} in the bathing medium (Bolton, 1979; van Breemen & Saida, 1989; Missiaen *et al.*, 1992; Somlyo & Somlyo, 1994). It is often assumed that the Ca^{2+} store is utilized only during the initial phasic response to agonists and plays a negligible role during the tonic increase in [Ca^{2+}]$_i$, because the tonic component is abolished after removal of extracellular Ca^{2+}. However, recent evidence suggests that this assumption may not hold under certain conditions and that the Ca^{2+} store is also involved in the generation of tonic phase. In this article I briefly review recent progress in the study of functions of intracellular Ca^{2+} stores in smooth muscle cells.

INTRACELLULAR Ca^{2+} RELEASE CHANNELS AND COMPARTMENTS OF Ca^{2+} STORES

Ca^{2+} can be released from the Ca^{2+} store of smooth muscle cells by caffeine, which is known as an activator of the Ca^{2+}-induced Ca^{2+} release (CICR) mechanism or the ryanodine receptor (RyR) in striated muscle cells (Endo, 1977). This suggested the presence of a CICR mechanism in the Ca^{2+} store of smooth muscle cells. Ca^{2+}-dependent release of Ca^{2+} was indeed found in permeabilized smooth muscle cells (Iino, 1989). The CICR channel in smooth muscle cells is also sensitive to ryanodine, and co-application of caffeine and ryanodine results in CICR channels being locked in the half-open state (Hwang & van Breemen, 1987; Iino *et al.*, 1988) as has been found in skeletal muscle. Indeed, mRNA for RyR has been recently detected in various smooth muscle tissues.

In permeabilized cells Ca^{2+} can also be released by IP_3 via the IP_3 receptors (IP_3R), and this is thought to be the major pathway for the agonist-induced Ca^{2+} mobilization (Berridge, 1993). While studying the properties of IP_3-induced Ca^{2+} release, I found that the activity of the IP_3R was biphasically dependent on the cytoplasmic concentration of Ca^{2+} (Iino, 1990). This mechanism confers the IP_3R with the property to function in a manner similar to the CICR channel. Indeed, both RyR and IP_3R have not only functional but also structural similarities and they appear to have evolved from the common ancestral Ca^{2+} release channel. The CICR activity of the IP_3R seems to be extremely important for signal transmission within the cells (see below).

RyR and IP_3R are distributed unevenly among the intracellular Ca^{2+} stores (Iino, 1989). Caffeine- and ryanodine-sensitive stores are also released by IP_3, but only a fraction (usually about half) of the IP_3-releasable Ca^{2+} store is sensitive to caffeine and ryanodine. The fraction of Ca^{2+} stores with RyR varies depending on the type of smooth muscle. In some tissues such as uterine smooth muscle, only a small fraction of compartment is sensitive to caffeine (Ashoori et al., 1985). The physiological roles of RyR in agonist-induced contractions are not fully understood, although RyR has been implicated in the amplification of Ca^{2+} signals subsequent to Ca^{2+} influx through voltage-sensitive Ca^{2+} channels in some types of cells (Ganitkevich & Isenberg, 1992; Grégoire et al., 1993). This amplification is supposed to induce transient outward current by activating Ca^{2+}-sensitive K channels (Sakai et al., 1988). Roles of RyR have also been proposed for the generation of stochastic Ca^{2+} rise in subplasmalemmal microdomains, and this is assumed to result in the opening of Ca^{2+}-sensitive K channels leading to spontaneous transient outward currents (Benham & Bolton, 1986).

AGONIST-INDUCED Ca^{2+} RELEASE IN SINGLE SMOOTH MUSCLE CELLS

In agonist-stimulated single smooth muscle cells, rapid upstroke of $[Ca^{2+}]_i$ is preceded by a slow rise of $[Ca^{2+}]_i$ (foot) which is reminiscent of a pacemaker potential observed prior to the generation of an action potential in excitable cells (Figure 1). Furthermore, using digital imaging of agonist-stimulated smooth muscle cells, we found generation of Ca^{2+} waves, i.e. propagation of the regenerative Ca^{2+} rise within the cells in the absence of extracellular Ca^{2+} (Iino et al., 1993). These results indicated the presence of a Ca^{2+}-mediated positive feedback mechanism in the generation of agonist-induced $[Ca^{2+}]$

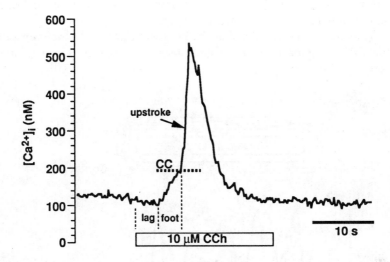

Figure 1 [Ca²⁺]ᵢ response in an agonist-stimulated single smooth muscle cell in the absence of extracellular Ca²⁺. Carbachol (CCh, 10 µM) was applied to a single cell obtained from guinea pig taenia caeci. As the slow rise in [Ca²⁺]ᵢ (foot) reached a critical concentration (CC), a rapid upstroke of [Ca²⁺]ᵢ was observed.

signals. Our results also indicated that the positive feedback mechanism involves IP₃R rather than RyR or phospholipase C (Iino *et al.*, 1993). We found an abrupt transition from the foot to upstroke around 160 nM [Ca²⁺]ᵢ; IP₃R has been shown to be activated by Ca²⁺ around this concentration (Iino, 1990).

Ca²⁺ OSCILLATIONS IN SMOOTH MUSCLE CELLS WITHIN VESSEL WALL

Analyses using smooth muscle tissues suggested that the Ca²⁺ stores are involved mainly in the initial phase of agonist-induced [Ca²⁺]ᵢ rise. However, only the average response of multiple cells has been observed in previous analyses of smooth muscle tissues. The advent of digital imaging techniques has enabled monitoring of [Ca²⁺]ᵢ change within single smooth muscle cells (Williams *et al.*, 1985). We applied this method to study [Ca²⁺]ᵢ in individual smooth muscle cells within the arterial wall (Iino *et al.*, 1994). Fluo-3-loaded rat tail artery was mounted over a glass capillary with a diagonal cross section and was observed using a confocal microscope (Figure 2A). There are four types of cells in the specimen. Endothelial cells constitute the innermost layer which is surrounded by a single layer of circular smooth muscle cells, and at the outermost layer the perivascular sympathetic nerve forms a network in the connective tissue cells. Using the confocal microscope we were able to distinguish clearly each cell layer and observe changes in $[Ca^{2+}]_i$ (Iino *et al.*, 1994).

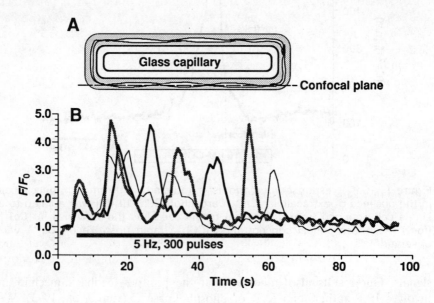

Figure 2 $[Ca^{2+}]_i$ measurement in individual vascular smooth muscle cells *in situ*. A, Schematic drawing of the cross-sectional view of rat tail artery mounted over a glass capillary. B, Changes in $[Ca^{2+}]_i$ in three different smooth muscle cells in response to electrical stimulation of the perivascular sympathetic nerve at 5 Hz (horizontal line).

Following stimulation of the perivascular sympathetic nerve by a train of electrical shocks, we found two phases in the $[Ca^{2+}]_i$ response in individual smooth muscle cells (Figure 2B). The first phase rose immediately after the initiation of electrical stimulation and fell in the next few seconds. The second phase developed after a delay of about 5s and consisted of intermittent rises in $[Ca^{2+}]_i$, or Ca^{2+} oscillations. Both phases were abolished after treatment of tetrodotoxin and were confirmed to be due to sympathetic activity. Only the second phase was blocked by an α-adrenergic antagonist.

Ca^{2+} oscillation was also observed when 0.1–1.0 μM noradrenaline was added to the bath. The increase in $[Ca^{2+}]_i$ propagated within the cell at a speed of about 20 μm s^{-1}. The Ca^{2+} oscillation was observed even in the absence of extracellular Ca^{2+}, although it was abolished after a few transients. Furthermore, Ca^{2+} oscillations were abolished when Ca^{2+} stores were depleted. Therefore, Ca^{2+} oscillations were produced by the intermittent release of Ca^{2+} from internal stores. The frequency of oscillation varied from cell to cell. Thus, at any point in time the increase in $[Ca^{2+}]_i$ was observed in only a fraction of cells. However, the average response of many cells appeared as if there was a tonic increase in $[Ca^{2+}]_i$. In the previous studies, as the tonic increase in $[Ca^{2+}]_i$ was dependent on the extracellular Ca^{2+}, it was thought to be a direct consequence of Ca^{2+} influx. However, $[Ca^{2+}]_i$ between oscillations returned to the resting level, which means that Ca^{2+} influx does not directly cause an increase in $[Ca^{2+}]_i$ but is required for the maintenance of Ca^{2+} oscillations.

LUMINAL Ca²⁺ MEASUREMENT – A NEW WAY TO STUDY Ca²⁺ STORES

The results described above show that Ca^{2+} waves and oscillations are of fundamental importance for the regulation of vascular contraction. It is therefore extremely important to elucidate the mechanism underlying the generation of Ca^{2+} oscillations. Recently, we succeeded in the real-time measurement of the luminal concentration of Ca^{2+} within the Ca^{2+} store of vascular smooth muscle cells (Hirose & Iino, 1994). The outline of this new measurement is described in the following paragraph.

First, we loaded cells with the acetoxymethyl ester of Furaptra, a low-affinity fluorescent Ca^{2+} indicator (Figure 3, upper panel). The dye entered not only the cytoplasm but also the intracellular organelles including IP_3-releasable stores. The cytoplasmic dye was released by permeabilization of the plasma membrane using β-escin. The remaining fluorescence responded to a Ca^{2+} concentration change in the store lumen with Ca^{2+} loading into and being released from the internal stores. The fluorescence change during Ca^{2+} loading was inhibited by cyclopiazonic acid while IP_3-induced Ca^{2+} release was blocked by heparin. The major advantages of this method are (1) measurement of the real-time change in Ca^{2+} concentration within the store lumen is possible, and (2) repeated measurements using the same preparation are possible, which facilitate comparison of the results obtained under different conditions.

Using this method we were able to show a Ca^{2+}-dependent increase in the rate of IP_3-induced Ca^{2+} release (Figure 3, lower panel), which is in agreement with my previous results (Iino, 1990). We also observed an apparently time-dependent decrease in the rate of Ca^{2+} release. Such phenomena have been thought to suggest the presence of an inactivation mechanism, a quantal Ca^{2+} release, or a luminal Ca^{2+} dependence of Ca^{2+}

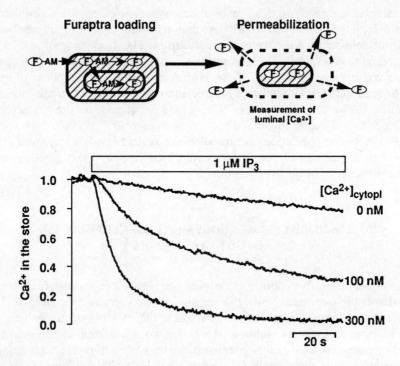

Figure 3 Luminal [Ca²⁺] measurement in permeabilized vascular smooth muscle cells. Upper panel: schematic drawing to show loading of Furaptra (F) into the lumen of intracellular organelles. Lower panel: cytoplasmic Ca²⁺ dependence of IP₃-induced Ca²⁺ release.

release rate. Because an inactivation mechanism, if present, may play a role in the determination of the interval between Ca²⁺ oscillations, we studied the mechanism that underlies the time-dependent decrease in the Ca²⁺ release rate. The decrease in the Ca²⁺ release rate did not recover even after removal of IP₃ and/or Ca²⁺. Thus, our results do not support the presence of an inactivation process. Recovery of the Ca²⁺ release rate was achieved only after reloading of the Ca²⁺ store. Our analyses suggested that the decrease in the Ca²⁺ release rate is due to the presence of multiple compartments with different IP₃R channel densities (Hirose & Iino, 1994).

PERSPECTIVES

Basic properties of the Ca²⁺ release channels and the compartments of the Ca²⁺ stores of smooth muscle cells have been characterized. Ca²⁺ release from intracellular Ca²⁺ stores takes place as Ca²⁺ oscillations, each of which propagates within the cell as a wave. Ca^{2+}-induced activation of IP_3R is the key mechanism underlying the Ca^{2+} wave. However, it is not yet clear what controls the interspike duration; neither is it known which Ca^{2+} influx pathway is required for the maintenance of the oscillations. Further studies are required to elucidate these mechanisms and to clarify the physiological roles of intracellular Ca^{2+} stores in other smooth muscle tissues.

REFERENCES

Ashoori, F., Takai, A. & Tomita, T. (1985). The response of non-pregnant rat myometrium to oxytocin in Ca-free solution. *Bri. J. Pharmacol.* **84**, 175–183.

Beenham, C. & Bolton, T. (1986). Spontaneous transient outward currents in single visceral and vascular smooth muscle cells of the rabbit. *J. Physiol.* **381**, 385–406.

Berridge, M.J. (1993). Inositol trisphosphate and calcium signalling. *Nature* **361**, 315–325.

Bolton, T. (1979). Mechanism of action of transmitters and other substances on smooth muscle. Physiolo. Rev. **59**, 606–718.

van Breemen, C. & Saida, K. (1989). Cellular mechanisms regulating [Ca^{2+}]i smooth muscle. *Annu. Rev. Physiol.* **51**, 315–329.

Endo, M. (1977). Calcium release from the sarcoplasmic reticulum. *Physiol. Rev.* **57**, 71–108.

Ganitkevich, V.Ya. & Isenbeerg, G. (1992). Contribution of Ca^{2+}-induced Ca^{2+} release to the [Ca^{2+}]i transients in myocytes from guinea pig urinary bladder. *J. Physiol.* **458**, 119–137.

Grégorie, G., Loirand, G. & Pacaud, P. (1993). Ca^{2+} and Sr^{2+} entry induced Ca^{2+} release from the intracellular Ca^{2+} store in smooth muscle cells of rat portal vein. *J. Physiol.* **474**, 483–500.

Hirose, K. & Iino, M. (1994). Heterogeneity of channel density in inositol-1,4,5-trisphosphate-sensitive Ca^{2+} stores. *Nature* **372**, 791–794.

Hwang, K.S. & van Breemen, C. (1987). Ryanodine modulation of ^{45}Ca efflux and tension in rabbit aortic smooth muscle. *Pflügers Arch.* **408**, 343-350.

Iino, M. (1989). Calcium-induced calcium release mechanism in guinea pig taenia caeci. *J. Gen. Physiol.* **94**, 363–383.

Iino, M. (1990). Biphasic Ca^{2+} dependence of inositol 1,4,5-trisphosphate-induced Ca release in smooth muscle cells of the guinea pig taenia caeci. *J. Gen. Physiol.* **95**, 1103–1122.

Iino, M., Kobayashi, T. & Endo, M. (1988). Use of ryanodine for functional removal of the calcium store in smooth muscle cells of the guinea pig. *Biochem. Biophys. Res. Commu.* **152**, 417-422.

Iino, M., Yamazawa, T., Miyashita, Y., Endo, M. & Kasai, H. (1993). Critical intracellular Ca^{2+} concentration for all-or-none Ca^{2+} spiking in single smooth muscle cells. *EMBO J.* **12**, 5287–5291.

Iino, M., Kasai, H. & Yamazawa, T. (1994). Visualization of neural control of intracellular Ca^{2+} concentration in single vascular smooth muscle cells *in situ*. *EMBO J.* **13**, 5026–5031.

Missaen, L., de Smedt, H., Droogmans, G., Himpens, B. & Casteels, R. (1992). Calcium ion homeostasis in smooth muscle. *Pharmacol. Therap.* **56**, 191–231.

Sakai, T., Teerada, K., Kitamura, K. & Kuriyama, H. (1988). Ryanodine inhibits the

Ca-dependent K current after depletion of Ca stored in smooth muscle cells of the rabbit ileal longitudinal muscle. *Br. J. Pharmacol.* **95**, 1089–1100.

Somlyo, A. & Somlyo, A. (1994). Signal transduction and regulation in smooth muscle. *Nature* **372**, 231–236.

Williams, D., Fogarty, K., Tsien, R. & Fay, F. (1985). Calcium gradients in single smooth muscle cells revealed by the digital imaging microscope using fura-2. *Nature* **318**, 558–561.

21

Partial Calcium Release through the Inositol 1,4,5-Trisphosphate Receptor

JAN B. PARYS
LUDWIG MISSIAEN
HUMBERT DE SMEDT
ILSE SIENAERT
RIK CASTEELS

*Laboratorium voor Fysiologie,
Campus Gasthuisberg O/N – K.U.Leuven,
Leuven, Belgium*

INTRODUCTION

Inositol 1,4,5-trisphosphate ($InsP_3$) is a very important and ubiquitous intracellular messenger. $InsP_3$ mediates Ca^{2+} release from intracellular Ca^{2+} stores by binding to its receptor ($InsP_3R$), a tetrameric channel protein (Berridge, 1993). $InsP_3$-induced Ca^{2+} release is involved in pharmacomechanical coupling in smooth muscle (Kobayashi *et al.*, 1989). The $InsP_3R$ proteins from bovine aorta (Chadwick *et al.*, 1990) and from rat vas deferens (Mourey *et al.*, 1990) were purified and characterized, and shown to be functionally similar to the $InsP_3R$ proteins present in other tissues.

One of the characteristics of the $InsP_3$-sensitive Ca^{2+} stores is that even a prolonged application of $InsP_3$ does not discharge the Ca^{2+} store completely. This partial release of Ca^{2+} was originally named 'quantal release' (Muallem *et al.*, 1989) and has since been demonstrated in many cell types, including smooth muscle (Missiaen *et al.*, 1992a). Although it is possible that an over-extensive fractionation of the endoplasmic reticulum leads to an overestimation of the 'quantal release' phenomenon after cell homogenization (Renard-Rooney *et al.*, 1993), the fact that partial Ca^{2+} release was demonstrated in intact cells (Muallem *et al.*, 1989; Bootman *et al.*, 1994) and in permeabilized cells with apparently intact endoplasmic

SMOOTH MUSCLE EXCITATION
ISBN 0-12-112360-X

reticulum (Short *et al.*, 1993) is indicative for a mechanism operating *in vivo*. This indicates that the Ca^{2+} store is not homogenous in composition and that Ca^{2+} diffusion between different subcompartments within the Ca^{2+} stores is somehow limited.

In physiological terms, the importance of the partial release phenomenon is that the Ca^{2+} stores can function as increment detectors, i.e. cells respond to each new stimulation by agonists with a new release of Ca^{2+}, independently of the background signal (Meyer & Stryer, 1990). Furthermore, although it was first believed that the partial release phenomenon was typical for $InsP_3$-induced Ca^{2+} release, it was recently demonstrated that Ca^{2+} release through the ryanodine receptor also occured quantally (Cheek *et al.*, 1993).

Notwithstanding $InsP_3$-induced Ca^{2+} release was extensively studied, the molecular mechanism underlying the 'quantal release' phenomenon is still not known and evidence for four different mechanisms have been presented. These mechanisms are now discussed.

VARIATIONS IN THE SENSITIVITY OF THE Ca^{2+} STORE UNITS TO $InsP_3$

Muallem *et al.* (1989) proposed that differences in $InsP_3$ sensitivity may be at the origin of the 'quantal release' phenomenon. In this model the various units for Ca^{2+} storage would each release their Ca^{2+} in an all-or-none manner, depending on the presence of $InsP_3Rs$ with different sensitivities to $InsP_3$.

The differences in sensitivity can be due to the expression, in each Ca^{2+} store unit, of different receptor isoforms, each with their own affinity for $InsP_3$. We performed a ratio polymerase chain reaction to determine in a quantitative way the expression of the various $InsP_3R$ isoforms in several muscle and nonmuscle cell types. In this way we demonstrated that most cell types co-express several $InsP_3R$ isoforms, e.g. A7r5 smooth muscle cells expressed for 73% type I receptors and for 26% type III receptors (De Smedt *et al.*, 1994). Moreover, in 76% of the type I receptors expressed in A7r5 smooth muscle cells the SI splice domain was included, while the SI domain was excluded in the remaining 24% (Parys *et al.*, 1995a). Differences in affinity of the $InsP_3$-binding site are until now the most apparent functional difference existing between various $InsP_3R$ isoforms. The general view is that the closely related $InsP_3Rs$ of type II (Südhof *et al.*, 1991), of type IV (Parys *et al.*, 1995a) and probably also of type V have the highest affinity for $InsP_3$. The type I receptor had a lower affinity. Interestingly, the peripheral splice isoform of $InsP_3R$-I of A7r5 cells had an affinity that was twice as high as the neuronal splice isoform (Parys *et al.*, 1995a). Lowest in affinity was the type III isoform (Newton *et al.*, 1994).

Differences in sensitivity can also be obtained by a differential post-translational modification of the InsP$_3$R proteins. Data obtained with purified InsP$_3$Rs reconstituted in liposomes suggest that differences occurring in the coupling domain of the receptor, e.g. at the level of the phosphorylation sites, may be important (Ferris *et al.*, 1992).

It may be difficult to envisage differences in affinity or sensitivity encompassing the whole range of possible responses (Meyer & Stryer, 1990), but mathematical modelling studies (Watras *et al.*, 1994) indicated that partial release could result, provided that the different InsP$_3$-binding polypeptides can assemble to heterotetramers and that the binding sites can reversibly switch from low-affinity active states to high-affinity inactive states. Although there is strong evidence that, at least in some cell types, InsP$_3$Rs can convert between a low- and a high-affinity state (Pietri *et al.*, 1990), the question of which affinity state correlates with an open channel has not been resolved.

REGULATION BY THE Ca^{2+} CONTENT OF THE STORES

Irvine (1990) proposed that partial release of Ca^{2+} might be caused by the presence of a regulatory Ca^{2+} binding site on, or associated with, the luminal part of the InsP$_3$R. The decrease of the luminal Ca^{2+} content occurring concomitantly with the Ca^{2+} release through the InsP$_3$-sensitive Ca^{2+} channel would inhibit further Ca^{2+} release. A stimulatory effect of luminal Ca^{2+} on InsP$_3$-induced Ca^{2+} release and on InsP$_3$ binding was demonstrated in smooth muscle cells (Missiaen *et al.*, 1992a,b, 1994; Nicholls *et al.*, 1993; Parys *et al.*, 1993; Loirand *et al.*, 1994; Bootman *et al.*, 1995), as well as in other cell types (Missiaen, 1991, 1992c; Nunn & Taylor, 1992; Oldershaw & Taylor, 1993; Tshipamba *et al.*, 1993; De Smedt *et al.*, 1994). The fact that no effect of luminal Ca^{2+} could be demonstrated in a number of other studies can be explained by the following. First, the effect of luminal Ca^{2+} is best observed at relatively low loading levels (Parys *et al.*, 1993), often not reached in other studies. Second, the effect of luminal Ca^{2+} is dependent on a number of experimental parameters, including cytosolic Ca^{2+} concentration (Missiaen *et al.*, 1994).

A major feature of the regulation of partial release by store content is that the release would not occur in an all-or-none fashion, but would instead continue in all store units until a new steady-state, depending upon the luminal and cytosolic Ca^{2+} concentration and also upon the InsP$_3$ concentration, would be reached. The regulation of InsP$_3$-induced Ca^{2+}

release by luminal and cytosolic Ca^{2+} and the relation between these regulatory mechanisms still need to be elucidated at the molecular level.

INACTIVATION OF THE InsP$_3$R

A time-dependent inactivation of the InsP$_3$-sensitive channel would also lead to partial Ca^{2+} release, if inactivation of the channel would occur before the Ca^{2+} stores are completely discharged. In earlier work no evidence for classical inactivation of the receptor was found, since the receptor remained fully sensitive to successive stimulation by higher InsP$_3$ concentrations (Meyer & Stryer, 1990). Recently, the idea that inactivation might play a role in partial Ca^{2+} release was suggested again by the observations that both the ryanodine receptor (Györke & Fill, 1993) and the InsP$_3$R (Hajnóczky & Thomas, 1994) can intrinsically inactivate. The function of InsP$_3$ and cytosolic Ca^{2+} in the process of InsP$_3$R inactivation is not yet understood, making it difficult to assess its role in partial release. It is tempting to speculate that the conformational changes of the receptor induced by cytosolic Ca^{2+} (Pietri *et al.*, 1990), the biphasic regulation of the InsP$_3$-induced Ca^{2+} flux by cytosolic Ca^{2+} observed in many tissues, including smooth muscle (Iino, 1990; Missiaen *et al.*, 1994; Bootman *et al.*, 1995), the existence of a slow-release phase of Ca^{2+} (Meyer & Stryer, 1990; Missiaen *et al.*, 1992a) and the inactivation of the channel by InsP$_3$ and Ca^{2+} (Hajnóczky & Thomas, 1994) are, at least in part, manifestations of the same process, but this must be analysed further. The fact that the regulation of the InsP$_3$R by cytosolic Ca^{2+} is strongly dependent on luminal Ca^{2+} (Missiaen *et al.*, 1994) and on InsP$_3$, Mg^{2+} and H^+ concentration (Bootman *et al.*, 1995) further adds to the complexity of the system. Currently, most data do not support a major role for inactivation in the process of partial Ca^{2+} release, at least in smooth muscle cells (Missiaen *et al.*, 1992a; Hirose & Iino, 1994; Parys *et al.*, 1995b).

EFFECT OF InsP$_3$R DENSITY

Meyer & Stryer (1990) proposed that differences in receptor density would also lead to partial release. Very recently, evidence was presented in vascular smooth muscle cells that differences in the density of the InsP$_3$-sensitive channels would allow some stores to deplete more rapidly than others (Hirose & Iino, 1994). It must be emphasized that an effect of InsP$_3$R density on partial Ca^{2+} release does not exclude any of the above-mentioned mechanisms, but that it can be considered as an additional mechanism that would reinforce any of the other mechanisms: i.e. variation in channel density could cause some store units to discharge more completely than others before the inhibiting effect of the decreasing luminal Ca^{2+} concentration would curtail further release.

CONCLUSIONS

Regulation of the $InsP_3R$ by luminal Ca^{2+} can provide an adequate explanation for partial release at low levels of store content. At higher levels of loading, the relative stimulatory effect of luminal Ca^{2+} decreases and eventually reaches a plateau. Partial release, however, is still observed. A simple explanation for this is that control by luminal Ca^{2+} acts in concert with one or more of the other mechanisms described above. Good candidates are the presence of $InsP_3R$ isoforms with different sensitivities for $InsP_3$ and perhaps also for cytosolic and/or luminal Ca^{2+}, and/or the presence of different receptor densities. These are factors that may be strongly cell type-dependent. The variable loading of the stores and the use of different cell types in different studies can thus explain the co-existence of the various hypotheses mentioned above.

Table 1 summarizes a number of regulatory parameters modulating the $InsP_3R$, which may be involved in the phenomenon of partial Ca^{2+} release. How these regulatory factors interact with the $InsP_3R$ at the molecular level has not been established. In order to clarify the molecular mechanism responsible for partial Ca^{2+} release, experiments to determine the regulation

Table 1 Overview of the effects and interactions of various factors modulating the $InsP_3R$, which may be involved in the phenomenon of partial Ca^{2+} release. See text for details and exact references.

	InsP₃ Receptor			
	Stimulation	Stimulation enhanced by	Inhibition	Inhibition enhanced by
$InsP_3$	YES	High cyt. Ca^{2+} High lum. Ca^{2+} Low Mg^{2+} High pH	Possible	High cyt. Ca^{2+}
Cyt. Ca^{2+}	YES	Low lum. Ca^{2+} Low Mg^{2+} High pH	YES`	Low $InsP_3$ Low Mg^{2+} High pH
Lum. Ca^{2+}	YES	Low cyt. Ca^{2+}	NO	–

Abbreviations: cyt., cytosolic; lum., luminal.

mechanisms of the InsP$_3$R, the kinetics of InsP$_3$-induced Ca^{2+} release and the molecular structure of the various InsP$_3$R isoforms must be performed. A multidisciplinary approach focusing on those points will resolve the complex nature of partial Ca^{2+} release and clarify the functioning of the various InsP$_3$R isoforms in complex spatio-temporal Ca^{2+} signalling.

REFERENCES

Berridge, M.J. (1993). Inositol trisphosphate and calcium signalling. *Nature* **361**, 315–325.

Bootman, M.D., Cheek, T.R., Moreton, R.B., Bennett, D.L. & Berridge, M.J. (1994). Smoothly graded Ca^{2+} release from inositol 1,4,5-trisphosphate-sensitive Ca^{2+} stores. *J. Biol. Chem.* **269**, 24783–24791.

Bootman, M.D., Missiaen, L., Parys, J.B., De Smedt, H. & Casteels, R. (1995). Control of inositol 1,4,5-trisphosphate-induced Ca^{2+} release by cytosolic Ca^{2+}. *Biochem. J.* **306**, 445–451.

Chadwick, C.C., Saito, A. & Fleisher, S. (1990). Isolation and characterization of the inositol trisphosphate receptor from smooth muscle. *Proc. Natl Acad. Sci. USA* **87**, 2132–2136.

Cheek, T.R., Moreton, R.B., Berridge, M.J., Stauderman, K.A., Murawsky, M.M. & Bootman, M.D. (1993). Quantal Ca^{2+} release from caffeine-sensitive stores in adrenal chromaffin cells. *J. Biol. Chem.* **268**, 27076–27083.

De Smedt, H., Missiaen, L., Parys, J.B., Bootman, M.D., Mertens, L., Van Den Bosch, L. & Casteels R. (1994). Determination of the relative amounts of inositol trisphosphate receptor mRNA isoforms by ratio polymerase chain reaction. *J. Biol. Chem.* **269**, 21691–21698.

Ferris, C.D., Cameron, A.M., Huganir, R.L. & Snyder, S.H. (1992). Quantal calcium release by purified reconstituted inositol 1,4,5-trisphosphate receptors. *Nature* **356**, 350–352.

Györke, S. & Fill, M. (1993). Ryanodine receptor adaptation: control mechanism of Ca^{2+}-induced Ca^{2+} release in heart. *Science* **260**, 807–809.

Hajnóczky, G. & Thomas, A.P. (1994). The inositol trisphosphate calcium channel is inactivated by inositol trisphosphate. *Nature* **370**, 474–477.

Hirose, K. & Iino, M. (1994). Heterogeneity of channel density in inositol-1,4,5-trisphosphate-sensitive Ca^{2+} stores. *Nature* **372**, 791–794.

Iino, M. (1990). Biphasic Ca^{2+} dependence of inositol 1,4,5-trisphosphate-induced Ca release in smooth muscle cells of the guinea pig taenia caeci. *J. Gen. Physiol.* **95**, 1103–1122.

Irvine, R.F. (1990). 'Quantal' Ca^{2+} release and the control of Ca^{2+} entry by inositol phosphates – a possible mechanism. *FEBS Lett.* **263**, 5–9.

Kobayashi, S., Kitazawa, T., Somlyo, A. V. & Somlyo, A. P. (1989). Cytosolic heparin inhibits muscarinic and α-adrenergic Ca^{2+} release in smooth muscle. Physiological role of inositol 1,4,5-trisphosphate in pharmacomechanical coupling. *J. Biol. Chem.* **264**, 17997–18004.

Loirand, G., Grégoire, G. & Pacaud, P. (1994). Photoreleased inositol 1,4,5-trisphosphate-induced response in single smooth muscle cells of rat portal vein. *J. Physiol. (London)* **479**, 41–52.

Meyer, T. & Stryer, L. (1990). Transient calcium release induced by successive increments of inositol 1,4,5-trisphosphate. *Proc. Natl Acad. Sci. USA.* **87**, 3841–3845.

Missiaen, L., Taylor, C.W. & Berridge, M.J. (1991). Spontaneous calcium release from inositol trisphosphate-sensitive calcium stores. *Nature* **352**, 241–244.

Missiaen, L., De Smedt, H., Droogmans, G. & Casteels, R. (1992a). Ca^{2+} release induced by inositol 1,4,5-trisphosphate is a steady-state phenomenon controlled by luminal Ca^{2+} in permeabilized cells. *Nature* **357**, 599–602.

Missiaen, L., De Smedt, H., Droogmans, G. & Casteels, R. (1992b). Luminal Ca^{2+} controls the activation of the Ins(1,4,5)P$_3$ receptor by cytosolic Ca^{2+}. *J. Biol. Chem.* **267**, 22961–22966.

Missiaen, L., Taylor, C.W. & Berridge, M.J. (1992c). Luminal Ca^{2+} promoting spontaneous Ca^{2+} release from inositol trisphosphate-sensitive stores in rat hepatocytes. *J. Physiol. (London)* **455**, 623–640.

Missiaen, L., De Smedt, H., Parys, J.B. & Casteels, R. (1994). Co-activation of inositol trisphosphate-induced Ca^{2+} release by cytosolic Ca^{2+} is loading-dependent. *J. Biol. Chem.* **269**, 7238–7242.

Mourey, R.J., Verma, A., Supattapone, S. & Snyder, S.H. (1990). Purification and characterization of the inositol 1,4,5-trisphosphate receptor protein from rat vas deferens. *Biochem. J.* **272**, 383–389.

Muallem, S., Pandol, S.J. & Beeker, T.G. (1989). Hormone-evoked calcium release from intracellular stores is a quantal process. *J. Biol. Chem.* **264**, 205–212.

Newton, C.L., Mignery, G.A. & Südhof, T.C. (1994). Co-expression in vertebrate tissues and cell lines of multiple inositol 1,4,5-trisphosphate (InsP$_3$) receptors with distinct affinities for InsP$_3$. *J. Biol. Chem.* **269**, 28613–28619.

Nicholls, J.A., Gillespie, J.I. & Greenwell, J.R. (1993). The time course of intracellular calcium movements in single human umbilical vein smooth-muscle cells. *Pflügers Arch. Eur. J. Physiol.* **425**, 225–232.

Nunn, D.L. & Taylor, C.W. (1992). Luminal Ca^{2+} increases the sensitivity of Ca^{2+} stores to inositol 1,4,5-trisphosphate. *Mol. Pharmacol.* **41**, 115–119.

Oldershaw, K.A. & Taylor, C.W. (1993). Luminal Ca^{2+} increases the affinity of inositol 1,4,5-trisphosphate for its receptor. *Biochem. J.* **292**, 631–633.

Parys, J.B., Missiaen, L., De Smedt, H. & Casteels, R. (1993). Loading dependence of inositol 1,4,5-trisphosphate-induced Ca^{2+} release in the clonal cell line A7r5. Implications for the mechanism of quantal Ca^{2+} release. *J. Biol. Chem.* **268**, 25206–25212.

Parys, J.B., De Smedt, H., Missiaen, L., Bootman, M.D., Sienaert, I. & Casteels, R. (1995a). Rat basophilic leukemia cells as model system for inositol 1,4,5-trisphosphate receptor IV, a receptor of the type II family: functional comparison and immunological detection. *Cell Calcium* **17**, 239–249.

Parys, J.B., Missiaen, L., De Smedt, H., Sienaert, I., Henning, R.H. & Casteels, R. (1995b). Quantal release of calcium in permeabilized A7r5 cells is not caused by intrinsic inactivation of the inositol trisphosphate receptor. *Biochem. Biophys. Res. Comm.* **209**, 451–456.

Pietri, F., Hilly, M. & Mauger, J.-P. (1990). Calcium mediates the interconversion between two states of the liver inositol 1,4,5-trisphosphate receptor. *J. Biol. Chem.* **265**, 17478–17485.

Renard-Rooney, D.C., Hajnóczky, G., Seitz, M.B., Schneider, T.G. & Thomas, A. P. (1993). Imaging of inositol 1,4,5-trisphosphate-induced Ca^{2+} fluxes in single permeabilized hepatocytes. Demonstration of both quantal and nonquantal patterns of Ca^{2+} release. *J. Biol. Chem.* **268**, 23601–23610.

Short, A.D., Klein, M.G., Schneider, M.F. & Gill, D.L. (1993). Inositol 1,4,5-

trisphosphate-mediated quantal Ca^{2+} release measured by high resolution imaging of Ca^{2+} within organelles. *J. Biol. Chem.* **268**, 25887–25893.

Südhof, T.C., Newton, C.L., Archer III, B.T., Ushkaryov, Y.A. & Mignery, G.A. (1991). Structure of a novel $InsP_3$ receptor. *EMBO J.* **10**, 3199–3206.

Tshipamba, M., De Smedt, H., Missiaen, L., Himpens, B., Van Den Bosch, L. & Borghgraef R. (1993). Ca^{2+} dependence of inositol 1,4,5-trisphosphate-induced Ca^{2+} release in renal epithelial $LLC\text{-}PK_1$ cells. *J. Cell. Physiol.* **155**, 96–103.

Watras, J., Moraru, I., Costa, D.J. & Kindman, L.A. (1994). Two inositol 1,4,5-trisphosphate binding sites in rat basophilic leukemia cells: relationship between receptor occupancy and calcium release. *Biochemistry* **33**, 14359–14367.

22

Modulation of Intracellular Ca²⁺ Concentration by the Endoplasmic Reticulum of Intact Endothelial Cells from Rabbit Pulmonary or Aortic Valves

LI LI
CORNELIS VAN BREEMEN

Department of Pharmacology & Therapeutics,
The University of British Columbia,
Faculty of Medicine,
Vancouver, Canada

SUMMARY

Intracellular Ca^{2+} signals of fura-2 loaded intact endothelial cells (EC) from rabbit aortic or pulmonary valves were measured using imaging fluorescence microscopy. Applications of agonists such as ATP or carbachol and an inhibitor of sarcoplasmic or endoplasmic reticulum (SR/ER) Ca^{2+}-ATPase (SERCA), cyclopiazonic acid (CPA), induced an increase in the intracellular free Ca^{2+} concentration ($[Ca^{2+}]_i$) that is maintained above the prestimulated level as long as agonist or CPA and extracellular Ca^{2+} are present. A proposed phospholipase C (PLC) inhibitor 2-nitro-4-carboxyphenyl-N,N-diphenyl-carbamate (NCDC) greatly reduced the maintained $[Ca^{2+}]_i$ increase caused by ATP, but not that induced by CPA, which was blocked by Ni^{2+}. This provides support for the hypothesis that the agonist- and CPA-stimulated maintained $[Ca^{2+}]_i$ increases were dependent on extracellular Ca^{2+} entry across the plasmalemma. To confirm the involvement of Ca^{2+} influx in this process, we measured Mn^{2+} quenching as an indicator of Ca^{2+} influx. In the presence of extracellular Mn^{2+}, fura-2 quenching at 360 nm was observed, indicating Mn^{2+} entry through the resting Ca^{2+} leak. The rate of quenching was increased by ATP stimulation and this increase was abolished when the EC were pretreated with NCDC. However, the rate of Mn^{2+} quenching was unaffected by CPA application. These results demonstrate that agonist-stimulated divalent cation influx is not caused by the discharge of ER Ca^{2+}. Abolition of Ca^{2+} uptake by the ER was postulated to be responsible for the CPA-induced elevation in $[Ca^{2+}]_i$.

INTRODUCTION

Cardiovascular endothelial cells release various substances which regulate cardiovascular functions (Adams et al., 1989). One of the substances released is endothelium-derived relaxing factor (EDRF) (Cherry et al., 1982), the production of which critically depends on the intracellular free Ca^{2+} concentration ($[Ca^{2+}]_i$) (Long & Stones, 1985). In the endothelium, $[Ca^{2+}]_i$ is regulated by ion transport mechanisms located in the plasmalemmal and endoplasmic reticulum (ER) membranes. $[Ca^{2+}]_i$ can be increased by Ca^{2+} release from the ER lumen through Ca^{2+} 'leak' channels, inositol trisphosphate (IP_3)-sensitive Ca^{2+} channels due to activation of plasmalemmal receptors coupled to phospholipase C (PLC) and Ca^{2+}-dependent cation channels on the ER membrane that are activated by a rise in $[Ca^{2+}]_i$ (Ca^{2+}-induced Ca^{2+} release, CICR) (Lesh et al., 1993). $[Ca^{2+}]_i$ can also be increased by Ca^{2+} entry across the plasmalemma through a non-selective Ca^{2+} 'leak', receptor-operated cation channels (ROC), through stretch-activated channels (SAC), Na^+–Ca^{2+} exchange (Adams et al., 1989; Li & van Breemen, 1995) and second messenger-operated cation channels (Lückhoff & Clapham, 1992). $[Ca^{2+}]_i$ can be decreased by Ca^{2+}-ATPase located on the plasmalemmal and ER membranes to pump Ca^{2+} towards extracellular space (ECS) or the ER lumen and Na^+–Ca^{2+} exchange on the plasmalemmal membrane to extrude Ca^{2+} towards ECS. This study focuses on the mechanisms whereby the ER modulates the $[Ca^{2+}]_i$ signals. By using ATP and CPA, we found that both substances release Ca^{2+} from the ER and contribute to an initial rise in $[Ca^{2+}]_i$. Although both agents also raised the steady state $[Ca^{2+}]_i$, only ATP enhanced the rate of Mn^{2+} entry. The results are discussed in terms of ROC and the 'superficial buffer barrier' (SBB) hypothesis.

METHODS

Tissue preparation

Adult New Zealand white rabbits weighing 2.0–2.5 kg were killed by CO_2 asphyxiation. The heart was excised. Both the aortic and pulmonary arteries were opened at their respective attachments to the left and right ventricles. The aortic and pulmonary valves were dissected and placed in physiological saline solution (PSS) (pH 7.4 at 37°C).

$[Ca^{2+}]_i$ measurement

The morphology and $[Ca^{2+}]_i$ measurement of ECs on both surfaces of the valve was described in previous studies (Laskey et al., 1994; Li & van Breemen, 1995). Briefly, the dissected valve was incubated in PSS with 1 μM of membrane-permeable fura-2 acetoxylmethyl ester (fura-2/AM) in the dark at room temperature for 60–75 min and subsequently transferred to PSS for a further 15 min. It was then mounted in a specially designed chamber perfused with warmed PSS (37°C) (15 μl s^{-1}) situated on the stage of an inverted microscope. Only the EC monolayers on both surfaces of valve were loaded with fura-2. The lower surface of the valve was exposed to alternating 340 nm and 380 nm (bandwidth 10 nm) of ultraviolet light (1 s^{-1}) passed through a 510 nm (bandwidth 40 nm) cut-off filter prior to acquisition by an ICCD camera (an intensified charge-coupled device, cohu 4810 series, San Diego, CA, USA). Fluorescence signals were recorded as digital image data using a Sun Sparc1$^+$ Workstation and Inovision acquisition and analysis software (Inovision, Research Triangle Park, NC, USA), which is controlled by a Data Translation frame grabber (DT3861) housed in a PC 80286 computer. Autofluorescence of the unloaded valve was minimal and background images were obtained from a region of the chamber away from the valve. Pairs of the fluorescence signal ratios collected every 7 s at 340 nm and 380 nm excitation wavelengths (F340/F380) were determined and plotted as background-subtracted ratios on-line during the experimental procedure as a relative indication of $[Ca^{2+}]_i$ according to the equation of Grynkiewicz et al. (1985). The resting $[Ca^{2+}]_i$ was calculated to be 90 ± 8 nM (n = 400 cells from six experiments). Mn^{2+} entry was measured by the slope of Mn^{2+} quenching of the fura-2 trace at 360 nm in Ca^{2+}-free PSS. Up to 64 regions of interest containing individual or groups of EC on the valve could be monitored simultaneously for changes in F340/F380 and fluorescence intensity at 360 nm. The single trace line shown in each figure was the average F340/F380 or intensity at 360 nm measured simultaneously in individual or groups of EC chosen in the field of the same valve preparation and is representative of similar responses obtained in at least five preparations. Chemicals were applied as indicated by the horizontal bars or arrows in each figure.

Solutions and chemicals

Normal PSS (N-PSS) contains (in mM): NaCl 140, KCl 5, CaCl$_2$ 1, MgCl$_2$ 1, Glucose 10, N-2-hydroxyethylpiperazine-N'-2-ethanesulfonic acid (HEPES) 5 (pH 7.4 at 37°C). In Ca^{2+}-free PSS, 0.2 mM ethylene glycol-bis(β-amino-ethyl ether) N,N,N',N'-tetraacetic acid (EGTA) replaced 1 mM CaCl$_2$.

Analytical grade reagents for PSS, ATP, CPA, 2-nitro-4-carboxyphenyl-*N,N*-diphenyl-carbamate (NCDC), $MnCl_2$, $NiCl_2$, carbachol (CCh) and dimethyl sulfoxide (DMSO) were obtained from Sigma (St Louis, MS, USA). Fura-2/AM was from Molecular Probes (Eugene, OR, USA). CPA was diluted from its respective stock solution in DMSO. NCDC was made fresh daily in 95% ethanol. Serial dilutions of all chemicals were made in PSS. The maximal concentration of any vehicle to which preparations were exposed was less than 0.1%, which had no effect on the fura-2 signal.

RESULTS

Effect of agonists on $[Ca^{2+}]_i$

Figure 1A shows that ATP (100 μM) in the presence of 1 mM extracellular Ca^{2+} induced an initially rapid but transient rise in $[Ca^{2+}]_i$ which peaked within 20 s and represents the release of Ca^{2+} from intracellular stores; followed by a prolonged $[Ca^{2+}]_i$ elevation lower than the initial peak which is due to Ca^{2+} influx. The prolonged $[Ca^{2+}]_i$ elevation was abolished immediately upon removal of extracellular Ca^{2+}. A similar pattern of $[Ca^{2+}]_i$ increase to that of ATP stimulation occurred with stimulation of 10 μM carbachol (CCh) and 4 μM bradykinin (BK) (data not shown). Applying CCh after ATP in the absence of extracellular Ca^{2+} did not cause a $[Ca^{2+}]_i$ transient, and vice versa, suggesting that ATP and CCh mobilize the same intracellular store (Figure 1B).

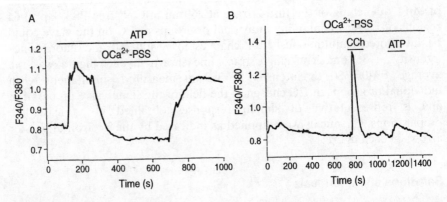

Figure 1. Representative traces of the average fluorescence ratio (F340/F380) signals of individual cells of rabbit valvular endothelial cells in response to agonists. Cells were exposed to: A, continuous ATP (100 μM) perfusion in N-PSS with the subsequent removal of extracellular Ca^{2+}; B, serial applications of ATP (100 μM) and carbachol (CCh, 10 μM) in $0Ca^{2+}$-PSS.

Effect of CPA on [Ca^{2+}]$_i$

CPA (10 µM), which interferes with ER Ca^{2+} accumulation through blockade of SERCA, induced a gradual increase in [Ca^{2+}]$_i$, reaching a sustained plateau within 3–6 min which was dependent on extracellular Ca^{2+} (Figure 2A). CPA could also prevent ER refilling, as indicated by the failure of CCh to induce a second [Ca^{2+}]$_i$ peak in N-PSS (Figure 2B).

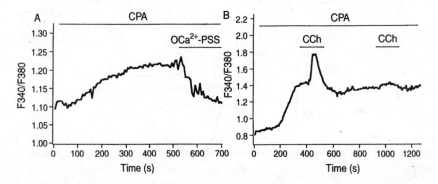

Figure 2 Representative trace of the average fluorescence ratio (F340/F380) signals of individual cells of rabbit valvular endothelial cells induced by SERCA inhibitor. Cells were exposed to 10 µM CPA. A, in N-PSS, followed by removal of extracellular Ca^{2+}; B, in N-PSS followed by subsequently serial applications of carbachol (CCh, 10 µM).

Effects of receptor-operated-Ca^{2+} channel (ROC) blockers on [Ca^{2+}]$_i$

The agonist- or CPA-induced elevation in steady-state [Ca^{2+}]$_i$ could be caused either by an increase in Ca^{2+} supply to or a decrease in Ca^{2+} removal from the cytoplasm.

The nature of the [Ca^{2+}]$_i$ increase was thus investigated by using Ca^{2+} channel blockers. NCDC (100 µM), a putative phospholipase C inhibitor and ROC blocker, was shown to greatly reduce the plateau level of the [Ca^{2+}]$_i$ increase induced by ATP, indicating that Ca^{2+} entry was linked to receptor activation (Figure 3A). The same dose of NCDC did not affect the ATP-induced [Ca^{2+}]$_i$ transient in 0Ca^{2+}-PSS, indicating that IP$_3$ was still generated (data not shown), and suggesting little inhibition of phospholipase. The CPA-induced [Ca^{2+}]$_i$ increase was, however, not blocked by NCDC (Figure 3B), but reversably inhibited by Ni^{2+}, a potent Ca^{2+} channel blocker (Figure 3C).

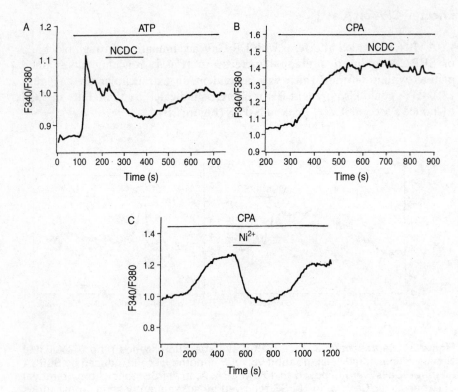

Figure 3 Effect of ROC blockers on the average fluorescence ratio (F340/F380) signals of individual cells of rabbit valvular endothelial cells. In N-PSS, cells were exposed to NCDC (100 μM) after stimulation with A, ATP (100 μM); B, CPA (10 μM). C, cells were exposed to 3 mM Ni^{2+} after stimulation with CPA (10 μM).

Mn^{2+} entry measurements

Using fura-2 to measure $[Ca^{2+}]_i$ provides only indirect evidence for the existence of Ca^{2+} entry pathways. To confirm the Ca^{2+} entry, we measured divalent cation influx by measuring fura-2 quenching by Mn^{2+} at 360 nm. Mn^{2+} (250 μM) entered the cell and progressively quenched the fura-2 fluorescence at 360 nm in a nearly linear manner. The slope of the linear part of the quenching trace is regarded as a measurement of the rate of Mn^{2+} entry into the EC. The decline of fluorescence intensity at 360 nm presumably reflects Mn^{2+} entry through the leak, together with a small level of photobleaching of intracellular fura-2. Figure 4A shows that, in addition to

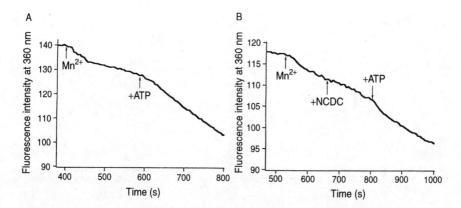

Figure 4 Representative traces showing the effect of ATP on the rate of Mn^{2+} quenching of fura-2 in individual cells of rabbit valvular endothelial cells. The rabbit cardiac valve was exposed to, respectively. A, N-PSS, Ca^{2+}-free PSS, 250 μM Mn^{2+} added to Ca^{2+}-free PSS and addition of 100 μM ATP to the preceding solution; B. N-PSS, Ca^{2+}-free PSS, 250 μM Mn^{2+} added to Ca^{2+}-free PSS, 100 μM NCDC and subsequent addition of 100 μM ATP to the preceding solution.

the leak pathway, Mn^{2+} also enters the EC through ROCs, as the rate of decline was increased by ATP. In agreement with the NCDC-induced reduction in plateau level of $[Ca^{2+}]_i$, the ATP mediated increased Mn^{2+} quenching rate was also inhibited by pretreatment with NCDC (Figure 4B), suggesting that ATP stimulates Mn^{2+} entry through a NCDC sensitive pathway.

CPA enhanced the steady-state $[Ca^{2+}]_i$, however, it appears not to do so by increasing Ca^{2+} entry through the plasmalemma, as reflected by its failure to increase the rate of Mn^{2+} entry (Figure 5A). It suggests that ER depletion by itself is not sufficient to cause an increase in plasmalemmal divalent cation permeability in intact ECs. Figure 5B shows that addition of Mn^{2+} 300 s after CPA application caused linear quenching of fura-2, but the rate of quenching was not changed in the following 300 s. After 600 s of CPA exposure, which was sufficiently long to deplete the ER (data not shown), subsequent ATP still increased the rate of quenching. Similar experiments were carried out with addition of Mn^{2+} at 170, 200, 400, 500, 600, and 800 s after CPA application; the quenching rate appeared not change within the time period of recording. It is concluded that ER depletion does not directly stimulate Ca^{2+} entry in a manner analogous to the effect of ATP.

We repeated each experiment at least five times and the average results of $[Ca^{2+}]_i$, and Mn^{2+} influx measurements are depicted in Figure 6.

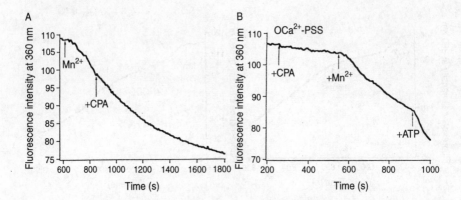

Figure 5 Representative trace showing the effect of CPA (10 μM) on the rate of Mn^{2+} quenching of fura-2 fluorescence in individual cells of rabbit valvular endothelial cells. The rabbit cardiac valve was exposed respectively to: A, N-PSS, Ca^{2+}-free PSS, 250 μM Mn^{2+} added to Ca^{2+}-free PSS and addition of 10 μM CPA to the preceding solution; B, N-PSS, Ca^{2+}-free PSS, 10 μM CPA added to Ca^{2+}-free PSS, 250 μM Mn^{2+} added to the preceding solution 300 s after exposure to CPA and addition of 10 μM ATP.

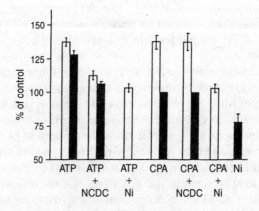

Figure 6 A summary of the effects of ATP and CPA on increasing steady state F340/F380 in N-PSS (open columns) and the rate of Mn^{2+} entry (closed columns) in the absence or presence of NCDC or Ni^{2+}. Values on the ordinate scale indicates the relative F340/F380 or Mn^{2+} entry rate compared with their respective control groups (100%). Each column represents mean ± SEM of five experiments.

DISCUSSION

The monolayers of EC covering the surface of the cardiac valves share at least some common functions with those of vascular endothelium. They possess pronounced secretory activities such as release of EDRF in response to vasoactive agents (Ku et al., 1990). The function of the endocardial surface of valves is related to several diseases such as thrombosis, hypertension, diabetes, etc. (Moncada et al., 1991; Shah, 1992). The study of valvular EC, particularly *in situ,* therefore has both physiological and pathological significance. The intact valvular endothelium used in this study, circumvents the problems of possible changes of ion transport mechanisms in cultured or dispersed cells owing to enzymatic treatment or subsequent culture procedures and permits the monitoring of individual cell $[Ca^{2+}]_i$ responses.

In this study we have compared the effects of the purinergic receptor agonist ATP and the SERCA inhibitor CPA on $[Ca^{2+}]_i$. Both agents deplete ER Ca^{2+} and cause maintained $[Ca^{2+}]_i$ elevation, which is dependent on the presence of extracellular Ca^{2+} (Figures 1 and 2). However, the mechanisms involved appear to be different. In the case of ATP, ER Ca^{2+} is released via stimulation of PLC and subsequent activation of IP_3 receptors; while CPA causes a slow Ca^{2+} release from the ER, via the leak, which is unopposed by the inhibited SERCA (Figure 3). Nevertheless the same intracellular Ca^{2+} stores was shown to be depleted by both agents (Figure 2B). The capacitative Ca^{2+} entry hypothesis (Casteels & Droogmans, 1981; Putney, 1990), which links ER depletion to stimulated Ca^{2+} influx in an obligatory manner, predict that both agents activated a common Ca^{2+} channel on the plasma membrane. We found that ATP stimulated Mn^{2+} entry (Figure 4A), but CPA did not (Figure 5). The putative ROC blocker NCDC abolished the stimulation Mn^{2+} entry by ATP (Figure 4B) and inhibited the ATP-induced increase in steady state $[Ca^{2+}]_i$, but it did not affect the CPA-induced $[Ca^{2+}]_i$ elevation (Figure 3A, B). The latter was abolished by Ni^{2+} (Figure 3C). These results are compatible with some reports (Gosnik & Forsberg, 1993; Lückhoff & Busse, 1990), but not with others (Morgan & Jacob, 1994; Schilling et al., 1992) on EC. The reason for these differences is not clear, but may be related to the preparation. A similar difference shows up between intact vascular smooth muscle (Chen & van Breemen, 1993) and A7r2 cells (a tissue culture cell line derived from rat smooth muscle) (Missiaen et al., 1990). It is known that tissue culture will alter the expression of receptors and transport mechanisms. The cultured EC thus may not accurately reflect *in vivo* physiology. ATP has been reported to open ROC (Johns et al., 1987). Our data support this view since the stimulated Mn^{2+} entry by ATP was blocked by NCDC. It is interesting to note that NCDC was more potent in inhibiting Ca^{2+} entry through ROC (maintained $[Ca^{2+}]_i$ increase) than inhibiting ER Ca^{2+} release (transient $[Ca^{2+}]_i$ increase) induced by ATP. Similar data were obtained in vascular smooth muscle cells (Rüegg *et al.*, 1989) when stimulated with vasopressin.

The elevation of $[Ca^{2+}]_i$ in response to CPA does not appear to result from the opening of ROCs but rather from inhibition of ER Ca^{2+} buffering. As discussed in a recent review (van Breemen *et al.*, 1995), steady state buffering of Ca^{2+} by ER at rest would require continuous unloading of ER Ca^{2+} to the ECS. Blockade of SERCA would interrupt the Ca^{2+} cycle between the SR and the plasmalemma and raise the $[Ca^{2+}]_i$ to a new steady-state level dependent only on the Ca^{2+} leak and plasmalemmal Ca^{2+} ATPase (PMCA). The component of ATP induced $[Ca^{2+}]_i$ elevation, which was resistant to NCDC, may be due to inhibition of ER Ca^{2+} buffering (Figure 3A). However, the possibility that depletion of the ER activates a highly specific Ca^{2+} channel, which is not permeant to Mn^{2+} (Hoth & Penner, 1992; van Renterghem & Lazdunski, 1994) is not excluded.

REFERENCES

Adams, D.J., Bareakeh, J., Laskey, R.E., & van Breemen, C. (1989). Ion channels and regulation of intracellular calcium in vascular endothelial cells. *FESEB J.* **3**, 2389–2400.

van Breemen, C., Chen, Q. & Laher, I. (1995). The superficial buffer barrier function of smooth muscle sarcoplasmic reticulum. *Trends Pharmacol. Sci.* **16** (3), 98–105.

Casteels, R. & Droogmans, G. (1981). Exchange characteristics of the noradrenaline-sensitive calcium store in vascular smooth muscle cells of rabbit ear artery. *J. Physiol.* **306**, 411–419.

Chen, Q. & van Breemen, C. (1993). The superficial buffer barrier in venous smooth muscle: sarcoplasmic reticulum refilling and unloading. *Br. J. Pharmacol.* **109**, 336–343.

Cherry, P.D., Furchgott, R.F., Zawadzki, J.V.& Jothianandan, D.J. (1982). Role of endothelial cells in relaxation of isolated arteries by bradykinin. *Proc. Natl Acad. Sci.USA* **79**, 2106–2110.

Demirel, E., Laskey, R.E., Purkerson, S. & van Breemen. C. (1993). The passive calcium leak in cultured porcine aortic endothelial cells. *Biochem. Biophy. Res. Commun* **191** (3), 1197–1203.

Gosnik, E.D., & Forsberg, E.J. (1993). Effects of ATP and bradykinin on endothelial cell Ca^{2+} homeostasis and formation of cGMP and prostacyclin. *Am. J. Physiol.* **265** (34), C1620–C1629.

Grynkiewicz, G., Poenie, M. & Tsien, R.Y. (1985). A new generation of Ca^{2+} indicators with greatly improved fluorescence properties. *J. Biol. Chem.* **260**, 3440–3450.

Hoth, M. & Penner, R. (1992). Depletion of intracellular calcium stores activates a calcium current in mast cells. *Nature* **355** (6358), 353–356.

Johns, A., Lategan, T.W., Lodge, N.J., Ryan, U.S., van Breemen, C. & Adams, D.J. (1987). Calcium entry through receptor-operated channels in bovine pulmonary artery endothelial cells. *Tissue Cell* **19** (6), 733–745.

Ku, D.D., Nelson, J.M., Caulfield, J.B. & Winn, M.J. (1990). Release of endothelium-derived relaxing factor from canine cardiac valves. *J. Cardiovasc. Pharmacol.* **16**, 212–218.

Laskey, R.E., Adams, D.J. & van Breemen, C. (1994). Cytosolic $[Ca^{2+}]_i$ measurements in endothelium of rabbit cardiac valve using imaging fluorescence microscopy. *Am. J. Physiol.* **266** (35), H2130–2135.

Lesh, R.E., Marks, A.R., Somlyo, A.V., Fleischer, S. & Somlyo, A.P. (1993). Antirynodine receptor antibody binding sites in vascular and endocardial endothelium. *Circ. Res.* **72** (2), 481–488.

Li, L. & van Breemen, C. (1995). Na^+–Ca^{2+} exchange in intact endothelium of rabbit cardiac valve. *Circ. Res.* **76** (3), 396–404.

Long, C.J. & Stones, T.W. (1985). The release of endothelium-derived relaxation factor is calcium-dependent. *Blood Vessels* **22**, 205–208.

Lückoff, A. & Busse, R. (1990). Refilling of endothelial calcium stores without bypassing the cytosol. *FEBS Lett* **276** (1–2), 108–110.

Lückoff, A. & Clapham, D. E. (1992). Inositol 1,3,4,5-tetrakisphosphate activates an endothelial Ca^{2+}-permeable channel. *Nature* **355**, 356–358.

Missiaen, L., Declerck, I., Droogmans, G., Plessers, L., de Smedt, H., Raeymaekers, L. & Casteels. R. (1990). Agonist-dependent Ca^{2+} and Mn^{2+} entry dependent on state of filling of Ca^{2+} stores in aortic smooth muscle cells of the rat. *J. Physiol.(London)* **427**, 171–186.

Moncada, S., Palmer, R.M.J. & Higgs, E.A. (1991). Nitric oxide: physiology, pathophysiology and pharmacology. *Pharmacol Rev.* **43**, 109–142.

Morgan, A.J. & Jacob, R. (1994). Ionomycin enhances Ca^{2+} influx by stimulating store-regulated cation entry and not by a direct action at the plasma membrane. *Biochem. J.* **300**, 665–672.

Putney, J.W., Jr (1990). Capacitative calcium entry revised. *Cell Calcium.* **11**(10), 611–624.

van Renterghem, C. & Lazdunski, M. (1994). Identification of the current activated by vasoconstrictors in vascular smooth muscle cells. *Pflügers Arch.* **429**, 1–6.

Rüegg, U.T., Wallnöfer, A., Weir, S., & Cauvin, C. (1989). Receptor-operated calcium-permeable channels in vascular smooth muscle. *J. Cardiovasc. Pharmacol.* **14** (Suppl. 6), S49–S58.

Schilling, W.P., Cabello, O.A., & Rajan, L. (1992). Depletion of the inositol 1,4,5-triphosphate-sensitive intracellular Ca^{2+} store in vascular endothelial cells activates the agonist-sensitive Ca^{2+}-influx pathway. *Biochem. J.* **284**, 521–530.

Shah, A.M. (1992). Vascular endothelium. *Br. J. Hosp Med.* **48** (9), 540–549.

23

Muscle and Non-muscle Properties of the Regulatory System for Cytosolic Ca^{2+} in Smooth Muscle Cells

L. RAEYMAEKERS
J. EGGERMONT
H. VERBOOMEN
F. WUYTACK
R. CASTEELS

*Laboratorium voor Fysiologie,
K. U. Leuven, Campus Gasthuisberg,
Leuven, Belgium*

INTRODUCTION

Ca^{2+} is peculiar as a second messenger in that its concentration is not regulated by synthesis and breakdown but by mechanisms mediating influx and efflux from the cytoplasmic compartment. The increase of [Ca^{2+}]$_i$ upon excitation of a cell results from the opening of Ca^{2+} channels in the plasma membrane (PM) and in the sarcoplasmic reticulum (SR) or endoplasmic reticulum (ER). Ca^{2+} pumps in the plasma membrane (PM) together with the Na$^+$/Ca^{2+} exchanger compensate the influx of Ca^{2+}, thereby allowing the cells to maintain a steady state with respect to total Ca^{2+} content. Ca^{2+} pumps in the membranes of the SR transport Ca^{2+} from the cytoplasm towards the lumen, where the accumulated Ca^{2+} is buffered by low-affinity Ca^{2+}-binding proteins. Both the SR and the PM transporters participate in returning the cell to the resting state at the end of a stimulus by decreasing [Ca^{2+}]$_i$ below 100 nanomolar.

Ca^{2+} pumps and Ca^{2+} channels also contribute to the fine tuning of cellular function by acting as targets for the action of second messengers and through the developmental- or tissue-dependent expression of functionally different isoforms. In addition, the high ER-luminal Ca^{2+} content built up by the SR Ca^{2+} pump represents a store of Ca^{2+} which can be released upon excitation of the cell, and also plays a role in the regulation of the synthesis, folding and sorting of proteins in the ER.

SMOOTH MUSCLE EXCITATION
ISBN 0-12-112360-X

The Ca^{2+} pumps, Ca^{2+} channels and Ca^{2+}-binding proteins exist in many different isoforms, often encoded by different gene families. Some of these isoforms are characteristically expressed in skeletal and (or) cardiac muscle and do not occur in nonmuscle cells. This overview will focus on the question of how far smooth-muscle cells resemble muscle cells or non-muscle cells with respect to the expression of proteins involved in the regulation of $[Ca^{2+}]_i$. Because these proteins have been better characterized in the SR than in the PM, the main part of this chapter will be devoted to the SR proteins.

Ca^{2+} PUMPS OF THE SARCOPLASMIC RETICULUM

Overview

Ca^{2+} transport in the SR is catalysed by five different protein isoforms, encoded by three different genes, *SERCA1*, *SERCA2* and *SERCA3*. SERCA2 is ubiquitously expressed, whereas SERCA1 and SERCA3 show a restricted tissue distribution. SERCA1 is expressed only in fast skeletal muscle. Alternative splicing generates an adult (SERCA1a) and a neonatal (SERCA1b) isoform. SERCA3 is expressed along with SERCA2 in platelets, in lymphoid cells, in mast cells and in some endothelial cells (Wuytack *et al.*, 1994). Alternative splicing of the *SERCA2* transcript generates two isoforms. In SERCA2b the last four amino acids of SERCA2a are replaced by a stretch of 49 amino acids. SERCA2b is probably ubiquitously expressed and can be considered as a 'housekeeping' isoform. The SERCA2a isoform is expressed only in cardiac muscle, slow skeletal muscle, and to some extent also in smooth muscle (Eggermont *et al.*, 1990b). The products of these alternatively spliced mRNAs differ in their functional properties. SERCA2b presents a higher affinity for Ca^{2+} (Verboomen *et al.*, 1992) but a lower turnover rate than SERCA2a (Verboomen *et al.*, 1994).

In cardiac muscle, the SERCA pump plays an important role in mediating the positive inotropic effect of β-receptor agonists. This effect is mediated via the phosphorylation of the small membrane-bound protein, phospholamban. Unphosphorylated phospholamban inhibits the pump, mainly by decreasing the apparent affinity of the Ca^{2+} pump for Ca^{2+}. Relief of the inhibition is brought about by phosphorylation by cyclic AMP-dependent protein kinase (cAK), cyclic GMP-dependent protein kinase (cGK) or Ca^{2+}/calmodulin-dependent protein kinase II. The role of unphosphorylated phospholamban bound to the SERCA pump is analogous to that of the calmodulin-binding domain of the PM Ca^{2+} pump (PMCA) which is autoinhibitory. Thus, the role of the phosphorylation of SERCA pump-associated phospholamban corresponds to that of binding of calmodulin to the PMCA pump (Chiesi *et al.*, 1991).

Number of SR Ca²⁺-transport sites in striated and in smooth muscle cells

The highest rate of Ca^{2+} uptake reported for purified SR from smooth muscle is at least one order of magnitude lower than that seen in isolated cardiac SR (Raeymaekers et al., 1985). A similar difference is found for the Ca^{2+}-stimulated ATPase activity and the steady-state level of phosphoprotein intermediate (Wuytack et al., 1984). This difference in activity is mainly due to the relatively low number of Ca^{2+}-transport sites in smooth-muscle SR, as shown by the scarceness of intramembrane particles in freeze-fractured SR membranes, by immunological results using antibodies directed against the cardiac and the nonmuscle isoform of the Ca^{2+} pump and by measurements of mRNA levels (for a review see Raeymaekers & Wuytack, 1993). In the smooth muscle of the rabbit stomach the difference in expression level compared with cardiac muscle was 70-fold at the protein level but only 3.5-fold at the mRNA level, suggesting that posttranscriptional steps contribute to the differences in expression level (Khan & Grover, 1993).

It can be concluded that with respect to the number of Ca^{2+} pump sites in the SR, smooth muscle cells resemble nonmuscle cells more than skeletal or cardiac muscle cells. Although considerable differences may exist between many smooth muscle types with respect to the number of the proteins involved in the regulation of $[Ca^{2+}]_i$, even the highest Ca^{2+} pump level that has been observed in smooth muscle is still far below that seen in cardiac muscle, which itself possesses less Ca^{2+} pump sites than skeletal-muscle cells.

It is interesting to note also that considerable differences exist between smooth-muscle types in the ratio of the number of SR to PM Ca^{2+} pump sites. This ratio was much higher in large blood vessels of the pig than in gastrointestinal muscles (Eggermont et al., 1988). It is not clear if this difference correlates with a relatively more important role of SR Ca^{2+} uptake, or a greater contribution of the Na^+/Ca^{2+} exchanger to Ca^{2+} extrusion in blood vessels.

Relative expression level of SERCA-pump isoforms

The expression of the different isoforms of SERCA Ca^{2+} pumps in smooth-muscle tissues was analysed both at the protein level using isoform-specific antibodies and at the level of their respective mRNAs. Before the identification of the different isoforms at the molecular level, it was found that the Ca^{2+}-transport ATPase from smooth muscle was immunologically more similar to that of cardiac and slow skeletal muscle than to that of fast skeletal muscle. Moreover, the Ca^{2+} pumps of fast skeletal muscle, and slow skeletal muscle and cardiac muscle could be discriminated by means of the tryptic fragments of the phosphorylated transport intermediate and this method confirmed the immunological results (Wuytack *et al.*, 1989b). Sequencing of cDNA revealed that the SR Ca^{2+} pump of smooth muscle is transcribed from the same gene (SERCA2) as in slow skeletal muscle and in cardiac muscle (Eggermont *et al.*, 1989). The Ca^{2+} pump of nonmuscle cells is transcribed from the same gene. It is, however, translated from an alternatively spliced mRNA giving rise to the SERCA2b (nonmuscle) isoform instead of the SERCA2a (muscle) isoform. Antibodies which discriminate between SERCA2a and SERCA2b were developed by Wuytack *et al.*, (1989a) and by Eggermont *et al.* (1990b). They were used in combination with nondiscriminating antibodies for the relative quantification of the SERCA2a/b isoforms in several smooth muscles of the pig. SERCA2b was the predominant isoform in all smooth-muscle tissues examined. This result was confirmed for several smooth muscles of the rabbit by discrimination of the SERCA2a and SERCA2b isoforms based on a small difference in electrophoretic migration resulting from the difference in molecular mass (Spencer *et al.*, 1991).

The analysis of mRNA levels in pig tissues revealed four classes of SERCA2-derived mRNAs. Class 1 (4.4 kb) encodes SERCA2a, whereas classes 2 (4.4 kb), 3 (8.0 kb)and 4 (5.6 kb) encode the b isoform. These four mRNA classes present a tissue-specific distribution. Class 4 is confined to neuronal cells. In pig smooth muscle all three remaining mRNA types are expressed (Eggermont *et al.*, 1990a). Any significance for the presence of three mRNA types that are translated into one single type of SERCA protein (e.g. differential stability of the messenger) remains speculative. Using an RNAase protection assay, Eggermont *et al.* (1990b) estimated that the SERCA2b messages (class 2 + class 3) accounted for 72-81% of the total SERCA2 mRNA in pig smooth muscles of stomach, longitudinal ileum, pulmonary artery and aorta, the remainder encoding SERCA2a. The analysis of mRNA from smooth muscles of the rabbit by Lytton *et al.* (1989) gave a value of 85% mRNA encoding SERCA2b in aorta and urinary bladder, and 95% in stomach and small and large intestine. Also Khan *et al.*, (1990) found almost exclusively the b-isoform mRNA in rabbit stomach smooth muscle. The slight difference in the values given by Eggermont *et al.* (1990b) may be related to the different animal species used; also rat uterus SERCA mRNA is predominantly SERCA2b.

Expression of phospholamban

In cardiac muscle, the increased activity of the Ca^{2+} pump of the SR as a consequence of the phosphorylation of phospholamban plays a key role in the positive chronotropic and inotropic action of β-receptor agonists (Luo *et al.*, 1994). The highest levels of expression of phospholamban are found in cardiac and in slow skeletal muscle, the two muscle types which express SERCA2a as the major Ca^{2+} pump isoform. Fast skeletal muscle which expresses SERCA1 does not contain phospholamban. Coexpression studies have shown, however, that phospholamban is able to interact with the SERCA1 pump (Fujii *et al.*, 1990).

Phospholamban has been detected in all vascular and gastrointestinal smooth muscles examined (animal species include rat, rabbit, dog, pig and cow), except in the aorta of the pig (for a review see Raeymaekers & Wuytack, 1993). The expression of phospholamban is down regulated in late-passage rat aortic cells in culture (Shanahan *et al.*, 1993). Although it is clear that the level of phospholamban in smooth-muscle cells, as that of the SERCA pump, is much lower than in cardiac muscle, there is less certainty on whether the ratio of the amount phospholamban/SERCA pump is similar or lower than in cardiac muscle. A lower value of this ratio would be the simplest explanation of the observation that the stimulation of the SR Ca^{2+} pump of smooth muscle by protein kinases is lower than that of cardiac SR. A similar ratio is found when comparing mRNA levels of SERCA and phospholamban in cardiac and smooth muscle (Eggermont *et al.*, 1990b) or when comparing protein levels by measuring the Ca^{2+}-stimulated ATPase activity and the level of phosphorylation of phospholamban (Raeymaekers *et al.*, 1990). However, a lower ratio is found in smooth muscle by using anti-SERCA and anti-phospholamban antibodies (Eggermont *et al.*, 1990b). A possible explanation for the discrepancy between the estimates of both gene products at the protein level and at the mRNA level could be a higher value of protein/mRNA ratio in cardiac muscle expressing mainly SERCA2a, compared with smooth muscle expressing mainly SERCA2b. Khan & Grover (1993) found evidence for a higher protein/mRNA ratio in cardiac muscle, whereas Wu & Lytton (1993) did not observe a significant difference in this respect between cardiac and smooth muscle.

The stimulation by cAK or cGK of the Ca^{2+} uptake in isolated SR vesicles from smooth muscle is smaller than that seen in cardiac SR vesicles (Raeymaekers *et al.*, 1990). This observation cannot be explained by an impaired interaction of the SERCA2b isoform with phospholamban compared with the SERCA2a isoform (Verboomen *et al.*, 1992). A lower ratio of phospholamban to Ca^{2+} pump would be the simplest explanation for this low degree of stimulation, but as explained above, this question has not yet been settled.

The phosphorylation of phospholamban in smooth-muscle cells *in vivo* has been demonstrated in rat aorta incubated with agents that increase cGMP (Cornwell *et al.*, 1991; Karczewski *et al.*, 1992). Phospholamban phosphorylation in response to cAMP-elevating agents has not yet been demonstrated in smooth-muscle cells.

Ca²⁺-BINDING PROTEINS OF THE SARCOPLASMIC RETICULUM

Overview

Proteins possessing many low-affinity Ca²⁺-binding sites are major constituents of the SR of striated muscle and of the ER of nonmuscle cells. The Ca²⁺-binding proteins identified in the lumen of the SR of skeletal and cardiac muscle are calsequestrin, sarcalumenin, the histidine-rich Ca²⁺-binding protein (HCP) and calreticulin. Calsequestrin is transcribed from two genes. One is typically expressed in skeletal muscle, the other one in cardiac muscle. The protein composition of the ER of nonmuscle cells differs from that of muscle SR (for a review see Milner *et al.*, 1992). Except for calreticulin, none of the SR-type Ca²⁺-binding proteins has been detected in mammalian non-muscle cells. Calreticulin in a minor component of the SR of striated muscle, whereas it is the major Ca²⁺-binding protein of the ER of nonmuscle cells.

Expression of SR-type Ca²⁺-binding proteins in smooth-muscle cells

Although the major Ca²⁺-binding protein of the SR of smooth-muscle cells is calreticulin, a typical protein of nonmuscle cells (Milner *et al.*, 1991), smooth-muscle cells also express SR-type Ca²⁺-binding proteins (Wuytack *et al.*, 1987; Raeymaekers *et al.*, 1993). A comparative study of the expression of SR-type Ca²⁺-binding proteins has been made in smooth muscles of the pig (Raeymaekers *et al.*, 1993). The cardiac form of calsequestrin, sarcalumenin and HCP were all expressed in the smooth muscle of the stomach at higher levels than in the other smooth muscles investigated. However, the amount of calsequestrin present in pig stomach smooth muscle was 20- to 30-fold lower than in pig cardiac (ventricular) muscle. This relatively low amount is not surprising in view of the low content of SR Ca²⁺-pump in smooth muscle. The SR from pig ileum contained calsequestrin and HCP, whereas sarcalumenin could not be detected. In the trachea, there was a cross-reacting band with the anti-calsequestrin serum only. In the SR from the vascular smooth muscles of the pulmonary artery and aorta, there was no reaction with any of the antibodies used. However, HCP is also abundant in arteriolar smooth-muscle cells of the rabbit (Pathak *et al.*, 1992). Cardiac calsequestrin has been detected only in trace amounts in the porcine uterus (Milner *et al.*, 1991).

It is also worth mentioning the 53 kDa glycoprotein. This protein is a quantitatively important component of skeletal and cardiac SR and has been proposed to be a regulator of the Ca²⁺ pump. The 53 kDa glycoprotein is transcribed from the same gene as sarcalumenin. It is smaller in size than sarcalumenin because it has lost the Ca²⁺-binding domain by an alternative splicing process. This glycoprotein has been detected in pig stomach and ileum smooth muscle. It is absent in pig trachea, aorta and pulmonary artery (Raeymaekers *et al.*, 1993).

THE PLASMALEMMAL Ca²⁺-PUMP

The plasmalemmal Ca^{2+} pump is encoded by at least four genes (PMCA1-4) which give rise to many more isoforms by alternative splicing at two sites (see Carafoli, 1994 for review). The expression of these isoforms has been studied mainly at the mRNA level, whereas at the protein level very little information is available. All 'or almost all' the PMCA mRNA in smooth-muscle cells codes for the PMCA1b isoform, which is the ubiquitously expressed 'house-keeping isoform' (De Jaegere *et al.*, 1990). In this respect smooth-muscle cells resemble non-excitable cells. Skeletal- and cardiac-muscle cells express, in addition to PMCA1b, other PMCA genes and splice variants, particularly PMCA1c, PMCA1d and PMCA4a (Hammes *et al.*, 1994).

DISCUSSION

Whereas smooth-muscle-specific isoforms of proteins of the contractile machinery, such as the smooth muscle-specific actin isoforms, have been well characterized, specific isoforms of the regulatory system for Ca^{2+} which are absent in striated muscle or nonmuscle cells have not been detected. From the data presented it is clear that with respect to the expression of Ca^{2+} pumps and Ca^{2+}-binding proteins, smooth-muscle cells present both muscle and nonmuscle properties, with the nonmuscle properties predominating. These muscle properties resemble more closely cardiac muscle than skeletal muscle: both the SERCA2a pump and calsequestrin, if present, are the variants typically expressed in the heart. An overview is given in Table 1. For comparison,

Table 1 Summary of the discussed properties of smooth muscle cells that have been studied with respect to their resemblance to muscle (+) or nonmuscle (−) cells

Property of smooth-muscle	Characteristic for muscle
Number of SR Ca²⁺-transport sites	−
Expression of SERCA isoforms	±
Expression of phospholamban	+
Expression of SR Ca²⁺-binding proteins	±
Plasmalemmal Ca²⁺-pump (PMCA)	−
SR Ca²⁺-release channels	−(mainly IP₃)
Type of intermediate filament	− in tonic smooth muscles (vimentin) + in phasic smooth muscle (desmin)

information on the expression of other muscle-specific proteins is included in this table.

Smooth-muscle cells also share with muscle and nonmuscle cells the protein components of the intermediate-filament system of the cytoskeleton, desmin and vimentin. This part of the cytoskeleton of sarcomeric muscle which includes the Z-line consists of desmin, whereas nonmuscle cells express vimentin. Smooth muscle cells of large arteries express vimentin as the major intermediate filament, whereas gastrointestinal smooth muscles express desmin. It has been proposed that this expression pattern correlates with, respectively, tonic and phasic contractile activity (Frank & Warren, 1981). The predominant expression of desmin in the gastrointestinal smooth muscles and of vimentin in the vascular muscles investigated in our study has been confirmed by Western blotting. It appears from our data, therefore, that the correlation between the type of contractile activity and the pattern of protein expression can be extended to the Ca^{2+}-binding proteins of the ER, although it should be kept in mind that only one animal species has been investigated. The Ca^{2+} stored in the SR of smooth muscle is known to play an important role in excitation–contraction coupling, especially during the initial phase of the contraction. The fact that the SR of striated muscles and the ER of non-muscle cells contain a different set of these proteins points to important functional differences between these proteins which may be related to the different mechanisms of initiation of Ca^{2+} release operating in these tissues. Most of the ER luminal nonmuscle type proteins possess the C-terminal amino-acid sequence Lys, Asp, Glu, Leu. The fact that the SR-type proteins calsequestrin, sarcalumenin, HCP and the 53 kDa glycoprotein do not have this ER-retention signal suggests the existence in smooth-muscle cells of a separate SR-like compartment, although less extensively developed than in sarcomeric muscles. Possibly, the properties of these proteins are better suited to the functional requirements or to interaction with other protein components of phasically contracting muscles than those of non-muscle Ca^{2+}-binding proteins. Conversely, the expression in smooth muscle of the cardiac Ca^{2+} pump splice variant SERCA2a does not appear to correlate with the expression of the other SR-type proteins. In this respect important questions that await clarification are which SR-type proteins are co-localized in smooth-muscle cells and whether or not these components constitute a separate compartment that is morphologically and functionally distinct from that of the non-muscle-type ER.

REFERENCES

Carafoli, E. (1994). Biogenesis: plasma membrane calcium ATPase: 15 years of work on the purified enzyme. *FASEB J.* **8**, 993–1002.
Chiesi, M., Vorherr, T., Falchetto, R., Waelchli, C. & Carafoli, E. (1991).

Phospholamban is related to the autoinhibitory domain of the plasma membrane Ca²⁺-pumping ATPase. *Biochemistry* **30**, 7978–7983.

Cornwell, T.L., Pryzwansky, K.B., Wyatt, T.A. & Lincoln, T.M. (1991). Regulation of sarcoplasmic reticulum protein phosphorylation by localized cyclic GMP-dependent protein kinase in vascular smooth muscle cells. *Mol. Pharmacol.* **40**, 923–931.

De Jaegere, S., Wuytack, F., Eggermont, J.A., Verboomen, H. & Casteels, R. (1990). Molecular cloning and sequencing of the plasma-membrane Ca²⁺ pump of pig smooth muscle. *Biochem. J.* **271**, 655–660.

Eggermont, J.A, Vrolix, M., Raeymaekers, L., Wuytack, F. & Casteels, R. (1988). Ca²⁺-transport ATPases of vascular smooth muscle. *Circu. Res.* **62**, 266–278.

Eggermont, J.A., Wuytack, F., De Jaegere, S., Nelles, L. & Casteels, R. (1989). Evidence for two isoforms of the endoplasmic-reticulum Ca²⁺ pump in pig smooth muscle. *Biochem. J.* **260**, 757–761.

Eggermont, J.A., Wuytack, F. & Casteels, R. (1990a). Characterization of the mRNAs encoding the gene 2 sarcoplasmic/endolplasmic-reticulum Ca²⁺ pump in pig smooth muscle. *Biochem. J.* **266**, 901–907.

Eggermont, J.A., Wuytack, F., Verbist, J. & Casteels, R. (1990b) Expression of endoplasmic-reticulum Ca²⁺-pump isoforms and of phospholamban in pig smooth-muscle tissues. *Biochem. J.* **271**, 649–653.

Frank, E. D. & Warren, L. (1981) Aortic smooth muscle cells contain vimentin instead of desmin. *Proc. Natl Acad. Sci. USA* **78**, 3020–3024.

Fujii, J., Maruyama, K., Tada,M. & MacLennan, D. H. (1990). Co-expression of slow-twitch/cardiac muscle Ca2(+)-ATPase (SERCA2) and phospholamban. *FEBS Lett.* **273**, 232–234.

Hammes, A., Oberdorf, S., Strehler, E. E., Stauffer, T., Carafoli, E., Vetter, H. & Neyses, L.. (1994). Differentiation-specific isoform mRNA expression of the calmodulin-dependent plasma membrane Ca²⁺-ATPase. *FASEB J.* **8**, 428–435.

Karczewski, P., Kelm, M., Hartmann, M. & Schrader, J. (1992). Role of phospholamban in NO/EDRF-induced relaxation in rat aorta. *Life Sci.* **5**, 1205–1210.

Khan, I. & Grover, A. K. (1993). Abundance of heteronuclear and messenger RNA for internal Ca pump in stomach smooth muscle and myocardium. *Cell Calcium* **14**, 17–23.

Luo, W., Grupp, I. l., Harrer, J., Ponniah, S., Grupp, G., Duffy, J. J., Doetschman, T. & Kranias, E. G. (1994). Targeted ablation of the phospholamban gene is associated with markedly enhanced myocardial contractility and loss of β-agonist stimulation. *Circation Research* **75**, 401–4019.

Lytton, J., Zarain-Herzberg, A., Periasamy, M. & MacLennan, D.H. (1989). Molecular cloning of the mammalian smooth muscle sarco(endo)plasmic reticulum Ca²⁺-ATPase. *J. Biol. Chem.* **264**, 7059–7065.

Milner, R. E., Baksh, S., Shemanko, C., Carpenter, M. R., Smillie, L., Vance, J. E., Opas, M. & Michalak, M. (1991). Calreticulin, and not calsequestrin, is the major calcium binding protein of smooth muscle sarcoplasmic reticulum and liver endoplasmic reticulum. *J. Biol. Chem.* **266**, 7155–7165.

Milner, R. E., Famulski, K. A. & Michalak, M. (1992). Calcium binding proteins in the sarcoplasmic/endoplasmic reticulum of muscle and nonmuscle cells. *Mol. Cellu. Biochem.* **112**, 1–13.

Pathak, R. K., Anderson, R. G. & Hofmann, S. L. (1992). Histidine-rich of striated muscle, is also abundant in arteriolar smooth muscle cells. *J. Muscle Res. Cell Motil.* **13**, 366–376.

Raeymaekers, L. & Wuytack, F. (1993). Ca^{2+} pumps in smooth muscle cells. *J. Muscle Res. Cell Motil.* **14**, 141–157.

Raeymaekers, L., Wuytack, F. & Casteels, R. (1985). Subcellular fractionation of pig stomach smooth muscle. A study of the distribution of the $(Ca^{2+}+Mg^{2+})$-ATPase activity in plasmalemma and endoplasmic reticulum. *Biochim. Biophys. Acta* **815**, 441–454.

Raeymaekers, L., Eggermont, J.A., Wuytack, F. & Casteels, R. (1990). Effects of cyclic nucleotide dependent protein kinases on the endoplasmic reticulum Ca^{2+} pump of bovine pulmonary artery. *Cell Calcium* **11**, 261–268.

Raeymaekers, L., Verbist, J., Wuytack, F., Plessers, L. & Casteels, R. (1993). Expression of Ca^{2+} binding proteins of the sarcoplasmic reticulum of striated muscle in the endoplasmic reticulum of pig smooth muscles. *Cell Calcium* **14**, 581–589.

Shanahan, C.M., Weissberg, P.L. & Metcalfe, J.C. (1993). Isolation of gene markers of differentiated and proliferating vascular smooth muscle cells. *Circu. Res.* **73**, 193–204.

Spencer, G.G., Yu, X., Khan, I. & Grover, A.K. (1991). Expression of isoforms of internal calcium pump in rabbit stomach smooth muscle and heart. *Biochim. Biophys. Acta* **1063**, 15–20.

Verboomen, H., Wuytack, F., De Smedt, H., Himpens, B., & Casteels, R. (1992). Functional difference between SERCA2a and SERCA2b Ca^{2+} pumps and their modulation by phospholamban. *Biochem. J.* **286**, 591–596.

Verboomen, H., Wuytack, F., Van den Bosch, L., Mertens, L., & Casteels, R., (1994). The functional importance of the extreme C-terminal tail in the gene 2 organellar Ca^{2+}-transport ATPase (SERCA2a/b). *Biochem. J.* **303**, 979–984.

Wu, K.-D. & Lytton, J. (1993). Molecular cloning and quantification of sarcoplasmic reticulum Ca^{2+}-ATPase isoforms in rat muscles. *Am. J. Physiol.* **264**, C333–C341.

Wuytack, F., Raeymaekers, L., Verbist, J., De Smedt, H. & Casteels, R. (1984). Evidence for the presence in smooth muscle of two types of Ca^{2+}-transport ATPase. *Biochem. J.* **224**, 445–451.

Wuytack, F., Raeymaekers, L., Verbist, J., Jones, L. R. & Casteels, R. (1987). Smooth-muscle endoplasmic reticulum contains a cardiac-like form of calsequestrin. *Biochim. Biophys. Acta* **899**, 151–158.

Wuytack, F., Eggermont, J.A., Raeymaekers, L., Plessers, L. & Casteels, R. (1989a). Antibodies against the non-muscle isoform of the endoplasmic reticulum Ca^{2+}-transport ATPase. *Biochem. J.* **264**, 765–769.

Wuytack, F., Kanmura, Y., Eggermont, J.A., Raeymaekers, L., Verbist, J., Hartweg, D., Gietzen, K. & Casteels, R. (1989b). Smooth muscle expresses a cardiac/slow muscle isoform of the Ca^{2+}-transport ATPase in its endoplasmic reticulum. *Biochem. J.* **257**, 117–123.

Wuytack, F., Papp, B., Verboomen, H., Raeymaekers, L., Dode, L., Bobe, R., Enouf, J., Bokkala, S., Authi, K. S., & Casteels, R. (1994). A sarco/endoplasmic reticulum Ca^{2+} ATPase 3-type Ca^{2+} pump is expressed in platelets, in lymphoid cells, and in mast cells. *J. Biol. Chem.* **269**, 1410–1416.

24

Effects of Protein Phosphatase Inhibitors on Smooth Muscles

AKIRA TAKAI

Department of Physiology,
School of Medicine,
Nagoya University,
Nagoya, Japan

INTRODUCTION

Protein phosphatases 1 and 2A (PP1 and PP2A) are two of the four major enzymes which dephosphorylate serine/threonine residues of proteins in eukaryotic cells (Cohen 1989; Shenolikar & Nairn, 1991). During the last decade these enzymes have been shown to be inhibited with different potency by several naturally occurring toxins, including okadaic acid (OA) (Takai *et al.*, 1987; Bialojan & Takai, 1988), calyculin-A (Ishihara *et al.* 1989), microcystin-LR (MCLR) (MacKintosh *et al.*, 1990), nodularin (Matsushima *et al.*, 1990), tautomycin (MacKintosh & Klumpp, 1990) and cantharidin (Li & Casida, 1992). They are now used as powerful tools for research of an increasingly wide variety of cellular events regulated by reversible protein phosphorylation.

The purpose of this chapter is to provide a brief overview of the findings obtained using the protein phosphatase inhibitors in the field of smooth muscle physiology, where their effects are probably most intensively studied. The applications of the protein phosphatase inhibitors in other biological systems have been reviewed elsewhere (Takai, 1988; Cohen *et al.*, 1990).

BIOCHEMICAL CHARACTERISTICS OF THE PROTEIN PHOSPHATASE INHIBITORS

For convenience of description I start out by giving some comments on the affinity and selectivity of the protein phosphatase inhibitors.

Table 1 gives the values of the dissociation constants K_i for the interaction

Table 1 Dissociation constants for the interaction of the purified catalytic submits of protein phosphateses 1 and 2A (PP1 and PP2A). The values for dissociation constants (K_i; means±SEM) obtained by dose-inhibition analyses are listed. Activities were measured using [^{32}P] phosphorylated chicken gizzard myosin light chains as substrate. Values are obtained by least-squares fitting of a theoretical function for tight-binding inhibitors to the dose-inhibition data. PP1/PP2A is the ratio of the K_i value for PP1 and that for PP2A; n denotes the total number of experiments (see Takai *et al.*, 1995)

Inhibitor	PP1		PP2A		
	K_i (pM)	n	K_i (pM)	n	PP1/PP2A
Okadic acid	153 000 ± 33 000	96	34 ± 2	126	4800
Microcystin-LR	50 ± 22	48	13 ± 8	72	3.8
Calyculin-A	980 ± 260	48	105 ± 36	48	9.3
Tautomycin	480 ± 60	48	28600 ± 4800	48	0.016

of okadaic acid, calyculin-A, microcystin-LR and tautomycin, which were estimated by dose-inhibition analyses with purified catalytic subunits of PP1 and PP2A (Takai *et al.*, 1992a, 1995). As most of these inhibitors act at very low concentrations comparable to, or lower than, the total enzyme concentration, E_t in the reaction mixture, the kinetic properties of 'tight-binding inhibitors' as defined by Henderson (1972) were duly considered to analyse the dose-inhibition data (Takai *et al.*, 1992a, 1995). It should be noted that the concentration required for 50% inhibition (ID_{50}), as often used in earlier reports to describe the affinity of the protein phosphatase inhibitors, is not an optimal parameter to use for comparison of the enzyme affinity of tight-binding inhibitors. When the binding of an inhibitor with an enzyme is very tight, the ID_{50} is dependent on the total enzyme concentration, E_t, and is not identical with K_i which is independent of E_t. In such cases, the dose-inhibition relationship tends to be shifted to the right as a result of a decrease in the free inhibitor concentration caused by binding with the enzyme and therefore the ID_{50} becomes larger than the K_i (Takai & Mieskes, 1991).

OA exhibits much higher affinity for PP2A than it does for PP1, whereas MCLR and calyculin-A inhibit these enzymes with similar potency (Table 1). The ratio of the K_i for PP1 to that for PP2A (PP1/PP2A ratio) is about 4800 for OA, 4 for MCLR and 9 for calyculin-A (Table 1). At present, tautomycin is the only naturally occurring toxin that is known to show higher affinity for PP1 than for PP2A. The PP1/PP2A ratio was 0.01:0.02 for this inhibitor. This value is considerably smaller than that (0.4) calculated from K_i values reported earlier (MacKintosh & Klumpp, 1990).

Of the other two major serine/threonine protein phosphatases, the Ca^{2+}/calmodulin-dependent protein phosphatase 2B (PP2B) is inhibited by these substances at much higher concentrations, whereas the Mg^{2+}-dependent protein phosphatase 2C (PP2C) exhibits no susceptibility (Bialojan & Takai, 1988; Ishihara et al., 1989; MacKintosh & Klumpp, 1990; MacKintosh et al., 1990). The following phosphatases are also insensitive to these toxins: acid and alkaline phosphatases, protein phosphatases that dephosphorylate tyrosine residues, and inositol trisphosphatase (Bialojan & Takai, 1988). No direct effect of these toxins has been reported for eight different protein kinases that have been tested, such as cyclic AMP or Ca^{2+}/calmodulin-dependent protein kinases, or protein kinase C (Takai et al., 1987; Haystead et al., 1989; Suganuma et al., 1988).

Because experiments with tight-binding inhibitors often have to be done with very low enzyme and inhibitor concentrations, the enzyme–inhibitor interaction tends to show a marked time-dependence (Cha, 1975, 1976). Takai et al., (1992b) have shown that the interaction of OA and PP2A is indeed very time-dependent. The inhibition of PP2A by MCLR or calyculin-A also exhibits a marked time dependence (A.T., unpublished observations). From the pre-steady-state time-course of OA–PP2A interaction, the rate constants for the binding of OA and PP2A is of the order of $10^7 M^{-1} s^{-1}$, a typical value for reactions involving relatively large molecules, whereas those for their dissociation have very low values in the range 10^{-4} to $10^{-3} s^{-1}$ (Takai et al., 1992b). It should be noted that these values of the rate constants were obtained with the enzyme freely dissolved in experimental buffers. The dissociation of a tight-binding inhibitor may be even slower than expected from the very small values of the rate constants for the dissociation when the reaction occurs in the cytosol, where movements of molecules are more or less restricted by cytoplasmic substances. Conversely, binding of the protein phosphatases with the tight-binding inhibitors in the cytoplasma will take place at a relatively fast rate with a time constant of the order of 0.1–1 s, because the intracellular concentrations of PP1 or PP2A usually lie in the range 0.1–1 µM (Cohen et al., 1990), which is much higher than the enzyme concentrations used in ordinary assay conditions.

PROTEIN PHOSPHATASE INHIBITION AND SMOOTH MUSCLE CONTRACTION

Okadaic acid was the first to be described as a specific protein phosphatase inhibitor acting on both PP1 and PP2A (Takai et al., 1987; Bialojan & Takai, 1988; Hescheler et al., 1988). It was the contractile effects on smooth muscle tissues of this toxin that provided the clue to the discovery of its inhibitory action on protein phosphatases (reviewed by Takai, 1988). In isolated vascular smooth muscle of human umbilical artery, rabbit aorta, and guinea pig taenia coli, Shibata *et al.* (1982) first demonstrated that okadaic acid caused a long-lasting and reversible contraction even under severe Ca^{2+}-deficient conditions. Ozaki *et al.* (1987a,b) showed that OA produced a marked leftward shift of the Ca^{2+}-tension relationship of saponin-skinned fibres of guinea pig taenia. The contractile effect of OA on skinned smooth muscle is well correlated with an increase of phosphorylated myosin light chains (Takai *et al.*, 1987; Bialojan *et al.*, 1988). OA strikingly slowed down relaxation and myosin dephosphorylation induced by Ca^{2+} removal following prior activation with a maximal concentration of Ca^{2+} (Bialojan *et al.*, 1988). All these effects of OA on chemically skinned smooth muscles are attributable to inhibition of the myosin light chain phosphatase activity (Takai 1988).

In permeabilized smooth muscle fibres, calyculin-A (Katsuyama & Morgan, 1993; Smith & Crichton, 1993), MCLR (Katsuyama & Morgan, 1993; Smith & Crichton, 1993) and tautomycin (Hori *et al.*, 1991; Gong *et al.*, 1992) causes contraction, increases 20 kDa myosin light chain phosphorylation, and inhibits the myosin phosphatase activity with the same potency sequence: MCLR > tautomycin ≅ calyculin-A > OA. This potency sequence is identical to the affinity sequence of these inhibitors for PP1 (Table 1), suggesting that the smooth muscle myosin light-chain phosphatase is a PP1.

In chicken gizzard, Alessi *et al.* (1992) have shown that the major protein phosphatase that dephosphorylates smooth muscle myosin is a hetrotrimeric enzyme comprising 37, 130 and 20 kDa components. The 37 kDa component is the catalytic subunit which is almost identical in amino acid sequence to the β-isoform of PP1 from mammalian skeletal muscle. The 130 kDa and 20 kDa components form a regulatory complex that enhances the activity of the catalytic subunit towards heavy meromyosin or the isolated smooth muscle myosin light chain and suppress its activity towards phosphorylase a, phosphorylase kinase and glycogen synthase. Like mammalian PP1, the activity of the catalytic subunit exhibits much higher sensitivity to MCLR than it does to OA (Alessi *et al.*, 1992). At least 80% of the smooth muscle protein phosphatase activity is associated with the myofibrillar pellet, indicating that the enzyme is bound to the contractile proteins (Alessi *et al.*, 1992). Interestingly, the heteromeric form of the avian PP1 is highly resistant to the intrinsic heat-stable inhibitory peptides, inhibitor-1 and inhibitor-2, which inhibit the activity of the catalytic subunit at nanomolar concentrations (Alessi *et al.*, 1992; Gong *et al.*, 1992).

Much less biochemical information is available for the myosin phosphatase activity of mammalian smooth muscles, although several protein phosphatases which dephosphorylate myosin light chains have been isolated from some restricted types of smooth muscle tissues such as bovine (DiSalvo *et al.*, 1982; Werth *et al.*, 1982) or porcine (Erdodi *et al.*, 1992) aorta. Takai *et al.*, (1989) examined the sensitivity of the protein phosphatase activity in crude extracts of the guinea pig ileum to OA and inhibitor-2, using phosphorylated myosin light chains as substrate. Their results suggest the presence of the following four distinct protein phosphatases in the muscle extracts. (1) A PP2A activity that has a very high affinity ($K_i \cong 40\,pM$) to OA, but is not affected by inhibitor-2. (2) A PP1 activity that has a relatively high affinity to OA ($K_i \cong 200\,nM$) and is very sensitive to inhibitor-2. (3) A PP2C activity that exhibits no sensitivity to both OA and inhibitor-2 and is characterized by a strict dependence on Mg^{2+} for activation. (4) A phosphatase activity that has a relatively high susceptibility to OA but is resistant to inhibitor-2. After the cell membrane is permeabilized by Triton X-100, more than 60% of this fraction remains and accounts for about 90% of the total activity, whereas the PP2A, PP1 and PP2C activities are nearly abolished. This is indicative that the inhibitor-2-resistant fraction is bound to some intracellular components (presumably to contractile protein). Although Takai *et al.* (1989) referred to this activity as 'a PP2A-like fraction' because of its resistance to inhibitor-2, it shows closer similarities to the oligomeric form of PP1 isolated from chicken gizzard, which is also resistant to inhibitor-2 (see above).

The protein phosphatase activities of other smooth muscles such as guinea pig taenia or rabbit main pulmonary artery exhibit similar sensitivity to OA and inhibitor-2, suggesting a similar phosphatase composition. As the inhibitor-2-resistant 'PP1-like' fraction (formerly called 'PP2A-like' fraction) is the only myosin light chain phosphatase activity remaining in skinned mammalian smooth muscles with reversible contractility (Takai *et al.*, 1989), it seems reasonable to speculate that this phosphatase activity dephosphorylates smooth muscle myosin to induce relaxation.

INHIBITORY EFFECT OF OKADAIC ACID ON SMOOTH MUSCLE CONTRACTION

In smooth muscle with intact plasma membrane, OA strongly and irreversibly inhibits the contractility at concentrations lower than those required to produce contraction (see Figure 1). No other protein phosphatase inhibitors are known to inhibit smooth muscle contraction in any concentration range examined. Inhibition of contractility by OA has been reported for various types of smooth muscles including pig coronary artery (Ashizawa *et al.*, 1989; Hirano *et al.*, 1989), dog basilar artery (Ashizawa *et al.*, 1989), rat (Abe & Karaki, 1993) and rabbit (Karaki *et al.*, 1989) aorta, guinea pig taenia caeci (Lang *et al.*, 1991) and vas deferens (Shibata *et al.*, 1991), rat uterus (Candenas *et al.*, 1992), and bovine iris (Wang *et al.*, 1994) and trachea

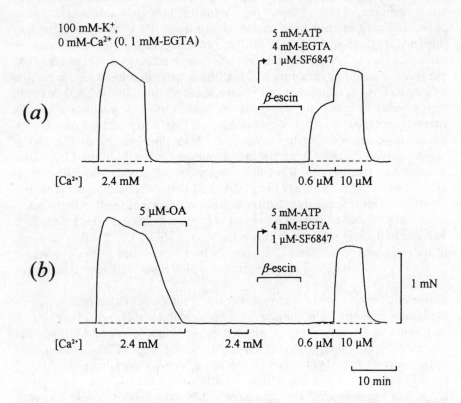

Figure 1 Inhibitory effect of okadic acid (OA) on the contractility of the taenia of guinea pig caecum (a) The muscle fibre was placed in a semi-closed glass chamber (1.0 ml volume) perfused with a peristaltic pump and equilibrated in a relaxing solution containing 100 mM KCl, 20 mM NaCl, 1.2 mM MgCl$_2$, 11.8 mM dextrose, 20 mM HEPES and 0.1 mM EGTA (pH 7.4 at 35°C). After steady mechanical responses to readmission of 2.4 mM Ca^{2+}, the fibre was permeabilized by incubation with 200 μM β-escin for 10 min in a solution with the following composition: 100 mM KCl, 2 mM MgCl$_2$, 20 mM HEPES, 5 mM ATP Na$_2$ and 4 mM EGTA (pH 7.0 at 35°C). SF6847 (1 μM), one of the most potent uncouplers (Bakker *et al.*, 1975), was added to inhibit regeneration of ATP by oxidative phosphorylation. The free Ca^{2+} concentration was increased by injecting CaCl$_2$ into the chamber after stopping perfusion. Reduction of the pH caused by reaction of EGTA with CaCl$_2$ added was compensated by adding NaOH. (b) An experiment with the same equipment as in (a). The contracture induced by Ca^{2+} readmission was irreversibly inhibited when 5 μM OA was applied. After permeabilization with β-escin, the fibre contracted in response to elevation of the free Ca^{2+} concentration. Note that only very small tension development was produced with 0.6 μM Ca^{2+} which produced a 60%-maximal contraction of the control fibre (see (a)).

(Tansey et al., 1990). Relaxant effects may also be observed prior to, or simultaneously with, contractions produced by higher concentrations of OA. Shibata et al. (1982) showed that the slow tension development caused by 50 μM OA in the guinea pig taenia was preceded by a complete cessation of the spontaneous mechanical activity. Obara et al. (1989) showed in their experiments on the smooth muscle of lamb trachea that both the tension development and the myosin phosphorylation produced by okadaic acid had a slow-time course which unchanged by either Ca^{2+}-depletion procedures or application of a calmodulin antagonist, W-7. This suggests that, in the presence of okadaic acid, the pathway involving Ca^{2+}/calmodulin-dependent myosin light-chain kinase was inactivated and myosin phosphorylation was catalysed by a Ca^{2+}/calmodulin-independent kinase.

There are several properties common to the relaxant effects of OA observed in different types of smooth muscles:

1. The inhibition is irreversible. In most smooth muscles examined, contractility once inhibited by OA does not recover even after washing for hours (Ashizawa et al., 1989).
2. The relaxant effect of OA is highly dependent on temperature. For example, Ashizawa et al. (1989) observed in the porcine coronary artery that 3 μM OA, which nearly abolished contracture induced by 40 mM K$^+$ in porcine coronary artery at 37°C, produced almost no change in the tension when applied at 30°C.
3. In most cases reported (but see Tansey et al. (1990)), the relaxant effect is not accompanied by a marked reduction of the intracellular free Ca^{2+} concentration, $[Ca^{2+}]_i$. Slight reduction of $[Ca^{2+}]_i$ has been observed on application of OA in some types of smooth muscle (Ashizawa et al., 1989; Hirano et al., 1989; Karaki et al., 1989). However, the $[Ca^{2+}]$ is reduced by only 10–20% even when the contraction is almost completely inhibited by OA.
4. Contractions induced by agonists or by high K$^+$ are both strongly inhibited by OA (Ashizawa et al., 1989; Karaki et al., 1989). OA also strongly inhibits the tension development produced by other protein phosphatase inhibitors such as tautomycin (A.T., unpublished observations).

These observations suggest that OA produces its inhibitory effects on various smooth muscles essentially by the same mechanism. However, there may be some tissue-specific factors in relaxant responses of each type of smooth muscle.

In porcine coronary artery, Hirano et al. (1989) investigated the effect of OA on the $[Ca^{2+}]$ tension relationship by the fura-2 method. They showed that OA inhibited the maximal levels of the contracture induced by high K$^+$ without changing the $[Ca^{2+}]_i$ for 50% activation. In the guinea pig taenia caeci, however, the Ca^{2+} sensitivity of the contractile system appears to be reduced when the contractility is inhibited by OA. In the experiments shown in Figure 1, the Ca^{2+} sensitivity of guinea pig taenia was examined after quick permeabilization with β-escin with or without pretreatment by 5 μM OA. The Ca^{2+}-tension relationship was markedly shifted to the right by the OA-treatment (see also Figure 2).

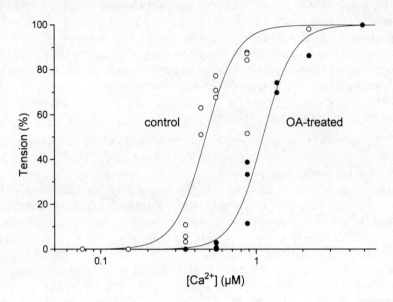

Figure 2 Reduction of Ca^{2+} sensitivity of smooth muscle contractile machinery after treatment with okadic acid (OA). In experiments similar to those shown in Figure 1, muscle fibres were permeabilized with β-escin and the magnitude of contractions produced by increasing the free Ca^{2+} concentration in the media ($[Ca^{2+}]$) were measured. Responses of fibres pretreated with 5 μM OA (OA-treated) are compared with those of untreated fibres (control). One fibre was used to examine one response to a submaximal $[Ca^{2+}]$ and one maximal $[Ca^{2+}]$ (= 10 μM) only. The values are normalized to the response to the maximal $[Ca^{2+}]$. Note the marked shift of the $[Ca^{2+}]$-tension relationship to the right in the OA-treated fibres.

In bovine tracheal muscle, Tansey *et al.* (1990) observed that myosin light chains remained highly phosphorylated when carbachol-induced contraction was completely inhibited by OA. In this case, the relaxation was associated with a decrease in the $[Ca^{2+}]_i$ measured with the fura-2 method. They speculated that OA inhibited the contraction of the tracheal muscle by reducing the $[Ca^{2+}]_i$ and/or by increasing phosphorylation of some protein other than myosin light chain.

In the guinea pig taenia caeci, OA-treatment resulted in a significant decrease in myosin light chain phosphorylation (Table 2). However, 15% of myosin light chains were still phosphorylated even when the contractility of the fibres was lost by OA treatment. It is unclear to what extent the decrease in myosin phosphorylation is related to the relaxation in this type of smooth muscle.

Table 2 Effect of pretreatment of guinea pig taenia caeci by okadaic acid (OA) on myosin light-chain phosphorylation. The relative amount of phosphorylated 20-kDa myosin light chains (PMLC) were analysed by two-dimensional gel electrophoresis (Bialojan *et al.*, 1988). The muscle strips were equilibrated in a Ca^{2+}-free, high K^+ solution (see the legend for Figure 1 for the composition) and stimulated by addition of 2.4 mM $CaCl_2$. They were fixed by trichloroacetic acid in acetone precooled with dry-ice just before or 100 s after the addition of 2.4 mM $CaCl_2$. Some fibres were immersed in a solution containing OA (1 or 10 μM) and 2.4 mM Ca^{2+} for 20 min. This treatment abolished the contractility of the fibre (Figure 1b). Note the significant ($p<0.001$) decrease in PMLC by pre-treatment with OA. Values are presented as mean ±SEM; *n* denotes the number of experiments

[OA] (μM)	$[Ca^{2+}]_o$ (mM)	PMLC (%)	*n*
0	0	<1	4
10	0	<1	4
10	2.4	35.0 ± 1.6	22
1	2.4	24.4 ± 1.1	9
10	2.4	14.2 ± 2.6	10

Because OA is the only protein phosphatase inhibitor that is known to exhibit much higher potency for PP2A than for PP1 (Table 1), it seems natural to speculate that its inhibitory effect on contraction unique to this toxin may be due to inhibition of PP2A, which results in an increase of phosphorylation of some regulatory protein. The irreversibility of the relaxant effect is possibly attributable to the very slow rate of dissociation of OA from PP2A (see above). Further experiments are necessary to elucidate the precise mechanism of the inhibitory effect of okadaic acid on intact smooth muscle fibres.

PROTEIN PHOSPHATASE INHIBITORS AND SMOOTH MUSCLE ELECTROPHYSIOLOGY

The relaxant effect of β-agonist on guinea pig and human airway smooth muscle is accompanied by marked hyperpolarization of the membrane (Honda *et al.*, 1986; Honda & Tomita, 1987). Kume *et al.*, (1989) studied the mechanism of this hyperpolarization by applying the patch-clamp technique on rabbit tracheal myocytes. They showed that Ca^{2+}-dependent K^+ channels of the tracheal myocytes were activated either by extracellular application of isoprenaline or by intracellular application of cAMP-dependent protein kinase. OA enhanced and prolonged the activating effects, supporting the notion that these channels are regulated by cAMP-dependent phosphorylation. Similar protocols were used to show that the Ca^{2+}-activated K^+ channels in myocytes of the canine proximal colon (Carl et al., 1991) and ATP-sensitive K^+ channels of gall-bladder smooth muscle cells (Zhang et al., 1994) are activated by cAMP-dependent protein kinase. Carl et al. (1991) showed that the combined use of okadaic acid and calyculin-A is effective for identifying the type of protein phosphatase responsible for de-phosphorylation of channel proteins.

In heart muscle, OA increases the duration of action potential and enhances the contraction (Kodama et al., 1986). It has now been established that this effect of OA is due to an increase in Ca^{2+}-influx through L-type Ca^{2+} channels by cAMP-dependent phosphorylation (Takai, 1988; Hescheler et al., 1988; Lee et al., 1991). In canine gastric and colonic smooth muscles, Ward et al. (1991) showed that calyculin-A and okadaic acid reduces the amplitude and duration of slow waves primarily by inhibiting the plateau component. They discussed the possibility that phosphorylation of Ca^{2+} channels of gastrointestinal smooth muscles may inhibit Ca^{2+} currents. Similar conclusions were drawn by Lang et al. (1991) and Obara & Yabu (1993) who examined the effect of OA and calyculin-A on the Ca^{2+} channel currents of single smooth muscle cells of the guinea pig taenia caeci.

CONCLUSIONS

In summary, I have reviewed recent findings obtained with the use of protein phosphatase inhibitors in the field of smooth muscle physiology. Several protein phosphatase inhibitors with different specificities are now available and their biochemical properties have been closely investigated. The use of the toxins of this category is steadily increasing, especially in this field. This is not surprising because protein phosphorylation is one of the central mechanisms by which smooth muscle function is regulated.

REFERENCES

Abe, A. & Karaki, H. (1993). Synergistic effects of cyclic AMP-related vasodilators and the phosphatase inhibitor okadaic acid. Jap. J. Pharmacol. **63**, 129–131.

Alessi, D., MacDougall, L.K., Sola, M.M., Ikebee, M. & Cohen, P. (1992). The control of protein phosphatase-1 by targetting subunits: The major myosin phosphatase in avian smooth muscle is a novel form of protein phosphatase-1. *Eur. J. Biochem.* **210**, 1023–1035.

Ashiwaza, N., Kobayashi, F., Tanaka, Y. & Nakayama, K. (1989). Relaxing action of okadaic acid, a black sponge toxin on the arterial smooth muscle. *Biochem. Biophys. Res. Comm.* **162**, 971–976.

Bakker, E.P., Arents, J.C., Hoebe, J.P.M. & Terada, H. (1975). Surface potential and the interaction of weakly acidic uncouplers of oxidative phosphorylation with liposomes and mitochondria. *Biochim. Biophys. Acta* **387**, 491–506.

Bialojan, C. & Takai, A. (1988). Inhibitory effect of a marine-sponge toxin, okadaic acid, on protein phosphatases: specificity and kinetics. *Biochem. J.* **256**, 283–290.

Bialojan, C., Rüegg, J.C. & Takai, A. (1988). Effects of okadaic acid on isometric tension and myosin phosphorylation of chemically skinned guinea pig taenia coli. *J. Physiol. (London)* **398**, 81–95.

Candenas, M.L., Norte, M., Gonzalez, R., Arteche, E., Fernandez, J.J., Borges, R., Boada, J., Adveenier, C. & Martin, J. D. (1992). Inhibitory and contractile effects of okadaic acid on rat uterine muscle. *Eur. J. Pharmacol.* **219**, 473–476.

Carl, A., Kenyon, J.L., Uemura, D., Fusetani, N. & Sanders, K.M. (1991). Regulation of Ca^{2+}-activated K^+ channels by protein kinase A and phosphatase inhibitors. *Am. J. Physiol.* **261**, C387–C392.

Cha, S. (1975). Tight-binding inhibitors: I. kinetic behavior. *Biochem. Pharmacol.* **24**, 2177–2185.

Cha, S. (1976). Tight-binding inhibitors: III. a new approach for the determination of competition between tight-binding inhibitors and substrates—inhibition of adenosine deaminase by coformycin. *Biochem. Pharmacol.* **25**, 2695–2702.

Cohen, P. (1989). The structure and regulation of protein phosphatases. *Annu. Rev. Biochem.* **58**, 453–508.

Cohen, P., Holmes, C.F.B. & Tsukatani, Y. (1990). Okadaic acid: a new probe for the study of cellular regulation. *Trends Biochem. Sci.* **15**, 98–102.

DiSalvo, J., Jiang, M.J., Vandenheede, J.R. & Merlevede, W. (1982). The ATPMg-dependent phosphatase is present in mammalian vascular smooth muscle. *Biochem. Biophys. Res. Commu.* **108**, 534–540.

Erdodi, F., Csortos, C., Sparks, L., Muranyi, A. & Gergely, P. (1992). Purification and characterization of three distinct types of protein phosphatase catalytic subunits in bovine platelets. *Arch. Biochem. Biophys.* **298**, 682–687.

Gong, M.C., Cohen, P., Kitazawa, T., Ikebe, M., Masuo, M., Somlyo, A.P. & Somlyo, A.V. (1992). Myosin light chain phosphatase activities and the effects of phosphatase inhibitors in tonic and phasic smooth muscle. *J. Biol. Chem.* **267**, 14662–14668.

Haystead, T.A., Sim, A.T., Carling, D., Honnor, R.C., Tsukitani, Y., Cohen, P. & Hardie, D.G. (1989). Effects of the tumour promoter okadaic acid on intracellular protein phosphorylation and metabolism. *Nature* **337**, 78–81.

Henderson, P.J.F. (1972). A linear equation that describes the steady-state kinetics of enzymes and subcellular particles interacting with tightly bound inhibitors. *Biochem. J.* **127**, 321–333.

Hescheler, J., Mieskes, G., Rüegg, J.C., Takai, A. & Trautwein, W. (1988). Effects of a protein phosphatase inhibitor, okadaic acid, on membrane currents of isolated guinea pig cardiac myocytes. *Pflügers Arch.* **412**, 248–252.

Hirano, K., Kanaide, H. & Nakamura, M. (1989). Effects of okadaic acid on cytosolic calcium concentrations and on contractions of the porcine coronary artery. *Br. J.*

Pharmacol. **98**, 1261–1266.

Honda, K. & Tomita, T. (1987). Electrical activity in isolated human tracheal muscle. *Jap. J. Physiol.* **37**, 333–336.

Honda, K., Satake, T., Takagi, K. & Tomita, T. (1986). Effects of relaxants on electrical and mechanical activities in the guinea pig tracheal muscle. *Br. J. Pharmacol.* **87**, 665–671.

Hori, M., Magae, J., Han, Y.G., Hartshorne, D.J. & Karaki, H. (1991). A novel protein phosphatase inhibitor, tautomycin: effect on smooth muscle. *FEBS Lett.* **285**, 145–148.

Ishihara, H., Martin, B.L., Braitigan, D.L., Karaki, H., Ozaki, H., Kato, Y., Fusetani, N., Watabe, S., Hasimoto, K., Uemura, D. & Hartshorne, D.J. (1989). Calyculin A and okadaic acid: inhibitors of protein phosphatase activity. *Biochem. Biophys. Res. Comm.* **159**, 871–877.

Karaki, H., Mitsui, M., Nagase, H., Ozaki, H., Shibata, S. & Uemura, D. (1989). Inhibitory effect of a toxin okadaic acid, isolated from the black sponge on smooth muscle and platelets. *Br. J. Pharmacol.* **98**, 590–596.

Katsuyama, H. & Morgan, K.G. (1993). Mechanisms of Ca^{2+}-independent contraction in single permeabilized ferret aorta cells. *Circ. Res.* **72**, 651–657.

Kodama, I., Kondo, N. & Shibata, S. (1986). Electromechanical effects of okadaic acid isolated from black sponge in guinea pig ventricular muscles. *J. Physiol. (London)* **378**, 359–373.

Kume, H., Takai, A., Tokuno, H. & Tomita, T. (1989). Regulation of Ca^{2+}-dependent K^+-channel activity in tracheal myocytes by phosphorylation. *Nature* **341**, 152–154.

Lang, R.J., Ozolins, I.Z. & Paul, R.J. (1991). Effects of okadaic acid and ATPγS on cell length and Ca^{2+}-channel currents recorded in single smooth muscle cells of the guinea pig taenia caeci. *Br. J. Pharmacol.* **104**, 331–336.

Lee, J.A., Takai, A. & Allen, D.G. (1991). Okadaic acid, a protein phosphatase inhibitor, increases the calcium transients in isolated ferret ventricular muscle. *Exp. Physiol.* **76**, 281–284.

Li, Y.M. & Casida, J.E. (1992). Cantharidin-binding protein: identification as protein phosphatase 2A. *Proc. Natl Acad. Sci. USA* **89**, 11867–11870.

Mackintosh, C. & Klumpp, S. (1990). Tautomycin from the bacterium *Streptomyces verticillatus*: another potent and specific inhibitor of protein phosphatases 1 and 2A. *FEBS Lett.* **277**, 137–140.

Mackintosh, C., Beattie, K.A., Klumpp, S., Cohen, P. & Codd, G.A. (1990). Cyanobacterial microcystin-LR is a potent and specific inhibitor of protein phosphatases 1 and 2A from both mammals and higher plants. *FEBS Lett.* **264**, 187–192.

Matsushima, R., Yoshizawa, S., Watanabe, M.F., Harada, K., Furusawa, M., Carmichael, W.W. & Fujiki, H. (1990). *In vitro* and *in vivo* effects of protein phosphatase inhibitors, microcystins and nodularin, on mouse skin and fibroblasts. *Biochem. Biophys. Res. Comm.* **171**, 867–874.

Obara, K. & Yabu, H. (1993). Dual effect of phosphatase inhibitors on calcium channels in intestinal smooth muscle cells. *Am. J. Physiol.* **264**, C296–C301.

Obara, K., Takai, A., Rüegg, J.C. & De Lanerolle, P. (1989). Okadaic acid, a phosphatase inhibitor, produces a Ca^{2+} and calmodulin-independent contraction of smooth muscle. *Pflügers Arch.* **414**, 134–138.

Ozaki, H., Ishihara, H., Kohama, K., Nonomura, Y., Shibata, S. & Karaki, H. (1987a). Calcium-independent phosphorylation of smooth muscle myosin light chain by okadaic acid isolated from black sponge (Halichondria okadai). *J. Pharmacol. Exp. Ther.* **243**, 1167–1173.

Ozaki, H., Kohama, K., Nonomura, Y., Shibata, S. & Karaki, H. (1987b). Direct activation by okadaic acid of the contractile elements in the smooth muscle of guinea pig taenia coli. *Naunyn-Schmiedeberg's Arch. Pharmacol* **335**, 356–358.

Shenolikar, S. & Nairn, A.C. (1991). Protein phosphatases: recent progress. *Adv. Second Messenger Phosphoprot. Res.* **23**, 1–121.

Shibata, S., Ishida, Y., Kitano, H., Ohizumi, Y., Habon, J., Tsukitani, Y. & Kikuchi, H. (1982). Contractile effects of okadaic acid, a novel ionophore-like substance from black sponge, on isolated smooth muscles under the condition of Ca deficiency. *J. Pharmacol. Exp. Ther.* **223**, 135–143.

Shibata, S., Satake, N., Morikawa, M., Kown, S.C., Karaki, H., Kurahashi, K., Sawada, T. & Kodama, I. (1991). The inhibitory action of okadaic acid on mechanical responses in guinea pig vas deferens. *Eur. J. Pharmacol.* **193**, 1–7.

Smith, G.L. & Crichton, C.A. (1993). Ca-EGTA affects the relationship between [Ca²⁺] and tension in alpha-toxin permeabilized rat anococcygeus smooth muscle. *J. Muscle Res. Cell Motil.* **14**, 76–84.

Suganuma, M., Fujiki, H., Suguri, H., Yoshizawa, S., Hirota, M., Nakayasu, M., Ojika, M., Wakamatsu, K., Yamada, K. & Sugimura, T. (1988). Okadaic acid: an additional non-phorbol-12-tetradecanoate-13-acetate-type tumor promoter. *Proc. Natl Acad. Sci. USA* **85**, 1768–1771.

Takai, A. (1988). Okadaic acid: protein phosphatase inhibition and muscle contractile effects. *J. Muscle Res. Cell Motil.* **9**, 563–565.

Takai, A. & Mieskes, G. (1991). Inhibitory effect of okadaic acid on the *p*-nitrophenyl phosphate phosphatase activity of protein phosphatases. *Biochem. J.* **275**, 233–239.

Takai, A., Bialojan, C., Troschka, M. & Rüegg, J.C. (1987). Smooth muscle myosin phosphatase inhibition and force enhancement by black sponge toxin. *FEBS Lett.* **217**, 81–84.

Takai, A., Troschka, M., Mieskes, G. & Somlyo, A.V. (1989). Protein phosphatase composition in the smooth muscle of guinea pig ileum studied with okadaic acid and inhibitor 2. *Biochem. J.* **262**, 617–623.

Takai, A., Murata, M., Torigoe, K., Isobe, M., Mieskes, G. & Yasumoto, T. (1992a). Inhibitory effect of okadaic acid derivatives on protein phosphatases: a study on structure-affinity relationship. *Biochem. J.* **284**, 539–544.

Takai, A., Ohno, Y., Yasumoto, T. & Mieskes, G. (1992b). Estimation of the rate constants associated with the inhibitory effect of okadaic acid on type 2A protein phosphatase by time-course analysis. *Biochem. J.* **287**, 101–106.

Takai, A., Sasaki, K., Nagai, H., Mieskes, G., Isobe, M., Isono, K. & Yasumoto, T. (1995). Inhibition of specific binding of okadaic acid to protein phosphatase 2A by microcystin-LR, calyculin-A and tautomycin: method of analysis of interactions of tight-binding ligands with target protein. *Biochem. J.* **306**, 657–665.

Tansey, M.G., Hori, M., Karaki, H., Kamm, K.E. & Stull, J.T. (1990). Okadaic acid uncouples myosin light chain phosphorylation and tension in smooth muscle. *FEBS Lett.* **270**, 219–221.

Wang, X.L., Akhtar, R.A. & Abdeel Latif, A.A. (1994). Studies on the properties of myo-inositol-1,4,5-trisphosphate 5-phosphatase and myo-inositol monophosphatase in bovine iris sphincter smooth muscle: effects of okadaic acid and protein phosphorylation. *Biochim. Biophys Acta* **1222**, 27–36.

Ward, S.M., Vogalis, F., Blondfield, D.P., Ozaki, H., Fusetani, N., Uemura, D., Publicover, N.G. & Sanders, K.M. (1991). Inhibition of electrical slow waves and Ca²⁺ currents of gastric and colonic smooth muscle by phosphatase inhibitors. *Am. J. Physiol.* **261**, C64–C70.

Werth, D.K., Haeberle, J.R. & Hathaway, D. R. (1982). Purification of a myosin phosphatase from bovine aortic smooth muscle. *J. Biol. Chem.* **257**, 7306–7309.

Zhang, L., Bonev, A.D., Mawe, G.M. & Nelson, M.T. (1994). Protein kinase A mediates activation of ATP-sensitive K⁺ currents by CGRP in gallbladder smooth muscle. *Am. J. Physiol.* **267**, G494–9.

25

Effects of Acidosis on Cytosolic Ca^{2+} Level, Ca^{2+} Sensitivity and Force in Vascular Smooth Muscle

SATOSHI KITAJIMA
HIROSHI OZAKI
HIDEAKI KARAKI

*Department of Veterinary Pharmacology,
Graduate School of Agriculture and Life Sciences,
University of Tokyo,
Tokyo, Japan*

SUMMARY

1. Effects of lowering extracellular pH (pH_o) and cytosolic pH (pH_i) on cytosolic Ca^{2+} levels ($[Ca^{2+}]_i$) and contractile force were examined in isolated rat aorta loaded with a fluorescent pH indicator, BCECF, or a fluorescent Ca^{2+} indicator, fura-2.

2. pH_i averaged 7.39 in a HEPES-buffered solution at pH_o 7.40. Decreasing pH_o to 6.50 decreased pH_i to 6.63 and increased $[Ca^{2+}]_i$, force and K_d of fura-2 for Ca^{2+}; a Ca^{2+} channel blocker, 1 μM verapamil, blocked the rise in $[Ca^{2+}]_i$ and partially inhibited contraction.

3. Depolarization with 70.4 mM external potassium ($[K^+]_o$), decreased pH_i from 7.39 to 7.33 and increased $[Ca^{2+}]_i$. In muscle depolarized with 27.7 mM $[K^+]_o$, decreasing pH_o from 7.40 to 6.50 decreased $[Ca^{2+}]_i$ without changing force development.

4. The $[Ca^{2+}]_i$-tension relationship, constructed by changing $[K^+]_o$ and pH_o, indicated that the Ca^{2+} sensitivity of contractile elements was increased at pH_o 6.50.

5. Addition of 10 mM NH_4Cl increased pH_i to 8.02 whereas removal of NH_4Cl decreased pH_i to 7.12. Both intracellular acidification and alkalization transiently increased $[Ca^{2+}]_i$ and force. The transient increase in $[Ca^{2+}]_i$ was observed also in the absence of extracellular Ca^{2+} (in the presence of 0.5 mM EGTA) or in the presence of 1 μM verapamil.

SMOOTH MUSCLE EXCITATION
ISBN 0-12-112360-X

6. These results suggest that extracellular acidosis induces intracellular acidosis and opens Ca^{2+} channel in the aorta at resting condition whereas it inhibits Ca^{2+} channels in high K^+-stimulated aorta. In addition, acidosis seemed to increase Ca^{2+} sensitivity of the contractile elements. It is also suggested that a sudden pH_i change in either direction releases Ca^{2+} from intracellular storage sites and induces a transient contraction.

INTRODUCTION

Changes in intracellular and extracellular pH levels (pH_i and pH_o, respectively) modulate functions of organelles, membrane permeability and conductance, cell-to-cell coupling, mechanical properties and energy metabolism in various types of cells, including smooth muscle (Wray, 1988). Several techniques have been employed to experimentally change pH_o and/or pH_i. These include changing the concentration of CO_2 or HCO_3^-, addition of H^+ or OH^-, and addition and subsequent removal of NH_4Cl (Karaki & Weiss, 1981). Using these techniques, it has been shown that changing pH_o and/or pH_i modulates contractile activity in smooth muscles. In carotid artery, extracellular alkalosis induces depolarization whereas extracellular acidosis induces hyperpolarization (Siegel & Schneider, 1981). Intracellular alkalosis and acidosis induce contraction in pulmonary artery (Krampetz & Rhoades, 1991). In mesenteric artery, intracellular alkalosis inhibits whereas intracellular acidosis enhances the contraction induced by noradrenaline (Nielsen *et al.*, 1991). In taenia caeci, extracellular acidosis enhances high K^+-induced contraction (Lofqvist & Nilsson, 1981). Because smooth muscle contraction is regulated primarily by the changes in cytosolic Ca^{2+} level ($[Ca^{2+}]_i$) and Ca^{2+} sensitivity of contractile element (Karaki, 1989), pH may affect either of these factors.

In the present study, we examined the effects of pH_i and pH_o on $[Ca^{2+}]_i$ and force in the isolated rat aorta. Results sugges that Ca^{2+} channel activity, Ca^{2+} release and the Ca^{2+} sensitivity of contractile elements are modulated by pH.

METHODS

Male Wistar rats (250–300 g) were stunned and bled and the thoracic aorta was dissected. After removing fat and connective tissues, the aorta was cut into helical strips approximately 2 mm wide and 8 mm long. Normal physiological salt solution contained (in mM): NaCl, 136.9; KCl, 5.4; $CaCl_2$, 1.5; $MgCl_2$, 1.0; HEPES, 20.0; glucose, 5.5; and EDTA, 0.01. High K^+ solution was made by replacing NaCl with equimolar KCl. Ca^{2+}-free solution was made by omitting CaCl$_2$ and adding 0.5 mM EGTA. These solutions were adjusted to the desired pH by adding NaOH or KOH at 37°C and aerated with 100% O$_2$.

pH$_i$ was measured according to Aalkjaer & Cragoe (1988) using a fluorescent indicator, BCECF (Rink et al., 1982), with a fluorimeter (CAF-100, Japan Spectroscopic, Tokyo, Japan). Muscle strips were treated with 5 μM acetoxymethyl ester of BCECF in the presence of 0.02% cremophor EL for 1–2 h at room temperature. The muscle strip was then held horizontally in a 7-ml bath attached to a fluorimeter. One end of the muscle strip was connected to a strain gauge transducer under a resting force of 10 mN. The muscle strip was illuminated alternatively (48 Hz) with two excitation wavelengths (450 nm and 500 nm) and the amount of 540 nm fluorescence induced by the 450 nm excitation and that induced by 500 nm excitation were measured. The ratio of these two was used as an indicator of pH$_i$. At the end of an experiment, the muscle strip was treated with a K$^+$–H$^+$ ionophore, nigericin, for calibration of pH$_i$ (Thomas et al., 1979).

[Ca^{2+}]$_i$ was measured as described by Ozaki et al. (1987) and Sato et al. (1988) using a fluorescent indicator, fura-2 (Grynkiewicz et al., 1985). Muscle strips were treated with 5 μM acetoxymethyl ester of fura-2 in the presence of 0.02% cremophor EL for 3–4 h at room temperature. The muscle strip was then attached to a fluorimeter (CAF-100) and illuminated alternately (48 Hz) with two excitation wavelengths (340 nm and 380 mm) and the levels of 500 nm fluorescence (F340 and F380) were measured. The ratio of these two (R340/380) was used as an indicator of [Ca^{2+}]$_i$ (Ozaki et al., 1987; Sato et al., 1988) taking the R340/380 in the resting muscle as 0% and that in 70.4 mM KCl-stimulated muscle as 100%.

Although Grynkiewicz et al., (1985) and Uto et al., (1991) reported that changes in pH in the range of 6.5–7.2 did not change the dissociation constant (K_d) of fura-2 for Ca^{2+}, Lattanzio (1990) reported some change. In the present experiment, therefore, we examined the effect of pH on fura-2 fluorescence. pH of the solution containing 2 mM EGTA, 20 mM PIPES, 80 mM KCl and 1 μM fura-2 was adjusted to 7.4, 7.2 or 6.6 at 37°C. Ca^{2+} concentration was adjusted to 200 nM by adding 1.51 mM [Ca^{2+}] at pH 7.4, 1.22 mM [Ca^{2+}] at pH 7.2 or 0.20 mM [Ca^{2+}] at pH 6.6, as reported by Fabiato (1981). As shown in Figure 1, decreasing pH from 7.4 to 7.2 showed almost no effect on the fura-2-Ca^{2+} fluorescence. Further decrease to pH 6.6, however, decreased F340 and increased F380. Increasing the Ca^{2+} concentration of the pH 6.6 solution to 250–300 nM made the F340 and F380 identical to those in the pH 7.4 solution containing 200 nM [Ca^{2+}]. Because Ca^{2+} concentration is proportional to K_d (Grynkiewicz et al., 1985), this result suggests that K_d increased by 1.25 to 1.5 times in the pH 6.6 solution. Change in pH to 8.5 also changed the fura-2 fluorescence (data not shown) and decreased K_d, as reported by Uto et al. (1991). Using R340/380 as an

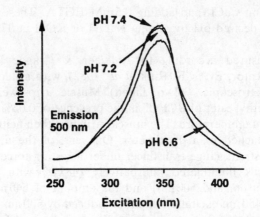

Figure 1 Effects of pH on the fura-2-Ca^{2+} fluorescence. Solution containing 1 μM fura-2 and 200 nM [Ca^{2+}] at different pH was excited at 250–450 nm and 500 nm emission was measured.

indicator, therefore, [Ca^{2+}]$_i$ measured at pH 6.5 is underestimate whereas [Ca^{2+}]$_i$ measured at pH 8.5 is overestimate. In some experiments, absolute [Ca^{2+}]$_i$ was calculated using the K_d value of 224 nM at pH$_i$ 7.4 (Grynkiewicz *et al.*, 1985) and 336 nM at pH$_i$ 6.6 based on the above results.

Following chemicals were used. Verapamil hydrochloride (Sigma Chemicals, St Louis, MO, USA) and ammonium chloride (Wako Pure Chemicals, Osaka, Japan) were dissolved in distilled water. Nigericin (Sigma) was dissolved in 100% ethanol. Acetoxymethyl esters of fura-2 and BCECF (Dojindo Laboratories) were dissolved in DMSO. HEPES and cremophor EL were obtained from Dojindo Laboratories and Nacarai Tesque, Kyoto, Japan, respectively.

The numerical data were expressed as mean ± SEM Differences were evaluated by Student's *t*-test or *F*-test, and p<0.05 was considered statistically significant.

RESULTS

Effects of pH$_o$ on pH$_i$ and force

Figure 2 shows an example of simultaneous measurements of pH$_i$ and force in the isolated rat aorta. Elevation of extracellular K$^+$ from 5.4 to 70.4 mM induced sustained contraction and decreased pH$_i$ from 7.39 ± 0.01 to 7.33 ± 0.01 (*P* <0.01, *n* = 8). Upon washing the muscle with normal solution, pH$_i$ returned to the control level in approximately 10 min. Increasing pH$_o$ from

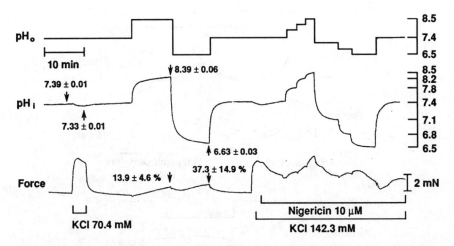

Figure 2 The effects of pH_o (upper trace) on pH_i (middle trace) and force (lower trace) in the isolated rat aorta. At the end of experiment, pH_i was calibrated by using a K^+–H^+ ionophore, nigericin, in Na^+-free, high K^+ solution at various pH.

7.40 to 8.50 increased pH_i to 8.39 $\pm$ 0.06 (n = 4) which reached a new steady level in approximately 10 min, and increased force to 13.9 $\pm$ 4.6% (n = 4). Decreasing pH_o from 8.50 to 6.50 decreased pH_i to 6.63 $\pm$ 0.03 (n = 4) in approximately 10 min, and transiently decreased force followed by an increase to 37.3 $\pm$ 14.9 %. At the end of the experiment, the muscle strip was treated with 142.3 mM K^+ solution containing 10 µM nigericin followed by the changes in pH_o to calibrate pH_i (Thomas *et al.*, 1979).

Effects of lowering pH_o on $[Ca^{2+}]_i$ and force

Figure 3A shows the effects of lowering pH_o on $[Ca^{2+}]_i$ (indicated by R340/380) and force in normal K^+ (5.4 mM) solution. Decrease in pH_o from 7.40 to 6.50 increased R340/380 by 19.46 $\pm$ 5.1% and force by 28.1 $\pm$ 5.8% (n = 4). The actual increase in $[Ca^{2+}]_i$ may be larger than that indicated by R340/380 (see Methods). Small oscillatory changes in $[Ca^{2+}]_i$ often superimposed on the basal increase in $[Ca^{2+}]_i$. The increase in $[Ca^{2+}]_i$ was completely inhibited by 1 µM verapamil. It has been shown that the same concentration of verapamil completely suppresses high K^+-induced increases in $[Ca^{2+}]_i$ (Sato *et al.*, 1988). Despite the complete inhibition of the rise in $[Ca^{2+}]_i$, verapamil only partially inhibited the contraction induced by low pH. The verapamil-insensitive portion of the contraction was inhibited by removing external Ca^{2+} (with 0.5 mM EGTA) with a further decrease in

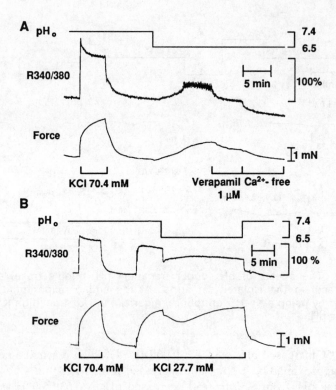

Figure 3 The effect of pH$_o$ (upper trace) on [Ca^{2+}]$_i$ (indicated by R340/380, middle trace) and force (lower trace) in the rat aorta in the presence of 5.4 mM [K$^+$]$_o$ (A) or 27.7 mM [K$^+$]$_o$ (B). 100% represents the 70.4 mM K$^+$-induced response.

[Ca^{2+}]$_i$ below the resting level. Contraction induced by low pH$_o$ was not affected by 1 μM phentolamine, suggesting that the contractile effect of low pH$_o$ is not due to release of endogenous catecholamines.

Figure 3B shows the effects of lowering pH$_o$ on [Ca^{2+}]$_i$ and force in high K$^+$-stimulated aorta. Addition of 27.7 mM [K$^+$]$_o$ induced a sustained increase in both R340/380 (80.5 ± 2.4%) and force (68.8 ± 3.7%, $n = 8$). Decrease in pH$_o$ from 7.40 to 6.50 decreased R340/380 to 55.6 ± 5.8% ($n = 4$) followed by slow and partial recovery. In response to the changes in R340/380, muscle force first decreased and then increased.

[Ca^{2+}]$_i$–force relationship

Figure 4 shows the effect of lowering pH$_o$ on [Ca^{2+}]$_i$ and force in the presence of different concentrations of K$^+$. Lowering pH$_o$ to 6.50 increased R340/380

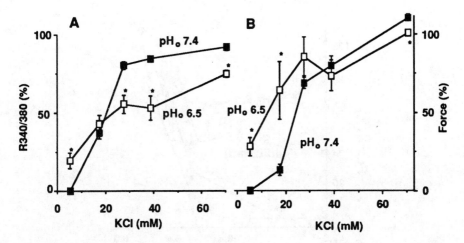

Figure 4 The effects of extracellular acidosis on [Ca²⁺]ᵢ (indicated by R340/380, A) and force (B) at various concentrations of K⁺. Values in the presence of 70.4 mM KCl at pH₀ 7.4 were taken as 100%. Each point represents mean ± SEM of four to eight experiments.

and force at normal K⁺ concentration (5.4 mM). In 17.5 mM K⁺ solution, lowering pH₀ augmented the high K⁺-induced contraction with little effect on the high K⁺-stimulated R340/380. When K⁺ concentration was increased to 27.7 mM or higher, lowering pH₀ decreased the high K⁺-stimulated R340/380 without or with a small decrease in force.

To know if pH changes the [Ca²⁺] sensitivity of the contractile elements, we calculated the absolute [Ca²⁺]ᵢ and examined the [Ca²⁺]ᵢ-force relationship. Data were obtained from the results in Figure 4A and B and [Ca²⁺]ᵢ was adjusted for the change in K_d (see Methods). As shown in Figure 5, there was a positive correlation between [Ca²⁺]ᵢ and force at each pH₀. In addition, the correlation curve at pH₀ 6.50 located to the left of the curve at pH₀ 7.40 $(P <0.05$ by F-test), suggesting that the Ca²⁺ sensitivity of the contractile elements is increased by lowering pH₀.

Effects of changing pHᵢ on [Ca²⁺]ᵢ and force

To determine the effects of acute change in pHᵢ on [Ca²⁺]ᵢ and force, we employed the ammonium pre-pulse method as described by Thomas (1974). Figure 6 shows the effects of NH₄Cl on pHᵢ and [Ca²⁺]ᵢ measured simultaneously with force. Addition of 10 mM NH₄Cl rapidly increased pHᵢ from 7.39 ± 0.01 to 8.02 ± 0.13 (n =8) and transiently increased R340/380 by

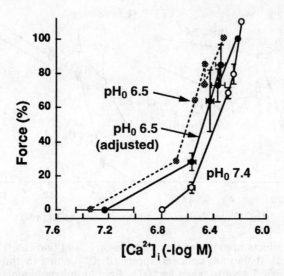

Figure 5 Relationship between absolute $[Ca^{2+}]_i$ (ordinate) and force (abscissa) in the presence of different concentrations of K^+ at pH_o of 7.40 (open circles) or 6.50 before (dotted line) and after adjustment of the change in K_d of fura-2 (closed circles). Contraction induced by 70.4 mM KCl at pH_o 7.40 was taken as 100%. Each point represents mean ± SEM of four to eight experiments.

36.3 ± 5.6 % ($n = 4$) (Figure 6A). The transient increments in pH_i and R340/380 were followed by a transient contraction (10.7 ± 3.0 %, $n = 8$). $[Ca^{2+}]_i$ in the presence of NH_4Cl may be smaller than that estimated from R340/380 (see Methods). In the presence of NH_4Cl, pH_i decreased to 7.52 ± 0.03 ($n = 4$) in 10 min. Both R340/380 and force also decreased to 3.3 ± 2.1% ($n = 4$) and 3.4 ± 0.9% ($n = 8$), respectively, in 10 min. Removal of NH_4Cl from the external medium rapidly decreased pH_i to 7.12 ± 0.06% ($n = 4$) and transiently increased R340/380 and force by 29.3 ± 4.1% ($n = 4$) and 11.3 ± 4.5% ($n = 8$), respectively.

To determine whether the transient increase in $[Ca^{2+}]_i$ induced by the addition or removal of NH_4Cl is due to Ca^{2+} release, we examined the effects of NH_4Cl in Ca^{2+}-free solution or in the presence of verapamil. In Ca^{2+}-free solution with 0.5 mM EGTA, the resting $[Ca^{2+}]_i$ gradually decreased (Figure 6B). NH_4Cl (10 mM), added 1 min after Ca^{2+} removal, caused a transient increase in R340/380 (32.8 ± 6.9%) and contraction (14.8 ± 3.5%, $n = 4$). Subsequent washout of NH_4Cl also induced a transient increase in R340/380 averaging 21.7 ± 1.9% ($n = 4$). However, the peak $[Ca^{2+}]_i$ was below the resting level. This change was not followed by contraction. In the presence of $1\,\mu M$ verapamil, addition and subsequent removal of NH_4Cl also induced transient increases in R340/380 and force to the levels that were not significantly different from those in the absence of verapamil ($n = 4$, data not shown).

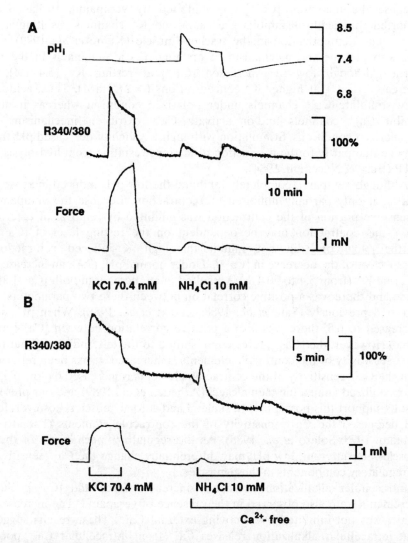

Figure 6 The effects of NH_4Cl. A, Effects on pH_i (upper trace), $[Ca^{2+}]_i$ (indicated by R340/380, middle trace) and force (lower trace). pH_i was measured in a preparation that differed from that used to measure $[Ca^{2+}]_i$ and force. B, Effects on $[Ca^{2+}]_i$ (upper trace) and force (lower trace) in the absence of external Ca^{2+} (with 0.5 mM EGTA).

DISCUSSION

Decrease in pH_o from 7.40 to 6.50 decreased pH_i from 7.39 to 6.63 in the isolated rat aorta. This change was followed by an increase in both $[Ca^{2+}]_i$ and force. Low pH_o appeared to open voltage-dependent Ca^{2+} channels because the increased $[Ca^{2+}]_i$ was inhibited by verapamil. It has been reported that acidosis inhibits Ca^{2+}-activated K^+ channels resulting in a membrane depolarization in the tracheal muscle (Kume *et al.*, 1990) and this also may be the mechanism of opening of Ca^{2+} channels in the rat aorta. Although low pH_o increased $[Ca^{2+}]_i$ at resting K^+ (5.4 mM), it decreased $[Ca^{2+}]_i$ at higher K^+ concentrations (≥ 27.7 mM). Thus, acidosis may stimulate Ca^{2+} channels under polarized condition whereas it may inhibit Ca^{2+} channels and/or activate Ca^{2+} extrusion mechanisms in depolarized conditions. Stimulation with high K^+ slightly decreased pH_i that may be due partly to the production of H^+ ions resulting from hydrolysis of ATP (Busa & Nuccitelli, 1984).

Although verapamil completely inhibited the low pH_o-induced increase in $[Ca^{2+}]_i$, it only partially inhibited the contraction. Because the verapamil-insensitive portion of the contraction was inhibited by removal of external Ca^{2+}, this contraction may be dependent on the resting level of $[Ca^{2+}]_i$. Further, low pH_o did not inhibit the high K^+-induced contractions irrespective of the decrease in $[Ca^{2+}]_i$. Under normal pH_o (7.4), an increase in external K^+ (from 5.4 to 70.4 mM) resulted in an increase in both $[Ca^{2+}]_i$ and force and there was a positive correlation between these two parameters, as reported previously (Sato *et al.*, 1988; Karaki *et al.*, 1988). When pH_o was decreased to 6.5, there was also a positive correlation between $[Ca^{2+}]_i$ and force. However, the $[Ca^{2+}]_i$-force curve shifted to the left, indicating that the Ca^{2+} sensitivity of the contractile elements is increased. It has been reported that the Ca^{2+} sensitivity of the contractile elements is increased by low pH_i in permeabilized guinea pig taenia caeci (Arheden *et al.*, 1989) and our present results support this possibility. In skeletal and cardiac muscles, however, low pH_i decreased the Ca^{2+} sensitivity of the contractile elements (Fabiato & Fabiato, 1978; Solaro *et al.*, 1988). As the regulatory mechanisms of these muscles are different, low pH_o may differentially change the Ca^{2+} sensitivity of regulatory components in these muscles.

Intracellular alkalization transiently increased force and $[Ca^{2+}]_i$. Such increments were also observed in the presence of verapamil. The increase in $[Ca^{2+}]_i$ was not inhibited by removing external Ca^{2+}. These results suggest that intracellular alkalization releases Ca^{2+} from intracellular Ca^{2+} pools. Similar result has been obtained in vascular smooth muscle cells (Siskind *et al.*, 1989). Intracellular acidification also induced transient contraction with transient increase in $[Ca^{2+}]_i$ and the increase in $[Ca^{2+}]_i$ was not inhibited by verapamil or removal of extracellular Ca^{2+}. These results suggest that intracellular acidosis has an effect similar to that of alkalosis in that it releases Ca^{2+} from intracellular Ca^{2+} stores.

In conclusion, it is suggested in the rat aorta that extracellular acidosis results in an intracellular acidosis that activates Ca^{2+} channels under resting conditions, although it inhibits Ca^{2+} channels under high K^+-stimulated conditions. Acidosis appeared to increase the Ca^{2+} sensitivity of the contractile elements. It is also suggested that sudden changes in pH_i in either direction release Ca^{2+} from intracellular storage sites and induce transient contraction

ACKNOWLEDGEMENTS

We thank Dr Kenton M. Sanders (University of Nevada, Reno) for his helpful advice on this paper. This study was supported by a Grant-in-Aid for Scientific Research from the Ministry of Education, Science and Culture of Japan.

REFERENCES

Aalkjaer, C. & Cragoe Jr, E.J. (1988). Intracellular pH regulation in resting and contracting segments of rat mesenteric resistance vessels. *J. Physiol.* **402**, 391–410.

Arheden, H., Arner, A. & Hellstrand, P. (1989). Calcium sensitivity and energetics of contraction in skinned smooth muscle of the guinea pig taenia coli at altered pH. *Pfluger's Arch.* **413**, 476–481.

Busa, W.B. & Nuccitelli, R. (1984). Metabolic regulation via intracellular pH. *Am. J. Physiol.* **246**, R409–R438.

Fabiato, A. (1981). Myoplasmic free calcium concentration reached during the twitch of an intact isolated cardiac cell and during calcium-induced release of calcium from the sarcoplasmic reticulum of a skinned cardiac cell from the adult rat or rabbit ventricle. *J. Gen. Physiol.* **78**, 457–497.

Fabiato, A. & Fabiato, F. (1978). Effects of pH on the myofilaments and the sarcoplasmic reticulum of skinned cells from cardiac and skeletal muscles. *J. Gen. Physiol.* **276**, 233–255.

Grynkiewicz, G., Poenie, M. & Tsien, R.Y. (1985). A new generation of Ca indicators with greatly improved fluorescence properties. *J. Biol. Chem.* **260**, 3340–3450.

Karaki, H. (1989). Ca^{2+} localization and sensitivity in vascular smooth muscle. *Trends Pharm. Sci.* **10**, 320–325.

Karaki, H. & Weiss, G.B. (1981) Effects of transmembrane pH gradient changes on potassium-induced relaxation in vascular smooth muscle. *Blood Vessels* **18**, 36–44.

Karaki, H., Sato, K. & Ozaki, H. (1988). Different effects of norepinephrine and KCl on cytosolic Ca^{2+}-tension relationship in vascular smooth muscle of rat aorta. *Euro. J. Pharmacol.* **151**, 325–328.

Krampetz, I.K. & Rhoades, R.A. (1991). Intracellular pH: effect on pulmonary arterial smooth muscle. *Am. J. Physiol.* **260**, L516–L521.

Kume, H., Takagi, K., Satake, T., Tokuno, H. & Tomita, T. (1990). Effects of intracellular pH on calcium-activated potassium channels in rabbit tracheal smooth muscle. *J. Physiol.* **424**, 445–457.

Lattanzio, F.A. (1990). The effects of pH and intracellular fluorescent calcium indicators as determined with chelex-100 and EDTA buffer systems. *Biochem. Biophys. Res. Comm.* **171**, 102–108.

Lofqvist, J. & Nilsson, E. (1981). Influence of acid-base change on carbachol- and potassium-induced contraction of taenia coli of the rabbit. *Acta Physiol. Scand.* **111**, 59–68.

Nielsen, H., Aalkjaer, C. & Mulvany, M.J. (1991). Differential contractile effects of changes in carbon dioxide tension on rat mesenteric resistance arteries precontracted with noradrenaline. *Pfluger's Arch.* **419**, 51–56.

Ozaki, H., Sato, K. & Karaki, H. (1987). Simultaneous recordings of calcium signals and mechanical activity using fluorescent dye fura 2 in isolated strips of vascular smooth muscle. *Jap. J. Pharmacol.* **45**, 429–433.

Rink, T.J., Tsien, R.Y. & Pozzan, T. (1982). Cytoplasmic pH and free Mg^{2+} in lymphocytes. *J. Cell Biol.* **95**, 189–196.

Sato, K., Ozaki, H. & Karaki, H. (1988). Changes in cytosolic calcium level in vascular smooth muscle strip measured simultaneously with contraction using fluorescent calcium indicator fura-2. *J. Pharmacol. Exp. Therap.* **246**, 294–300.

Siegel, G. & Schneider, W. (1981). Anions, cations, membrane potential, and relaxation. In *Vasodilation* (Leusen, I. & Vanhoutte, P.M. eds), pp. 285–298. Raven Press, New York.

Siskind, M.S., McCoy, C.E., Chobanian, A. (1989). Regulation of intracellular calcium by cell pH in vascular smooth muscle cells. *Am. J. Physiol.* **256**, C234–C240.

Solaro, R.J., Lee, J.A., Kentish, J.C. & Allen, D.G. (1988). Effects of acidosis on ventricular muscle from adult and neonatal rats. *Circ. Res.* **63**, 779–787.

Thomas, R.C. (1974). Intracellular pH of snail neurons measured with a new pH-sensitive glass electrode. *J. Physiol.* **238**, 159–180.

Thomas, J.A., Buchbaum, R.N., Zimniak, A. & Racker, E. (1979). Intracellular pH measurements in Ehrlich ascites tumor cells utilizing spectroscopic probes generated *in situ*. *Biochemistry* **18**, 2210–2218.

Uto, A., Arai, H. & Ogawa, Y. (1991). Reassessment of fura-2 and the ratio method for determination of intracellular Ca^{2+} concentrations. *Cell Calcium* **12**, 29–37.

Wray, S. (1988). Smooth muscle intracellular pH: measurement, regulation, and function. *Am. J. Physiol.* **254**, C213–C225.

26

pH and Smooth Muscle Function

SUSAN WRAY*
CLARE AUSTIN*
MICHAEL J. TAGGART*
THEODOR V. BURDYGA**

*The Physiological Laboratory,
The University of Liverpool,
Liverpool, UK

**AV Palladine Institute of Biochemistry,
Kiev, Ukraine

INTRODUCTION

If Ca^{2+} is the cation that most workers would regard as being of primary importance to smooth muscle functioning, then close behind it comes H^+, i.e. pH. The importance of pH to smooth muscle functioning has been appreciated for over a century with, for example, the observation by Gaskell (1880) that acidification of the plasma caused a profound vasodilation. Since then many other reports have appeared noting alteration of smooth muscle function with pH change (Wray, 1988). As with Ca^{2+}, the body and the cell have developed both long- and short-term mechanisms for regulating the pH; an indication of the importance to the organism of maintaining its value within strict limits. Nevertheless pH will change under physiological conditions e.g. exercise, and pathophysiological conditions e.g. vascular occlusion. Prolonged periods of abnormal pH may cause tissue damage but the purpose of this article is to consider how acute changes of pH alter smooth muscle function, and what mechanisms underlie the functional changes. Although changes of intracellular pH (pH_i) and extracellular pH (pH_o) are both of importance, space does not permit a review of both and this chapter focuses on pH_i. The functional effects of pH_o alteration may not necessarily be the same as those of pH_i alteration (Taggart et al., 1994) and the mechanisms of its effect may (Austin & Wray, 1993) or may not (Klöckner & Isenberg, 1994; Heaton et al., 1992) be similar; thus, the findings

SMOOTH MUSCLE EXCITATION
ISBN 0-12-112360-X

described in this chapter should not be extrapolated to pH_o. Finally, although smooth muscle cells may perform other specialized functions, for example secretion of extracellular matrix components, the function considered in this chapter is the ability to produce force, i.e. contraction. pH_i is capable of having profound effects on the contractile ability of smooth muscle and is one of the most important physiological modulators of its contraction. It is also possible that it may play a role in some pathological processes.

METHODOLOGY

In order to correlate directly a change of pH_i with a change of force produced by smooth muscle, it is necessary to measure them simultaneously. The main way pH_i has been measured in smooth muscle cells has been with pH-sensitive fluorescent indicators; particularly BCECF (dual excitation, single emission) or SNARF (single excitation, dual emission) (Buckler & Vaughan-Jones, 1990). These indicators can be loaded into cells in their membrane permeant form and then used for several hours to measure pH_i. The records can be calibrated in situ or in vitro using nigericin (a K^+-H^+ ionophore), both methods giving good agreement or in situ, by adding known amounts of a weak acid or base to null the pH_i change and hence calculate what its value must have been (Eisner et al., 1989).

If the pH-indicator is loaded into a muscle strip or ring then simultaneous force measurements can also be obtained and an example of this, from rat uterus, is shown in Figure 1. This was the first time simultaneous recordings of force and pH_i had been made in the myometrium and such techniques revealed that pH_i transients were produced by the spontaneous contractions (Taggart & Wray, 1993a). If single cells are used then it may be possible to measure change in length and relate this to force, or to grow the cells on a substrate that will be 'wrinkled' when the cell contracts and relate the degree of wrinkling to force.

Nuclear Magnetic Resonance (NMR) spectroscopy can be used to measure pH_i. Its advantages are that it can provide in vivo measurements of pH_i, along with other muscle metabolites and force (Harrison et al., 1994). This facility is not however readily available and can have a poor time resolution; it is not therefore a routine technique.

The buffering of pH_o is a requirement for many in vitro studies and is usually done either by incorporating HCO_3^- in the solution and gassing with CO_2/O_2 or by adding a buffering chemical such as HEPES or MOPS. Two points should be noted: (1) all buffers have a pH optimum and therefore the K_d of the buffer should be appropriate to the pH range to be investigated; (2) if pH_o is altered by alteration of CO_2/HCO_3^- buffer, then changes of CO_2 will

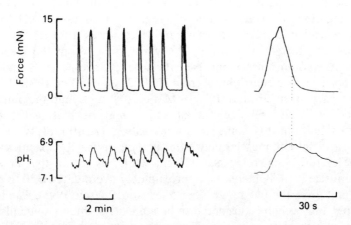

Figure 1 Simultaneous measurement of spontaneous contractions (top trace) and intracellular pH (pH$_i$, bottom trace) in rat myometrium. The averaged contraction and pH$_i$ from the data is shown on the right (n = 8). The dotted line indicates the peak of the acidification, which lags the contraction by 15 s. pH$_i$ measured from the emission signals of the pH-sensitive fluorophore carboxy-SNARF. Reproduced from Taggart & Wray (1993a) with permission.

cause a rapid alteration of pH$_i$ as it crosses the cell membrane, which will therefore mean that the effects of alteration of pH$_o$ and pH$_i$ are being studied, not pH$_o$ alone. Alterations to pH$_i$ are most often made by the introduction of weak acids, e.g. butyrate or bases e.g. NH$_4$Cl to the perfusate.

RESTING VALUES OF pH$_i$, BUFFERING POWER AND pH REGULATION IN SMOOTH MUSCLE

A sufficient number of smooth muscles have now been examined for it to be reasonable to draw some overall conclusions. Thus, it appears that pH$_i$ is around 7.1 ± 0.1 in smooth muscles, at 37°C and with a pH$_o$ of 7.4. As temperature falls, pH$_i$ becomes alkaline and pH$_o$ alteration will be reflected in a change in pH$_i$ (Austin & Wray, 1993). There is still some uncertainty over whether different steady-state values of pH$_i$ occur in HCO$_3^-$/CO$_2$ buffered systems compared with those buffered by, for example, HEPES. It is probably fair to say that if there are differences, they are small. This is of course a different issue from whether a HCO$_3^-$/CO$_2$ buffering system increases the buffering power of the cell.

Buffering power (β) is defined as the amount of H$^+$ (moles) required to produce a pH unit change in one litre of solution i.e. the bigger β, the smaller will be the change in pH_i produced by an acidic or alkaline load. Subsequent to buffering of the H^+ load (or loss) pH_i regulation will restore pH_i to resting levels. β is usually divided into that part which arises from HCO_3^-/CO_2 and the remainder, termed intrinsic β ($β_i$), which arises from the intracellular proteins. In smooth muscles much of the total β arises from $β_i$ and indeed some reports find no contribution from HCO_3^-/CO_2 (Aickin, 1994). Values of $β_i$ found vary from around 10–60 mM per pH unit, but the number of investigations is still relatively small and it may be that methodological differences account for some of the variation (Austin & Wray, 1995). Nevertheless, smooth muscles may differ in their buffering capacities and this could be of functional relevance. Recent work has shown that in vascular smooth muscle cells, $β_i$ increased approximately fivefold, from 30 to 150 mM per pH unit, over the pH_i range 7.5–6.5 (Austin &Wray, 1995). The increase in $β_i$ as pH_i falls may be considered to be a means of attenuating falls in pH_i, which cause vasodilation, before pH regulation restores pH_i to resting values.

Much work is still being undertaken to establish the mechanism, and importance of, the pH_i regulating processes present in smooth muscle cells. All cells appear to have the Na^+/H^+ exchanger which will remove H^+ from

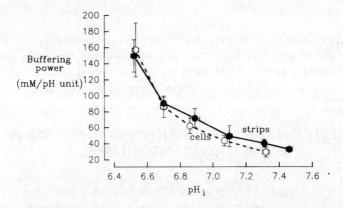

Figure 2 The relationship between pH_i and $β_i$ in mesenteric vascular smooth muscle strips (solid line and symbols) and single cells (dashed line and open symbols). All points are the means obtained from between 4 and 17 measurements. The data were grouped in $0.2 pH_i$ ranges from 6.4–6.6 up to 7.4–7.6 and the mean pH_i values in each group are plotted. The horizontal error bars indicate the size of the SEM. The vertical bars indicate the size of the SEM on the determinations of $β_i$. It can be seen that in both strips and cells as pH_i decreases, $β_i$ increases and similar values of $β_i$ are found in single cells and strips over the pH_i range examined. The steady-state range of pH_i values were obtained by alteration of external pH_o, and acute pH_i changes were obtained by addition of the weak base trimethylamine. Reproduced from Austin & Wray (1995) with permission.

the cell. A variety of anion exchangers have been identified e.g. Cl^-/HCO_3^- some of which are linked to Na^+. Their distribution may well be cell specific (Aalkjaer, 1990). In conclusion, it appears that the smooth muscle cell is well endowed with a variety of mechanisms to regulate pH_i and restore pH_i to resting values within a minute or so, from any physiological pH excursion.

FUNCTIONAL EFFECT OF pH_i ALTERATION

To summarize the ensuing discussion, no simple answer can be given to such questions as what does a fall in pH_i do to contraction in smooth muscle? The answer may depend on one or more of the following variables: (most importantly), which smooth muscle, how was pH_i altered, what kind of preparation, what time-scale, what buffer, and was pH_o altered? Even for a related group of smooth muscles, e.g. phasic or vascular or genito-urinary, the situation is still the same – no common response. All that can be said categorically is that, as far as can be established, changes of pH_i affect contraction in every smooth muscle studied to date. This emphasizes the point made earlier, that pH can have profound effects on smooth muscle function and hence an understanding of its effects is important to our overall knowledge of smooth muscle performance in health and disease. To illustrate the diverse effects of pH_i on smooth muscle we will discuss two preparations that we have examined in some detail: the uterus and the ureter.

pH_i AND THE UTERUS

The smooth muscle of uterus, the myometrium, is spontaneously active. This activity can be augmented by hormonal and neuronal signals (Wray, 1993). Irrespective of which of these mechanisms is used, pH_i affects the force produced. In both rat and human myometrium a fall in pH_i will reduce or even abolish spontaneous force production (Taggart &Wray, 1993b; Parratt et al., 1994) as shown in Figure 3.

Intracellular alkalinization will increase force; notably, by increasing the frequency of contraction. The uterus has been shown to alter its contractile pattern to pH_i changes as small as 0.04 pH unit (Taggart & Wray, 1993a). It has been demonstrated in vivo that uterine ischaemia in rats decreases pH_i by as much as 0.3 pH unit and abolishes contraction (Harrison et al., 1994). Thus any change of pH_i during labour may influence the ability of the uterus to contract and thereby influence the outcome of labour (Parratt et al., 1994; Wray, 1994).

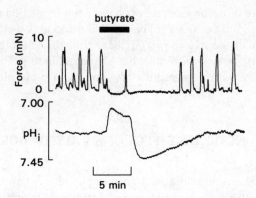

Figure 3 The effect of acidification produced by application of the weak acid butyrate, on spontaneous contractions of isolated rat uterus. Reproduced from Taggart & Wray (1993b) with permission.

pH_i IN THE URETER

The ureters conduct urine from the kidneys to the bladder. The pH of normal urine can vary between pH 4.5 to 8.0. The smooth muscle cells of the urinary tract and bladder may experience changes of pH, for example if the urinary Pco_2 varies, or if the urothelium lining is damaged and becomes more permeable. The ureters do not contract spontaneously but require stimulation, and their contractile pattern depends upon the configuration of the underlying action potential (Shuba, 1977). As with the myometrium, changes of pH_i have been shown to alter markedly the contractile force developed by the ureters. However, unlike the uterus, studies of both rat and human ureteric smooth muscle have shown that intracellular acidification will increase electrically evoked phasic contractions (Cole *et al.*, 1990; Burdyga *et al.*, 1995). This response may be a protective mechanism to deal with acidic urine, which can drop to below pH 5.0. This pH_o may be transmitted, in part, to the smooth muscle cells and increase contractility. This may then speed up the passage of urine through the tract and prevent damage. The rat ureter responds to an intracellular alkalinization with a marked reduction in contraction. A typical example of these effects is shown in Figure 4.

Thus comparison of Figures 3 and 4 provides a clear demonstration of the different functional responses of different smooth muscles to pH_i alteration. The obvious next question to be addressed is what mechanisms can account for the functional differences, i.e. how are H^+ acting to alter force in the two situations?

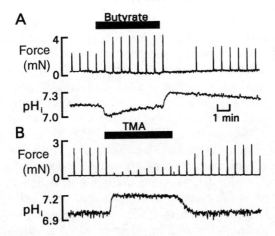

Figure 4 Simultaneous measurements of force (top traces) and intracellular pH (pH$_i$) (bottom traces) in guinea pig ureter. In A, the cytoplasm was acidified by application of 40 mM butyrate for the period indicated by the solid bar, while in B, the cytoplasm was alkalinized by the addition of trimethylamine (TMA, 40 mM). The external pH was 7.4 throughout. The tissue was loaded with carboxy-SNARF, and the fluorescence signals at 590 and 640 mm recorded to obtain the measurement of pH$_i$ and the preparation electrically stimulated to produce force. Reproduced from Burdyga *et al.* (1996) with permission.

HOW DOES pH$_i$ ACT TO ALTER FORCE?

The effect of pH$_i$ alteration shown in Figures 3 and 4 is on force, which is the final step in a sequence of events which starts with excitation of the cell membrane, progresses to a rise in intracellular Ca^{2+} ([Ca^{2+}]$_i$) and phosphorylation of myosin light chains and ends with the cyclic interactions of phosphorylated myosin with actin to generate force, as detailed elsewhere in this volume. Thus, there are many regulatory points in excitation–contraction coupling where H$^+$ may act, and consideration of this allows us to begin understanding possible explanations for pH$_i$ alteration to lead to opposite effects on contraction in different smooth muscle. For example if H$^+$ has a more pronounced inhibitory effect on Ca^{2+} entry in one smooth muscle but a stimulatory effect on say myosin light chain kinase on another, then inhibition of contraction may occur in the former and potentiation in the latter. To date there has been no systematic analysis pH$_i$ modulation of each step in excitation-contraction coupling for any smooth muscle, but rather different preparations have revealed influences of H$^+$ at certain steps.

SENSITIVITY

One way of analyzing the effects of pH_i is to firstly decide whether H^+ are acting to alter $[Ca^{2+}]_i$ or alter the relation between $[Ca^{2+}]_i$ and tension at the contractile machinery, i.e. sensitivity, or both. To investigate sensitivity changes it is usual to work on a permeabilized (skinned) preparation so that the environment around the myofilaments can be accurately controlled and manipulated. The effect of changes of pH_i can then be examined at constant $[Ca^{2+}]_i$ and its effect on force determined. This therefore bypasses any earlier effects pH_i may have had in intact preparations, which may have altered $[Ca^{2+}]_i$. Permeabilizing smooth muscle is not without technical problems. For example, if large holes are made in the surface membrane, are some normal control constituents lost from the cell? When pH_i is altered, have corrections been made for the effects this will have on the ionization and binding constants of other cellular constituents; most Ca^{2+} buffers are pH sensitive.

Results from a variety of different preparations and techniques have tended to indicate no major effect of pH_i on the Ca^{2+}-tension relationship. Little effect on Ca-sensitivity of acid or alkaline pH_i, was seen in the uterus (Crichton et al, 1993). However, in permeabilized myometrium the effect of acidic pH was to potentiate Ca^{2+}-activated force, and alkaline pH depressed force (Crichton *et al.*, 1993). Recall that in intact preparations (Figure 3) acidification depressed force and alkalinization potentiated it. Thus, by keeping $[Ca^{2+}]_i$ constant in the permeabilized preparation we have unmasked a positive effect of H^+ on force. It appears likely that this may arise because acidic pH_i inhibits the phosphatase which dephosphorylates myosin; thus the balance between phosphorylated and unphosphorylated myosin is disturbed and force increased. This study also suggests that in the intact preparation the effect of H^+ is on $[Ca^{2+}]_i$ since when $[Ca^{2+}]$ is maintained there is no decrease in force. We shall therefore now turn to how pH_i may alter $[Ca^{2+}]_i$.

EFFECTS OF pH_i ON $[Ca^{2+}]_i$

Normally, in smooth muscle, the intracellular $[Ca^{2+}]$ will rise as a result of surface membrane excitation. The excitation may arise (1) spontaneously in the membrane of some smooth muscles e.g. in the myometrium, due to the action of pacemaker cells, or (2) following stimulation by an agonist, e.g. in mesenteric blood vessels. Agonists may also alter the excitatory pattern in spontaneously active smooth muscles. As will be reviewed elsewhere in this volume, agonists can act via receptor – or voltage-operated channels. The receptor-operated channels may lead to some Ca^{2+} entry directly, or may cause a degree of depolarization which in turn leads to voltage-gated Ca^{2+} entry. The functional role of Ca^{2+}-induced Ca^{2+}-release (CICR) from the sarcoplasmic reticulum (SR) still remains to be fully elucidated in many smooth muscles. The size of the SR varies between smooth muscles, as does their dependence upon external Ca^{2+} entry for contraction. It seems reasonable to suggest that such variations underlie much of the functional diversity of smooth muscle and that a continuum will exist – from those where agonists causing IP_3 production and thereby SR Ca^{2+} release and contraction, to those where agonists cause voltage-gated Ca^{2+} entry and IP_3 production and/or CICR and hence contraction.

In studies of several cell types, including some smooth muscle, pH_i has been shown to affect many of the membrane currents which will be involved in excitation of the surface membrane. In general intracellular acidification appears to inhibit many K^+ and Ca^{2+} channels (Moody, 1984), but the appropriate studies have not always been made on smooth muscle and invariably functional data is absent. It is hard to relate, for example, patch-clamp studies of a particular channel, whose density is not known, on a cultured preparation whose phenotype may no longer be contractile, to a more physiological situation. We will now examine what is known about pH_i on Ca^{2+} in uterus and ureter.

pH_i, Ca^{2+} AND THE UTERUS

Recent studies using Ca^{2+}-sensitive indicators in intact myometrial preparations have shown that acidification abolishes the normal Ca^{2+} transient. Thus, there is no rapid rise of $[Ca^{2+}]_i$ and contraction does not occur (Heaton & Wray, 1994).

In many preparations a slow, small rise in baseline Ca^{2+} occurred with the acidification. This may arise from Ca^{2+} being displaced from common intracellular binding sites when $[H^+]$ is increased (Wray, 1993). This slow, small rise of Ca^{2+} does not cause contraction and therefore either may not be of the correct 'form' to stimulate contraction or may occur in a compartment not freely available or sensed by the myofilaments; imaging of Ca^{2+} in cells could throw light on such processes.

The inhibition of the normal Ca^{2+} transient with intracellular acidification may, in turn, result from H^+ preventing depolarization of the membrane, and hence the opening of the L-type Ca^{2+} channels, or by inhibiting the Ca^{2+} current. There is no direct evidence to help distinguish between the two hypotheses. Indirect evidence suggests that the inhibition is at the level of the surface membrane excitation, rather than the Ca^{2+} current, as depolarization with high K^+ overcomes the effect of H^+ on contraction. However, more direct measurements need to be made.

In summary, in the uterus the data are consistent with H^+ depressing the excitability of the surface membrane and abolishing the Ca^{2+}-transient. Thus, spontaneous contractions fail early on in the excitation–contraction pathway. The permeabilized myometrial preparation indicated that if Ca^{2+} was maintained then H^+ can potentiate force, possibly by inhibition of the phosphatase which dephosphorylates myosin. In depolarized myometrial preparations, acidification does not depress force, presumably because the block to excitation at the surface membrane has been overcome.

pH_i, $[Ca^{2+}]_i$ AND THE URETER

As H^+ potentiated force in the ureter, one would predict that they also potentiated the Ca^{2+}-transient in this preparation. Recent work has shown this to be the case; acidification of the cytoplasm led to an increase in force and the amplitude of Ca^{2+} transient, and alkalinization decreased its magnitude (Burdyga *et al.*, 1995). Parallel studies have shown that the effects of acidification were to increase the duration and amplitude of the action potential, whereas alkalinization shortened the action potential and reduced its amplitude. The effects of acidification on the action potential resembled the effects of the K^+ channel blocker tetraethyl ammonium (TEA). When the ability of pH_i alteration to change tension when K^+ channels were blocked by TEA was investigated, it was found that there was little or no effect on force under these conditions.

Thus, in summary, it appears that when pH_i is altered in the ureter, the action potential is modulated probably by alteration of K^+ currents. These changes will in turn influence $[Ca^{2+}]_i$ and thereby contraction.

CONCLUSIONS

1. Changes of pH_i can have profound effects on contraction in smooth muscles and these may be of clinical significance.
2. The effects of pH_i alteration are specific to the smooth muscle and the method of stimulation; the effects cannot be generalized.
3. H^+ can act on many stages of excitation–contraction coupling in smooth muscle. Major functional differences may lie in the different susceptibility to H^+ of these stages in different smooth muscles. Many details of these processes have not been elucidated.

ACKNOWLEDGEMENTS

This work was supported by grants from the MRC, BHF and Wellcome Trust and Physiological Society.

REFERENCES

Aalkjaer, C. (1990). Regulation of intracellular pH and its role in vascular smooth muscle function. *J. Hyperten.* **8**, 197–206.

Aickin, C.C. (1994). Regulation of intracellular pH in the smooth muscle of the guinea pig ureter: Na⁺ dependence. *J. Physiol.* **479**, 301–316.

Austin, C. & Wray, S. (1993). Extracellular pH signals affect rat vascular tone by rapid transduction into intracellular pH changes. *J. Physiol.* **466**, 1–8.

Austin, C. & Wray, S. (1995). An investigation of intrinsic buffering power in rat vascular smooth muscle cells. *Pflüger's Arch.* **429**, 325–331.

Buckler, K.J. & Vaughan-Jones, R.D. (1990). Application of a new pH-sensitive fluorophore (carboxy-SNARF-1) for intracellular pH measurements in small, isolated cells. *Pflüger's Arch.* **417**, 234–239.

Burdyga, T.V., Taggart, M.J. & Wray, S. (1996). An investigation into the mechanism whereby intracellular pH affects tension in guinea pig ureteric smooth muscle. *J. Physiol.* **494**, (in press).

Cole, R.S., Fry, C.H. & Shuttleworth, K.E.D. (1990). Effects of acid-base changes on human ureteric smooth muscle contractility. *Br. J. Urol.* **66**, 257–264.

Crichton, C.A., Taggart, M.J., Wray, S. & Smith, G.L. (1993). Effects of pH and inorganic phosphate on force production in α-toxin-permeabilized isolated rat uterine smooth muscle. *J. Physiol.* **465**, 629–645.

Eisner, D.A., Kenning, N.A., O'Neill, S.C., Pocock, G., Richards, C.D. & Valdeolmillos, M. (1989). A novel method for absolute calibration of intracellular pH indicators. *Pflüger's Arch.* **413**, 553–558.

Gaskell, W.H. (1880). On the tonicity of the heart and blood vessels. *J. Physiol.* **3**, 48–75.

Harrison, N., Larcombe-McDouall, J.B., Earley, L. & Wray, S. (1994). An *in vivo* study of the effects of ischaemia on uterine contraction, intracellular pH and metabolites in the rat. *J. Physiol.* **476**, 349–354.

Heaton, R.C. & Wray, S. (1994). Intracellular acidification increases intracellular [Ca²⁺] but decreases force in isolated rat uterine smooth muscle. *J. Physiol.* **477**, 42–43P.

Heaton, R.C., Taggart, M.J. & Wray, S. (1992). The effects of intracellular and extracellular alkalinization on conditions of the isolated uterus. *Pflüger's Arch.* **422**, 24–30.

Klockner, U. & Isenberg, G. (1994). Calcium channel current of vascular smooth muscle cells: extracellular protons modulate gating and single channel conductance. *J. Gen. Physiol.* **103**, 665–678.

Moody, W. (1984). Effects of intracellular H⁺ on the electrical properties of excitable cells. *Annu. Rev. Neurosci.* **7**, 257–278.

Parratt, J., Taggart, M. & Wray, S. (1994). Abolition of contractions in the myometrium by acidification *in vitro*. *Lancet* **344**, 717–718.

Shuba, M.F. (1977). The effect of sodium-free and potassium-free solutions, ionic current inhibitors and ouabain on electrophysiological properties of smooth muscle. *J. Physiol.* **264**, 837–851.

Taggart, M.J. & Wray, S. (1993a). Occurrence of intracellular pH transients during spontaneous contractions in rat uterine smooth muscle. *J. Physiol.* **472**, 23–31.

Taggart, M. & Wray, S. (1993b). Simultaneous measurements of intracellular pH and contraction in uterine smooth muscle. *Pflüger's Arch.* **423**, 527–529.

Taggart, M., Austin, C. & Wray, S. (1994). A comparison of the effects of intracellular and extracellular pH on contraction in isolated rat portal vein. *J. Physiol.* **475**, 285–292.

Wray, S. (1988). Smooth muscle intracellular pH: measurement, regulation and function. *Am. J. Physiol.* **254**, C213–C225.

Wray, S. (1993). Uterine contraction and physiological mechanisms of modulation. Am. J. Physiol. 264, C1–C18. Wray, S. (1988). Smooth muscle intracellular pH: measurement, regulation and function. *Am. J. Physiol.* **254**, C213–C225.

Wray, S. (1994). Hypoxia in the uterus. NIPS **9**, 88–92.

27

Metabolic Modulation of Excitation–Contraction Coupling in Smooth Muscle

RICHARD J. PAUL
JOHN LORENZ

Department of Molecular and Cellular Physiology,
University of Cincinnati,
College of Medicine,
Cincinnati, USA

Studies of the relations between smooth muscle metabolism and its electrophysiological properties have been long associated with the smooth muscle school championed by Dr. Edith Bülbring and colleagues (Bülbring & Golenhofen, 1967). Dr Tadao Tomita and his colleagues (Tomita, 1992; Nakayama & Tomita, 1989) continue this strong tradition and have long been in the forefront of the field studying the regulation and coordination of metabolism and smooth muscle contractility. In this chapter, we review recent evidence linking glycolytic metabolism through ion pumps and channels to Ca^{2+} homeostasis and modulation of excitation–contraction coupling in smooth muscle.

While metabolism is ultimately linked to muscle performance, the coupling between metabolism and smooth muscle function is more immediate than in its skeletal muscle counterpart. This is due to different function and energetic strategies. Skeletal muscle is characterized by a large pool of phosphocreatine (PCr) which rapidly resynthesizes ATP. With rapid contraction speeds, this pool is utilized first and generally only after the muscle relaxes is the PCr pool restored which underlies the so-called 'oxygen debt' phenomenon. Conversely, most smooth muscles are characterized by small reserves of ATP and PCr. For tonic smooth muscle, the high-energy phosphagen pool would not be of sufficient magnitude to permit the peak of an isometric contraction to be obtained (Paul, 1980). Hence, smooth muscle adopts a 'pay as you go' plan, requiring a moment by moment synthesis of ATP and a close coordination of contractile ATP

SMOOTH MUSCLE EXCITATION
ISBN 0-12-112360-X

utilization with synthesis is paramount for normal function.

Thus, an understanding of smooth muscle energy metabolism is an important facet of our knowledge of the regulation of smooth muscle contractility. Although the variation among smooth muscle types is often more extensive than that between striated and smooth muscle, there are some generalizations that can be made. Smooth muscle is primarily an oxidative tissue with perhaps greater than 80% of its ATP requirements met by mitochondrial oxidative phosphorylation (Paul, 1980). Although its mitochondrial content is low compared with cardiac or slow skeletal muscle, its capacity is similar to fast skeletal muscle and is more than sufficient to support the relatively modest requirements of its contractile protein ATPase. Compared with fast striated muscle, the actin–myosin associated ATPase in smooth muscle is two to three orders of magnitude lower, despite the ability of smooth muscle to generate and maintain isometric forces equal to or larger than skeletal muscle. The molecular basis of the high economy of force maintenance of smooth muscle is primarily attributable to its low actin-activated myosin ATPase activity; however, other factors such as longer effective sarcomere lengths and 'latch' mechanisms also contribute (de Lanerolle & Paul, 1991). Oxidative metabolism is well-coordinated with isometric force. Under normal physiological conditions, the rate of oxidative phosphorylation is linearly related to isometric force (Paul, 1987). However, for cases in which myosin regulatory chain light chain phosphorylation is high, J_{O_2} increases more sharply with force (Wingard et al., 1994). This information is essential to understanding crossbridge regulation and the 'latch state', in which both shortening velocity and ATP utilization are reduced two- to threefold while isometric force is maintained in prolonged contractions (Hai & Murphy, 1988; Paul, 1990).

Despite the primary oxidative nature of smooth muscle, a most unusual feature of smooth muscle metabolism is the substantial production of lactate under fully oxidative conditions. In early studies, this was thought to be an artefact of tissue preparation for inadequate mitochondrial capacity. It now appears that this aerobic glycolysis is a physiological reflection of enzyme organization in smooth muscle, and may be common to a wide variety of cell types (Ishida et al., 1994). While this aerobic glycolysis accounts for a relatively small fraction of the total ATP requirements, it appears to play an inordinately important role in fuelling processes connected with excitation–contraction coupling in smooth muscle. Underlying its role in E-C coupling is the localization of glycolytic enzymes to the plasma membrane and sarcoplasmic reticulum, Key players in excitation–contraction coupling. Moreover, there is now a growing body of evidence suggesting that the cell membrane and immediate subsarcolemmal region form a functionally distinct compartment (Chen & van Breemen, 1993; Moore et al., 1993). We hypothesized that localized glycolytic enzyme cascades appear to preferentially support the energy requirements of this compartment (Paul *et al.*, 1979; Lynch & Paul, 1983) as well as that of the sarcoplasmic reticulum (Ishida *et al.*, 1994).

Before describing the evidence supporting this hypothesis, it is worth demonstrating that the sensitivity of smooth muscle to various stimuli can be dramatically dependent on the nature of the exogenous substrate. Figure 1 shows concentration–isometric force response curves of porcine carotid artery for norepinephrine stimulation with glucose or β-hydroxybutyrate (a pure oxidative substrate).

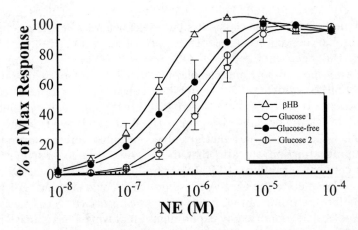

Figure 1 The dependence on the type of the exogenous substrate for the concentration–isometric force response curves for norepinephrine (NE) stimulation in porcine carotid artery. Sensitivity increases in the absence of glucose. Addition of β-hydroxybutyrate, a substrate for oxidative metabolism, does not affect the shift in sensitivity, whereas further addition of glucose restores the initial control levels. Note that maximum isometric forces were similar. Adapted from Zhang & Paul (1994).

While the global ATP and PCr energy stores were not affected by substrate conditions (including no exogenous substrate), the sensitivity of active isometric force to norepinephrine was enhanced in the absence of glucose (Zhang & Paul, 1994). It is worth pointing out that the maximum isometric forces obtained were similar, reinforcing the fact that the tissue was not energy limited in a global sense, as the ATP required for force maintenance would be expected to be the major factor in ATP utilization. Nonetheless, sensitivity to stimulation was dramatically altered in the absence of glucose, despite available oxidative substrate and global ATP. In a series of experiments studying Ca^{2+} metabolism, we (Zhang & Paul, 1994) showed that the presence of glucose was essential for normal Ca^{2+}

homeostasis. Our hypothesis is that ATP supplied by membrane-associated glycolysis fuels a local pool of ATP which supports the ion-pumps and channel function underlying E-C coupling.

There are a number of lines of evidence supporting this hypothesis. In intact smooth muscle, lactate production is correlated with the activity of the Na-pump (Paul *et al.*, 1979). Indeed, more recent studies have quantified this relationship. Activation of the Na^+-pump by addition of K^+ to K^+-depleted arteries was associated with an immediate activation of glycolysis which is stoichiometrically linked to K^+-uptake (Campbell & Paul, 1992). Oxidative metabolism could be activated, but only after the aerobic glycolytic capacity of the artery was saturated. This is exactly the opposite of what might be expected on the basis of the classic Pasteur effect, whereas lactate production under aerobic conditions is expected to occur only after oxidative metabolism has been saturated.

Using a purified smooth muscle plasmalemmal vesicle preparation as a model system for studying the coupling between membrane level glycolysis and ion transport activity, we showed that Ca^{2+} pump activity could be supported by glycolytic substrates alone (Paul *et al.*, 1989; Hardin *et al.*, 1992). This indicated not only that glycolytic enzymes were associated with this membrane fraction but also that the enzyme cascade was functional, acting in concert to produce ATP. Importantly, this endogenous ATP was functionally coupled to the Ca^{2+}-ATPase in that it could support Ca^{2+} pump activity before diffusing away from the vesicle surface. This functional linkage was further supported by experiments employing a hexokinase-based 'ATP trap' in the solution bathing the plasmalemmal vesicles. In the presence of the ATP trap, Ca^{2+} uptake could still be supported by glycolytic substrate (but not by ATP) suggesting a close spatial arrangement of the Ca^{2+} ATPase and glycolytic enzymes. The existence of a functionally distinct metabolic compartment involving the energetics of membrane-associated processes can also be demonstrated in intact smooth muscle. Using isotopic (Lynch & Paul, 1983) and more recently ^{13}C-NMR techniques (Hardin & Kushmerick, 1994), it was shown that lactate originates solely from exogenous glucose whereas the glycogen stores are oxidized. As the intermediate metabolites involved in glycolysis and glycogenolysis would be similar, this implies that at least two functionally distinct glycolytic compartments exist (Lynch & Paul, 1986). Thus despite the absence of well-defined borders, such as those associated with mitochondria, the plasmalemmal compartment maintains a biochemically distinct environment.

While ion pump energetics represent one possible link between metabolism and excitation–contraction coupling, the ATP-dependence of ion channel function represents another intriguing connection. Here too, there is a growing literature suggesting that glycolysis and oxidative metabolism might differentially affect electrical activity. In chick embryo heart cells, for example, Hasin *et al.* (1984) showed that cyanide treatment had a profound negative inotropic effect with corresponding changes in the action potential amplitude and duration, while having only a moderate effect on the diastolic membrane potential. Conversely 2-deoxy-D-glucose (an inhibitor of glycolysis) caused a marked reduction in the diastolic potential with little effect on contractility or action potentials. Weiss & Lamp (1987) also reported differential effects of substrate on K^+-channel currents in cardiac myocytes, with glycolytic substrates being more effective than oxidative substrate in inhibiting ATP-dependent K^+-channel activity in the presence of an ATP trap. Similarly, in rat portal vein, Ekmehag (1989) showed that exposure to cyanide substantially inhibited force production while having relatively little effect on membrane resting potential or action potentials. Furthermore, in contrast to the insubstantial effect in the presence of glucose, treatment with cyanide in the presence of β-hydroxybutyrate (substituted for glucose) caused a marked hyperpolarization. They concluded that the decrease in mechanical activity during respiratory inhibition was largely independent of membrane activity and that increases in glycolysis prevented more pronounced changes in membrane potential. In another example, the ATP dependence of K^+-channels has been proposed as the mechanism underlying hypoxic vasodilatation in coronary vessels (Daut *et al.*, 1990) and hypoxic vasoconstriction in pulmonary vessels (Yuan *et al.*, 1993). In a related study using isolated renal microvessels, vasodilatation produced either by diazoxide (a K^+-channel opener) or 2-deoxy-D-glucose could be reversed by glibenclamide, a selective blocker of ATP-sensitive K^+-channels (Lorenz *et al.*, 1992). It is interesting that the ATP dependence of these channels in vitro is much lower than the global ATP levels in hypoxia, as measured by NMR or freeze-clamping techniques. Again, this would suggest that ion channels are responding to local, compartmentalized ATP concentrations.

Less well understood, but potentially more directly involved in excitation–contraction coupling is the ATP sensitivity of Ca^{2+} channel activity. Ohya & Sperelakis (1989a,b, 1991) investigated these mechanisms in a series of papers using whole-cell and single channel recordings of Ca^{2+} current. Using whole-cell voltage clamp and intracellular perfusion on freshly isolated cells from guinea pig mesenteric artery, they demonstrated that increasing intracellular ATP levels from 0.3 mM to 5 mM resulted in a more than twofold increase in the peak Ca^{2+} channel current, which was dependent on the ATP concentration between 0.1 and 5 mM. In a separate study on VSM cells from guinea pig portal vein, these investigators studied the effect of ATP on single channel currents using the cell-attached configuration; intracellular composition was modified by permeabilizing the cell membrane and altering bath composition. They demonstrated that the number of channels available for opening and/or their open probability was a strong function of the ATP concentration. These results are supported in a recent study by Okashiro *et al.*(1992). Using whole-cell voltage clamp and intracellular perfusion they found that decreasing intracellular ATP from 5 mM to 0 mM dramatically decreased Ca^{2+} current. When 5 mM ATP was reintroduced to the cell, the Ca^{2+} current only partially recovered and then only transiently, supporting the notion that ATP alone is unable to fully maintain Ca^{2+} currents at high levels.

In a more recent study (Lorenz & Paul, 1995), we studied the effects of endogenous versus exogenous sources of ATP on Ca^{2+}-channel currents in freshly dissociated rat portal vein. We also found that the peak amplitude of the Ca^{2+} channel current was highly dependent on the ATP concentration in the patch pipette. Moreover, by measuring these currents over extended periods of time (at least 30 min), we also demonstrated that the stability of the current appears to depend more heavily on the integrity of glycolytic metabolism within the cell. The presence of both ATP and glycolytic substrates in the patch pipette resulted in very high and remarkably stable Ca^{2+}-channel currents, in contrast to ATP alone as shown in Figure 2. To verify further a specific role for metabolism in this phenomenon, we showed that metabolic inhibition with cyanide and iodoacetate, despite the continued presence of ATP, resulted in an increase in the rate of current run-down

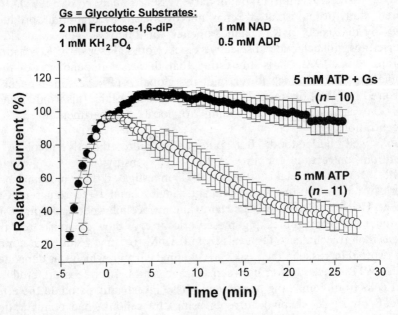

Figure 2 Stabilizing effects of glycolytic substrates on whole-cell Ca^{2+}-channel in rat portal vein cells. Note that ATP alone is not sufficient to prevent run-down of currents.

(Lorenz & Paul, 1994). We postulated that some product of metabolism *per se* is at least partly responsible for the observed stabilization of Ca^{2+} currents.

Given that in the whole-cell configuration the cell interior is bathed by the pipette solution, the sensitivity of Ca^{2+}-channel currents to endogenous metabolism further supports a functional membrane compartment in which local ATP produced by membrane–associated glycolysis, can affect Ca^{2+}-channel activity before being diluted by the patch pipette solution.

One may question why glycolytic substrates or PCr, which also have to diffuse from the pipette, are more effective than ATP itself in supporting membrane-associated energy requirements. There are a number of possibilities, clearly all speculative, on why this type of cellular enzyme organization has evolved. The first explanation is that the ATP produced by endogenous systems is colocalized with the ion channels or pumps and a pass-down or form of tunneling mechanism is involved, whereby metabolically synthesized ATP is directly supplied to pumps or channels. A higher effective local concentration of ATP in the vicinity of the channel is another way of describing these types of mechanism. It may also be possible that the function of colocalized production of ATP is to ensure that the ADP concentration, a known inhibitor of some types of ion channel activity, is maintained at low levels. A separation of different metabolic cascades with the functions they support lends itself better to independent regulation, as similar metabolic intermediates may be involved in the cell signaling pathway. This may also provide a basis for this compartmentalized enzyme organization (Lynch & Paul, 1988). Taken as a whole, these data suggest that the subsarcolemmal space is a more separate environment than generally envisioned. The juxtaposition of transporters, channels and glycolytic enzymes suggest that not only ion concentrations, but also high-energy phosphagens and metabolism may significantly differ from that of the average cytosolic values.

We have shown that glycolytic metabolism is particularly critical to normal excitation–contraction coupling, despite being only a minor player in total ATP production. Both ion pumps and channels are likely involved. This modulation of excitation–contraction coupling by glycolysis may be an important facet in the pathophysiology of many diseases in which smooth muscle is the end effector, with diabetes and hypertension being likely examples.

ACKNOWLEDGEMENTS

Supported by NIH HL23240 and the American Heart Association National Center.

REFERENCES

Bülbring, E. & Golenhofen, K. (1967). Oxygen consumption by the isolated smooth muscle of the guinea pig taenia coli. *J. Physiol.* **193**: 213–224.

Campbell, J.D. & Paul, R.J. (1992). The nature of fuel provision for the Na^+-K^+-ATPase in vascular smooth muscle. *J. Physiol.* **447**:67–82.

Chen, Q. & van Breemen C. (1993). The superficial buffer barrier in venous smooth muscle: sarcoplasmic reticulum refilling and unloading. *Br. J. Pharmacol.* **109**, 336–343.

Daut, J., Maier-Rudolph, W., Von Beckerath, N., Mehrke, G., Gunther, K. & Goedel-Merner, L. (1990). Hypoxic dilation of coronary arteries is mediated by ATP-sensitive potassium channels. *Science* **247**: 1341–1344.

de Lanerolle, P. & Paul, R.J. (1991). Myosin phosphorylation/dephosphorylation and the regulation of airway smooth muscle contractility. *Am. J. Physiol.* **261** (*Lung Cell. Molec. Physiol.* **5**), L1–L14.

Ekmehag, B.L. (1989). Electrical and mechanical responses to inhibition of cell respiration in smooth muscle of the rat portal vein. Acta Physiol. Scand. 137: 41–51.

Hai, C.-M. & Murphy, R.A. (1988). Cross-bridge phosphorylation and regulation of latch state in smooth muscle. *Am. J. Physiol.* **254**, C99–106.

Hardin, C.D. & Kushmerick, M.J. (1994). Simultaneous and separable flux of pathways for glucose and glycogen utilization studied by ^{13}C-NMR. *J. Mol. Cell. Cardiol.* **26,** 1197–1210.

Hardin, C., Raeymaekers, L. & Paul, R.J. (1992). Comparison of endogenous and exogenous sources of ATP in fueling Ca uptake in smooth muscle plasma membrane vesicles. *J. Gen. Physiol.* **99**, 21–40.

Hasin, Y., Doorey, A. & Barry, W.H. (1984). Electrophysiologic and mechanical effects of metabolic inhibition of high-energy phosphate production in cultured chick embryonic ventricular cells. *J. Mol. Cell. Cardiol.* **16**, 1009–1021.

Ishida, Y, Riesinger, I. Wallimann, T. & Paul, R.J. (1994). Compartmentation of ATP synthesis and utilization in smooth muscle: Roles of aerobic glycolysis and creatine kinase. In Saks V., Ventura-Clapier, R. Cellular Energetics: Role of Coupled Creatine Kinases. *Mol. Cell. Bioch.* **133/134,** 39–50.

Lorenz, J.N. & Paul, R.J. (1994). Glycolytic ATP enhances Ca^{2+} current in vascular smooth muscle (VSM). cells. *Hypertension.* **24,** 383 (Abstract).

Lorenz, J.N. & Paul, R.J. (1995). Dependence of Ca^{2+} channel currents on the glycolytic production of ATP in vascular smooth muscle. *J. Physiol.* (submitted).

Lorenz, J. N., Schnermann, J., Brosius, F.C., Briggs, J.P. & Furspan P. B. (1992). Intracellular ATP can regulate afferent arteriolar tone via ATP-sensitive K^+ channels in the rabbit. *J. Clin. Invest.* **90,** 733–740.

Lynch, R.M. & Paul, R.J. (1983). Compartmentation of glycolysis and glycogenolysis in vascular smooth muscle. *Science* **222,** 1344–1346.

Lynch, R.M. & Paul, R.J. (1986). Compartmentation of carbohydrate metabolism in vascular smooth muscle: Evidence for at least two functionally independent pools of glucose-6-phosphate. *Biochim. Biophys. Acta* **887,** 315–318.

Lynch, R.M. & Paul, R.J. (1988). Functional compartmentation of carbohydrate metabolism. In *CRC Reviews Microcompartmentation* (Jones, D. ed), pp. 17–35. CRC Press, Boca Raton.

Moore, E.D., Effer, E.F., Philipson, K.D., Carrington, W.A., Fogarty, K.E., Lifshitz, L.M. & Fay, F.S. (1993). Coupling of the Na^+/Ca^{2+} exchanger, Na^+/K^+ pump and sarcoplasmic reticulum in smooth muscle. *Nature (London).* **365, 657**–660.

Nakayama, S., and Tomita, T. (1989). Intracellular phosphorus compounds during metabolic inhibition in the smooth muscle of guinea pig taenia caeci. *Prog. Clin. Biol. Res.* **315**, 429–438.

Ohya, Y. & Sperelakis N. (1989a). ATP regulation of the slow calcium channels in vascular smooth muscle cells of guinea pig mesenteric artery. *Circ. Res.* **64**, 145–154.

Ohya, Y. & Sperelakis, N. (1989b). Modulation of single slow (L-type). calcium channels by intracellular ATP in vascular smooth muscle cells. *Pflügers Arch.* **414**, 257–264.

Ohya, Y. & Sperelakis, N. (1991). Agonist modulation of voltage-dependent calcium channels in vascular smooth muscles. In *Electrophysiology and Ion Channels of Vascular Smooth Muscle and Endothelial Cells* (Sperelakis, N. & Kuriyama, H. eds), pp. 39–46. Elsevier Publishers, Amsterdam.

Okashiro, T., Tokuno, H., Fukumitsu, T., Hayashi, H. & Tomita, T. (1992). Effects of intracellular ATP on Ca^{2+} current in freshly dispersed single cells of guinea pig portal vein. *Exp. Physiol.* **77**, 719–31.

Paul, R.J. (1980). The chemical energetics of vascular smooth muscle. Intermediary metabolism and its relation to contractility. In *Handbook of Physiology, Section on Circulation II* (Bohr, D.F., Somlyo, A.P. & Sparks, H.V. eds), pp. 201–235 Am. *Physiol. Soc.* Bethesda, MD.

Paul, R.J. (1987). Smooth muscle: Mechanochemical Energy Conversion, relations between metabolism and contractility. In *Physiology of the Gastrointestinal Tract* (Johnson, L.R. *et al.*, eds), 2nd edition, Vol. 1, pp. 483–506. Raven Press, New York.

Paul, R.J. (1990). Smooth muscle energetics and theories of cross-bridge regulation. *Am. J. Physiol.* **258**, C369–375.

Paul, R.J., Bauer, M. & Pease, W. (1979). Vascular smooth muscle: Aerobic glycolysis linked to Na-K transport processes. *Science* **206**, 1414–1416.

Paul, R.J., Hardin, C., Wuytack, F., Raeymaekers, L. & Casteels, R. (1989). An endogenous glycolytic cascade can preferentially support Ca uptake in smooth muscle plasma membrane vesicles. *FASEB J.* **3**, 2298–3201.

Tomita, T. (1992). Advance in smooth muscle electrophysiology. *Jap. J. Pharmacol.* **58** (Suppl. 2), 1P–6P.

Weiss, J.M. & Lamp, S.T. (1987). Glycolysis preferentially inhibits ATP-sensitive K^+ channels in isolated guinea pig myocytes. *Science* **238**, 67–69.

Wingard, C.J., Paul, R.J. & Murphy, R.A. (1994). Dependence of ATP consumption on cross-bridge phosphorylation in swine carotid smooth muscle. *J. Physiol.* 111–117.

Yuan, X.J., Goldman, W.F., Tod, M.L. Rubin, L.J. & Blaustein, M.P. (1993). Hypoxia reduces potassium currents in cultured rat pulmonary but not mesenteric arterial myocytes. *Am. J. Physiol.* **264**, L116–L123.

Zhang, C. & Paul, R.J. (1994). Excitation-contraction coupling and relaxation in porcine carotid arteries are specifically dependent on glucose. *Am. J. Physiol.* **267**, H1996–H2004.

28

Ca²⁺-induced Ca²⁺ Release in Single Isolated Smooth Muscle Cells

V. Ya. GANITKEVICH

Department of Physiology,
University of Cologne,
Cologne, Germany

Ca^{2+}-induced Ca^{2+} release (CICR) from sarco(endo)plasmic reticulum (SR) is believed to be one of the mechanisms by which extracellular signals are processed in the cytosol (Berridge, 1993). Its importance for excitation–contraction coupling in cardiac preparations is well documented (Bers, 1991). In smooth muscle, however, the situation is less clear (Somlyo & Somlyo, 1994). During a single action potential, Ca^{2+} entry into the smooth muscle cell appears to be large enough to provide the necessary amount of Ca ions for contractile activation. However, because of the presence of many Ca^{2+}-binding sites in the cytosol that possess sufficient binding capacity, and fast enough on-rate to bind almost all Ca^{2+} entering the cell, less than 1% of Ca ions commonly remain ionized. Thus, questions arise about additional sources of Ca^{2+} influx into cytosol and among these sources the prime candidate is Ca^{2+} efflux from the SR mediated by the CICR mechanism. For a long time it has been known that Ca release channels, sensitive to ryanodine and caffeine, are expressed in smooth muscle. Ryanodine has been commonly found to modify the contractile state of visceral and vascular smooth muscle (van Breemen & Saida, 1989). Caffeine triggers a 'force transient' in a variety of smooth muscle cells in the absence of extracellular Ca^{2+} which is indicative of the presence of a CICR mechanism in these cells (Endo, 1977; Saida, 1982). Caffeine is known to sensitize the ryanodine receptors to Ca^{2+} (Iino, 1989) so that CICR is activated at low (resting) levels of free Ca^{2+}. Caffeine induced Ca^{2+} efflux in skinned preparations (Yamamoto & van Breemen, 1985). Later, CICR in skinned fibres was demonstrated directly (Iino, 1989). For activation by Ca^{2+}, the release channels required an ionized Ca concentration of $1\,\mu M$ or more. The ryanodine receptor from smooth muscle has been isolated, incorporated into

SMOOTH MUSCLE EXCITATION
ISBN 0-12-112360-X

artificial membranes and activation of ryanodine receptors by Ca^{2+} has been directly demonstrated both for vascular (Herrmann-Frank et al., 1991) and for visceral (Xu et al., 1994) smooth muscle. Channel openings were induced by micromolar concentrations of Ca^{2+}, concentrations comparable with studies in skinned muscles. On this basis, the physiological role of CICR was questioned because force activation occurs at lower levels of free Ca than appear to be necessary to activate CICR (Iino, 1989).

In the last few years, ideas about participation of CICR in excitation–contraction coupling in smooth muscle have been changed as new methods have been developed. The conclusion, whether CICR is of physiological importance, depends, however, on the method of stimulation. Caffeine diffuses quickly all over the cell (when applied quickly enough) and binds to the release channels nearly synchronously. This is unlike the physiological situation where Ca^{2+} diffusion in a highly buffered milieu should be slowed down at least by a factor of 100 compared with diffusion in solution. Thus, the results that demonstrate the large cytosolic Ca^{2+} increment by means of 'synchronized' activation of ryanodine-receptors by caffeine do not necessarily tell us anything about how CICR can be activated by calcium influx with I_{Ca} or by action potential. Similarly, the observation that ryanodine modifies contraction of many smooth muscles does not demonstrate how ryanodine receptors are involved in excitation–contraction coupling: the effects could result partly from modified Ca^{2+} handling in the cytoplasm.

Physiologically, the trigger Ca^{2+} for activation of CICR derives through the plasmalemmal Ca^{2+} channels. Both theoretical considerations (Stern, 1992; Kargacin, 1994) and direct measurements (Neher & Augustine, 1992; Chow et al., 1994) suggest that during Ca^{2+} current flow, close to the membrane local $[Ca^{2+}]_i$ values easily exceeding $1\,\mu M$ could be reached. These would be not detected during whole-cell measurements using high-affinity fluorescence indicators like Fura-2 or Indo-1, because indicators would be locally saturated. In addition, these Ca^{2+}-indicators produce considerable buffering of cytoplasmic Ca^{2+} changes because of their high affinity, and because of their mobility are expected to attenuate putative Ca^{2+} gradients (Zhou & Neher, 1993). However, localized high levels of Ca^{2+} could be detected by Ca^{2+}-activated K^+ currents and recently a late outward current, with properties that would be expected if it was due to CICR, has been recorded in single ileal smooth muscle cells suggesting that I_{Ca} can activate CICR in these cells (Zholos et al., 1992). Using Indo-1 as a Ca^{2+}-indicator in voltage-clamped bladder cells of guinea pig, CICR triggered by a maximal I_{Ca} (steps to 0 mV) was demonstrated directly (Ganitkevich & Isenberg, 1992). The contribution of CICR in the depolarization-induced increment of free Ca^{2+} was estimated from the effects of ryanodine or caffeine treatment. It was shown that CICR contributes to the 'phasic' component of the Ca^{2+} transient evoked by I_{Ca}. Ca^{2+} release from the SR triggered by I_{Ca} was demonstrated also in portal vein myocytes (Gregoire *et al.*, 1993). Among the divalent cations permeating through plasmalemmal Ca^{2+} channels, Sr^{2+} ions can substitute for Ca^{2+} in triggering Ca^{2+} release in portal vein (Gregoire *et al.*, 1993), but Ba^{2+} ions in coronary myocytes cannot (V.Ya.G. & G. Isenberg, unpublished data).

CICR is expected to receive trigger Ca^{2+} not only from inflowing Ca^{2+} but also from released Ca^{2+} and in this case it is expected to be regenerative (all-or-none). This is not the case in cardiac preparations where CICR is clearly graded. Recent experimental evidence has suggested that gradation of CICR in cardiac cells results from graded recruitment of release units, each of which respond in all-or-none fashion (Cheng *et al.*, 1993; Wier *et al.*, 1994, Isenberg & Han, 1994; Sham *et al.*, 1995). We are far from understanding the release process in smooth muscle. CICR lasting longer than the duration of the pulse, i.e. showing regenerative properties, was demonstrated in portal vein myocytes (Gregoire *et al.*, 1993). In bladder cells, the Ca^{2+} increments evoked by 160-ms steps were shown to be graded by membrane potential, along a bell-shaped curve, similar to that of calcium current (Ganitkevich & Isenberg, 1991).

In urinary bladder myocytes bathed in 10 mM Ca^{2+}, potential steps from the holding potential -80 mV to -30, -20 and 0 mV evoked Ca^{2+} increments of progressively larger amplitude (Figure 1; for experimental procedures see Ganitkevich & Isenberg, 1991, 1992). In this cell, at -30 mV, [Ca^{2+}]$_i$ rises slowly to a peak of 400 nM which was reached 2.5 s after the start of

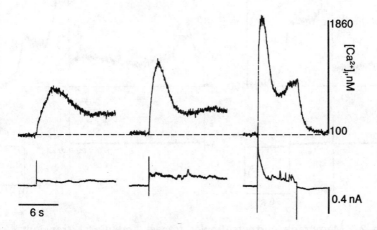

Figure 1 Membrane currents (lower traces) and [Ca^{2+}]$_i$ transients (upper traces) in response to voltage steps from a holding potential -80 mV to -30 mV (left traces), -20 mV (middle traces) and 0 mV (right traces). Myocyte from urinary bladder, K$^+$-rich intracellular solution, 36°C, 10 mM [Ca^{2+}]$_o$.

depolarization and then decayed to some tonic level. During the step to −20 mV, a peak of 610 nM was reached 1 s after start of depolarization. At 0 mV, a peak of 1860 nM was reached 0.4 s after the start of the pulse. This 'phasic' component of these Ca^{2+} transients was removed by ryanodine and was insensitive to heparin; it can thus be attributed to CICR triggered by Ca^{2+} influx. It is clear from Figure 1 that larger depolarization induced accordingly larger Ca^{2+} release. This appeared as progressively larger peaks reached during the pulses (the peak is not the measure of release, but rather the point where Ca^{2+} influx into cytoplasm equals Ca^{2+} removal from cytoplasm) and increased rates of rise of $[Ca^{2+}]_i$ during the transient (rate of rise is proportional to the number of simultaneously open release channels under conditions when reuptake does not superimpose).

In 3.6 mM $[Ca^{2+}]_i$, steps to −30 mV were usually subthreshold for inducing Ca^{2+} release (Figure 2A). $[Ca^{2+}]_i$ was sustained at 170 nM for 6 s during a step to −30 mV. Following a further step to 0 mV larger I_{Ca} was activated and $[Ca^{2+}]_i$ responded with phasic elevation (attributed to CICR) superimposed on a sustained increment. In other cells, a clearly distinguishable 'hump' in the $[Ca^{2+}]_i$ increment due to CICR was observed (Figure 2B). Stepping 18 s later to 0 mV evoked a maximal I_{Ca} which triggered full-sized Ca^{2+} release. This results shows that CICR in bladder myocytes is graded by Ca^{2+} influx. It

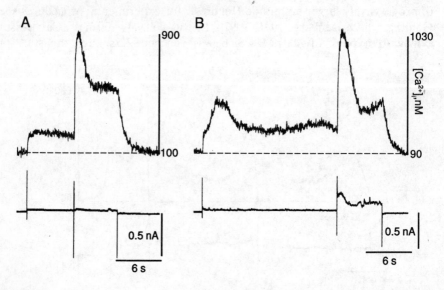

Figure 2   Membrane currents (lower traces) and $[Ca^{2+}]_i$ transients (upper traces) in two myocytes (A and B) from urinary bladder during steps to −30 mV (first current transient) followed by steps to 0 mV (second current transient). Holding potential −60 mV, K⁺-rich intracellular solution, 36°C, 3.6 mM $[Ca^{2+}]_o$.

should be noted, that $[Ca^{2+}]$ increments were measured globally (from the whole cell). Thus, the signals do not discriminate between partial Ca^{2+} release from a single pool or localized release (when only parts of SR are involved). The second possibility appears more likely for the following reasons. It has become clear in the last few years that Ca^{2+}, which is extensively buffered in the cytosol, act as a local second messenger. This contrasts with IP_3, the diffusion of which is not extensively buffered (Allbritton *et al.*, 1992; Kasai & Petersen, 1994). Ca^{2+} influx thus is expected to trigger localized CICR close to the membrane at first. Whether CICR remains localized or will propagate throughout the cell will depend on several factors.

The greater the influx of Ca^{2+} into the cell, the greater the increase of cytosolic Ca^{2+} and the greater the number of putative release sites which will be activated simultaneously. With more Ca^{2+} flowing into the cytosol, the cytoplasmic buffer becomes more saturated and this will enhance diffusion of free Ca^{2+} to the neighbouring release sites. For suboptimal triggers (small depolarizations) the result, (whether CICR will propagate) depends on the load of SR units, the distance between them, and the quantity, affinity and mobility of cytoplasmic Ca^{2+}-buffer (Kargacin & Fay, 1991; Nowycky & Pinter, 1993). Thus, the result can differ between cells owing to different loading with Indo-1. CICR could become regenerative when it receives trigger Ca^{2+} in addition to Ca^{2+} influx from released Ca^{2+}.

In some bladder cells CICR occurring in a regenerative way was observed. Figure 3 demonstrates that a $[Ca^{2+}]_i$ increment to a prominent peak of 1030 nM was reached within 2 s during the first clamp step to -20 mV. Then

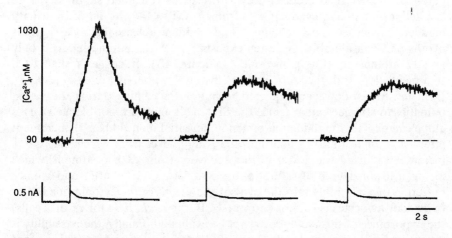

Figure 3 Example of regenerative Ca^{2+} release in bladder myocyte. $[Ca^{2+}]_i$ transients (upper traces) and membrane currents (lower traces) during three 6 s steps to -20 mV.

$[Ca^{2+}]_i$ fell and at the end of a 6 s step reached 170 nM. The second and third depolarizations evoked nearly identical $[Ca^{2+}]_i$ increments with much smaller peaks of 400 nM. Six seconds after the start of depolarization $[Ca^{2+}]_i$ reached 280 nM. Presumably, I_{Ca} remains almost constant over this period (as suggested by the similarity of the second and third response). If the trigger is not modified, then this result suggests that during the first $[Ca^{2+}]_i$ transient SR releases more Ca^{2+} (at the beginning of a step) and buffers influx to a larger extent (by the end of the step) during the first pulse compared with the other two. The regenerative response during the first depolarization in Figure 3 can be explained if Ca^{2+} released from SR participates in further CICR. Presumably, reduction of the SR Ca^{2+} load after the first response (due to plasmalemmal Ca^{2+} extrusion) results in a reduced gain of CICR during the following $[Ca^{2+}]_i$ responses. In this aspect CICR in smooth muscle could resemble that in cardiac cells where SR Ca^{2+} load has been shown to affect the gain of CICR (Han et al., 1994). Thus, experimental evidence suggests that in addition to the maximal trigger (I_{Ca} at 0 mV) CICR can be triggered also during smaller depolarizations which evoke smaller I_{Ca}. However, with no voltage-steps occurring in vivo, the question arises whether CICR can be triggered by a single action potential. Figure 4A shows $[Ca^{2+}]_i$ transients and action potentials in a spontaneously firing (at approx. 1 Hz) bladder myocyte. $[Ca^{2+}]_i$ was elevated and fluctuated between 230 nM and 430 nM in response to each action potential. Thus, the $[Ca^{2+}]_i$ increment induced by single action potential is considerably lower than can be evoked by voltage-steps activating maximal I_{Ca}. When 10 μM acetylcholine was then rapidly applied to the cell, $[Ca^{2+}]_i$ rapidly increased to 2000 nM. Following wash-out, action potentials slowly recovered. However, transients remained suppressed (the last action potential elevates $[Ca^{2+}]_i$ from 70 nM to 140 nM only). In urinary bladder myocytes, acetylcholine- and caffeine-releaseable Ca^{2+} pools overlapped considerably, i.e. after exposure to ACh caffeine induced only greatly attenuated $[Ca^{2+}]_i$ increment (Figure 4B). It suggests that ACh treatment deprived the caffeine-sensitive Ca^{2+} pool of releasable Ca^{2+}. Depleted SR is, however, expected to buffer Ca^{2+} influx during the action potential to a larger extent (since the SR Ca^{2+} pumps are not blocked). This alone can explain the reduction of action potential induced $[Ca^{2+}]_i$ increment after ACh application. In addition, the $[Ca^{2+}]_i$ level from which the $[Ca^{2+}]_i$ increments started was lower during recovery from ACh treatment, which means a lower degree of saturation of cytoplasmic Ca^{2+}-buffer and greater buffering of Ca^{2+} influx into the cytosol. As the K_d of the cytoplasmic buffer in bladder myocytes is yet not known (see Berlin et al., 1994 for cardiac cells) the importance of this factor could not be evaluated. Finally, the possibility is open that local (or partial) CICR contributes to the action potential induced $[Ca^{2+}]_i$ increments and this contribution is removed by partial Ca^{2+} store depletion. Despite being inconclusive, this experiment suggest that a single action potential is unable to trigger full-sized CICR in bladder myocytes. It would be interesting to see whether full-sized CICR can be triggered in smooth muscle generating action potentials with plateau (like ureter). In smooth muscles, which usually do not generate action potentials (like

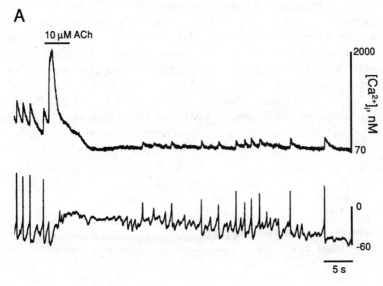

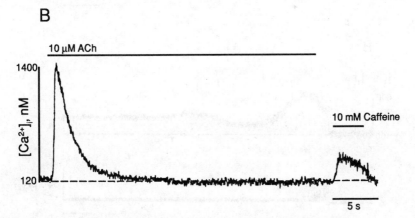

Figure 4 A, $[Ca^{2+}]_i$ transients (upper trace) and membrane potential (lower trace) under current-clamp conditions. Bladder myocyte, 3.6 mM $[Ca^{2+}]_o$; K⁺-rich intracellular solution. ACh, 10 µM was applied to the cell where indicated. B, Overlap between ACh- and caffeine-releaseable Ca²⁺ pool in bladder myocyte. Holding potential −50 mV, the duration of ACh (10 µM) and caffeine (10 mM) applications is indicated.

epicardial coronary artery of guinea pig), we also tested how efficient depolarization and I_{Ca} were in activating CICR (Ganitkevich & Isenberg, 1995).

When the membrane potential of a coronary myocyte bathed in 2.5 mM $[Ca^{2+}]_o$ was stepped from a holding potential of -50 mV to 0 mV, $[Ca^{2+}]_i$ was incremented by about only 100 nM (Figure 5). In some cells this was followed by a slow 'creep' (Figure 5 B). At 0 mV, $[Ca^{2+}]_i$ then stayed at low elevated level (Figure 5A), or fluctuated (Figure 5B). Fluctuations were especially seen in cells demonstrating 'creep' and after prominent creep $[Ca^{2+}]_i$ often fell transiently to a level lower than that before depolarization. $[Ca^{2+}]_i$ fluctuations indicate the involvement of SR Ca^{2+} release in $[Ca^{2+}]_i$ responses, because they cannot be explained by a form of I_{Ca} which rapidly activates and inactivates to a small steady-state level. Essentially similar

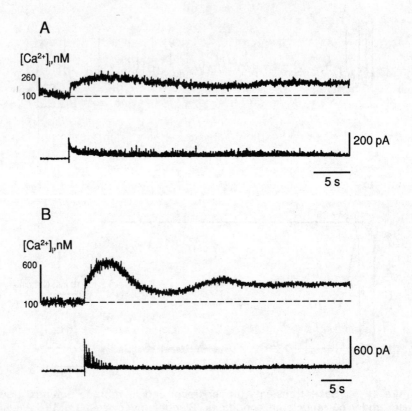

Figure 5 Effect of stepping of the membrane potential from -50 mV to 0 mV on $[Ca^{2+}]_i$ and membrane current of two coronary myocytes (A and B). Upper trace shows $[Ca^{2+}]_i$, lower traces shows membrane current; 36°C, 2.5 mM $[Ca^{2+}]_o$; K$^+$-rich intracellular solution.

responses were recorded with intracellular heparin $(5\,mg\,ml^{-1})$, which excludes the possibility of an involvement of IP_3 receptors in generation of these $[Ca^{2+}]_i$ responses and suggests that they are generated through CICR. As is clear from Figure 5, the $[Ca^{2+}]_i$ responses to maximal trigger (maximal I_{Ca} occurring close to $0\,mV$ with $2.5\,mM\ [Ca^{2+}]_o$) are much smaller in coronary myocytes than in urinary bladder (Figure 1). Maximal I_{Ca} in bladder cells triggers a $[Ca^{2+}]_i$ increment with a peak comparable to that of the caffeine-induced transient (Ganitkevich & Isenberg, 1992). The increment of $[Ca^{2+}]_i$ induced by maximal I_{Ca} (6-s pulses to $0\,mV$) in coronary cells constitutes only $10 \pm 6\%$ $(n = 3)$ of the caffeine-induced increment. Thus, depolarizations with maximal trigger for CICR failed to activate full-sized Ca^{2+} release in coronary myocytes in contrast to bladder cells. Because of the apparent similarity of the $[Ca^{2+}]_i$ responses of coronary cells to steps to $0\,mV$ activating a maximal I_{Ca} (Figure 5) and responses of bladder cells during steps to $-30\,mV$ activating small I_{Ca} (Figure 2) we suggested that this inefficacy of I_{Ca} in coronary cells to trigger a large CICR can be due to a low density of Ca^{2+} channels in this vascular preparation. Indeed, when measured with Cs^+-filled electrodes, the density of peak I_{Ca} in coronary cells was -0.80 ± 0.17 $\mu A \times cm^{-2}$ $(n = 8)$ a value typical for electrically inexcitable vascular myocytes under physiological conditions. To test this hypothesis, the density of peak I_{Ca} can be artificially increased by elevating extracellular $[Ca^{2+}]$ to $10\,mM$ and the addition of $1\,\mu M$ of Ca^{2+}-agonist Bay K 8644. Under these conditions the density of peak I_{Ca} was augmented to -2.6 ± 1.1 $\mu A \times cm^{-2}$ $(n = 14)$. When tested by paired measurements in the same cells, this intervention increased $[Ca^{2+}]_i$ increment induced by 6-s pulses to $0\,mV$ by a factor of 3.3 ± 0.8 $(n = 8)$. However, even when augmented with elevated $[Ca^{2+}]_o$ and by Bay K 8644, in paired experiments the I_{Ca}-induced $[Ca^{2+}]_i$ increments were only $30 \pm 10\%$ of the caffeine-induced $\Delta[Ca^{2+}]_i$ $(n = 8)$. To further increase the density of peak I_{Ca}, experiments with intracellular dialysis of trypsin were performed. Trypsin was shown to increase the amplitude of vascular L-type I_{Ca} (Klöckner, 1988; Obejero-Paz et al., 1991). Cell dialysis of trypsin $(1\,mg\,ml^{-1})$ increased the density of peak I_{Ca} within $3\,min$ up to $12.5\,\mu A \times cm^{-2}$. Steps to $0\,mV$ now induced large $[Ca^{2+}]_i$ increments with peak often over $1\,\mu M$ (Figure 6A), values comparable with the peak of caffeine-induced $[Ca^{2+}]_i$ transients. Ryanodine $(10\,\mu M)$ treatment reduced these $[Ca^{2+}]_i$ increments to about one-third that approximately two-thirds of the Ca^{2+} influx into the cytosol stems from SR Ca^{2+} release through the CICR mechanism. With K^+-filled electrodes in trypsin-treated cells, a hump of outward current appeared (Figure 6B) which was attributed to CICR occurring with high degree of synchronization within the cell.

In conclusion, the CICR mechanism is present in both bladder and coronary myocytes and CICR is graded by I_{Ca}. Under physiological

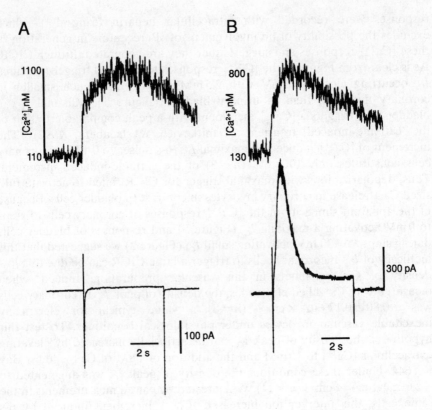

Figure 6 Large $[Ca^{2+}]_i$ transients in coronary myocytes induced by I_{Ca} augmented with 10 mM $[Ca^{2+}]_o$, 1 mM Bay K8644 and intracellular perfusion of trypsin (1 mg ml^{-1}) for 2 min. A, Cs$^+$-rich and B, K$^+$-rich intracellular solution.

conditions, however, I_{Ca} in coronary myocytes does not provide a sufficient trigger for full-sized CICR. It is likely that with low trigger efficacy, CICR remains localized close to the membrane and does not propagate throughout the cell.

REFERENCES

Allbritton, N.L., Meyer, T. & Stryer, L. (1992). Range of messenger action of calcium ion and inositol 1,4,5-trisphosphate. *Science* **258**, 1812–1815.
Berlin, J.R., Bassani, J.W.M. & Bers,D.M. (1994). Intrinsic cytosolic calcium buffering properties of single rat cardiac myocytes. *Biophys. J.* **67**, 1775–1787.
Berridge, M.J. (1993). Inositol trisphosphate and calcium signalling. *Nature* **361**, 315–325.

Bers, D.M. (1991). *Excitation–Contraction Coupling and Cardiac Contractile Force.* Kluwer Academic Publishers, Dodrecht.

van Breemen, C. & Saida, K. (1989). Cellular mechanisms regulating $[Ca^{2+}]_i$ in smooth muscle. *Annu. Rev. Physiol.* **51**, 315–329.

Cheng, H., Lederer, W.J. & Cannell, M.B. (1993). Calcium sparks: elementary events underlying excitation-contraction coupling in heart muscle. *Science* **262**, 740–744.

Chow,R.H., Klingauf, J. & Neher, E. (1994). Time course of Ca^{2+} concentration triggering exocytosis in neuroendocrine cells. *Proc. Natl Acad.Sci. USA* **91**, 12765–12769.

Ganitkevich, V.Ya., & Isenberg, G. (1991). Depolarization-mediated intracellular calcium transients in isolated smooth muscle cells of guinea pig urinary bladder. *J. Physiol.* **435**, 187–205.

Ganitkevich, V.Ya. & Isenberg, G. (1992). Contribution of Ca^{2+}-induced Ca^{2+} release to the $[Ca^{2+}]$ transients in myocytes from guinea pig urinary bladder. *J. Physiol.* **458**, 119–137.

Ganitkevich, V.Ya. & Isenberg, G. (1995). Efficacy of I_{Ca} as trigger of SR Ca^{2+} release in myocytes from the guinea pig coronary artery. *J. Physiol.* **484**, 287–306.

Gregoire,G., Loirand, G. & Pacaud, P. (1993). Ca^{2+} and Sr^{2+} entry induced Ca^{2+} release from the intracellular Ca^{2+} store in smooth muscle cells of rat portal vein. *J. Physiol.* **474**, 483–500.

Han, S. Schiefer, A. & Isenberg, G. (1994). Ca^{2+} load of guinea pig ventricular myocytes determines efficacy of brief Ca^{2+} currents as trigger for SR Ca^{2+} release. *J. Physiol.* **480**, 411–422.

Herrmann-Frank, A., Darling, E. & Meissner, G. (1991). Functional characterization of the Ca^{2+}-gated Ca^{2+} release channel of vascular smooth muscle sarcoplasmic reticulum. *Pflügers Archiv.* **418**, 353–359.

Endo, M. (1977). Calcium release from the sarcoplasmic reticulum. *Physiol. Rev.* **57**, 71–108.

Iino, M. (1989). Calcium-induced calcium release mechanism in guinea pig taenia caeci. *J. Gen. Physiol.* **94**, 363–383.

Isenberg, G. & Han, S. (1994). Gradation of Ca^{2+} induced Ca^{2+} release by clamp step duration in potentiated guinea pig ventricular myocytes. *J. Physiol.* **480**, 423–438.

Kargacin, G.J. (1994). Calcium signaling in restricted diffusion spaces. *Biophys. J.* **67**, 262–272.

Kargacin, G. & Fay, F.S. (1991). Ca^{2+} movement in smooth muscle cells studied with one- and two-dimensional diffusion models. *Biophys J.* **60**, 1088–1100.

Kasai, H. & Petersen, O.H. (1994). Spatial dynamics of second messengers: IP_3 and cAMP as long-range and associative messengers. *Trends Neurosci.* **17**, 95–101.

Klöckner, U. (1988) Isolated coronary smooth muscle cells. Increase in the availability of L-type Ca^{2+} channels by intracellularly applied peptidases. *Pflügers Archiv.* **412**, R82.

Neher, E. & Augustine, G.J. (1992). Calcium gradients and buffers in bovine chromaffin cells. *J. Physiol.* **450**, 273–301.

Nowycky, M. & Pinter, M. (1993). Time courses of calcium and calcium-bound buffers following calcium influx in a model cell. *Biophys. J.* **64**, 77–91.

Obejero-Paz, C.A., Jones, S.W. & Scarpa, A. (1991). Calcium currents in the A7r5 smooth muscle-derived cell line. Increase in current and selective removal of voltage-dependent inactivation by intracellular trypsin. *J. Gen. Physiol.* **98**, 1127–1140.

Saida, K. (1982). Intracellular Ca release in skinned smooth muscle. *J. Gen. Physiol.* **80**, 191–202.

Sham, J.S.K., Cleemann, L. & Morad, M. (1995). Functional coupling of Ca^{2+} channels and ryanodine receptors in cardiac myocytes. *Proc. Natl Acad. Sci. USA* **92**, 121–125.

Somlyo, A.P. & Somlyo, A.V. (1994). Signal transduction and regulation in smooth muscle. *Nature* **372**, 231–236.

Stern, M.D. (1992). Buffering of calcium in the vicinity of a channel pore. *Cell Calcium* **13**, 183–192.

Wier, W.G., Egan, T.M., Lopez-Lopez, J.R. & Balke, C.W. (1994). Local control of excitation-contraction coupling in rat heart cells. *J. Physiol.* **474**, 463–471.

Xu, L., Lai, F.A., Cohn, A., Etter, E., Guerrero., A., Fay, F.S. & Meissner, G. (1994). Evidence for a Ca^{2+}-gated ryanodine-sensitive Ca^{2+} release channel in visceral smooth muscle. *Proc. Natl Acad. Sci. USA* **91**, 3294–3298.

Yamamoto, H. & van Breemen, C. (1985). Inositol-1,4,5-trisphosphate releases calcium from skinned cultured smooth muscle cells. *Biochem. Biophys. Res. Comm.* **130**, 270–274.

Zholos, A.V., Baidan, L.V. & Shuba, M.F. (1992). Some properties of Ca^{2+}-induced Ca^{2+}-release mechanism in single visceral smooth muscle cell of the guinea pig. *J. Physiol.* **457**, 1–25.

Zhou, Z. & Neher, E. (1993). Mobile and immobile calcium buffers in bovine adrenal chromaffin cells. *J. Physiol.* **469**, 245–273.

29

Regulation of Ca-dependent K Current and Action Potential Shape by Intracellular Ca Storage Sites in Some Types of Smooth Muscle Cells

YUJI IMAIZUMI
SATOSHI HENMI
NORIHIRO NAGANO
KATSUHIKO MURAKI
MINORU WATANABE

*Department of Chemical Pharmacology,
Faculty of Pharmaceutical Sciences,
Nagoya City University,
Nagoya, Japan*

INTRODUCTION

In the last decade, mechanisms underlying the diversity of membrane excitability in various types of smooth muscles have been revealed based on measurements of macroscopic currents from whole-cell and single channel currents from membrane patches. Substantial voltage-dependent Ca currents through mainly L-type channels have been recorded in single cells isolated from smooth muscles, which have relatively high membrane excitability and elicit action potentials (APs) spontaneously or in response to electrical stimulation, such as urinary bladder, portal vein, taenia caeci, ileum, stomach fundus, vas deferens, ureter etc. It is clear that the density and characteristics of Ca channels in the plasma membrane are the most important determinant of membrane excitability of the myocyte (Kitamura *et al.*, 1989a).

Although in all types of smooth muscle cells examined, Ca-dependent K current (I_{K-Ca}) is the major or one of the main components of outward current elicited by depolarization, the current is especially large in highly excitable smooth muscle cells. As the I_{K-Ca} upon depolarization is blocked by

SMOOTH MUSCLE EXCITATION
ISBN 0-12-112360-X

low concentrations of tetraethylammonium (TEA), charybdotoxin or iberiotoxin but not by apamin, the current is due to activation of large-conductance K (BK) channels (Bolton & Beech, 1992). The density of BK channels is extremely high in all types of smooth muscle cells examined. Changes in BK channel activity, therefore, greatly modulate total membrane current and cellular excitability. In addition to Ca^{2+} influx, Ca^{2+} release from intracellular storage sites may also strongly affect BK channel activity. The present study is focused on the relationship between functions of intracellular Ca storage sites and membrane excitability with respect to the regulation of I_{K-Ca}.

CONTRIBUTION OF I_{K-Ca} TO ACTION POTENTIAL REPOLARIZATION AND AFTERHYPERPOLARIZATION

Typical recordings of APs and membrane currents in single smooth muscle cells isolated from taenia caeci, ileal longitudinal layer, vas deferens and urinary bladder of the guinea pig at room temperature are shown in Figures 1 and 2. APs in these cells had rapid repolarization and clear after-hyperpolarization (AHP), when the pipette solution contained mainly KCl and also low concentrations of EGTA. The initial inward and following outward currents were recorded upon depolarization under voltage-clamp in these cells. The fast transient outward current was almost abolished when the pipette solution contained 10 mM EGTA and a delayed rectifier type outward current remained in taenia caeci cells (Figure 1Ab) and in other cells as well (not shown). Under these conditions, correspondingly, the AP rate of fall and the AHP amplitude were markedly reduced (Figure 1Ab, upper trace). Application of a Ca channel blocker (0.1 mM Cd^{2+}, 1 mM Mn^{2+} or 3 μM nifedipine) abolished and markedly reduced both the inward current and the fast transient outward current, respectively. The delayed rectifier K current at 0 mV in the presence of 0.1 mM Cd^{2+} was much smaller than the peak I_{K-Ca} observed before application of Cd^{2+} and was not sensitive to 2 mM 4-aminopyridine (4-AP) and 100 nM charybdotoxin. Ca-independent transient outward current (A-type K current) was observed only in vas deferens cells among these cells and was markedly reduced by addition of 2 mM 4-AP. It has been considered, therefore, that the fast I_{K-Ca} upon depolarization is one of the main repolarizing current of AP in smooth muscle cells isolated from stomach (Mitra & Morad, 1985), urinary bladder (Klöckner & Isenberg, 1985), longitudinal muscle layer of ileum (Ohya *et al.*, 1986) and taenia caeci (Yamamoto *et al.*, 1989). It is also the case in vas deferens cells because the AP rate of fall was slower when the pipette solution contained 5 mM EGTA.

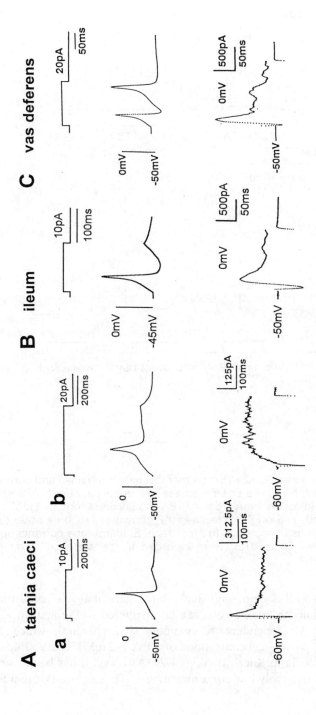

Figure 1 Action potentials (APs) recorded under current clamp (upper traces) and membrane currents under voltage-clamp (lower traces) in single smooth muscle cells isolated from three kinds of guinea pig tissues. Each pair of APs and current was recorded from the same cell. The pipette solution contained low (0.05–0.3 mM) EGTA, except in Ab where it contained 10 mM EGTA. A, Taenia caeci; B, ileal longitudinal layer; C, vas deferens. All recordings were performed at room temperature.

A   urinary bladder

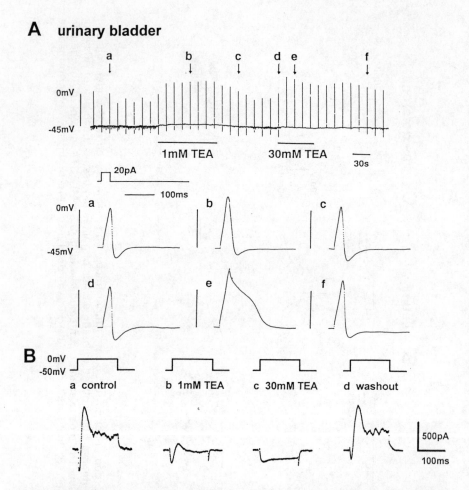

Figure 2   Effects of 1 and 30 mM TEA on membrane potential (A) and currents (B) in a single smooth muscle cell of guinea pig urinary bladder. APs were elicited by current injection every 15 s. A, TEA at concentrations of 1 mM and 30 mM were applied. The original traces of AP shown at fast time scale (a–f) were recorded at times indicated in the top trace. B, Membrane currents upon depolarization from −50 to 0 mV were recorded in the same cell after the procedure shown in A.

It has also been well documented that a large part of $I_{K\text{-}Ca}$ elicited upon depolarization in smooth muscle cells can be attributed to the activation of large conductance Ca-dependent K channels (BK channel), which are selectively blocked by low concentrations of TEA (<2 mM), charybdotoxin, and iberiotoxin (Garcia & Kaczorowski, 1992). Although it has been shown that application of relatively low concentrations of TEA (<5 mM), quinidine and charybdotoxin, (BK channel blockers) results in an increase in frequency and a decrease in AHP amplitude of spontaneous AP firing in ileal circular and longitudinal strips (Bauer & Kuriyama, 1982; Nakao et al., 1986, Uyama et al., 1993), direct evidence indicating the contribution of BK channel activation to AP shape has not been clearly shown in single cells. Figure 2 shows that 1 mM TEA reduced the AP rate of fall and the amplitude of AHP and increased the AP amplitude in a single cell from urinary bladder. Duration of AP was extensively prolonged when 30 mM TEA was applied. Accordingly, under voltage-clamp, $I_{K\text{-}Ca}$ upon depolarization was markedly reduced by 1 mM TEA and the net current was inward throughout the depolarization in the presence of 30 mM TEA. Application of 0.1 μM apamin, which is a selective blocker of small conductance Ca-dependent K channels, affected neither AP shape nor $I_{K\text{-}Ca}$ upon depolarization. Qualitatively similar results about the contribution of BK channel activation on AP shape were obtained in cells from taenia caeci, vas deferens and ileal longitudinal layer of the guinea pig. These results indicate that the suppression of $I_{K\text{-}Ca}$ changes AP shape and, as a consequence, increases Ca^{2+}-influx during APs and membrane excitability.

ACTIVATION OF $I_{K\text{-}Ca}$ BY Ca-INDUCED Ca RELEASE MECHANISM

The activation of a fast transient $I_{K\text{-}Ca}$ upon depolarization discussed above may be due to not only Ca-influx through voltage-dependent Ca channels but also Ca release from intracellular storage sites, presumably sarcoplasmic/endoplasmic reticulum (ER/SR; Ca-induced Ca release; CICR). CICR through ryanodine receptor in smooth muscle has been demonstrated in reconstituted channels (Xu et al., 1994). Evidence supporting this hypothesis has been accumulated in several types of smooth muscle cells (small intestine: Ohya et al., 1987, Sakai et al., 1988, Suzuki et al., 1992; ureter: Imaizumi et al., 1989, 1990; urinary bladder: Suzuki et al., 1992), while CICR may not be very important in induced contraction in smooth muscle (Iino, 1989). It has been reported that application of caffeine transiently increases and, thereafter, markedly reduces $I_{K\text{-}Ca}$ upon depolarization in smooth muscle cells of small intestine (Ohya et al., 1987). The transient $I_{K\text{-}Ca}$ upon depolarization is susceptible to ryanodine (Sakai et al., 1988). Correspondingly, it can be assumed that AP repolarization and AHP are mainly due to activation of BK channels via CICR. Figure 3 shows effects of caffeine on APs and membrane current in single cells from guinea pig ileal longitudinal layer. Application of 5 mM caffeine elicited a phasic hyperpolarization and, thereafter, abolished repetitive spontaneous transient hyperpolarizations. Moreover, the AP rate of fall and AHP amplitude were

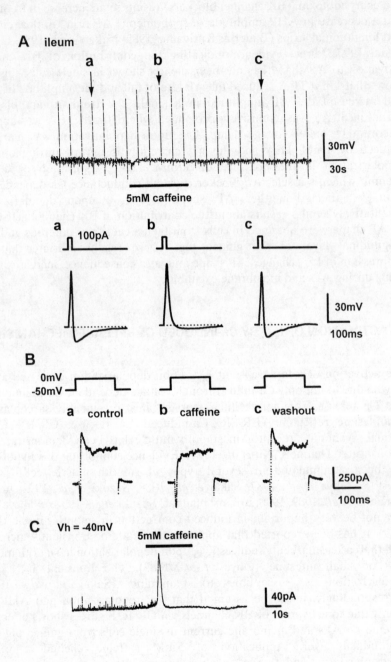

markedly reduced and AP amplitude was increased. The effect of caffeine disappeared within 2 min after washout. I_{K-Ca} upon depolarization was transiently (<20) increased just after the application of 5 mM caffeine (not shown) and thereafter markedly reduced (Figure 3B).

Stimulation of receptors by an agonist which couples with phospholipase C (PLC), such as acetylcholine (ACh) and substance P, also transiently increased I_{K-Ca} and then markedly reduced it, as has been reported in intestinal smooth muscle cells of the rabbit (Benham & Bolton, 1986). Qualitatively, the same effects of norepinephrine (NE) on I_{K-Ca} have been observed in cells from vas deferens (Takeda et al., 1991). The decrease in I_{K-Ca} by NE was inhibited by addition to the recording pipette of low molecular weight heparin (mol. wt. = 3000–5000), which blocks inositol trisphosphate (IP_3)-binding to its receptor on sarcoplasmic reticulum (SR) (Kobayashi et al., 1989b). In the same cells loaded with heparin, application of 5 mM caffeine showed biphasic effect on I_{K-Ca} in the same manner as in the absence of heparin (Takeda et al., 1991). These observations suggest that agonists, which enhance IP_3 formation by activation of PLC and release Ca^{2+} from SR, may have similar effects on I_{K-Ca} to those of caffeine. The decrease in I_{K-Ca} by caffeine or agonists is not mainly the result of decrease in Ca channel current (I_{Ca}) via Ca-induced inactivation of Ca channels, as I_{K-Ca} was almost abolished when the peak I_{Ca} amplitude was reduced only by about 20% in the presence of caffeine. BK channel activity in excised patch was unaffected by 10 mM caffeine. Moreover, I_{K-Ca} did not recover even when an addition of Bay K 8644 increased I_{Ca} by 40 % in the presence of caffeine. It is more likely that an exhaustion of stored Ca after a large Ca release results in a marked decrease in I_{K-Ca}.

Spontaneous transient outward current (STOC) is also due to activation of BK channels by cyclical Ca release from and uptake to local intracellular storage sites (Benham & Bolton, 1986; Imaizumi et al., 1989). STOCs are transiently enhanced and, thereafter, abolished by caffeine (Figure 3C, ileal longitudinal smooth muscle cell) or by agonists in several types of smooth muscle cells (Bolton & Lim, 1989; Komori & Bolton, 1989). The transient enhancement and subsequent suppression of STOCs by caffeine under

---

Figure 3 Effects of 5 mM caffeine on membrane potential (A) and currents (B and C) under current- and voltage-clamp modes, respectively, in single cells isolated from longitudinal layer of the guinea pig ileum. A, AP was elicited by current injection every 15 s. The APs indicated by a, b, and c in upper trace are shown on a faster time scale in the lower trace. The resting membrane potential was about −45 mV. B, The transient outward current upon depolarization from −50 to 0 mV was markedly reduced by the application of 5 mM caffeine. A and B were recorded in the same cell. C, Spontaneous transient outward currents and effects of 5 mM caffeine on them were examined at a holding potential of −40 mV in another cell.

voltage-clamp were in good agreement with the generation of phasic hyperpolarizations and the suppression of spontaneous repetitive hyperpolarizations under current clamp, respectively (Figure 3A, C). In the presence of 5 mM caffeine, addition of 10 μM ACh did not elicit outward current.

Based upon these observations, it can be suggested that, when an AP occurs, stored Ca is released by Ca^{2+} influx through voltage-dependent Ca channels via CICR mechanism and, at least in part, contributes to activation of I_{K-Ca} which is responsible for AP repolarization and AHP. During exposure to an agonist or caffeine, stored Ca is released transiently and, thereafter, may be exhausted, resulting in the marked decrease in I_{K-Ca}. Alternatively, Ca release might be suppressed after a large release by negative feedback mechanism. An inhibition of further Ca release via activation of protein kinase C by NE has been suggested (Kitamura *et al.*, 1992). Moreover, direct inhibition of BK channel activities by muscarinic stimulation via GTP binding protein has also been suggested (Kume & Kotlikoff, 1992). It can be concluded that the decrease in I_{K-Ca} prolongs AP duration and reduces AHP and, thereby, may result in the increase in Ca^{2+}-influx during APs and membrane excitability.

Ca-DEPENDENT K CURRENT AND Ca-PUMP IN SARCOPLASMIC RETICULUM

Recently, specific inhibitors of Ca-ATPase in ER/SR – thapsigargin (TG), cyclopiazonic acid (CPA) and 2,5-di(*t*-butyl)-1,4-benzohydroquinone – have been introduced. These inhibitors are useful as a pharmacological tool to reduce Ca-uptake into the ER/SR and deplete stored Ca. CPA effectively suppressed ATP-dependent Ca-uptake into the SR, which was monitored by the peak amplitude of phasic contraction induced by caffeine or IP_3 following the Ca-uptake at pCa 6.3 in skinned ileal longitudinal strips ($IC_{50} = 0.6$ μM) (Uyama *et al.*, 1992). These agents reduce the amount of stored Ca and may, thereby, affect I_{K-Ca} in smooth muscle cells.

Application of 5 μM CPA markedly reduced the initial transient outward current upon depolarization from -50 to 0 mV for 150 msec every 15 s in cells from ileal longitudinal layer and urinary bladder of the guinea pig as shown in Figure 4 (Suzuki *et al.*, 1992). The effect of CPA was, at least in part, removed by washout. The reduction of I_{K-Ca} depended upon the concentration of CPA (Figure 4Ba). The CPA-sensitive component of outward current was almost identical to I_{K-Ca} which was sensitive to 2 mM TEA (Figure 4Bb). Application of 1–300 nM TG also reduced the I_{K-Ca}, but its effect was irreversible. The IC_{50}s of CPA on I_{K-Ca} were approximately 3

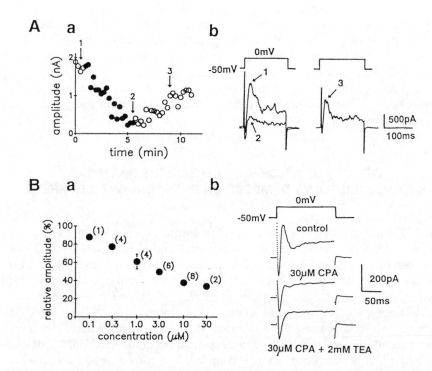

Figure 4 Effects of CPA on outward currents in smooth muscle cells isolated from urinary bladder (A) and ileum (B). Cells were depolarized once every 15 s. A, The peak amplitude of outward current was measured and plotted against time. Open and closed symbols indicate the amplitude in the absence and presence of 5 μM CPA, respectively. Recordings shown in (b) were obtained at the time correspondingly indicated by numbers in (a). B, The relationship between the concentration of CPA and the relative amplitude of outward current normalized by that of the control. The number of observations is shown in parenthesis. (From Suzuki *et al.*, 1992 with permission).

and 5 μM in cells from ileal longitudinal layer and vas deferens, respectively. That of TG in vas deferens cell was approximately 30 nM, indicating that the potency of TG in terms of IC_{50} for $I_{K\text{-}Ca}$ inhibition was about 100 times higher than that of CPA.

Voltage-dependent Ca channel current and delayed rectifier K current in cells from ileum and urinary bladder were not affected significantly by 10 μM CPA (Suzuki *et al.*, 1992) and by 0.3 μM TG. The A-type transient K current in vas deferens cells was affected neither by 10 μM CPA nor 0.3 μM TG. I_{Ca} was slightly reduced by CPA and TG at concentrations higher than 30 and 1 μM, respectively. Moreover, the single channel activity of BK channel was not affected by 10 μM CPA (Suzuki *et al.*, 1992) or 0.3 μM TG. These data indicate that the decrease in I_{K-Ca} by CPA and TG may be due to the decrease in the rate of Ca-uptake to SR by the inhibition of Ca-ATPase but not by the direct block of K or Ca channels. Application of $10\,\mu M$ CPA decreased AHP and increased spontaneous AP frequency in ileal longitudinal strips just as charybdotoxin did (Uyama *et al.*, 1993). It can be postulated that the activity of the Ca-pump in SR indirectly but significantly correlates with the membrane excitability via the regulation of I_{K-Ca} in these smooth muscle cells.

EFFECTS OF A NOVEL Ca-RELEASER, 9-METHYL-7-BROMOEUDISTOMIN D (MBED), ON Ca-DEPENDENT K CURRENT

MBED is a derivative of eudistomin D, a natural marine product and has a chemical structure similar to that of caffeine (Figure 5). It has been shown that MBED releases Ca^{2+} from SR in skinned skeletal muscle fibre in a similar manner to caffeine but is 100 times more effective ($ED_{50} = 10\,\mu M$) (Kobayashi *et al.*, 1989a; Seino *et al.*, 1991). It has been suggested that MBED competes with caffeine at the same binding site on the ryanodine receptor of skeletal muscle. In skinned fibres from ileal longitudinal layer and mesenteric artery of the guinea pig, application of 30 mM caffeine elicited a phasic contraction in a relaxing solution containing 0.1 mM EGTA (pCa = ~7.5), when the SR of the skinned fibres was preloaded with Ca in pCa 6.3 solution. Surprisingly, application of $1\text{–}100\,\mu M$ MBED did not elicit a contraction under the same conditions and did not affect significantly the magnitude of subsequent contraction induced by 30 mM caffeine (Imaizumi *et al.*, 1993).

Application of $30\,\mu M$ MBED, however, transiently enhanced and thereafter markedly reduced the I_{K-Ca} upon depolarization in a similar manner as caffeine did in single cells isolated from urinary bladder (Figure 5A, B) and ileal longitudinal layer (Imaizumi *et al.*, 1993). Moreover, application of $30\,\mu M$ MBED at a holding potential of $-40\,mV$ transiently enhanced STOCs and thereafter suppressed them (Figure 5C). These effects of MBED were removed by washout. The discrepancy between effects of MBED on contraction in skinned fibre and on I_{K-Ca} in single cells cannot be attributed to the difference between multi and single cell preparations because a substantial contraction was induced by 10 mM caffeine but not by $100\,\mu M$ MBED in a single urinary bladder cell. Ca current and delayed rectifier K current were not affected by $30\,\mu M$ MBED. BK channel activity in excised patch was also unaffected by $30\,\mu M$ MBED. These results suggest that MBED effectively releases Ca^{2+} from SR available for the activation of BK channels but not from that for contractile system.

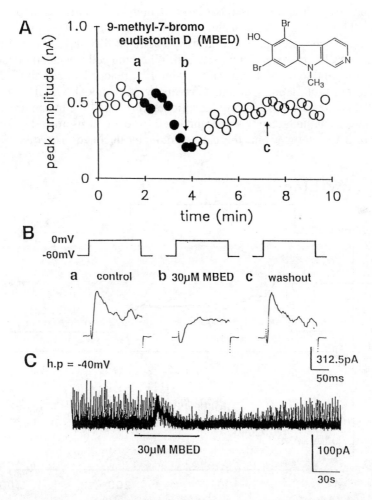

Figure 5 Effects of 30 μM MBED on membrane currents in single smooth muscle cells isolated from urinary bladder of the guinea pig. A, Cells were depolarized from −60 to 0 mV for 150 ms once every 15 s. Open and closed symbols indicate amplitude of peak outward currents in the absence and presence of 30 μM MBED, respectively, and are plotted against time. The inset shows the chemical structure of MBED. B, Traces shown in Ba, b and c were recorded at the time indicated correspondingly in A. C, Spontaneous transient outward currents (STOCs), which were recorded at holding potential of −40 mV, were transiently enhanced by application of 30 μM MBED and thereafter suppressed. (From Imaizumi *et al.*, 1993 with permission).

DISSOCIATION BETWEEN INDO-1 SIGNAL AND Ca-DEPENDENT
K CURRENT UPON DEPOLARIZATION

Figure 6 shows simultaneous recordings of membrane currents and indo-1 signal as the indication of intracellular Ca^{2+} concentration ($[Ca^{2+}]_i$) (the ratio of fluorescent intensity measured at wavelengths of 405 and 485 nm) from a single urinary bladder smooth muscle cell. When the cell was depolarized for 150 ms from −60 to 0 mV, the transient large I_{K-Ca} reached a peak about 20 ms after the start of depolarization. Conversely, the indo-1 signal increased about 10 ms after the start of depolarization and reached the maximum about 100 ms later. The high $[Ca^{2+}]_i$ was maintained for over 50 ms after the cell was repolarized to −60 mV and thereafter gradually declined. The dissociation

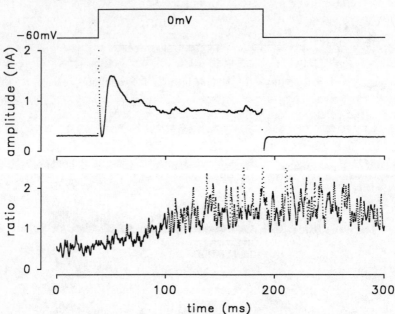

Figure 6 Membrane currents (upper trace) and indo-1 signal (lower trace) were recorded simultaneously from a smooth muscle cell isolated from urinary bladder. The cell was loaded with indo-1 by diffusion from the pipette solution which contained 50 μM indo-1. The excitation wavelength was 360 nm. Indo-1 signal was shown as the ratio of fluorescent intensity detected at two wave lengths, 405 and 485 nm (F_{405}/F_{485}). The cell was depolarized from −60 to 0 mV once every 15 s. The ratio values of 0.5 and 2.0 correspond to about 100 and 700 nM $[Ca^{2+}]_i$, respectively.

between the peak of $I_{K\text{-}Ca}$ and that of indo-1 signal suggests that the increase in $[Ca^{2+}]_i$ just beneath the cell membrane which is available for activation of BK channels cannot be detected by indo-1 under these conditions. Alternatively, BK channels are inactivated after the peak of $I_{K\text{-}Ca}$ by an unknown mechanism, whereas $[Ca^{2+}]_i$ increases. It is, however, unlikely that the decay of $I_{K\text{-}Ca}$ is due to the inactivation of BK channels, since such rapid inactivation of BK channels has not been reported in cell-attached and excised patch modes in smooth muscle cells.

CONCLUSIONS

It is confirmed that the major ionic current responsible for the repolarization and AHP of an evoked AP at room temperature is $I_{K\text{-}Ca}$ through BK channels in smooth muscle cells isolated from urinary bladder, vas deferens, ileal longitudinal layer, and taenia caeci of the guinea pig, whereas the amplitude of $I_{K\text{-}Ca}$ and its contribution to AP shape somewhat varies with the cell type. The contribution of delayed rectifier K current might be larger at 37°C, especially in intestinal cells.

Evidence supporting the hypothesis that a Ca-induced Ca release (CICR) mechanism is involved in the activation of $I_{K\text{-}Ca}$ during depolarization in some smooth muscle cells has been accumulated using caffeine and ryanodine (Ohya et al., 1987; Sakai et al., 1988; Kitamura et al., 1989b; Ganitkevich & Isenberg, 1991, 1992; Zholos et al., 1992). It has, however, not been shown that CICR is triggered by an AP and that subsequent activation of $I_{K\text{-}Ca}$ contributes, at least in part, to AP repolarization and AHP. The effects of caffeine on AP shape in this study are in good agreement with the results in voltage-clamp experiments and, thereby, the hypothesis. Moreover, the results obtained using CPA (Suzuki et al., 1992; Uyama et al., 1993) and TG gave further evidence which is consistent with the hypothesis.

Taken together, the application of several substances, which reduce or exhaust stored Ca, such as caffeine, ryanodine, agonists which activates PLC and inhibitors of Ca-ATPase, decreased $I_{K\text{-}Ca}$ upon depolarization and, thereby, decreased the AP rate of fall and the AHP amplitude in four types of smooth muscle cells.

MBED induced Ca release and consequently activated BK channels in single cells, just as caffeine did, but surprisingly did not elicit Ca release in skinned fibre (Imaizumi et al., 1993). Although the mechanism underlying this difference has not yet been clarified, the following explanation may be the most likely. Because the hydrophilicity of MBED is much lower than that of caffeine, MBED applied from outside may affect preferentially to Ca releasing channels in SR just beneath the cell membrane (superficial SR) and, therefore, selectively depletes stored Ca which is particularly available for BK channel activation. Alternatively, there might be two distinctive types of Ca-releasing channels which are resolved by sensitivity to MBED but are both sensitive to caffeine in these smooth muscles. Although three types of c-DNAs encoding ryanodine receptor proteins have been described (Sorrentino & Volpe, 1993), the characteristics of non-muscle type ryanodine receptor (RyR3) (Hakamata et al., 1992) which may be predominant RyR in smooth muscles, have not yet been clarified.

In the present study, a fast transient I_{K-Ca} was elicited by a relatively short depolarization, for 100–200 ms from -60 to 0 mV. The current reached a peak within 30 msec after the start of depolarization and declined progressively to a steady level within about 100 ms from the peak under whole-cell clamp mode, as has been shown by other groups (Benham & Bolton, 1986; Ohya et al., 1986, 1987; Yamamoto et al., 1989). Although the decline of I_{K-Ca} during a depolarization appeared to be slightly slower under nystatin-perforated patch clamp than the standard whole-cell clamp, the time to peak of I_{K-Ca} was identical under these two recording conditions. Therefore, the transient nature of I_{K-Ca} upon depolarization was not the artifact due to 0.05–0.3 mM EGTA added to the pipette solution or to the dilution of cytosolic factor controlling the I_{K-Ca} decline.

The I_{K-Ca} upon depolarization were clearly dissociated from the increase in intracellular Ca^{2+} concentration ($[Ca^{2+}]_i$) measured with fluorescent Ca^{2+} indicator. Some dissociation between I_{K-Ca} and fura-2 or indo-1 signal has also been suggested in coronary arterial smooth muscle cell (Stehno-Bittel & Sturek, 1992; Ganitkevich & Isenberg, 1995). Moreover, a fast Ca-dependent Cl current (I_{Cl-Ca}), which may also be activated via CICR mechanism upon depolarization, has been reported in cardiac myocytes and, interestingly, the activation of I_{Cl-Ca} is faster than the elevation of indo-1 signal (Sipido et al., 1993). The dissociation between the signals measured with different means may be consistent with the results obtained using MBED. I_{K-Ca} is a good indicator of $[Ca^{2+}]_i$ just beneath the cell membrane and indo-1 signal represents averaged $[Ca^{2+}]_i$ in whole cytoplasm.

The density of BK channels is extremely high in all types of smooth muscle cells examined. For example, the amplitude of macroscopic BK channel current at 0 mV in single cell of the guinea pig urinary bladder would be over 100 nA, if all BK channels open simultaneously. The measured peak I_{K-Ca} upon depolarization to 0 mV was approximately 2 nA, indicating that a very small part of BK channels are activated under the conditions. Based upon the assumption that the I_{K-Ca} activation is due to CICR from superficial SR, it is likely that only a very limited part of plasma membrane area is covered with superficial SR. Existence of superficial SR and its functional importance in Ca buffering and releasing system have been suggested in several smooth muscle cells (Sturek et al., 1992; Chen et al., 1992, Xiong et al., 1992; Etter et *al.*, 1994; van Breeman *et al.*, 1995). As in cardiac muscle (Cheng *et al.*, 1993), Ca^{2+} sparks by Ca^{2+} release from local superficial SR upon depolarization may have important roles in smooth muscle cells, partly via activation of I_{K-Ca}. Ca^{2+} sparks as Ca^{2+} release under resting state have been reported in vascular smooth muscle cells (Nelson *et al.*, 1995). In addition to the superficial SR, there may be SR available for Ca release more deep inside the cell (deep SR) which mainly contributes to activation of contractile proteins. The Ca release from deep SR can be monitored by Ca-indicators (Ganitkevich & Isenberg, 1991, 1992, 1995; Stehno-Bittel & Sturek, 1992). Sequential Ca release from SR in superficial and deep areas might be functional in E–C coupling triggered by an AP in some of these smooth muscles. In quiescent smooth muscles such as coronary artery, however, CICR may not be triggered by Ca^{2+} current upon depolarization but by excess Ca^{2+} influx or by caffeine (Ganitkevich & Isenberg, 1995).

In conclusion, it is assumed in the present study that superficial SR, which may be distributed sparsely (as spots), has important roles in the regulation of action potential shape and membrane excitability via the control of BK channel activity by CICR mechanism in some types of smooth muscle cells.

ACKNOWLEDGEMENTS

This work was supported by a Grant in Aid for Scientific Research from the Japanese Ministry of Education, Science and Culture to Y.I.

REFERENCES

Bauer, V. & Kuriyama, H. (1982). The nature of non-cholinergic, non-adrenergic transmission in longitudinal and circular muscles of the guinea pig ileum. *J. Physiol.* **332**, 375–391.

Benham, C.D. & Bolton, T.B. (1986). Spontaneous transient outward currents in single visceral and vascular smooth muscle cells of the rabbit. *J. Physiol.* **281**, 385–406.

Bolton, T.B. & Beech, D.J. (1992). Smooth muscle potassium channels: their electrophysiology and function. In *Potassium Channel Modulators* (Weston, A.H. & Hamilton, T.C., eds), pp. 144–180. Blackwell Scientific Publications, Oxford.

Bolton,T.B. & Lim, S.P. (1989). Properties of calcium stores and transient outward currents in single smooth muscle cells of rabbit intestine. *J. Physiol.* **409**, 385–401.

van Breemen, C., Chen, Q. & Laher, I. (1995). Superficial buffer barrier function of smooth muscle sarcoplasmic reticulum. *T:PS.* **16**, 98–105.

Chen, Q., Cannell, M. & van Breemen, C. (1992). The superficial buffer barrier in vascular smooth muscle. *Can. J. Physiol. Pharmacol.* **70**, 509–514

Cheng, H., Lederer, W.J. & Cannell, M.B. (1993). Calcium sparks: elementary events underlying excitation – contraction coupling in heart muscle. *Science.* **262,** 740–744.

Etter, E.F., Kuhn, M.A. & Fay, S. (1994). Detection of changes in near-membrane Ca^{2+} concentration using a novel membrane-associated Ca^{2+} indicator. *J. Biol. Chem.* **269,** 10141–10149.

Ganitkevich, V.Y. & Isenberg, G. (1991). Depolarization-mediated intracellular calcium transients in isolated smooth muscle cells of guinea pig urinary bladder. *J. Physiol.* **435,** 187–205.

Ganitkevich, V.Y. & Isenberg, G. (1992). Contribution of Ca^{2+}-induced Ca^{2+} release to the $[Ca^{2+}]i$ transients in myocytes from guinea pig urinary bladder. *J. Physiol.* **458,** 119–137.

Ganitkevich, V.Y. & Isenberg, G. (1995). Efficacy of peak Ca^{2+} currents (I_{Ca}) as trigger of sarcoplasmic reticulum Ca^{2+} release in myocytes from the guinea pig coronary artery. *J. Physiol.* **484,** 287–306.

Ganitkevich, V.Y. & Isenberg, G. (1996). Dissociation of sarcolemmal from grobal cytosolic $[Ca^{2+}]$ in myocytes from guinea pig coronary artery. *J. Physiol.* **490,** 305–318.

Garcia, M.L. & Kaczorowski, G.J. (1992). High conducatnce calcium-activated potassium channels: molecular pharmacology, purification and regulation. In *Potassium Channel modulation.* (Weston, AH. & Hamilton, T.C., eds), pp. 76–109. Blackwell Science Publications, Oxford.

Hakamata, Y., Nakai, J., Takeshima, H. & Imoto, K. (1992). Primary structure and distribution of a novel ryanodine receptor calcium release channel from rabbit brain. *FEBS Lett.* **312,** 229–235.

Iino, M. (1989) Calcium-induced calcium release mechanism in guinea pig taenia caeci. *J. Gen. Physiol.* **94,** 363–383.

Imaizumi, Y., Muraki, K. & Watanabe, M. (1989). Ionic currents in single smooth muscle cells from the ureter of the guinea pig. *J. Physiol.* **411,** 131–159.

Imaizumi, Y., Muraki, K. & Watanabe, M. (1990). Characteristics of transient outward currents in single smooth muscle cells from the ureter of the guinea pig. *J. Physiol.* **427,** 301–324.

Imaizumi, Y., Henmi, S., Uyama, Y., Watanabe, M. & Ohizumi, Y. (1993). Effects of 9-methyl-7-bromoeudistomin D (MBED), a powerful releaser, on smooth muscles of the guinea pig. In *Molecular Basis of Ion Channels and Receptors Involved in Nerve Excitation, Synaptic Transmission and Muscle Contraction. Ann. New York Acad. Sci.* **707,** 546–549.

Kitamura, K., Inoue, Y., Inoue, R., Ohya, Y., Terada, K, Okabe, K. & Kuriyama,H. (1989a). Properties of the inward ionic currents and their regulating agents in smooth muscle cells. *Gen. Physiol. Biophys.* **8,** 289–312.

Kitamura, K., Sakai, T., Kajioka, S. & Kuriyama, H. (1989b). Activation of the Ca dependent K channel by Ca released from the sarcoplasmic reticulum of mammalian smooth muscles. *Biomed. Biochim. Acta* 48, (5–6), S364–369.

Kitamura, K., Xiong, Z., Teramoto, M., Kuriyama, H. (1992). Roles of inositol trisphosphate and protein kinase C in the spontaneous outward current modulated by calcium release in rabbit portal vein. *Pflügers Arch.* **421,** 539–551.

Klöckner, U. & Isenberg, G. (1985). Action potentials and net membrane currents of isolated smooth muscle cells (Urinary bladder of the guinea pig). *Pflügers Arch.* **405,** 329–339.

Kobayashi, J., Ishibashi, M., Nagai, U. & Ohizumi, Y. (1989a). 9-Methyl-7-bromoeudistomin D, a potent inducer of calcium release from sarcoplasmic reticulum of skeletal muscle. *Experientia* **45,** 782–783.

Kobayashi, S., Kitazawa, T., Somlyo, A.V., & Somlyo, A.P. (1989b) Cytosolic heparin inhibits muscarinic and alpha-adrenergic Ca^{2+}-release in smooth muscle. *J. Biol. Chem.* **264**, 17997–18004.

Komori, S. & Bolton, T.B. (1989). Actions of guaninenucleotides and cyclic nucleotides on calcium stores in single patch-clamped smooth muscle cells from rabbit portal vein. *Bri. J. Pharmacol.* **97**, 973–982.

Kume, H. & Kotlikoff, M.I. (1992). Muscarinic inhibition of single KCa channels in smooth muscle cells by a pertussis-sensitive G protein. *Am. J. Physiol.* 261, C1204–C1209.

Mitra, R & Morad, M (1985). Ca^{2+} and Ca^{2+}-activated K^+ currents in mammalian gastric smooth muscle cells. *Science* 229, 269–272.

Nakao, K., Inoue, R., Yamanaka, K. & Kitamura, K. (1986). Actions of quinidine and apamin on after-hyperpolarization of the spike in circular smooth muscle of the guinea pig. *Naunyn-Schmiedebergs' Arch. Pharmacol.* **344**, 508–513.

Nelson, M.T., Cheng, H., Rubart, M., Santana, L.F., Bonev, A.D., Knot, H.J. & Lederer, W.J. (1995). Relaxation of arterial smooth muscle by calcium sparks. *Science.* **270**, 633–637.

Ohya, Y., Terada, K., Kitamura, K. & Kuriyama, H. (1986). Membrane currents recorded from a fragment of rabbit intestinal smooth muscle cell. *Am. J. Physiol.* **251**, C335–C346.

Ohya, Y., Kitamura, K. & Kuriyama, H. (1987). Cellular calcium regulates outward currents in rabbit intestinal smooth muscle cell. *Am. J. Physiol.* **252**, C401–C410.

Sakai, T., Terada, K., Kitamura, K. & Kuriyama, H. (1988). Ryanodine inhibits the Ca-dependent K current after depletion of Ca stored in smooth muscle cells of the rabbit ileal longitudinal muscle. *Br. J. Pharmacol.* **95**, 1089–1100.

Seino, A., Kobayashi, M., Kobayashi, J., Fang, Y-I., Ishibashi, M., Nakamura, H., Momose, K. & Ohizumi, Y. (1991). 9-Methyl-7-bromoeudistomin D, a powerful radio-labelable Ca^{++} releaser having caffeine-like properties, acts on Ca^{++}-induced Ca^{++} release channels of sarcoplasmic reticulum. *J. Pharmacol. Exp. Therap.* **256**, 861–867.

Sipido, K., R., Callewaert, G. & Carmeliet, E. (1993). $[Ca^{2+}]_i$ transients and $[Ca^{2+}]_i$-dependent chloride current in single purkinje cells from rabbit heart. *J. Physiol.* **468**, 641–667.

Sorrentino, V. & Volpe, P. (1993). Ryanodine receptors: how many, where and why? *Trends Pharmacol. Sci.* **14**, 98–103.

Stehno-Bittel, L. & Sturek, M. (1992). Spontaneous sarcoplasmic reticulum calcium release and extrusion from bovine, not porcine, coronary artery smooth muscle. *J. Physiol.* 451, 49–78.

Sturek, M., Kunda, K. & Hu, Q. (1992). Sarcoplasmic reticulum buffering of myoplasmic calcium in bovine coronary artery smooth muscle. *J. Physiol.* **451**, 25–48.

Suzuki, M., Muraki, K., Imaizumi, Y. & Watanabe, M. (1992). Cyclopiazonic acid, an inhibitor of sarcoplasmic reticulum Ca^{2+}-pump, reduces Ca^{2+}-dependent K^+ current in smooth muscle cells. *Br. J. Pharmacol.* **107**, 134–140.

Takeda, M., Imaizumi, Y. & Watanabe, M. (1991). Effects of noradrenaline and heparin on outward current in single smooth muscle cells of the guinea pig vas deferens. *Eur. J. Pharmacol.* **193**, 375–378.

Uyama, Y., Imaizumi, Y. & Watanabe, M. (1992). Effects of cyclopiazonic acid, a novel Ca^{2+}-ATPase inhibitor, on contractile responses in skinned ileal smooth muscle. *Br. J. Pharmacol.* **106**, 208–214.

Uyama, Y., Imaizumi, Y. & Watanabe, M. (1993). Cyclopiazonic acid, an inhibitor of Ca^{2+}-ATPase in sarcoplasmic reticulum, increases excitability in ileal smooth muscle. *Br. J. Pharmacol.* **110**, 565–572.

Xiong, Z., Kitamura, K. & Kuriyama, H. (1992). Evidence for contribution of Ca^{2+} storage sites on unitary K^+ channel currents in inside-out membrane of rabbit portal vein. *Pflügers Arch.* **420**, 112–114.

Xu, L., Lai, A., Cohn, A., Etter, E., Guerrero, A., Fay, F.S. & Meissner, G. (1994). Evidence for a Ca^{2+}-gated ryanodine-sensitive Ca^{2+} release channel in visceral smooth muscle. *Proc. Natl Acad. Sci. USA.* **91**, 3294–3298.

Yamamoto, Y., Hu, S.L. & Kao, C.Y. (1989). Outward current in single smooth muscle muscle cells of the guinea pig taenia coli. *J. Gen. Physiol.* **93**, 551–564.

Zholos, A. V., Baisan, L. V. & Shuba, M. F. (1992). Some properties of $Ca^{(2+)}$-induced Ca^{2+} release mechanism in single visceral smooth muscle cell of the guinea pig. *J. Physiol.* **457**, 1–25.

30

Intracellular Ca²⁺ Release: A Basis for Electrical Pacemaking in Lymphatic Smooth Muscle

D. F. VAN HELDEN
P-Y. VON DER WEID
M. J. CROWE

Faculty of Medicine and Health Sciences,
University of Newcastle,
Callaghan, Australia

SUMMARY

Many lymphatic vessels act like 'primitive' hearts to actively propel lymph. Pumping occurs when action potential-induced phasic constrictions of the muscle transiently reduce vessel volume causing a net forward movement of lymph through frequently occurring unidirectional valves. Studies on small lymphatic vessels that occur in the mesentery of the guinea pig have provided insight into the pacemaker mechanism underlying the generation of action potentials and thus constrictions. Pacemaking occurs through depolarizing currents, termed spontaneous transient inward currents (STICs), generated by synchronized 'quantal' release of an intracellular activator which is likely to be Ca²⁺ released from inositol 1,4,5-trisphosphate (InsP₃) receptor- operated intracellular stores. This pacemaker mechanism provides an elegant control system. Factors which are known to increase intracellular concentration of InsP₃ and/or [Ca²⁺]ᵢ (e.g. noradrenaline, stretch) increase the pumping rate whereas factors known to decrease InsP₃ and/or [Ca²⁺]ᵢ (e.g. endothelial-derived nitric oxide, isoprenaline) reduce pumping rate. We suggest that this pacemaker mechanism is not a unique property of lymphatic smooth muscle but underlies rhythmic spontaneous electrical activity in many other cell types.

SMOOTH MUSCLE EXCITATION
ISBN 0-12-112360-X

ROLE OF LYMPHATICS

Lymphatic vessels are ubiquitous throughout most of the body at densities similar to that of blood vessels. While they are absent in the brain there is evidence for channels which allow drainage from the central nervous system into the lymphatic system (Casley-Smith, 1983; Castenholz et al., 1991). The lymphatic circulation is essential to life and subserves many roles. A key role of the lymphatics is to maintain tissue fluid homeostasis through removing proteins, cell debris and other particles with the accompanying fluid which accumulates in the interstitium. The lymphatic circulation is fundamental in immunity providing the linking pathway for circulation of immune competent cells and transporting antigenic substances to lymphoid tissues (e.g. the lymph nodes). Furthermore, this system is essential in wound healing and in combating local infections (Yoffey & Courtice, 1970). Interestingly, the lymphatics provide the pathway by which toxins, including those injected through venomous bites, are transported from the interstitium to the circulation. It is the belated recognition of this fact which has led to marked changes in first aid procedures related to life-threatening evenomation with efforts now made to prevent lymph flow but not blood flow.

Tissue fluid enters the lymphatic system through the initial lymphatics which are blind-ended tubes comprised of endothelial cells without smooth muscle. This can occur because adjacent endothelial cells are frequently linked by open junctions (Casley-Smith, 1972) through which particulate matter including very large particles (e.g. 150 nm diameter), together with the interstitial fluid in which the particles lie, can enter the vessel. Compression of the initial lymphatic vessels closes the endothelial junctions and propels lymph forward into the collecting lymphatics where luminal unidirectional valves (also formed by endothelial cells) are present at close spacing. The result of this process is collection and net propulsion of lymph fluid containing the particulate matter which, if left in the interstitium, would lead to insurmountable osmotic imbalance (see Casley-Smith, 1983).

The collecting lymphatic vessels differ from the initial lymphatics in that most have smooth muscle in their outer walls (except within skeletal muscle beds where external compression can propel lymph; see Aukland & Reed, 1993). Like small blood vessels, the wall of these vessels has an intima, media and adventitia, respectively, comprised of a monolayer of endothelial cells, a thin layer of smooth muscle cells and a layer of connective tissue containing the nerves which innervate the smooth muscle (Yoffey & Courtice, 1970). Only recently has it been accepted that the phasic constrictions of the smooth muscle is a primary mechanism by which lymph is propelled centrally. This contractile behaviour is remarkably heart-like in that the phasic constrictions of the smooth muscle transiently compress the chambers, formed by adjacent valves, propelling lymph in a pulsatile manner. Furthermore, as intrinsic pumping of the smooth muscle occurs in the walls of a great number of vessel chambers, in series and in parallel, the intrinsic lymphatic pump is both robust and can achieve substantial pressures (>40 mmHg; Werner, 1965).

Factors which affect pacemaker rate are distension consequent to vessel filling (Florey, 1927a,b; Smith, 1949), modulatory factors released from the endothelium (Yokoyama & Ohhashi, 1993; Crowe et al., 1994; Reeder et al., 1994), circulating hormones and humoral substances (Florey, 1927a,b; Mawhinney & Roddie, 1973; McHale & Roddie, 1983), arachidonate metabolites (Johnston & Gordon, 1981; Johnston & Feuer, 1983) and nerves (McHale et al., 1980, 1991; Allen et al., 1988). Lymphatic innervation of the smooth muscle involves sympathetic, parasympathetic and sensory nerves. All nerves are present at low density compared with the innervation of adjacent blood vessels (Todd & Bernard, 1973; Alessandrini et al., 1981; Ohhashi et al., 1982; Guarna et al., 1991; Wang et al., 1994). As for the vasculature, the nerves exhibit specific peptides which can be used for their identification with the repertoire of peptides often similar to that of the innervation to adjacent blood vessels. For example, guinea pig or rat mesenteric lymphatics have sympathetic nerves which contain neuropeptide Y (NPY) and sensory nerves with both substance P and calcitonin gene related peptide (Guarna et al., 1991; Wang et al., 1994), a repertoire of peptides also found in the corresponding innervation of the mesenteric arteries/arterioles and veins. Functional information on the role of these different nerve types has so far only been provided for the sympathetic nerves which are excitatory causing an increase in the frequency of phasic constrictions (McHale et al., 1980, 1991).

THE LYMPHANGION

The studies of Horstmann (1952, 1959) and Mislin (1972, 1983) on the collecting vessels of the guinea pig mesentery (the lacteals) led Mislin to adopt the term 'lymphangion' to define the smallest functional unit of the intrinsic lymphatic pump. In essence, a lymphangion is defined to be a single chamber bounded by two adjacent valves (see Figure 1) with smooth muscle in the vessel wall. In the guinea pig preparation, individual chambers sometimes actively pump independently from adjacent chambers. Such behaviour is due to total or partial discontinuities in the syncytial smooth muscle cells in the region of valves (Horstmann, 1952, 1959; Crowe & van Helden, 1992). However, contractile activity of adjacent lymphangions can be coordinated by phasic constrictions propelling the contents of one chamber unidirectionally with the resulting distension activating downstream lymphangions (Horstmann, 1952, 1959). While this description of the

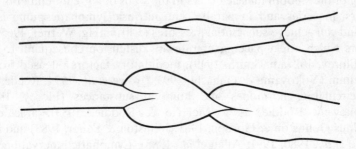

Figure 1 Lymphatic vessels in the guinea pig mesentery (ileal region). Vessels are composed of multiple chambers (lymphangions) each separated by unidirectional valves. These chambers show great variation in shape and size. The largest diameter of the central 'heart' in the lower vessel is 234 μm.

contractile behaviour of lymphangions often applies to the guinea pig lacteals, larger vessels such as bovine mesenteric lymphatics generally exhibit approximately synchronous constrictions involving groups of two or more adjacent chambers. Thus, the term lymphangion probably needs a broadened description to refer to one or a group of chambers. The important message is that lymphatic smooth muscle functions in discrete units comprised of one or more chambers. Each lymphangion or groups of lymphangions act like 'primitive' hearts to pump lymph. As can readily be demonstrated, increased fluid load causes an increase in the frequency of constrictions (Florey, 1927a, b; Smith, 1949; Hall *et al.*, 1965). However, when the frequency becomes too high, vessel filling is compromised and the stroke volume of the lymphangion is diminished (e.g. see McGeown *et al.*, 1987; van Helden *et al.*, 1995).

PACEMAKER POTENTIALS

The pacemaker mechanisms underlying lymphatic pumping should have as their output an electrical event (pacemaker potential) which generates each action potential/phasic constriction of a lymphangion. Studies on large lymphatic vessels (bovine mesenteric lymphatics) have demonstrated that the pacemaker mechanisms underlying lymphatic constrictions relate to a slow depolarization leading to generation of action potentials, this process repeating (Kirkpatrick & McHale, 1977; Ward *et al.*, 1991). Such a potential is characteristic of voltage-dependent channel mechanisms as occur in the heart. However, detailed studies on this pacemaker potential have been hampered by the electrical characteristics of the syncytial smooth muscle present within lymphangions. Pacemaker activity in large vessels is difficult to study because of uncertainties in the electrical distance of the pacemaker cells from the site at which recordings are made in the smooth muscle. Thus, the pacemaker potential which generates each action potential cannot readily be distinguished from the potential change which underlies propagation of the action potential itself. A method to overcome this problem is to cut vessels into electrically short segments, as has been used to advantage for other purposes in studies of arteriolar (Hirst & Neild, 1978) and venous (van Helden, 1988 a,b) smooth muscle.

The circularly-oriented smooth muscle in lymphangions has the passive electrical properties of a one-dimensional cable. When small vessels of diameter of <250 μm are cut into short lengths of <300 μm, the smooth muscle behaves as if it was approximately isopotential with the simplified equivalent circuit of a resistor and capacitor in parallel. Such segments respond to injection of a constant current with an exponential voltage response (van Helden, 1993). The consequence of this vessel-sculpting procedure is that electrical events generated anywhere within the smooth muscle cause similar potential changes in all cells within the syncytium of electrically coupled cells (van Helden, 1991). Therefore, pacemaker potentials, if present, should be directly measurable when recording from any of the smooth muscle cells within a short segment which exhibits spontaneous action potentials/phasic constrictions.

The results of recording smooth muscle membrane potential in a spontaneously active segment of guinea pig mesenteric lymphatic vessel are shown in Figure 2. This segment was considered to be electrically short as the voltage transient resulting from application of a current pulse was exponential (not shown). The important finding exhibited in Figure 2 is the occurrence of spontaneous transient depolarizations (STDs) which were either subthreshold or of sufficient amplitude, either individually or through summation, to generate an action potential. While action potentials were of similar amplitude and each always caused a phasic constriction, STDs were of variable amplitude and did not themselves cause constriction. To date, we have recorded from more than 300 cut segments and have recorded STDs in about 95% of these. Those segments that showed no STD activity did not exhibit spontaneous constrictions. Spontaneous constrictions were observed in some 20% of the segments showing STDs. These exhibited large STDs at moderate to high frequency, some of which either directly or through summation exceeded the threshold potential for generation of an action potential (moving the membrane potential positive to about −50 mV). STDs in the other segments were individually too small and occurred at low frequencies so that action potential threshold could not be reached. Where tested, action potentials could always be generated by current injection through the microelectrode. Taken together, these findings support the premise that STDs are the pacemaker potentials underlying generation of

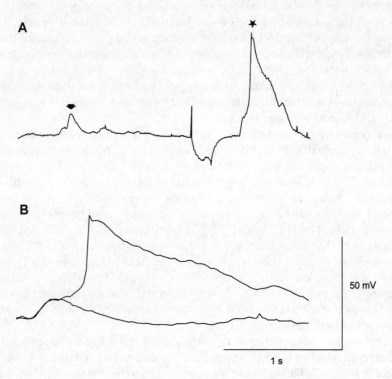

Figure 2 STDs underlie generation of action potentials. A, Recording of the membrane potential from the smooth muscle of a lymphatic segment. The record exhibits STDs (e.g. arrow) and an action potential (asterisk). The downward deflection was due to injection of a current pulse (0.1 nA). B, The action potential and large STD of A (marked by asterisk and arrow respectively) have been superimposed demonstrating that STDs underlie generation of action potentials. The resting potential of the segment was −63 mV.

action potentials and hence spontaneous constrictions in guinea pig mesenteric lymphatic vessel segments.

Some lymphangions in intact guinea pig mesenteric lymphatics are particularly small (length <500 μm; diameter <200 μm). Like short segments, small lymphangions should have smooth muscle which is electrically short (although not necessarily isopotential) allowing both action potentials and underlying pacemaker potentials to be recorded. Membrane potential was recorded from small lymphangions in intact lymphatic vessels before, during and after spontaneous constrictions. Only lymphangions which constricted independently of adjacent chambers were chosen. These chambers constricted uniformly indicating that the smooth muscle behaved as if it was reasonably isopotential. As for isolated segments such lymphangions exhibited STDs and action potentials which generated phasic constrictions. The initial phase of the action potential (the foot) had the same time course as the rising phase of STDs consistent with the premise that STDs underlie pacemaking in small lymphangions (see Figure 3A and also Figure 3; van Helden, 1993). The likelihood that this mechanism also underlies pacemaking in large lymphatics is considered below.

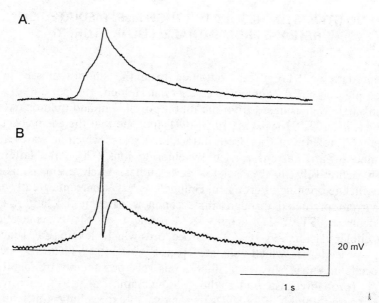

Figure 3 Comparison of action potentials recorded in a small (A) and large (B) lymphangion. Action potentials recorded in the smooth muscle of a small and large lymphatic vessel (diameter approximately 200 μm and 500 μm; resting membrane potentials −55 mV and −65 mV respectively). The STD-like bump at the foot of the action potential in A should be compared with the slow depolarization in B.

PROPERTIES OF THE PACEMAKER POTENTIALS (STDs) AND THEIR UNDERLYING CURRENTS (STICs)

STDs are likely to be generated within lymphatic smooth muscle as they occur in denervated or de-endothelialized vessels (van Helden, 1993). Such activity is not unique to lymphatic smooth muscle and occurs more generally. For example, myogenic depolarizing activity was reported in the rabbit portal vein (Holman et al., 1968) and in the guinea pig mesenteric vein (Suzuki, 1981) although the origin of the STDs was not determined. Subsequently, detailed studies on STDs were made in short segments of mesenteric vein where STDs and the underlying spontaneous transient inward currents (STICs) were investigated in detail (van Helden, 1991). STICs have also been observed in enzymatically isolated smooth muscle cells from the rabbit portal vein and rabbit pulmonary artery using the perforated patch recording method (Wang *et al.*, 1992; Hogg *et al.*, 1993).

DO STICs/STDs RESULT THROUGH InsP₃-MEDIATED Ca²⁺ RELEASE FROM INTRACELLULAR STORES?

Present data on STICs/STDs obtained from the smooth muscle in both guinea pig veins and lymphatic vessels (van Helden, 1989a,b,c, 1991, 1993) and in single cells isolated from the rabbit portal vein and pulmonary artery (Wang *et al.*, 1992; Hogg *et al.*, 1993, 1994) indicate that the events occur due to 'quantal' release of Ca^{2+} from intracellular stores which activates a Ca^{2+}-activated inward current carried by chloride ions (Cl_{Ca}); the latter were shown definitively in the isolated cell studies. Each event is likely to represent the opening of groups of channels as larger currents greatly exceed the current predicted through single channels of even the largest known conductances. STIC/STD activity is dependent on the concentration of intracellular calcium ions $[Ca^{2+}]_i$ as procedures which elevate $[Ca^{2+}]_i$ increase, while procedures which chelate $[Ca^{2+}]_i$ inhibit, STIC/STD activity. Extracellular entry of Ca^{2+} facilitates this role presumably by maintaining $[Ca^{2+}]_i$ (probably just under the plasmalemma) at a sufficiently high concentration. Inhibition of STDs by removal of extracellular Ca^{2+} can occur without depletion of the Ca^{2+} stores as store release can be stimulated by agonists such as noradrenaline well after inhibition of STIC/STD activity through exposure to Ca^{2+} free or Ca^{2+} ion substituted solutions.

STIC/STD activity is enhanced by stimulation of receptors such as α_1-adrenoceptors which are known to mobilize InsP₃ in other smooth muscles (Somlyo *et al.*, 1985; Hashimoto *et al.*, 1986) and also in smooth muscle of the guinea pig mesenteric vein (S. Woolridge, S. Bunn & D.F.v.H., unpublished observations). InsP₃ releases stored Ca^{2+} by directly opening InsP₃ receptors present in the membrane of the Ca^{2+} stores, a process which is enhanced by the positive feedback effect of Ca^{2+}-induced Ca^{2+} release (Berridge, 1993). Confirmation of a direct role of Ca^{2+} release through InsP₃ receptors comes from experiments with caffeine, which at high concentrations (>5 mM) blocks STICs/STDs. As well as its role in stimulating ryanodine receptors, caffeine is known to block release of Ca^{2+} through InsP₃ receptors (Parker & Ivorra, 1991; Berridge, 1993). Taken together, the findings are consistent with the hypothesis that STICs/STDs result from quantal release of Ca^{2+} through activation of one or more InsP$_3$ receptor channels with the released Ca²⁺ opening groups of calcium-activated chloride channels. The release sites must be located very near the membrane and alter [Ca²⁺]$_i$ at very localized regions as STICs/STDs never directly cause constriction and the rise phase of STICs measured in single cells is relatively rapid (30 ms; Hogg et al., 1993). Further to this, we have undertaken studies to monitor lymphatic smooth muscle Ca²⁺ levels using the confocal microscope. While readily detecting [Ca²⁺]$_i$ changes associated with action potentials within smooth muscle cells in intact vessels, we have only rarely observed localized STD related [Ca²⁺]$_i$ changes (M.J.C. & D.F.v.H., unpublished observations). Difficulty to observe changes in [Ca²⁺]$_i$ is consistent with the now growing body of evidence that Ca²⁺ release caused by various stimulatory substances occurs within localized regions near the smooth muscle plasma membrane (e.g. see Stehno-Bittel & Sturek, 1992; Yamaguchi et al., 1995; van Breemen, 1995). These regions could be very localized indeed, as would be the case if release occurs from the junctional sarcoplasmic reticulum which can be as close as 12–18 nm from the plasma membrane (Somlyo & Somlyo, 1991).

SPONTANEOUS TRANSIENT OUTWARD CURRENTS (STOCs) ANALOGY TO STICs

Spontaneous transient outward currents (STOCs), as first reported in single smooth muscle cells by Benham & Bolton (1986), have been observed in many enzymatically isolated smooth muscle cells. The mechanism underlying generation of STICs/STDs appears to be entirely analogous to that for STOCs, the primary difference being that STOCs involve opening Ca²⁺-activated potassium (K$_{Ca}$) channels. Detailed studies on STOCs indicate that these events arise through quantal release of Ca²⁺ from InsP$_3$-sensitive stores with the activity dependent on [Ca²⁺]$_i$, [Ca²⁺]$_o$ and InsP$_3$ (Benham and Bolton, 1986; Ohya et al., 1987; Komori & Bolton, 1991). As for STICs, STOCs must involve very localized release of Ca²⁺ as direct visualisation of localized changes of [Ca²⁺]$_i$ corresponding to STOCs has yet to be made. It is curious that STOCs, while seen in many enzymatically isolated smooth muscle cells, are rarely manifest in intact tissues. It may be that the enzyme treatment and/or perfusion associated with the whole cell or perforated patch recording procedures either expose K$_{Ca}$ channels or enhance their sensitivity (Wang et al., 1992) to the localized Ca²⁺ release while diminishing the viability, or sensitivity of Cl$_{Ca}$ channels. Support for this premise comes from studies on smooth muscle of the rabbit portal vein where STD type activity but not spontaneous transient hyperpolarizations were observed in intracellular voltage recordings from intact vessels (Holman et al., 1968). By comparison, only STOCs were recorded in single enzymatically isolated cells from this preparation when recordings were made using the whole-cell recording technique (Ohya et al., 1988; Beech & Bolton, 1989; Hume & Leblanc, 1989). Hume & Leblanc (1989) in studies on smooth muscle cells isolated from the rabbit portal vein found that STOC activity was not present but developed after achieving whole-cell voltage clamp, yet, both STICs and STOCs were recorded when the perforated-patch method was utilized (Wang et al., 1992; Hogg et al., 1993). Importantly, in some cases a quantal event was observed to activate an outward followed by inward current indicating that K_{Ca} and Cl_{Ca} channels lie in close proximity (Hogg et al., 1993).

While normally recorded in intact smooth muscle, STOC-related hyperpolarizations have been measured through microelectrode recording in an intact longitudinal smooth muscle of the guinea pig ileum in response to ACh (Cousins et al., 1995). Nondissociated neurones also exhibit a STOC-like activity termed spontaneous miniature outward currents (SMOCs) as reported in bullfrog ganglia cells with recordings made under two electrode voltage clamp (Adams et al., 1985). Regardless of their physiological relevance, detailed investigations on STOCs have given great insight into the intracellular mechanisms which underlie this activity. Most importantly, the fact that STICs appear to show the same underlying mechanism makes information obtained on STOCs directly relevant to understanding STICs.

PULSATILE Ca²⁺ RELEASE IN OTHER TISSUES

Activity involving 'pulsatile' (quantal) release of Ca^{2+} from intracellular stores has been reported in a number of tissues (for review see Berridge, 1993). Invertebrate photoreceptors exhibit an electrical depolarizing activity termed 'bumps' which can occur spontaneously but normally occurs in response to light, with a single photon believed to activate a single bump. Events occur through activation of intracellular messengers (Lillywhite, 1977), each event opening groups of channels (Wong, 1978). These events, although generally of shorter duration, are similar in appearance to STDs. Intracellular release of Ca^{2+} from $InsP_3$ receptor-operated stores has been implicated as underlying these bumps (Fein et al., 1984; Minke & Selinger, 1992).

Xenopus oocytes and secretory cells such as pancreatic acinar cells also exhibit spontaneous inward currents caused by the opening of groups of Cl_{Ca} channels through localized release of Ca^{2+} from $InsP_3$ receptor-operated stores (Parker & Miledi, 1986; Wakui et al., 1989). Indeed, studies on Xenopus oocytes have now provided direct visualization of quantal Ca^{2+} release viewed as spontaneous localized increases ('quantal puffs') of $[Ca^{2+}]_i$ (Parker & Yao, 1991; Yao et al., 1995). This breakthrough has resulted through both experimental technique, (e.g. injection of a poorly metabolized $InsP_3$ analogue) and through morphological advantages. For example, oocytes have Ca^{2+} release sites which occur some $5\,\mu m$ from the plasma membrane with activation of $InsP_3$ receptors causing an increase in $[Ca^{2+}]_i$ in a substantial localized volume.

Ca²⁺ WAVES AND THEIR PROPAGATION

Direct visualization of cells undergoing spontaneous calcium release was first made on hepatocytes (Woods *et al.*, 1986) where periodic oscillatory increases in $[Ca^{2+}]_i$ were observed. This activity has subsequently been directly visualized in many cell systems including endothelial cells (Hallam *et al.*, 1988), secretory cells (Petersen *et al.*, 1991) and oocytes (Lechleiter *et al.*, 1991; Parker & Yao, 1991).

Xenopus oocytes provide an excellent system to study mechanisms underlying the generation and propagation of Ca^{2+} waves. Current evidence indicates that increases in intracellular $InsP_3$ levels in the presence of $[Ca^{2+}]_i$ (or *vice versa*) activate localized quantal release of Ca^{2+} which, under sufficient stimulation, generate spiralling Ca^{2+} waves within the oocyte (Lechleiter *et al.*, 1991; Parker & Yao, 1991; Yao & Parker, 1994). Both quantal release and calcium waves are all or none events with both likely to depend on an interplay between $[Ca^{2+}]_i$ and $[InsP_3]_i$ in opening $InsP_3$ receptors and releasing stored Ca^{2+} into the cytosol. Critical to this process is the positive feedback caused by the release of Ca^{2+}, a phenomenon which can happen in both $InsP_3$ or ryanodine receptor operated stores and is generally referred to as Ca^{2+}-induced Ca^{2+} release. While there is positive reinforcement of the release process at low $[Ca^{2+}]_i$, inactivation occurs at high local or cytoplasmic $[Ca^{2+}]_i$ (Iino, 1990; Finch *et al.*, 1991; Bezprozvanny *et al.*, 1991; Iino & Endo, 1992; Yao *et al.*, 1995). Thus, the build-up of cytosolic Ca^{2+} inhibits further release with removal of the cytosolic Ca^{2+} occurring through reuptake into Ca^{2+} stores or active extrusion out of the cell (Berridge, 1993).

DO PROPAGATING Ca²⁺ WAVES UNDERLIE PACEMAKING IN LARGE LYMPHANGIONS ?

Our studies have shown that spontaneous action potentials are generated by STDs in lymphatic smooth muscle of cut segments or small lymphangions. Both these systems have a common property, namely the input resistance of the syncytium of smooth muscle cells is relatively high (range 20–100 MΩ). If it is assumed that a 20 mV STD is required to generate an action potential then the underlying steady-state current required to achieve this would be in the order of 0.25 to 1 nA. Voltage clamp measurements of STICs recorded in venous segments from guinea pig mesentery held near −60 mV showed a spectrum of current amplitudes typically less than 0.3 nA, although in a few cases larger STICs up to 0.9 nA were recorded (van Helden, 1991). Studies on enzymatically isolated rabbit portal vein smooth muscle cells demonstrated that STICs in single cells exhibited an amplitude range at −50 mV of about 0.002 to 0.2 nA (typical range 0.01–0.03 nA; Wang *et al.*, 1992). The larger maximum size of STICs in intact venous segments may reflect a tissue difference. However, an alternative explanation is that in intact tissues synchronized release of Ca^{2+} occurs involving groups of electrically coupled smooth muscle cells.

The basis for pacemaking in large lymphangions which should have lower input resistances is yet to be confirmed. If STICs underlie such pacemaking then they could only do so through a mechanism which generated substantial inward current (e.g. synchronization of STIC activity both within and across adjacent cells). A mechanism by which this could be achieved is through propagating Ca^{2+} waves. The conduction velocity of such waves recorded in oocytes or secretory cells has been shown to range between 3–95 μm s^{-1} (see Lechleiter *et al.*, 1991; Nathanson *et al.*, 1992; Stricker et al, 1992). Furthermore, there is ample evidence of propagation of calcium waves across the gap junctions of various cell syncytia (Charles *et al.*, 1991; Boitano *et al.*, 1992). Therefore synchronization of STD activity could occur through propagation of a Ca^{2+} wave to synchronously activate STICs both within a single cell and between a local group of electrically coupled smooth muscle cells. The conduction velocity range of Ca^{2+} waves could produce kinetics consistent with the time course of large STICs recorded in syncytial smooth muscle cells (van Helden, 1991). However, while this proposal is interesting, the fact that we rarely observed calcium waves in lymphatic smooth muscle (M.J.C. & D.F.v.H., unpublished observations) indicates that: (1) the cytosolic $[Ca^{2+}]_i$ is either much lower than the $[Ca^{2+}]_i$ change caused by an action potential which is readily observed by confocal microscopy (see above); (2) the Ca^{2+} wave occurs in a restricted space just under the plasmalemma as directly demonstrated in oocytes (Yao *et al.*, 1995) but markedly scaled down so that it is difficult to visualize the Ca^{2+} wave; or (3) an alternative synchronizing mechanism operates. While we cannot be absolutely certain on the mechanism by which synchronization may occur there is evidence that it does. For example, we have observed synchronization underlying STD activity in lymphatic smooth muscle in response to agonist-induced enhancement of STDs (van Helden & Bull, 1995). Such synchronization occurred periodically – there was a summation of STD activity followed by a quiet period which repeated cyclically. Synchronization of STDs has also been observed in intact veins under continued nerve stimulation (D.F.v.H., unpublished observations) and also in veins in response to distension (Figure 4).

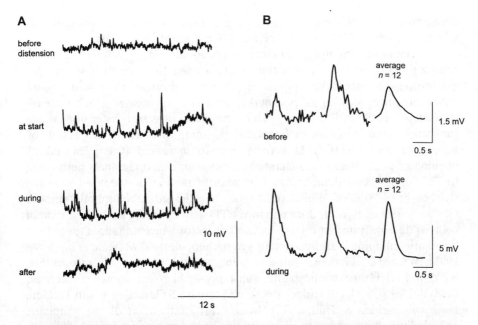

Figure 4 Recordings of membrane potential during local distension of a small vein. A, Continuous recording sampled before distension, with the onset of distension, during maximal and after maximal distension (downward sequence). B, Sample STDs and the average of 12 STDs (rightmost records) recorded before and during maximal distension. The maximal distension was estimated to be 5% of the vessel diameter (diameter 140 μm). The resting membrane potential during the recording varied between −61 and −57 mV.

Insight into a basis for synchronization comes from the rapidly increasing literature on cells which exhibit Ca²⁺ oscillations (for review see Berridge, 1993). Probably the most direct analogy comes from studies on oocytes which have provided direct evidence that quantally released Ca²⁺ from InsP₃ stores markedly enhances the probability of release from adjacent stores when they are nearby (<about 2 μm; Yao *et al.*, 1995). These authors also showed that the probability of release at any fixed site was approximately random except at intervals less than a few seconds where there was a relative refractory period. The tendency for STDs to synchronize in an approximately cyclical manner fit these observations. Thus, it can be postulated for lymphatic smooth muscle that quantal release enhances the probability of adjacent quantal release (namely, gradual depolarization) until a threshold is reached at which there is an explosive increase in the number of synchronized events (a large depolarization generating action potentials). The subsequent refractory period terminates the process and so the cycle continues. This process may explain pacemaking in large lymphatic vessels where a slow

depolarization is observed to precede generation of each action potential (Kirkpatrick & McHale, 1977; McHale, 1990; see also Figure 3B).

A mechanism involving calcium-induced calcium release from $InsP_3$ receptor operated Ca^{2+} stores represents a compelling control system for generation of pacemaker potentials. Such a mechanism would ensure enhancement or slowing of pacemaker activity by processes which increase or decrease $InsP_3$ and/or $[Ca^{2+}]_i$. Thus, the effect of vessel distension, which can cause large increases in lymphatic pumping, may exert this action by generating more STIC/STD activity due to increased $[Ca^{2+}]_i$ caused by opening of stretch-activated channels. Stretch-activated channels permeable to Ca^{2+} have been demonstrated in smooth muscle of the toad stomach (Kirber *et al.*, 1988). While yet to be investigated in lymphatic smooth muscle, vessel distension does enhance STD activity in the smooth muscle of veins as demonstrated in Figure 4. Another factor which enhances the rate of lymphatic pumping is stimulation of sympathetic nerves (McHale *et al.*, 1980, 1991). We have found that noradrenaline and the putative co-transmitters, NPY and adenosine triphosphate, substances which are known to increase $InsP_3$ and/or $[Ca^{2+}]_i$ (Berridge, 1993), all increase STD activity (van Helden, 1993; van Helden & Bull, 1995). In contrast, stimulation of the lymphatic endothelium slows the rate of pumping (Yokoyama & Ohhashi, 1993), an effect which is in part due to direct inhibition of STDs possibly owing to a decrease in $[Ca^{2+}]_i$ (Crowe *et al.*, 1994).

CONCLUSION

This review has addressed the proposal that electrical pacemaking in lymphatic smooth muscle occurs through intracellular release of an activator substance. Present data indicates that this activator is Ca^{2+} released through $InsP_3$ receptors on intracellular Ca^{2+} stores located close to the plasma membrane. The ability of such a mechanism to synchronize and self-inhibit its activity within and across coupled cells provides a powerful current source with repetitive cyclical behaviour characteristic of an electrical pacemaker. It is proposed that this mechanism not only underlies pacemaking in lymphatic vessels but operates in many other cells.

REFERENCES

Adams, P.R., Brown, D.A., Constanti, A., Clark, R.B. & Satin, L. (1985). Calcium-activated potassium channels in bullfrog sympathetic ganglion cells. In *Calcium in Biological Systems* (Rubin, R.P., Weiss, G.B. & Putney, J.W. eds), pp. 181–191.

Plenum Publishing Corporation, New York.

Aleessandrini, C., Gerli, R., Sachhi, G., Ibba, L., Pucci, A.M. & Fruschelli, C. (1981). Cholinergic and adrenergic innervation of mesenterial lymph vessels in guinea pig. *Lymphology* 14, 1–6.

Allen, J.M., McCarron, J.G., McHale, N.G. & Thornbury, K.D. (1988). Release of [³H]-noradrenaline from the sympathetic nerves to bovine mesenteric lymphatic vessels and its modification by alpha-agonists and antagonists. *Br. J. Pharmacol.* 94, 823–833.

Aukland, K. & Reed, R.K. (1993). Interstitial-lymphatic mechanisms in the control of extracellular fluid volume. *Physiol. Rev.* 73, 1–78.

Beech, D.J. & Bolton, T.B. (1989). Two components of potassium current activated by depolarization of single smooth muscle cells from the rabbit portal vein. *J. Physiol. (London)* 418, 293–309.

Benham, C.D. & Bolton, T. B. (1986). Spontaneous transient outward currents in single visceral and vascular smooth muscle cells of the rabbit. *J. Physiol. (London)* 381, 385–406.

Berridge, M.J. (1993). Inositol trisphosphate and calcium signalling. *Nature.* 361, 315–325.

Bezprozvanny, I., Watras, J. & Ehrlich, B.E. (1991). Bell-shaped calcium-response curves of Ins(1,4,5)P3- and calcium-gated channels from endoplasmic reticulum of cerebellum. *Nature.* 351, 751–754.

Boitano, S., Dirksen, E.R. & Sanderson, M.J. (1992). Intercellular propagation of calcium waves mediated by inositol trisphosphate. *Science.* 258, 292–295.

van Breemen, C. (1995). Superficial buffer barrier function of smooth muscle sarcoplasmic reticulum. *TIPS.* 16, 98–105..

Casley-Smith, J R. (1972). The role of the endothelial intercellular junctions in the functioning of the initial lymphatics. *Angiologica* 9, 106–131.

Casley-Smith, J R. (1983). The structure and functioning of blood vessels, interstitial tissues and lymphatics . In *Lymphangiology* (Foldi, M. & Casley-Smith, J.R., eds). pp. 27–164. F.K. Schattauer Verlag, Stuttgart.

Castenholz, A., Hauck, G. & Rettburg, U. (1991). Light and electron microscopy of the structural organization of the tissue-lymphatic fluid drainage system in the mesentery: an experimental study. *Lymphology* 24, 82–92.

Charles, A.C., Merrill, J.E., Dirksen, E.R. & Sanderson, M. J. (1991). Intercellular signaling in glial cells: calcium waves and oscillations in response to mechanical stimulation and glutamate. *Neuron* 6, 983–992.

Cousins, H.M., Edwards, F.R. & Hirst, G.D.S. (1995). Neurally released and applied acetylcholine on longitudinal muscle of the guinea pig ileum. *Neuroscience* 65, 193–207.

Crowe, M.J. & van Helden, D.F. (1992). Lymphatic chambers in the guinea pig mesentery. *Proc. Aust. Physiol. Pharmacol. Soc.* 23, 207P.

Crowe, M.J., von der Weid, P.-Y. & van Helden, D.F. (1994). Endothelium-dependent modulation of lymphatic pumping in the guinea pig mesentery. *Proc. Aust. Physiol. Pharmacol. Soc.* 25, 146P.

Fein, A., Payne, R., Corson, D.W., Berridge, M.J. & Irvine, R. F. (1984). Photoreceptor excitation and adaptation by inositol 1,4,5-trisphosphate. *Nature.* 311, 157–160.

Finch, E.A., Turner, T.J. & Goldin, S.M. (1991). Calcium as a coagonist of inositol 1,4,5-trisphosphate-induced calcium release. *Science* 254, 443– 446.

Florey, H.W. (1927a). Observations on the contractility of lacteals. Part I. *J. Physiol. (London)* 62, 267–272.

Florey, H.W. (1927b). Observations on the contractility of lacteals. Part II. *J. Physiol. (London)* **63**, 1–18.

Guarna, M., Pucci, A.M., Alessandrini, C., Volpi, N., Fruschelli, M., D'Antona, D. & Fruschelli, C. (1991). Peptidergic innervation of mesenteric lymphatics in guinea pigs: an immunocytochemical and pharmacological study. *Lymphology* **24**, 161–167.

Hall, J.G., Morris, B. & Woolley, G. (1965). Intrinsic rhythmic propulsion of lymph in the unanaesthetized sheep. *J. Physiol. (London)* **180**, 336–349.

Hallam, T.J., Jacob, R. & Merritt, J.E. (1988). Evidence that agonists stimulate bivalent-cation influx into human endothelial cells. *Biochem. J.* **255**, 179–184.

Hashimoto, T., Hirata, M., Itoh, T., Kanmura, Y. & Kuriyama, H. (1986). Inositol 1,4,5-trisphosphate activates pharmacomechanical coupling in smooth muscle of the rabbit mesenteric artery. *J. Physiol. (London)* **370**, 605–618.

van Helden, D.F. (1988a). Electrophysiology of neuromuscular transmission in guinea pig mesenteric veins. *J. Physiol. (London)* **401**, 469–488.

van Helden, D.F. (1988b). An alpha-adrenoceptor-mediated chloride conductance in mesenteric veins of the guinea pig. *J. Physiol. (London)* **401**, 489–501.

van Helden, D.F. (1989a). Noradrenaline-induced transient depolarizations in the smooth muscle of isolated guinea pig mesenteric lymphatics. *J. Physiol. (London)* **418**, 173P.

van Helden, D.F. (1989b). Parallels between alpha-adrenoceptor mediated depolarizations and photoreceptor `bumps'. *Neurosci. Lett. Suppl.* **34**, S162.

van Helden, D.F. (1989c). Spontaneous activity in the smooth muscle of lymphatic vessels of the guinea pig mesentery. *Int. Congr. Physiol. Sci.* **9**, P4386.

van Helden, D.F. (1991). Spontaneous and noradrenaline-induced transient depolarizations in the smooth muscle of guinea pig mesenteric vein. *J. Physiol. (London)* **437**, 511–541.

van Helden, D.F. (1993). Pacemaker potentials in lymphatic smooth muscle of the guinea pig mesentery. *J. Physiol. (London)* **471**, 465–479.

van Helden, D.F. & Bull, N. (1995). Neuropeptide Y enhances pacemaking in smooth muscle of guinea pig mesenteric lymphatics. *Proc. Aust. Physiol. Pharmacol. Soc.* **26**, 185.

van Helden, D.F., von der Weid, P.-Y. & Crowe, M.J. (1995). Electrophysiology of lymphatic smooth muscle. In *Interstitium, Connective Tissue and Lymphatics* (Reed, R.K., McHale, N.G., Bert, J.L., Winlove, C.P. & Laine, G. A., eds), pp. 221–236. London: Portland Press.

Hirst, G.D.S. & Neild, T.O. (1978). An analysis of excitatory junction potentials recorded from arterioles. *J. Physiol. (London)* **280**, 87–104.

Hogg, R.C., Wang, Q., Helliwell, R.M. & Large, W.A. (1993). Properties of spontaneous inward currents in rabbit pulmonary artery smooth muscle cells. *Pflugers Arch.* **425**, 233–240.

Hogg, R.C., Wang, Q., & Large, W.A. (1994). Effects of Cl channel blockers on Ca-activated chloride and potassium currents in smooth muscle cells from rabbit portal vein. *Br. J. Pharmacol.* **111**, 1333–1341.

Holman, M.E., Kasby, C.B., Suthers, M.B. & Wilson, J.A.F. (1968). Some properties of the smooth muscle of rabbit portal vein. *J. Physiol. (London)* **196**, 111–132.

Horstmann, E. (1952). Uber die funktionelle struktur der mesenterialen lymphgefasse. *Morphologisches Jahrbuch* **91**, 483–510.

Horstmann, E. (1959). Beobachtungen zur motorik der lymphgefasse. *Pflugers Arch.* **269**, 511–519.

Hume, J.R. & Leblanc, N. (1989). Macroscopic K^+ currents in single smooth muscle cells of the rabbit portal vein. *J. Physiol. (London)* **413**, 49–73.

Iino, M. (1990). Biphasic Ca²⁺ dependence of inositol 1,4,5-trisphosphate-induced Ca release in smooth muscle cells of the guinea pig taenia caeci. *J. Gen. Physiol.* **95**, 1103–1122.

Iino, M. & Endo, M. (1992). Calcium-dependent immediate feedback control of inositol 1,4,5-triphosphate-induced Ca²⁺ release. *Nature* **360**, 76–78.

Johnston, M.G. & Feuer, C. (1983). Suppression of lymphatic vessel contractility with inhibitors of arachidonic acid metabolism. *J. Pharmacol. Exp. Ther.* **226**, 603–607.

Johnston, M.G. & Gordon, J.L. (1981). Regulation of lymphatic contractility by arachidonate metabolites. *Nature* **293**, 294–297.

Kirber, M.T., Walsh, J.V. & Singer, J.J. (1988). Stretch-activated ion channels in smooth muscle: A mechanism for the initiation of stretch-induced contraction. *Pflugers Arch.* **412**, 339–345.

Kirkpatrick, C.T. & McHale, N.G. (1977). Electrical and mechanical activity of isolated lymphatic vessels. *J. Physiol. (London)* **272**, 33P–34P.

Komori, S. & Bolton, T.B. (1991). Calcium release induced by inositol 1,4,5-trisphosphate in single rabbit intestinal smooth muscle cells. *J. Physiol. (London)* **433**, 495–517.

Lechleiter, J., Girard, S., Peralta, E. & Clapham, D. (1991). Spiral calcium wave propagation and annihilation in *Xenopus laevis* oocytes. *Science.* **252**, 123–126.

Lillywhite, P.G. (1977). Single photon signals and transduction in an insect eye. *J. Comp. Physiol.* **122**, 189–200.

Mawhinney, J.D. & Roddie, I. C. (1973). Spontaneous activity in isolated bovine mesenteric lymphatics. *J. Physiol. (London)* **229**, 339–348.

McGeown, J.G., McHale, N.G., Roddie, I. C. & Thornbury, K. (1987). Peripheral lymphatic responses to outflow pressure in anaesthetised sheep. *J. Physiol. (London)* **383**, 527–536.

McHale, N.G. (1990). Lymphatic innervation. *Blood Vessels* **27**, 127–136.

McHale, N.G. & Roddie, I.C. (1983). The effect of intravenous adrenaline and noradrenaline infusion of peripheral lymph flow in the sheep. *J. Physiol. (London)* **341**, 517–526.

McHale, N.G., Roddie, I.C. & Thornbury, K.D.(1980). Nervous modulation of spontaneous contractions in bovine mesenteric lymphatics. *J. Physiol. (London)* **309**, 461–472.

McHale, N.G., Harty, H.R. & Thornbury, K.D. (1991). Excitatory neurotransmission in isolated sheep mesenteric lymphatic vessels. *Proc. Physiolog. Soc.* **432**, 9P.

Minke, B. & Selinger, Z. (1992). Inositol lipid pathway in fly photoreceptors: Excitation, calcium mobilisation and retinal degeneration. *Prog. Retinal Res.* **11**, 99–124.

Mislin, H. (1972). Die Motorik der Lymphgefasse und die Regulation der Lymphherzen. In *Handbuch der Allgemeinen Pathologie 3rd Edn* (Meessen, H., ed.), vol 6, pp. 219–238. Springer Verlag, Berlin.

Mislin, H. (1983). The lymphangion. In *Lymphangiology* (Foldi, M. & Casley-Smith, J. R. eds), pp. 165–175. F.K. Schattauer Verlag, New York, Stuttgart.

Nathanson, M.H., Padfield, P.J., O'Sullivan, A.J., Burgstahler, A.D. & Jamieson, J. D. (1992). Mechanism of Ca²⁺ wave propagation in pancreatic acinar cells. *J. Biol. Chem.* **267**, 18118–18121.

Ohhashi, T., Kobayashi, S., Tsukahara, S. & Azuma, T. (1982). Innervation of bovine mesenteric lymphatics: from the histochemical point of view. *Microvas. Res.* **24**, 377–385.

Ohya, Y., Kitamura, K. & Kuriyama, H. (1987). Cellular calcium regulates outward currents in rabbit intestinal smooth muscle cell. *Am. J. Physiol.* **252**, C401–C410.

Ohya, Y., Terada, K., Yamaguchi, K., Inoue, R., Okabe, K., Kitamura, K., Hirata, M. & Kuriyama, H. (1988). Effects of inositol phosphates on the membrane activity of smooth muscle cells of the rabbit portal vein. *Pflugers Arch.* **412**, 382–389.

Parker, I. & Ivorra, I. (1991). Caffeine inhibits inositol trisphosphate-mediated liberation of intracellular calcium in *Xenopus* oocytes. *J. Physiol. (London)* **433**, 229–240.

Parker, I. & Miledi, R. (1986). Changes in intracellular calcium and in membrane currents evoked by injection of inositol trisphosphate into *Xenopus* oocytes. *Proc. R. Soc. (London) B. Biol. Sci.* **228**, 307–315.

Parker, I. & Yao, Y. (1991). Regenerative release of calcium from functionally discrete subcellular stores by inositol trisphosphate. *Proc. R. Soc. (London) B. Biol. Sci.* **246**, 269–274.

Petersen, O.H., Gallacher, D.V., Wakui, M., Yule, D.I., Petersen, C.C. & Toescu, E.C. (1991). Receptor-activated cytoplasmic Ca^{2+} oscillations in pancreatic acinar cells: generation and spreading of Ca^{2+} signals. *Cell. Calcium.* **12**, 135–144.

Reeder, L.B., Yang, L.H. & Ferguson, M.K. (1994). Modulation of lymphatic spontaneous contractions by EDRF. *J. Surg. Res.* **56**, 620–625.

Smith, R.O. (1949). Lymphatic contractility: A possible mechanism of lymphatic vessels for the transport of lymph. *J. Exp. Med.* **90**, 497–509.

Somlyo, A.P. & Somlyo, A.V. (1991). Smooth muscle structure and function. In *The heart and cardiovascular system* (Fozzard, H.A., ed.), pp. 1295–1324. Raven Press, New York.

Somlyo, A.V., Bond, M., Somlyo, A.P. & Scarpa, A. (1985). Inositol trisphosphate induced calcium release and contraction in vascular smooth muscle. *Proc. Natl Acad. Sci. USA* **82**, 5231–5235.

Stehno-Bittel, L. & Sturek, M. (1992). Spontaneous sarcoplasmic reticulum calcium release and extrusion from bovine, not porcine, coronary artery smooth muscle. *J. Physiol. (London)* **451**, 49–78.

Stricker, S.A., Centonze, V.E., Paddock, S.W. & Schatten, G. (1992). Confocal microscopy of fertilization-induced calcium dynamics in sea urchin eggs. *Dev. Biol.* **149**, 370–380.

Suzuki, H. (1981). Effects of endogenous and exogenous noradrenaline on the smooth muscle of guinea pig mesenteric vein. *J. Physiol. (London)* 321, 495–512.

Todd, G.L. & Bernard, G.R. (1973). The sympathetic innervation of the cervical lymphatic duct of the dog. *Anatomical Record* **177**, 303–316.

Wakui, M., Potter, BV. & Petersen, O.H. (1989). Pulsatile intracellular calcium release does not depend on fluctuations in inositol trisphosphate concentration. *Nature.* **339**, 317–320.

Wang, Q., Hogg, R.C. & Large, W.A. (1992). Properties of spontaneous inward currents recorded in smooth muscle cells isolated from the rabbit portal vein. *J. Physiol. (London)* **451**, 525–537.

Wang, X.Y., Wong, W.C. & Ling, E.A. (1994). Studies of the lymphatic vessel-associated neurons in the intestine of the guinea pig. *J. Anat.* **185**, 65–74.

Ward, S.M., Sanders, K.M., Thornbury, K D. & McHale, N.G. (1991). Spontaneous electrical activity in isolated bovine lymphatics recorded by intracellular microelectrodes. *J. Physiol. (London)* **438**, 168P.

Werner, B. (1965). Thoracic duct cannulation in man. I. Surgical technique and a clinical study on 79 patients. *Acta Chir. Scand.* **353**, 1–32.

Wong, F. (1978). Nature of light-induced conductance changes in ventral photoreceptors of Limulus. *Nature* **276**, 76–79.

Woods, N.M., Cuthbertson, K.S.R. & Cobbold, P.H. (1986). Repetitive transient rises in cytoplasmic free calcium concentration in single rat hepatocytes. *Nature* **319**, 600–602.

Yamaguchi, H.,Kajita, J. & Madison, J.M. (1995). Isoproterenol increases peripheral intracellular calcium and decreases inner intracellular calcium in single airway smooth muscle cells. *Am. J. Physiol.* **268**, C771–C779.

Yao, Y. & Parker, I. (1994). Ca²⁺ influx modulation of temporal and spatial patterns of inositol trisphosphate-mediated Ca²⁺ liberation in *Xenopus* oocytes. *J. Physiol. (London)* **476**, 17–28.

Yao, Y., Choi, J. & Parker, I. (1995). Quantal puffs of intracellular calcium evoked by inositol trisphosphate in Xenopus oocytes. *J. Physiol. (London)* **482**, 533–553.

Yoffey, J.M. & Courtice, F.C. (1970). *Lymphatics, Lymph and Lymphomyeloid Complex*. Academic Press, New York.

Yokoyama, S. & Ohhashi, T. (1993). Effects of acetylcholine on spontaneous contractions in isolated bovine mesenteric lymphatics. *Am. J. Physiol.* **264**, H1460–H1464.

31

Hormonal Influences on Contraction of Uterine Smooth Muscle

HELENA C. PARKINGTON
H. A. COLEMAN

Department of Physiology,
Monash University,
Clayton, Victoria,
Australia

INTRODUCTION

Strong, coordinated contractions of uterine smooth muscle are required in order to effect successful labour. Failure of such contractions to occur may give rise to abnormal labour necessitating chemical and/or physical intervention. Prostaglandins (PGs) and oxytocin are likely to play a pivotal role in stimulating uterine activity during labour. The aim of this chapter is to discuss the response of uterine smooth muscle to these two hormones.

CONTRACTION IN SMOOTH MUSCLE

There is general consensus that contraction is initiated in smooth muscle when Ca^{2+} binds with calmodulin which then complexes with, and activates myosin light-chain kinase (MLCK). This kinase phosphorylates the 20 kDa light chain of myosin exposing an ATPase domain. In concert with actin, ATP is split to release the energy necessary for the relative movement of myosin against actin resulting in muscle shortening or tension development. While an initial increase in cytoplasmic calcium, $[Ca^{2+}]_i$, and myosin phosphorylation appear to be obligatory for the initiation of contraction, the processes involved in the maintenance of contraction of longer duration in response to some hormones are less clearly defined.

The responses of smooth muscle to hormones and neurotransmitters, in

SMOOTH MUSCLE EXCITATION
ISBN 0-12-112360-X

general, are initial rises in $[Ca^{2+}]_i$ and phosphorylation of myosin which are associated with force development or shortening. However, within minutes, the concentrations of both $[Ca^{2+}]_i$ and phosphorylated myosin decline, while tension remains high, or may even continue to increase slowly (Kamm & Stull, 1989). The changes in $[Ca^{2+}]_i$ are likely to reflect release of the ion from intracellular stores within the endoplasmic reticulum (ER) and influx of Ca^{2+} across the plasma membrane (see below), in concert with Ca^{2+}-removal mechanisms stimulated, at least in part, by the initial rise in Ca^{2+}. Cleavage of the phosphate from the light chain by MLC phosphatases can account for the decline in the levels of phosphorylated myosin that follows the initial peak. Murphy and colleagues proposed that dephosphorylation of myosin while still attached to actin results in a considerable reduction in the rate of detachment of myosin from actin and hence tension is maintained with minimal cross-bridge cycling (Aksoy et al., 1982). They called this the latch state of myosin–actin interaction. This hypothesis has been challenged and expanded and alternative propositions include the possibility of cooperative interactions between phosphorylated and unphosphorylated myosin, and actin-dependent mechanisms.

In human myometrium stimulatory hormones induce an initial peak in myosin phosphorylation that subsequently declines to lower levels (Word et al., 1990), similar to observations in other smooth muscles.

CALCIUM INFLUX THROUGH VOLTAGE-OPERATED CALCIUM CHANNELS

One of the most conspicuous routes of Ca^{2+} influx into many smooth muscle tissues under normal physiological conditions is that which occurs through voltage-operated calcium channels (VOCCs). More than one type of VOCC has been described in smooth muscle tissues. These can be distinguished by their voltage dependence, single channel conductance, relative permeability to divalent cations and profile of pharmacological blockade. The main VOCC in uterine smooth muscle is the so-called L-type channel (Mironneau, 1974; Ohya & Sperelakis, 1989; Miyoshi et al., 1991). Voltage clamp studies of myometrium from pregnant rats have demonstrated that the inward Ca^{2+} current is blocked by members of the dihydropyridine class of drug, such as nifedipine (Amédée et al., 1987; Ohya & Sperelakis, 1989; Miyoshi et al., 1991). Such blockade is a major distinguishing feature of this channel type.

Spontaneous contractions of uterine smooth muscle in vivo are highly sensitive to members of this class of drug. A bolus injection, or continuous infusion of nifedipine into anaesthetized rats was an order of magnitude more effective in suppressing uterine contractions compared with its

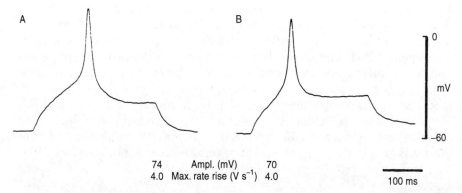

| | 74 | Ampl. (mV) | 70 |
| | 4.0 | Max. rate rise (V s⁻¹) | 4.0 |

Figure 1 A spike action potential evoked by a depolarizing current step in control solution had an amplitude of 74 mV and a maximum rate of rise of 4.0 V s⁻¹ (A). A spike evoked in the same cell in the presence of $PGF_{2\alpha}$ (10^{-6} M) had an amplitude of 70 mV and a maximum rate of rise of 4.0 V s⁻¹ (B). Records from circular myometrium of guinea pig during mid pregnancy.

suppression of cardiovascular parameters (Downing & Hollingsworth, 1988). Moreover, the dihydropyridines have been used to suppress untimely uterine contractions and suspend premature labour in women (Keirse, 1992) suggesting a significant role for VOCCs in the response to agents such as PGs, oxytocin and other hormones involved in the process of labour.

Oxytocin increases the amplitude of the inward Ca^{2+} current in rat myometrium by about 30% (Mironneau, 1976). In contrast, PGE_1 enhances contraction with no increase, or even a small inhibitory effect on the Ca^{2+} current through VOCCs in this tissue. $PGF_{2\alpha}$ appears to have little effect on the amplitude or maximum rate of rise of the dihydropyridine-sensitive action potential in guinea pig myometrium (Figure 1). It is interesting to consider the differences in the responses to oxytocin and PGs in terms of mechanism. Oxytocin has been shown to mobilize membrane phospholipids and to invoke the production of diacylglycerol which gives rise to the activation of protein kinase C (see below). Phorbol esters and the synthetic diacylglycerol, dioctanoyl-glycerol which stimulates protein kinase C, have been found to increase the Ca^{2+} current through L-type VOCCs in toad stomach and in vascular smooth muscle (Vivaudou et al., 1988; Fish et al., 1988). No stimulation of diacylglycerol was found in the response to $PGF_{2\alpha}$, at least for human myometrium (Schrey et al., 1988).

Only action potentials consisting of simple spikes are recorded in the longitudinal myometrium of rats and the opening of VOCCs underlies these events since they are blocked by dihydropyridines. A complex action potential consisting of spikes and plateau occurs spontaneously (i.e. in the absence of hormone) in the circular muscle layer of rat uterus (Osa &

Kawarabayashi, 1977; Bengtsson *et al.*, 1984; Chamley & Parkington, 1984). These differences in electrical activity are associated with differences in the duration and strength of contraction (Bengtsson *et al.*, 1984; Chamley & Parkington, 1984). The contraction associated with the plateau-type action potential is prolonged for as long as the duration of the plateau. While the spike component of the complex action potential is highly sensitive to blockade by dihydropyridines, the plateau is considerably less sensitive. Modulation of this action potential, and the currents underlying it, by oxytocin or PGs have not been studied. It is noteworthy that the plateau gives way to a burst of simple spikes at term (Osa & Kawarabayashi, 1977; Bengtsson *et al.*, 1984) suggesting an enhanced importance of VOCCs at this time.

RECEPTOR-ACTIVATED CALCIUM INFLUX

It is clear that the contractile responses of many smooth muscles to hormones are much more resistant to blockade by Ca^{2+} channel antagonists than are spontaneous, electrically evoked or K^+-induced contractions, which are dependent only on an increase in the probability of opening of VOCCs. The existence of 'receptor-operated calcium channels' was first formally suggested in independent reviews by Bolton and by van Breemen and colleagues (Bolton, 1979; van Breemen *et al.*, 1979) and experimental verification has been keenly sought ever since.

Acetylcholine activates a cation channel in guinea pig ileum (Benham *et al.*, 1985; Inoue *et al.*, 1987) via direct coupling between the receptor, a GTP-binding protein (G-protein) and the ion channel (Inoue & Isenberg, 1990; Zholos & Bolton, 1994). Among vascular smooth muscles, noradrenaline induces a cation current in rabbit ear artery (Amédée et al, 1990). An ion channel in portal vein has a selectivity ratio for Ca^{2+}/Na^+ of 21/1, but this channel is activated by $[Ca^{2+}]_i$ acting as a cytoplasmic second messenger (Loirand *et al.*, 1991). ATP activates a poorly selective cation channel in vascular smooth muscle, not involving cytoplasmic second messengers. This channel conducts a small amount of Ca^{2+}, with a selectivity ratio for Ca^{2+}/Na^+ of 3/1 (Benham & Tsien, 1987).

In longitudinal myometrial strips from pregnant mice, exogenous ATP evokes some 25 mV depolarization that is accompanied by a modest increase in membrane conductance (Ninomiya & Suzuki, 1983). Voltage clamp studies of the effects of exogenous ATP on rat myometrial cells on day 19 of pregnancy revealed an inward current that reversed at around 0 mV. The amplitude of the current was reduced to around 40% by day 21 of pregnancy, the day before delivery, an effect that was mimicked by oestrogen treatment of day 19 pregnant rats (Honoré *et al.*, 1989). Circulating oestrogen levels increase sharply on days 20–21 of pregnancy in rats and hence this steroid may be responsible for the changes in response to ATP that take place at term. Interactions between Ca^{2+} and ATP make determination of the Ca^{2+} permeability of this channel difficult.

We have found that $PGF_{2\alpha}$ also evokes substantial depolarization (to approximately $-17\,mV$) in the longitudinal myometrium of guinea pigs (Figure 2). Similar effects of histamine and carbachol have been reported in guinea pig ileum (Bolton *et al.*, 1981). The sustained depolarization and accompanying sustained contraction that occur in the myometrium at mid pregnancy are largely resistant to nifedipine (Figure 2). The extent of the depolarization and the resistance of the contraction to nifedipine are much reduced at term, again suggesting a possible increased significance of VOCCs at this time.

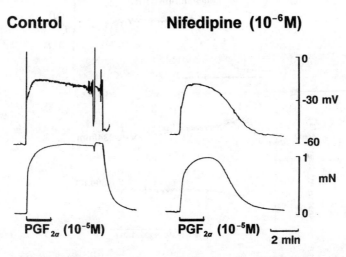

Control   **Nifedipine (10^{-6}M)**

$PGF_{2\alpha}$ (10^{-5}M) $PGF_{2\alpha}$ (10^{-5}M)   2 min

Figure 2 In a longitudinal strip of guinea pig myometrium obtained at mid pregnancy, $PGF_{2\alpha}$ (10^{-5} M for 2 min) evoked a spike followed by a plateau of depolarization which was accompanied by a large, sustained contraction. Nifedipine (10^{-6} M) abolished the spike leaving the plateau and most of the contraction.

Although $PGF_{2\alpha}$ also induces sustained, dihydropyridine-resistant depolarization in the circular muscle layer of guinea pig myometrium, this is only to -45 to $-40\,mV$. Furthermore, depolarization occurs only at mid pregnancy and is absent at term. This observation may be added to the list of differences between the longitudinal and circular muscle layers of the uterus.

The development of fluorescent probes that are sensitive to the concentration of free Ca^{2+}, and the use of the probes fura-2 and indo-2 in the measurement of $[Ca^{2+}]_i$ in cells has given a fresh impetus to smooth muscle research and has increased our understanding of the mechanisms of contraction. We have used the fura-2 technique to study how $[Ca^{2+}]_i$ changes during exposure to $PGF_{2\alpha}$ in guinea pig myometrium at mid and late pregnancy (Figure 3). From a resting level of approximately 100 nM, $PGF_{2\alpha}$ induces a transient increase in $[Ca^{2+}]_i$ to around 850 nM. Within 1 min $[Ca^{2+}]_i$ declines to a level of around 300 nM, where it remains during the entire duration of a 3-min exposure to $PGF_{2\alpha}$ (Hart et al., 1993). This response in myometrium is remarkably similar to the response of airways smooth muscle

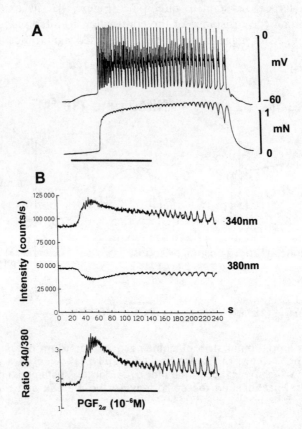

Figure 3 $PGF_{2\alpha}$ (10^{-6} M for 2 min) evoked depolarization, action potential discharge (upper trace) and contraction (lower trace) (A) in the longitudinal myometrium of guinea pig obtained at mid pregnancy. In a different preparation (B), 2 min application of the PG evoked an increase in the 340 nm signal and a decrease in the 380 nm signal emitted by fura-2. The ratio, 340/380, indicating an increase in $[Ca^{2+}]_i$, underwent oscillations that were likely to result from Ca^{2+} entry during action potentials.

to histamine (Murray & Kotlikoff, 1991). The transient component of the rise in $[Ca^{2+}]_i$ in myometrium is reduced to around 650 nM in the presence of nifedipine, and is abolished by a combination of nifedipine (10^{-6} M) and thapsigargin (10^{-5} M), which blocks Ca^{2+} uptake into the ER. These observations indicate that the transient component of $[Ca^{2+}]_i$ results from Ca^{2+} influx through VOCCs and release of Ca^{2+} from intracellular stores, in particular, the store that is accessed by inositol trisphosphate ($Ins(1,4,5)P_3$) (see below). In contrast, the sustained component of the increase in $[Ca^{2+}]_i$ is entirely resistant to a combination of nifedipine and thapsigargin. There is a decline in the amplitude of the sustained depolarization and in the level of the sustained increase in $[Ca^{2+}]_i$ by term, suggesting that receptor-operated Ca^{2+} influx assumes less importance in delivering Ca^{2+} for contraction in guinea pig myometrium as term approaches. A switch from a significant role for receptor-operated Ca^{2+} entry at mid pregnancy to a greater reliance on Ca^{2+} influx through VOCCs at term would explain the effectiveness of the dihydropyridines in suppressing uterine contractions during labour (Keirse, 1992).

MOBILIZATION OF INTRACELLULAR CALCIUM

The interaction between many stimulatory hormones and their receptors results in the activation of a G-protein which stimulates phospholipase C within the plasma membrane. This lipase mobilizes membrane phospholipids by cleaving phosphatidylinositol bisphosphate to form $Ins(1,4,5)P_3$, a hydrophilic agent that acts as a cytoplasmic second messenger, and diacylglycerol, a lipophilic moiety that remains in the membrane and activates protein kinase C. $Ins(1,4,5)P_3$ interacts with its receptor on the endoplasmic reticulum (ER), which becomes an ion channel that allows Ca^{2+} to flow from the ER into the cytoplasm down its considerable chemical gradient. Ca^{2+} released from the ER is thought to deliver Ca^{2+} close to the contractile apparatus to facilitate a rapid velocity of shortening or development of tension. Emptying of the stores may evoke Ca^{2+} influx across the plasma membrane by a mechanism that has yet to be clarified in smooth muscle.

Uterine smooth muscle contains an $Ins(1,4,5)P_3$-sensitive store (rat, Savineau et al., 1988; guinea pig, Coleman et al., 1988). Oxytocin mobilizes $Ins(1,4,5)P_3$ production in uterine smooth muscle (Marc et al., 1986; Ruzycky & Triggle, 1987; Ruzycky & Crankshaw, 1988; Schrey et al., 1988) but PG has not been found to stimulate $Ins(1,4,5)P_3$ in myometrium, at least in women (Schrey et al., 1988). It is interesting that the coupling between the G-protein and phospholipase C, and hence the capacity for $Ins(1,4,5)P_3$ production, decreases during pregnancy in guinea pigs (Arkinstall & Jones, 1990). Similar to the apparent decline in the significance of receptor-operated Ca^{2+} influx at term discussed above, we have found that the contraction possible in response to release of store also declines to negligible levels at term in both layers of guinea pig myometrium (Coleman et al., 1988).

The ER may not be homogeneous. Thus, in some tissues a rise in $[Ca^{2+}]_i$, for example, following influx across the plasma membrane, may release additional Ca^{2+} from some regions of the ER and in this way amplify the original Ca^{2+} signal. This Ca^{2+}-induced Ca^{2+} release mechanism may also exist in uterine smooth muscle of rat (Savineau et al., 1988).

CYTOPLASMIC CALCIUM

Although the evidence implicating a pivotal role for Ca^{2+} in the initiation of contraction in smooth muscle is overwhelming, several groups have reported that a variety of hormones can evoke sustained contraction of rat uterine smooth muscle following prolonged (hours) deprivation of $[Ca^{2+}]_o$ (Edman & Schild, 1962; Sakai et al., 1983; Ashoori et al., 1985; Mironneau et al., 1984). This may be a manifestation of the Ca^{2+}-independent contraction suggested by others (Somlyo & Somlyo, 1994). A similar mechanism may occur in guinea pig myometrium. When Ca^{2+} is omitted from and EGTA added to the perfusing solution $[Ca^{2+}]_i$ falls to very low levels within 5 min yet $PGF_{2\alpha}$ induces a contraction that is similar in amplitude to that which occurs in control, Ca^{2+}-containing solution.

SENSITIVITY OF THE CONTRACTILE APPARATUS TO CALCIUM

Circular myometrium from guinea pigs at term develops tonic tension in response to $PGF_{2\alpha}$ in the absence of depolarization. This tension is resistant to nifedipine and to removal of $[Ca^{2+}]_o$. $[Ca^{2+}]_i$ remains unchanged or increases to levels that are barely detectable above resting $[Ca^{2+}]_i$ (Figure 4) (Coleman et al., 1995). Increasing $[Ca^{2+}]_o$ in tissues depolarized with 100 mM K^+ results in graded increments in tension and $[Ca^{2+}]_i$. When this procedure is repeated in the presence of $PGF_{2\alpha}$ the $[Ca^{2+}]_i$-tension curve is shifted to the left, indicating a greater contraction at a given concentration of $[Ca^{2+}]_i$ in myometrium. A similar increase in the sensitivity of the contractile apparatus to Ca^{2+} has been observed in other smooth muscles.

The identification and study of increases in the sensitivity of the contractile apparatus to Ca^{2+} (sensitization) have been facilitated by the use of a toxin from Staphylococcus aureus, α-toxin, which creates holes in the plasma

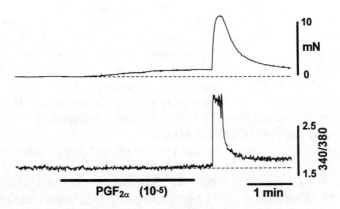

Figure 4 In circular myometrium obtained from a guinea pig during late pregnancy, $PGF_{2\alpha}$ (10^{-5} M for 3 min) evoked an increase in tension, after a delay, (upper trace) with a minimal increase in $[Ca^{2+}]_i$ (lower trace). Shortly after removal of $PGF_{2\alpha}$ an increase in $[Ca^{2+}]_i$ and contraction occurred spontaneously.

membrane such that $[Ca^{2+}]_i$ can be clamped at the concentration of $[Ca^{2+}]_0$, while hormone receptors, G-proteins, lipases and all but the smallest of cytoplasmic components remain intact (Nishimura & van Breemen, 1989; Himpens *et al.*, 1990). The mechanisms involved in sensitization have been studied in vascular smooth muscle (Nishimura & van Breemen, 1989; Himpens *et al.*, 1990; Hirata *et al.*, 1992; Jensen *et al.*, 1992) and visceral smooth muscles (Oishi *et al.*, 1992; Sato *et al.*, 1994). The involvement of protein kinase C has been suggested. The physiological activation of this kinase occurs in the presence of diacylglycerol and Ca^{2+}. Diacylglycerol appears in the membrane following the mobilization of membrane phospholipids, as described previously. Phorbol esters, tumour-promoting agents that activate protein kinase C, mimic the sensitization evoked by hormones in some tissues. Calphostin C and staurosporine, which inhibit protein kinase C, block the sensitizing actions of hormones in some smooth muscles (Nishimura & van Breemen, 1989; Katsuyama & Morgan, 1993). However, these drugs failed to prevent sensitization in guinea pig stomach (Oishi *et al.*, 1992) or rabbit mesenteric artery (Hirata *et al.*, 1992). In these last two studies the evidence suggested that one of the smaller, monomeric G-proteins, rho p21, may be involved. In guinea pig myometrium, neither calphostin C nor staurosporine block the sensitization induced by $PGF_{2\alpha}$ or oxytocin.

Some evidence indicates that sensitization of the contractile apparatus to Ca^{2+} may occur owing to increased levels of myosin phosphorylation per unit Ca^{2+}. The level of phosphorylated myosin is a balance between the activities of MLCK and MLC phosphatase. Convincing evidence implicates a decrease in the activity of MLC phosphatases in the dissociation between tension and $[Ca^{2+}]_i$ in smooth muscle (Somlyo & Somlyo, 1994). The mechanism involves a G-protein, since GTP-γS mimics, and GDP-βS inhibits, the actions of hormones by increasing the amplitude of contraction in the presence of a constant level of $[Ca^{2+}]_i$. It has been suggested that the activity of the phosphatase(s) involved may be suppressed by protein kinase II, a kinase which requires concentrations of Ca^{2+}/calmodulin for activation that are in excess of those required to activate MLCK.

It has been reported that the contraction of rat myometrium in response to oxytocin in Ca^{2+} free solution is not accompanied by an increase in the levels of phosphorylated myosin (Oishi et al., 1991) and this may be a manifestation of the Ca^{2+}-independent contraction suggested by others (see above); involvement of magnesium has been suggested (Ashoori et al., 1985).

The less than perfect correlation between $Ins(1,4,5)P_3$ production/$[Ca^{2+}]_i$ and sensitization involving diacylglycerol/protein kinase C observed in some smooth muscle tissues in response to hormones has been noted. It must be emphasized here that, while mobilization of phospholipids such as phosphatidylserine, phosphatidylethanolain ethanolamine by lipases other than phospholipase C can give rise to diacylglycerol without $Ins(1,4,5)P_3$, only phosphatidyl inositol gives rise to both diacylglycerol and $Ins(1,4,5)P_3$.

INTERACTIONS BETWEEN PROSTAGLANDIN AND OXYTOCIN

Oxytocin evokes substantial depolarization in uterine smooth muscle (rats and mice, Osa & Taga, 1973; Osa & Kawarabayashi, 1977; guinea pig, Hart et al., 1993). The response of the longitudinal myometrium of guinea pigs to oxytocin at mid pregnancy is remarkably similar to the response to $PGF_{2\alpha}$: a transient burst of spike action potentials is accompanied by a transient increase in $[Ca^{2+}]_i$ to approximately 600 nM, which includes components of Ca^{2+} influx through VOCCs and store release. The subsequent sustained depolarization is associated with a sustained increase in $[Ca^{2+}]_i$, also to around 300 nM. The fact that the sustained depolarization and the sustained component of the increase in $[Ca^{2+}]_i$ in responses to $PGF_{2\alpha}$ and oxytocin were so similar prompted us to test the possibility that both hormones might act via the same mechanism. In the presence of maximal concentrations of either hormone, addition of a maximal concentration of the other caused no change in the sustained increase in $[Ca^{2+}]_i$, suggesting the possibility of a common mechanism (Hart et al., 1993). However, an additional contraction was observed when the second hormone was added in all cases. This is likely to be due to an increase in the sensitivity of the contractile apparatus to $[Ca^{2+}]_i$.

POSSIBLE MECHANISMS INVOLVED IN RECEPTOR-MEDIATED
INCREASE IN CYTOPLASMIC CALCIUM

The pathway(s) involved in the sustained increase in $[Ca^{2+}]_i$ evoked by $PGF_{2\alpha}$ and oxytocin in mid pregnant longitudinal myometrium of guinea pig have not been determined directly. The possibility was considered that emptying the ER of its store of Ca^{2+} might induce Ca^{2+} influx, as occurs in several other cell types. Both hormones release intracellular stores of Ca^{2+} during mid pregnancy, a time when the sustained increase in $[Ca^{2+}]_i$ is largest. However, removal of hormone, in the continued presence of thapsigargin to prevent refilling, results in cessation of the sustained increase in $[Ca^{2+}]_i$ and the contraction.

Hormones, and the second messenger systems that they stimulate, are capable of modulating the activity of various ion pumps and exchangers in a wide variety of smooth muscles (O'Donnell & Owen, 1994). An elevated $[Ca^{2+}]_i$ might be maintained as a result of inhibition of the Ca^{2+}-ATPase extrusion pump in the plasma membrane. It has been suggested that PGs suppress the activity of this pump in rat myometrium (Deliconstantinos & Fotiou, 1986). The mobilization of membrane phospholipids by oxytocin is likely to lead to activation of protein kinase C. This kinase has been reported to stimulate the plasma membrane Ca^{2+} extrusion pump in vascular smooth muscle (Furukawa et al., 1989).

We have considered the possibility that a slowing or reversal of Na^+/Ca^{2+} exchange may be involved in the sustained increase in $[Ca^{2+}]_i$ in response to $PGF_{2\alpha}$ and oxytocin. The depolarization induced by these two hormones would favour operation of this exchanger in reverse mode, that is, to extrude Na^+ and facilitate Ca^{2+} entry. However, reverse mode would tend to hyperpolarize the membrane and hence is difficult to reconcile with the sustained depolarization that occurs. Moreover, incubation in ouabain $(10^{-5} M)$ for 30 min to increase Na^+_i had little effect on the depolarization or contraction in response to $PGF_{2\alpha}$. Likewise, lowering $[Na^+]_o$ had little effect on $[Ca^{2+}]_i$ or contraction evoked by either $PGF_{2\alpha}$ or oxytocin, although the depolarization was decreased by approximately one-third.

The receptor-activated channel in a number of tissues is sensitive to blockade by low concentrations of gadolinium or SK&F 96365. SK&F 96365 was without effect on the depolarization, contraction or increase in $[Ca^{2+}]_i$ in response to either hormone in uterine smooth muscle. In the presence of nifedipine, gadolinium was only effective in reducing the depolarization and contraction in response to $PGF_{2\alpha}$ when present at greater than 1 mM, and as such, was less potent than cadmium or nickel. SK&F 96365 and gadolinium are not universally effective at inhibiting receptor-activated ion channels in smooth muscle and hence the possible involvement of such a channel that is insensitive to these blockers can not be ruled out at this stage.

Hormones have been shown to alter the mode of activity of ion channels in other tissues (Naranjo & Brehm, 1993) and VOCCs appear to have more than one mode of activity in the smooth muscle of bladder (Nakayama & Brading, 1993). Thus, it may be that PGs and oxytocin modulate VOCCs in such a way as to make them insensitive to blockade by nifedipine and the other dihydropyridines and verapamil that have been tested. If this process were slow to develop it could accommodate the slow rate of rise in $[Ca^{2+}]_i$. We have previously reported the likely transformation of an essentially voltage-dependent mechanism by PGs in guinea pig myometrium very early in pregnancy (Coleman & Parkington, 1988).

IN CONCLUSION

PGs and oxytocin have an important role in the functioning of uterine smooth muscle, especially during labour. Inhibitors of PG synthesis and antagonists of the oxytocin receptor can delay normal and preterm labour. These two hormones can influence the contractile state of the myometrium by a variety of mechanisms, including release of Ca^{2+} from the ER, increasing the sensitivity of the contractile apparatus to Ca^{2+}, activation or modulation of ion channels, and possible effects on ion pumps and exchangers. With so many possible mechanisms interacting during the response of the myometrium to oxytocin and PG it is clear that much work is needed before the mechanisms underlying the responses are well understood. In this regard, it is worthwhile stating that closer attention to the kinetics and time courses of events is likely to be crucial in coming to a final understanding of the events controlling contraction in this fascinating tissue. Despite the uncertainties, it is clear that Ca^{2+} influx has a central role in determining contractile activity. During mid pregnancy, influx is through VOCCs and receptor mediated mechanisms. At term, Ca^{2+} influx through VOCCs appears to dominate. The principal effect of PGs and oxytocin at term appears to be their ability to increase the sensitivity of the contractile apparatus to Ca^{2+}, thus priming the uterus for maximal contraction when $[Ca^{2+}]_i$ rises. This, together with the increase in cell-to-cell coupling that occurs at term, transforms the uterus into an organ that contracts forcefully and in a coordinated manner to expel the fetus and effect successful birth.

REFERENCES

Aksoy, M.O., Murphy, R.A. & Kamm, K.E. (1982). Role of Ca^{2+} and myosin light chain phosphorylation in regulation of smooth muscle. *Am. J. Physiol.* **242**, C109–C116.

Amédée, T., Mironneau, C. & Mironneau, J. (1987). The calcium channel current of pregnant rat single myometrial cells in short-term primary culture. *J. Physiol.* **392**, 253–272.

Amédée, T., Benham, C.D., Bolton, T.B., Byrne, N.G. & Large, W.A. (1990). Potassium, chloride and non-selective cation conductances opened by noradrenaline in rabbit ear artery cells. *J. Physiol.* **423**, 551–568.

Arkinstall, S.J. & Jones, C.T. (1990). Pregnancy suppresses G protein coupling to phosphoinositide hydrolysis in guinea pig myometrium. *Am. J. Physiol.* **259**, E57–E65.

Ashoori, F., Takai, A. & Tomita, T. (1985). The response of non-pregnant rat myometrium to oxytocin in Ca^{2+}-free solution. *Br. J. Pharmacol.* **84**, 175–183.

Bengtsson, B., Chow, E.M.H. & Marshall, J.M. (1984). Activity of circular muscle of rat uterus at different times in pregnancy. *Am. J. Physiol.* **246**, C216–C223.

Benham, C.D., Bolton, T.B. & Lang, R.J. (1985). Acetylcholine activates an inward current in single mammalian smooth muscle cells. *Nature* **316**, 345–346.

Benham, C.D. & Tsien, R.W. (1987). A novel receptor-operated Ca^{2+}-permeable channel activated by ATP in smooth muscle. *Nature* **328**, 275–278.

Bolton, T.B. (1979). Mechanism of action of transmitters and other substances on smooth muscle. *Physiol. Rev.* **59**, 606–718.

Bolton, T.B., Clark, J.P., Kitamura, K. & Lang, R.J. (1981). Evidence that histamine and carbachol may open the same ion channels in longitudinal smooth muscle of guinea pig ileum. *J. Physiol.* **320**, 363–379.

van Breemen, C., Aaronson, P.I. & Loutzenhiser, R. (1979). Sodium–calcium interactions in mammalian smooth muscle. *Pharmacol. Rev.* **30**, 167–208.

Chamley, W.A. & Parkington, H.C. (1984). Relaxin inhibits the plateau component of the action potential in the circular myometrium of the rat. *J. Physiol.* **353**, 51–65.

Coleman, H.A. & Parkington, H.C. (1988). Induction of prolonged excitability in myometrium of pregnant guinea pigs by prostaglandin $F_{2\alpha}$. *J. Physiol.* **399**, 33–47.

Coleman, H.A., McShane, P.G. & Parkington, H.C. (1988). Gestational changes in the utilization of intracellularly stored calcium in the myometrium of guinea pigs. *J. Physiol.* **399**, 13–32.

Coleman, H.A., McKinlay, D.M. & Parkington, H.C. (1995). Different mechanisms for the initiation of contraction in response to prostaglandin $F_{2\alpha}$ in myometrium during pregnancy in guinea pigs. *Proc. Aust. Physiol. Pharmacol. Soc.* **26**, 93P.

Deliconstantinos, G. & Fotiou, S. (1986). Effect of prostaglandins E_2 and $F_{2\alpha}$ on membrane calcium binding, Ca^{2+}/Mg^{2+}-ATPase activity and membrane fluidity in rat myometrial plasma membranes. *J. Endocrinol.* **110**, 395–404.

Downing, S.J. & Hollingsworth, M. (1988). Nifedipine kinetics in the rat and relationship between its serum concentrations and uterine cardiovascular effects. *Br. J. Pharmacol.* **95**, 23–32.

Edman, K.A.P. & Schild, H.O. (1962). The need for calcium in the contractile responses induced by acetylcholine and potassium in the uterus. *J. Physiol.* **161**, 424–441.

Fish, R.D., Sperti, G., Colucci, W.S. & Clapham, D.E. (1988). Phorbol ester increases the dihydropyridine-sensitive calcium conductance in a vascular smooth muscle cell line. *Circ. Res.* **62**, 1049–1054.

Furukawa, K., Tawada, Y. & Shigekawa, M. (1989). Protein kinase C activation stimulates plasma membrane Ca^{2+} pump in cultured vascular smooth muscle cells. *J. Biol. Chem.* **264**, 4844–4849.

Hart, J.D., Coleman, H.A. & Parkington, H.C. (1993). Prostaglandin $F_{2\alpha}$ and oxytocin activate a common calcium-permeable channel in uterine smooth muscle of guinea pigs. *Proc. Aust. Physiol. Pharmacol. Soc.* **24**, 130P.

Himpens, B., Kitazawa, T. & Somlyo, A.P. (1990). Agonist-dependent modulation of Ca^{2+} sensitivity in rabbit pulmonary artery smooth muscle. *Pflügers Arch.* **417**, 21–28.

Hirata, K., Kikuchi, A., Sasaki, T., Kuroda, S., Kaibuchi, K., Matsuura, Y., Seki, H., Saida, K. & Takai, Y. (1992). Involvement of rho p21 in the GTP-enhanced calcium ion sensitivity of smooth muscle contraction. *J. Biol. Chem.* **267**, 8719–8722.

Honoré, E., Martin, C., Mironneau, C. & Mironneau, J. (1989). An ATP-sensitive condutance in cultured smooth muscle cells from pregnant rat myometrium. *Am. J. Physiol.* **257**, C297–C305.

Inoue, R. & Isenberg, G. (1990). Acetylcholine activates nonselective cation channels in guinea pig ileum through a G protein. *Am. J. Physiol.* **258**, C1173–C1178.

Inoue, R., Kitamura, K. & Kuriyama, H. (1987). Acetylcholine activates single sodium channels in smooth muscle cells. *Pflügers Arch.* **410**, 69–74.

Jensen, P.E., Mulvany, M.J. & Aalkjaer, C. (1992). Endogenous and exogenous agonist-induced changes in the coupling between $[Ca^{2+}]_i$ and force in rat resistance arteries. *Pflügers. Arch.* **420**, 536–543.

Kamm, K.E. & Stull, J.T. (1989). The function of myosin and myosin light chain kinase phosphorylation in smooth muscle. *Annu. Rev. Physiol.* **51**, 299–313.

Katsuyama, H. & Morgan, K.G. (1993). Mechanisms of Ca^{2+}-independent contraction in single permeabilized ferret aorta cells. *Circ. Res.* **72**, 651–657.

Keirse, M.J.N.C. (1992). Inhibitors of prostaglandin synthesis for treatment of preterm labour. In *Prostaglandins and the Uterus* (Drife J.O. & Calder, A.A., eds), pp. 277–296. Springer-Verlag, London.

Loirand, G., Pacaud, P., Baron, A., Mironneau, C. & Mironneau, J. (1991). Large conductance calcium-activated non-selective cation channel in smooth muscle cells isolated from rat portal vein. *J. Physiol.* **437**, 461–475.

Marc, S., Leiber, D. & Harbon, S. (1986). Carbachol and oxytocin stimulate the generation of inositol phosphates in the guinea pig myometrium. *FEBS Lett.* **201**, 9–14.

Mironneau, C., Mironneau, J. & Savineau, J.P. (1984). Maintained contractions of rat uterine smooth muscle incubated in a Ca-free medium. *Br. J. Pharmacol.* **82**, 735–743.

Mironneau, J. (1974). Voltage clamp analysis of the ionic currents in uterine smooth muscle using the double sucrose gap method. *Pflügers Arch.* **352**, 197–210.

Mironneau, J. (1976). Effects of oxytocin on ionic currents underlying rhythmic activity and contraction in uterine smooth muscle. *Pflügers Arch.* **363**, 113–118.

Miyoshi, H., Urabe, T. & Fujiwara, A. (1991). Electrophysiological properties of membrane currents in single myometrial cells isolated from pregnant rats. *Pflügers Arch.* **419**, 386–393.

Murray, R.K. & Kotlikoff, M.I. (1991). Receptor-activated calcium influx in human airway smooth muscle cells. *J. Physiol.* **435**, 123–144.

Nakayama, S. & Brading, A.F. (1993). Evidence for multiple open states of the Ca^{2+} channels in smooth muscle cells isolated from the guinea pig detrusor. *J. Physiol.* **471**, 87–105.

Naranjo, D. & Brehm, P. (1993). Modal shifts in acetylcholine receptor channel gating confer subunit-dependent desensitization. *Science* **260**, 1811–1814.

Ninomiya, J.G. & Suzuki, H. (1983). Electrical responses of smooth muscle cells of the mouse uterus to adenosine triphosphate. *J. Physiol.* **342**, 499–515.

Nishimura, J. & van Breemen, C. (1989). Direct regulation of smooth muscle contractile elements by second messengers. *Biochem. Biophys. Res. Commun.* **163**,

929–935.

O'Donnell, M.E. & Owen, N.E. (1994). Regulation of ion pumps and carriers in vascular smooth muscle. *Physiol. Rev.* **74**, 683–721.

Ohya, Y. & Sperelakis, N. (1989). Fast Na^+ and slow Ca^{2+} channels in single uterine muscle cells from pregnant rats. *Am. J. Physiol.* **257**, C408–C412.

Oishi, K., Takano-Ohmuro, H., Minakawa-Matsuo, N., Suga, O., Karibe, H., Kohama, K. & Uchida, M.K. (1991). Oxytocin contracts rat uterine smooth muscle in Ca^{2+}-free medium without any phosphorylation of myosin light chain. *Biochem. Biophys. Res. Commun.* **176**, 122–128.

Oishi, K., Mita, M., Ono, T., Hashimoto, T. & Uchida, M.K. (1992). Protein kinase C-independent sensitization of contractile proteins to Ca^{2+} in alpha-toxin-permeabilized smooth muscle cells from the guinea pig stomach. *Br. J. Pharmacol.* **107**, 908–909.

Osa, T. & Taga, F. (1973). Electrophysiological comparison of the action of oxytocin and carbachol on pregnant mouse myometrium. *Jpn. J. Physiol.* **23**, 81–96.

Osa, T. & Kawarabayashi, T. (1977). Effects of ions and drugs on the plateau potential in the circular muscle of pregnant rat myometrium. *Jpn. J. Physiol.* **27**, 111–121.

Ruzycky, A.L. & Triggle, D.J. (1987). Effects of 17β-estradiol and progesterone on agonist-stimulated inositol phospholipid breakdown in uterine smooth muscle. *Eur. J. Pharmacol.* **141**, 33–40.

Ruzycky, A.L. & Crankshaw, D.J. (1988). Role of inositol phospholipid hydrolysis in the initiation of agonist-induced contractions of rat uterus:effects of domination by 17-beta-estradiol and progesterone. *Can. J. Physiol. Pharmacol.* **66**, 10–17.

Sakai, K., Yamaguchi, T., Morita, S. & Uchida, M. (1983). Agonist-induced contraction of rat myometrium in Ca-free solution containing Mn. *Gen. Pharmacol.* **14**, 391–400.

Sato, K., Leposavic, R., Publicover, N.G., Sanders, K.M. & Gerthoffer, W.T. (1994). Sensitization of the contractile system of canine colonic smooth muscle by agonists and phorbol ester. *J. Physiol.* **481**, 677–688.

Savineau, J.P., Mironneau, J. & Mironneau, C. (1988). Contractile properties of chemically skinned fibres from pregnant rat myometrium: existence of an internal Ca store. *Pflügers Arch.* **411**, 296–303.

Schrey, M.P., Cornford, P.A., Read, A.M. & Steer, P.J. (1988). A role for phosphoinositide hydrolysis in human uterine smooth muscle during parturition. *Am. J. Obstet. Gynecol.* **159**, 964–970.

Somlyo, A.V. & Somlyo, A.P. (1968). Electromechanical and pharmacomechanical coupling in vascular smooth muscle. *J. Pharmacol. Exp. Ther.* **159**, 129–145.

Somlyo, A.P. & Somlyo, A.V. (1994). Signal transduction and regulation in smooth muscle. *Nature* **372**, 231–236.

Vivaudou, M.B., Clapp, L.H., Walsh, J.V. & Singer, J.J. (1988). Regulation of one type of Ca^{2+} current in smooth muscle cells by diacylglycerol and acetylcholine. *FASEB J.* **2**, 2497–2504.

Word, R.A., Kamm, K.E., Stull, J.T. & Casey, M.L. (1990). Endothelin increases cytoplasmic calcium and myosin phosphorylation in human myometrium. *Am. J. Obstet. Gynecol.* **162**:1103–1108.

Zholos, A.V. & Bolton, T.B. (1994). G-protein control of voltage dependence as well as gating of muscarinic metabotropic channels in guinea pig ileum. *J. Physiol.* **478**, 195–202.

32

A Simple Mathematical Model of the Spontaneous Electrical Activity in a Single Smooth Muscle Myocyte

R. J. LANG
C. A. RATTRAY-WOOD
Department of Physiology,
Monash University,
Clayton, Victoria,
Australia

INTRODUCTION

Since the mid 1980s, the development of the techniques of recording single channel and whole-cell membrane currents has led to the identification and characterization of at least two voltage-activated Ca^{2+} channels and up to eight K^+-selective channels in a number of visceral and vascular smooth muscles (Bolton & Beech, 1992). Particular Ca^{2+} and K^+ channels have been distinguished by their conductances and kinetics of activation and inactivation, and also by the action of a number of 'specific' channel openers and blockers. For example, the two Ca^{2+} channel populations ('T' and 'L'-type) have been distinguished by their differing kinetic behaviour and by their respective sensitivity/insensitivity to dihydropyridine channel blockers/ activators (Aaronson *et al.*, 1988); the small and large conductance ('SK' and 'BK') Ca^{2+}-activated K^+ channels are distinguished by their relative sensitivity to apamin and charybdotoxin respectively; cromakalim-activated/ATP-sensitive K^+ channels are blocked by glibenclamide; voltage-activated transiently-opening K^+ channel currents(I_{Kt}) are selectively blocked by 4-aminopyridine (4-AP) (Vogalis & Lang, 1994) and delayed rectifier-type K^+ channel currents (I_{Kdel}) are blocked by relatively-high concentrations of tetraethylammonium (TEA), although in some smooth muscles I_{Kdel} is also reduced by 4-AP. Over the last 6 years, we have been characterizing, at both the single and whole-cell current level, the distinguishing properties of the membrane ionic channels in four visceral smooth muscles of the guinea pig:

SMOOTH MUSCLE EXCITATION
ISBN 0-12-112360-X

the ureter, taenia caeci, pulmonary artery and circular muscle of the proximal colon. We have found that all four smooth muscle types expressed 'L-type' Ca^{2+} and 'BK' K^+ channels; the ureter and proximal colon cells also expressed I_{Kt} channels, while I_{Kdel} channels were well expressed in cells from the proximal colon and pulmonary artery, but less so in the taenia caeci (Gow & Lang, 1989; Lang, 1989, 1990; Lang & Paul, 1991; Vogalis et al., 1993; Vogalis & Lang, 1994).

In this report, we present a simple mathematical model of the electrical activity of an idealised single smooth muscle cell which consists of (1), a membrane capacitance; (2), a voltage-activated Ca^{2+} conductance (g_{Ca}) which is inactivated by Ca^{2+} itself at an internal binding site; (3), a voltage-activated delayed rectifier K^+ conductance (g_{Kdel}); (4), a voltage- and Ca^{2+}-activated ('BK') K^+ conductance (g_{KCa}); and (v), a background 'leak' conductance (g_{leak}). Essential to this model is a feed-back mechanism by which Ca^{2+} accumulates in a submembrane space to decrease and increase g_{Ca} and g_{KCa}, respectively (Standen & Stanfield, 1982; Chay 1990). Rather than having mathematical descriptions of various Na^+:K^+ and Na^+:Ca^{2+} pumps or exchanger currents to describe the cell's capacity to buffer Ca^{2+}, we have simply assumed that the inner core of the cell has a relatively large apparent volume. Among many predictions, this model has revealed that (1), limiting the rate of Ca^{2+} diffusion from the submembrane compartment has profound effects on the generation of the whole-cell Ca^{2+} and 'BK' channel currents; (2), relatively small changes in the individual Ca^{2+} and K^+ conductances/currents can result in marked changes in the waveform of the action potentials generated; and (3), the reversal potential and relative amplitude of the 'leak' conductance can markedly affect the frequency and duration of spontaneously discharging action potentials. Some of these results have been presently previously in brief (Rattray-Wood & Lang, 1991).

METHODS

The Cell

The smooth muscle myocyte was assumed to consist of two cones placed base-to-base with a combined length of 200 μm and a maximum diameter of 12 μm. The surface area of the cell was set to be 5×10^{-5} cm^2, which gives a total membrane capacitance (C_m) of 50 pF per cell using a specific membrane capacitance of 1 μF cm^{-2}. The membrane was described by an equivalent circuit in which a capacitance is connected in parallel to a number of channel-mediated currents. The differential equation which described the membrane potential (V)(mV) is

$$\Delta V / \Delta t = -(I_{Ca} + I_{Kdel} + I_{KCa} + I_{leak}) / C_m$$

where I_{Ca}, I_{Kdel} and I_{KCa}, respectively, represent the time- and voltage-dependent whole-cell current flow through dihydropyridine-sensitive Ca^{2+} channels, 'delayed rectifier' K^+ channels and 'BK' channels.

I_{leak}

The background 'leak' current (I_{leak}), was modelled as the sum of any voltage- and time-independent channel currents across the cell membrane and described by

$$I_{leak} = g_{leak} (E_{leak} - V)$$

where g_{leak} is equal to the specific membrane conductance at the resting membrane potential (G_{leak}) multiplied by the cell surface area and E_{leak} is the equilibrium potential of I_{leak}. Typical values of g_{leak} used were 200–2000 pS per cell (equivalent to G_{leak} = 4–40 µS cm^{-2} or R_m = 25–250 kΩ cm^2) which gave rise to membrane time constants of 20–250 ms (Holman et al., 1990); E_{leak} was varied between −20 and −60 mV.

The movement of Ca²⁺

The cell was envisaged to have a submembrane compartment which had no significant buffering capacity and whose internal border acted as a semipermeable barrier to the diffusion of Ca^{2+}. The width of this submembrane compartment was assumed to be constant throughout the cell; both the plasma membrane and the intracellular diffusion barrier were assumed to be homogeneous. The rate of diffusion of Ca^{2+} ions across the submembrane barrier (CompLoss) was calculated to be a variable somewhat slower than the rate of Ca^{2+} diffusion through water (7×10^{-6} cm^2 s^{-1}). Internal to the submembrane space, the core compartment was assumed to contain myoplasmic Ca^{2+}-binding proteins which act as a high-capacity Ca^{2+} 'sink'. This was modelled by assigning the core compartment an apparent volume (APVOL) many times ($\times$ 1000–100000) greater than its physical volume (Standen & Stanfield, 1982). At the commencement of each simulation, the Ca^{2+} concentration in the core compartment ($[Ca^{2+}]_{core}$) and in the submembrane compartment ($[Ca^{2+}]_{sub}$) were assumed to be in equilibrium at 0.1 µM. The Ca^{2+} concentration external to the plasma membrane ($[Ca^{2+}]_{out}$) (2.5 mM) was assumed to be well-stirred and of infinite volume. Changes in $[Ca^{2+}]_{core}$ were therefore calculated according to the equation:

$$\Delta[Ca^{2+}]_{core} / \Delta t = [Ca^{2+}]_{sub} (CompLoss/SACC) (CV/APVOL)$$

where SACC and CV respectively represent the surface area and volume of the core compartment. This predicts a linear (rather than sigmoidal) relationship between Ca^{2+} influx and the rate of increase of both $[Ca^{2+}]_{sub}$ and $[Ca^{2+}]_{core}$. This is approximately true if $[Ca^{2+}]_{core}$ does not increase greatly over the time course of a simulation, as was the case in all simulations described in this paper.

I_{Ca}

The rise time of the whole-cell Ca^{2+} channel currents (I_{Ca}) was modelled with a standard Hodgkin–Huxley activation kinetic process ('d'), using activation curves obtained experimentally. The decay of I_{Ca}, however, was modelled as having two inactivation kinetic processes: (1) f, consisting of two voltage- and time-dependent inactivation steps (called f_{fast} and f_{slow}) with time constants τ_{Fast} and τ_{slow} ; and (2), h_{Ca}, dependent on Ca^{2+} binding to an internal site. Ca^{2+} binds to this site with a variable equlibrium dissociation constant (K_{Ca}) which was varied (0.01–10 μM) (Standen & Stanfield; 1982). I_{Ca} was therefore described by

$$I_{Ca} = g_{Ca}\, dfh_{Ca}\,(\,V - E_{Ca/K})$$

where $E_{Ca/K}$ was the experimentally observed reversal potential of I_{Ca} (-40 to -60 mV), due, in part, to the outward flow of K^+ through these Ca^{2+} channels at potentials positive of $E_{Ca/K}$. Thus

$$\Delta d\,/\,\Delta t = \alpha_{Ca^{2+}}(\,1 - d\,) - d\beta_{Ca^{2+}}$$

where
$$\alpha_{Ca^{2+}} = 13(\,V + 15\,)\,/\,(\,1 - \exp\{\,-(V + 15)/3\})$$
$$\beta_{Ca^{2+}} = 31\exp(\,-0.04(\,V + 15\,)).$$

In addition,
$$f = f_{fast}\,f_{slow}$$

where
$$\Delta f_{fast}/\,\Delta t = \alpha_{fast}(\,1 - f_{fast}\,) - \beta_{fast}f_{fast}$$
$$\Delta f_{slow}\,/\,\Delta t = \alpha_{slow}(\,1 - f_{slow}\,) - \beta_{slow}f_{slow}$$
$$\alpha_{fast} = K_{inact}\,/\,\tau_{fast}$$
$$\beta_{fast} = (\,1 - K_{inact}\,)\,/\,\tau_{fast}$$
$$\alpha_{slow} = K_{inact}\,/\,\tau_{slow}$$
$$\beta_{slow} = (\,1 - K_{inact}\,)/\,\tau_{slow}$$
$$K_{inact} = 1\,/\,(\,1 + \exp\{(V + 40.5\,)\,/\,13.1\,\}).$$

Finally,
$$h_{Ca} = 1\,/\,(\,(\,1 + [Ca^{2+}]_{sub}\,)\,/\,K_{Ca}\,).$$

I_{Kdel}

The time course of the activation of I_{Kdel} at various potentials (between -60 and $+40$ mV) was simultaneously fitted to exponential equations raised to the second power, using standard Hodgkin & Huxley analysis (Volk *et al.*,

1991), such that

$$I_{Kdel} = g_{Kdel} n^2 (V - E_K)$$

where $$\Delta n / \Delta t = a_{Kdel} (1 - n) - \beta_{Kdel} n$$

and $$\alpha_{Kdel} = -1.26(V + 8.821) / (\exp(-0.386(V + 8.821)) - 1)$$
$$\beta_{Kdel} = 17.02 \exp(-0.022(V + 60)).$$

I_{KCa}

Whole-cell I_{KCa} currents were calculated from voltage- and Ca^{2+}-dependent probability of opening curves (h_{KCa}) according to

$$I_{KCa} = g_{KCa} h_{KCa} (V - E_K).$$

These h_{KCa} curves were Boltzmann equations of the form

$$h_{KCa} = 1 / (1 + \exp((K_n - V)/ S_{KCa}))$$

where $$K_n = K_{VCa} [Ca^{2+}]_{sub} + 119.44$$

represents the potential of half-maximal activation of a single 'BK' channel at any given $[Ca^{2+}]_{sub}$; K_{VCa} reflects the shift of these activation curves per tenfold change in $[Ca^{2+}]_{sub}$. S_{KCa} is a slope factor, which varied according to

$$S_{KCa} = 14.372 [Ca^{2+}]_{sub} + 11.566.$$

RESULTS

Simulations of I_{Ca}, I_{Kdel} and I_{KCa}

The mathematical descriptions of I_{Ca}, I_{Kdel} and I_{KCa} were first used to generate whole-cell currents in our idealized cell that were realistic simulations of the currents recorded in single cells of the guinea pig ureter, taenia caeci, proximal colon and pulmonary artery, as well as many other smooth muscles. Figure 1A illustrates typical whole-cell I_{Ca} generated by the model when the half-maximal voltage for d was set at $-15\,mV$ and the equilibrium dissociation constant (K_{Ca}) for h_{Ca} varied between 0.1 and 10 μM. These changes in K_{Ca} were meant to estimate the changes in I_{Ca} amplitude (without allowing for any changes of surface charge effects!) when other divalent ions (Ba^{2+} or Sr^{2+}) with lower affinities for the inactivation binding site were substituted for Ca^{2+}. It can be seen in Figure 1B that the current-voltage (I–V) relationships generated by these simulations resemble the I–V curves recorded experimentally in a number of smooth muscles (Aaronson et al., 1988; Lang, 1990; Lang & Paul, 1991). The time course of I_{Ca} at different K_{Ca}

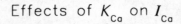

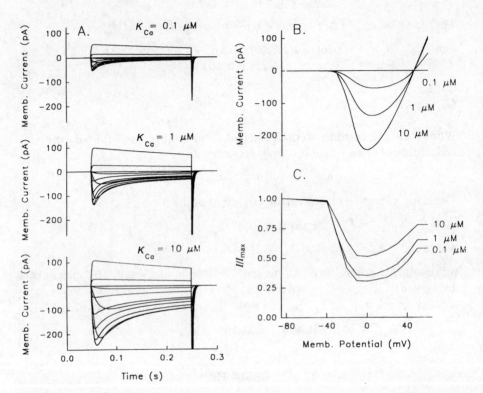

Figure 1 A, Simulated I_{Ca} currents recorded upon depolarization to every 10 mV between −40 and +60 mV with K_{Ca} of 0.1, 1 and 10 µM; holding potential −80 mV. B, Predicted *I–V* relationships of I_{Ca} using these three values of K_{Ca}. C, Predicted voltage dependence of the relative inactivation of a test I_{Ca} (at 0 mV), expressed as a fraction of its value in the absence of a conditioning depolarisation (I/I_{max}), plotted against conditioning pulse amplitude.

could also be adjusted to match published data by varying the volume of the submembrane space or *CompLoss*. The adjustments of these parameters were best made using classical twinpulse experimental protocols, using depolarizing pulses of varying amplitudes and intervals (Yamamoto *et al.*, 1989; Matsuda *et al.*, 1990). For example, in Figure 1C the submembrane volume, *CompLoss* and K_{Ca} were adjusted until the relative inactivation (I/I_{max}) of the second of a pair of pulses (0.1 s duration and 50 ms apart) was maximum near the peak of the *I–V* curve and increased when K_{Ca} was reduced, resembling similar previously published data (Yamamoto *et al.*, 1989; Matsuda *et al.*, 1990).

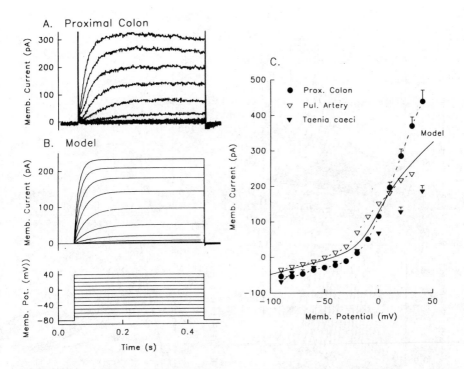

Figure 2 Comparison of the whole-cell I_{Kdel} in a single cell of the circular muscle of the guinea pig proximal colon (A). with the model-generated I_{Kdel} (B, upper panel) every 10 mV between −70 and +40 mV (B, lower panel) holding potential −80 mV. C, Comparison of the predicted I–V plot of I_{Kdel} with those obtained from single cells of the guinea pig proximal colon, taenia caeci and pulmonary artery.

Whole-cell I_{Kdel} were recorded every 10 mV between −80 and +40 mV in single cells of the proximal colon ($n = 7$), pulmonary artery ($n = 3$) and taenia caeci ($n = 3$) in the presence of a Ca^{2+}-entry blocker (Cd^{2+} or nifedipine), 2 µM TEA and 2-5 mM 4-AP (Vogalis *et al.*, 1993). In Figure 2A, it can be seen that the time course of the model-generated whole-cell I_{Kdel} was similar to the whole-cell I_{Kdel} recorded in a single cell of the proximal colon. There was also good agreement between the I–V relationship of the model-generated I_{Kdel} and the I–V plots of I_{Kdel} measured in the proximal colon, taenia caeci and pulmonary artery (Figure 2B).

'BK' channels recorded in membrane patches excised from many smooth muscles are sensitive to both membrane depolarization and the internal concentration of Ca^{2+} ($[Ca^{2+}]_i$); the voltage range of activation at a particular $[Ca^{2+}]_i$ and the shift of this voltage range with a $\Delta [Ca^{2+}]_i$, however, vary considerably. For example, the $[Ca^{2+}]_i$ which gave a membrane potential of

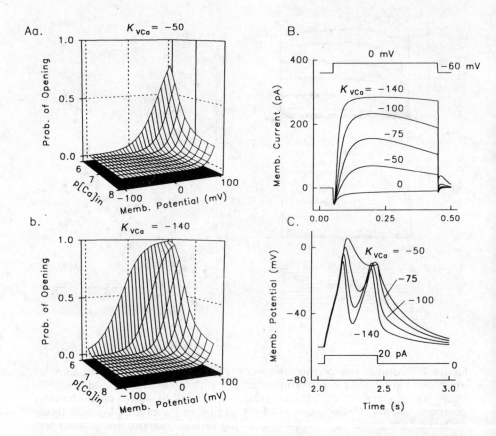

Figure 3 A, Three-dimensional plots of the probability of opening for 'BK' channels against membrane potential and internal Ca^{2+} concentration (p[Ca]$_{in}$), with K_{VCa} values of -50 (Aa. and -140 (Ab). mV. B, Whole-cell I_{KCa} currents (at 0 mV). predicted when K_{VCa} was varied between -50 and -140 mV, superimposed on I_{Ca}. C, Predicted effects of varying K_{VCa} on the repolarizing phase of an action potential triggered with a depolarizing current of 20 pA. In B and C, I_{Ca} was held constant and the holding potential was -60 mV.

half-maximal activation at 0 mV was 0.5 µM, 0.75–1 µM and 1 µM respectively for 'BK' channels excised from cells of the rabbit jejunum (Benham *et al.*, 1986), dog colon (Carl & Sanders, 1989) and guinea pig taenia caeci (Hu *et al.*, 1989; McPhee & Lang, 1994). In addition, these curves shifted, respectively 30–60, 134 and 25 mV with a tenfold $\Delta [Ca^{2+}]_i$.

In Figure 3A, three-dimensional curves of probability of 'BK' channel opening (h_{KCa}) against both membrane potential and $[Ca^{2+}]_i$ (p[Ca]$_{in}$) are plotted, using K_{VCa} values of -50 (Figure 3Aa) and -140 (Figure 3Ab) mV. These curves mimic published data reasonably well, reflecting both the differing leftward shifts and decrease in the slope of these h_{KCa} curves as $[Ca^{2+}]_i$ increases. As K_{VCa} increased, the amplitude of the whole-cell I_{KCa}, triggered under voltage clamp and assuming a constant I_{Ca}, also increased (Figure 3B). Such an increasing I_{KCa} induced more rapid repolarization of the action potentials triggered under simulated current clamp (Figure 3C).

Simulations of 'plateau-like' action potentials

Judicious adjustments of the parameters in our model allowed us to generate spontaneous action potentials of varying waveforms in the idealized myocyte.

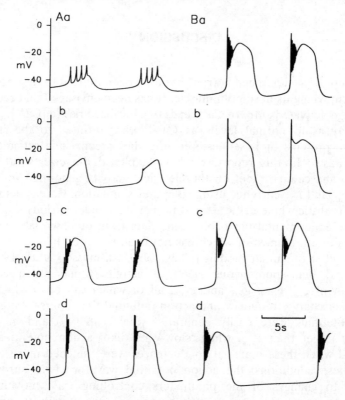

Figure 4 A, Various spontaneous action potential waveforms could be generated by varying the width of the submembrane space (0.2–1.2 μm) and the *CompLoss* (3000–40 000), keeping maximal g_{Ca}, g_{KCa}, g_{Kdel} and g_{leak} constant at 1800, 480, 540 and 15 nS per cell respectively. B, Particular aspects of the time course or frequency of simulated 'slow-waves' (Ba) could be modified by selectively changing g_{KCa} (decreased by 25%) (Bb), g_{Kdel} (decreased by 90%) (Bc) and g_{leak} (increased by 30%) (Bd).

It proved easy to generate 'spike-like' action potentials using relatively large values of g_{Ca} and g_{KCa} or g_{Kdel} (compared with g_{leak}) (data not shown). 'Slow wave-like' action potentials could also be generated by decreasing these membrane conductances relative to g_{leak} and by allowing Ca^{2+} to accumulate in the submembrane space. In Figure 4Aa–d, these four spontaneous waveforms were generated by changing the submembrane volume and/or the *CompLoss*, but keeping g_{Ca}, g_{KCa}, g_{Kdel} and g_{leak} constant. In contrast, the effects of systematically changing the membrane conductances on a spontaneous 'slow wave' simulation (Figure 4Ba) are illustrated in Figure 4B where g_{KCa} (Figure 4Bb), g_{Kdel} (Figure 4Bc) were decreased 25 and 90% respectively, and g_{leak}(Figure 4Bd) increased 30%.

DISCUSSION

The concept of a 'superficial barrier' has long been utilized to describe Ca^{2+} economy/movements in smooth muscle. It has been envisaged that receptor- and voltage-activated entry of Ca^{2+} leads to a localized rise in $[Ca^{2+}]_{sub}$ which slowly returns to normal levels as Ca^{2+} either diffuses to the internal contractile proteins or is sequestered into the sarcoplasmic reticulum via Ca^{2+} ATPases. In this report, we have explored the effects of such a submembrane compartment on the electrical activity generated by whole-cell I_{Ca}, I_{Kdel} and I_{KCa} currents, using computer simulation. Care was taken to generate realistic whole-cell Ca^{2+} and K^+ currents under various single- and twin-pulse experimental protocols, using data from our own laboratory or from the literature, most of which has not been reviewed here. In common with a number of similar models (Chay, 1990; Rasmusson *et al.*, 1990), we have found that spontaneous electrical activity represents a complex interaction of g_{Ca}, g_{Kdel}, g_{leak} and g_{KCa}, all of which can be modulated to influence discharge frequency and action potential time course. 'Spike-like' action potentials were easily generated when g_{Ca}, g_{Kdel} and g_{KCa} were relatively larger than g_{leak}, while 'slow-wave like' action potentials were generated when these maximal conductances were matched more equally. Under these conditions, the action potential waveform was surprisingly sensitive to changes of the parameters controlling Ca^{2+} movement, a phenomenon we had not previously suspected. Our integrative approach using computer simulations of characterized membrane channel currents now allows us to relate observed membrane electrical events with measured changes in $[Ca^{2+}]_i$, and, therefore, muscle contraction. We intend to extend our model by including: (1), mathematical descriptions of K^+/Na^+ and Ca^{2+} pumps/exchangers on both the plasmalemmal and sarcolemmal membranes;

(2), receptor- and Ca^{2+}-activated release mechanisms of stored Ca^{2+}; and by (3), connecting our cell to a syncytium with similar/graded electrical properties and additional internal and extracellular compartments/clefts. In this way, we hope to describe accurately the electrical activity recorded in intact smooth muscles.

ACKNOWLEDGEMENTS

This work was supported by the N.H. and M.R.C. (Australia)

REFERENCES

Aaronson P.I., Bolton T.B., Lang R.J. & MacKenzie I. (1988) Calcium currents in single isolated smooth muscle cells from the rabbit ear artery in normal-calcium and high-barium solutions. *J. Physiol.* **405**, 57–75

Benham C.D., Bolton T.B., Lang R.J. & Takewaki T. (1986). Calcium-activated potassium channels in single dispersed smooth muscles cells of rabbit jejunum and guinea pig mesenteric artery. *J. Physiol.* **371**, 45–67

Bolton T.B. & Beech D.J. (1992). Smooth muscle potassium channels: their electrophysiology and function. In *Frontiers in Pharmacology & Therapeutics: Potassium Channel Modulators: Pharmacological Molecular and Clinical Aspects.* (Weston A.H. & Hamilton T.C. eds). Blackwell Scientific Publications, Oxford.

Carl A. & Sanders K.M. (1989). Ca^{2+}-activated K channels of canine colonic myocytes. *Am. J. Physiol.* **257**, C470–C480

Chay T.R. (1990). Effect of compartmentalised Ca^{2+} ions on electrical bursting activity of pancreatic β-cells. *Am. J. Physiol.* **258**, C955–C965

Gow R.M. & Lang R.J. (1989). Division of the K^+ current in single cells from the guinea pig pulmonary artery into three components. *Neurosci. Let. Suppl.* **34**, S87

Holman M.E., Neild T.O. & Lang R.J. (1990). On the passive properties of smooth muscle. In Frontiers in Smooth Muscle Research, Emil Bozler International Symposium. *Prog. Clin. Biol. Res.* **327**, 379-398

Hu S.L., Yamamoto Y. & Kao C.Y. (1989). The Ca^{2+}-activated K^+ channel and its functional roles in smooth muscle cells of the guinea pig taenia coli. *J. Gen. Physiol.* **94**, 833–847

Lang R.J. (1989). Identification of the major membrane currents in freshly dispersed single smooth muscle cells of guinea pig ureter. *J. Physiol.* **412**, 375–395

Lang R.J. (1990). The whole-cell Ca^{2+}-channel current in single smooth muscle cells of the guinea pig ureter. *J. Physiol.* **423**, 453–473

Lang R.J. & Paul R.J. (1991). Effects of 2,3-butanedione monoxime on whole-cell Ca^{2+} channel currents in single cells of the guinea pig taenia caeci. *J. Physiol.* **433**, 1–24

Matsuda J.J., Volk K.A. & Shibata E.F. (1990). Calcium currents in isolated rabbit coronary arterial smooth muscle myocytes. *J. Physiol.* **427**, 657–680

McPhee G.J. & Lang R.J. (1994). Effects of nitric oxide donors, nitrosocysteine and sodium nitroprusside, on the activity of the Ca^{2+}-activated K^+ ('B-K'). channels in the guinea pig taenia caeci. *Aust. Physiol. and Pharmacol. Soc.* **25**, 214P

Rasmusson R.L., Clark J.W., Giles W.R., Shibata E.F. & Campbell D.L. (1990). A mathematical model of a bullfrog pacemaker cell. *Am. J. Physiol.* **259**, H352–H369

Rattray-Wood C.A. & Lang R.J. (1991). A mathematical model of a single smooth muscle cell showing spontaneous electrical activity. *Aust. Physiol. and Pharmacol. Soc.* **22**, 173P

Standen N.B. & Stanfield P.R. (1982). A binding site model for calcium channel inactivation that depends on calcium entry. *Proc. Roy. Soc. (Lond.) Ser. B* **217**, 101–110

Vogalis F. & Lang R.J. (1994). Identification of single transiently-opening ('A-type'). K^+ channels in guinea pig colonic myocytes. *Pflügers Arch.* **429**, 160–164

Vogalis F., Lang R.J., Bywater R.A.R. & Taylor G.S. (1993). Voltage-gated ionic currents in smooth muscle cells of the guinea pig proximal colon. *Am. J. Physiol.* **264**, C527–C536

Volk K.A., Matsuda J.J. & Shibata E.F. (1991). A voltage-dependent potassium current in rabbit coronary artery smooth muscle cells. *J. Physiol.* **439**, 751–768

Yamamoto Y., Hu S.L & Kao C.Y. (1989). Inward current in single smooth muscle cells of the guinea pig taenia coli *J. Gen. Physiol.* **93**, 521–550

33

The Relationship between the Electrophysiological Properties of Lower Urinary Tract Smooth Muscles and their Function *in vivo*

A. F. BRADING
N. TERAMOTO
S. NAKAYAMA
N. BRAMICH
R. INOUE
K. FUJII
J. MOSTWIN

Department of Pharmacology,
University of Oxford,
Oxford, UK

1. The electrophysiological properties of guinea pig detrusor smooth muscle are described, including the spontaneous electrical activity, and the effects of channel blocking drugs. The cells possess L type Ca channels and several types of K channel.
2. The L-type Ca channels have at least two open states, the normal one being rapidly inactivating, but large depolarizations induce long channel openings which may play a role in allowing influx of calcium ions during agonist activation.
3. Different K channels are involved in the spike repolarization and after-hyperpolarization. K-channel activating drugs suppress spontaneous spike activity.
4. The detrusor smooth muscles are poorly coupled electrically and respond to two excitatory transmitters, (acetylcholine and ATP) using different cellular mechanisms, and with activation of different receptor-operated channels.
5. Smooth muscle from the pig urethra shows little sign of any voltage sensitive Ca channel activity. No spikes are produced, but spontaneous

hyper-polarizations are seen. The cells possess at least three types of K channel, two of which are both voltage dependent and exquisitely sensitive to intracellular Ca ions. The third is activated by K^+-channel activating drugs. At present little is known of the cellular mechanisms involved in the neuronal control of urethral tone.

The enormous diversity apparent in the properties and behaviours of smooth muscles isolated from different organs reflect the different roles that they are required to play to allow the organs to perform their various functions. In the urinary tract this is well displayed, as the smooth muscles within the walls of the tract show widely different properties depending on their location. In the bladder wall the smooth muscles are adapted and arranged to give the wall great compliance, and allow filling of the bladder at low pressure, with the concomitant rearrangement and thinning of the muscle bundles (Uvelius & Gabella, 1980). The smooth muscle also has to be able to contract with a sustained and synchronous contraction until the bladder is emptied. Conversely, the smooth muscles of the urethra must produce continuous tone most of the time, to ensure that the lumen is occluded and urine does not leak out. This must occur not only when the bladder is filling, but also when intra-abdominal pressure rises, such as during exercise, coughing and sneezing. At the appropriate time the urethral smooth muscle must relax to allow micturition to take place. If these normal patterns of smooth muscle behaviour are altered, for instance if the bladder smooth muscle contracts inappropriately, or the urethral smooth muscle does not maintain tone, urinary incontinence can result.

Investigations on the electrical properties of the smooth muscles that have been undertaken by members of the Oxford Continence Group over the last decade will be discussed within the framework of their functional significance. The work has been strongly influenced by the insight gained into the electrical properties of smooth muscle by Edith Bülbring and Tadao Tomita, and our group has been very fortunate to have had the interest and support of Professor Bülbring during her last years, and of having the active involvement of Professor Tomita, who spent a year working with the group.

METHODS

Smooth muscle was obtained from guinea pigs and pigs. Most of the pig tissues were obtained from Landrace or Large-White/Landrace crosses killed at a local abattoir; some was from Göttingen or Yucatan mini-pigs after terminal anaesthesia. Smooth muscle from the bladder wall (detrusor) was dissected after removal of the urothelium. For experiments with intact tissue, strips of smooth muscle were dissected following the direction of muscle bundles as viewed under a binocular microscope. Isolated myocytes were prepared from detrusor smooth muscle and from smooth muscle dissected from the proximal urethral wall. Enzymatic digestion was carried out either in Ca^{2+}-free solution using collagenase and pronase (Inoue & Brading, 1990; Nakayama & Brading, 1993a), or using papein (Clapp & Gurney, 1991).

Electrophysiological methods included conventional microelectrode recordings, double-sucrose gap recordings, whole-cell voltage clamp, and single channel recording using patch-clamp techniques, under various ionic conditions.

Most experiments on tissue strips were carried out using a modified Krebs' solution of the following composition (in mM) NaCl 120, KCl 5.9, $NaHCO_3$ 15.4, $MgCl_2$ 1.2, NaH_2PO_4 1, $CaCl_2$ 2.5, glucose 11, equilibrated with 97% O_2, 3% CO_2. The bath and pipette solutions for the patch-clamp experiments are given in the figure legends. For microelectrode studies contractile activity was abolished either by addition of 12 g sucrose per 100 ml solution, or by addition of 10^{-7}M nifedipine.

RESULTS AND DISCUSSION

Properties of the detrusor

Detrusor smooth muscle shows spontaneous electrical and mechanical activity. Microelectrode recordings from strips of guinea pig detrusor show spikes with a rather symmetrical rising and falling phase, followed by an after hyperpolarization (Figure 1; Mostwin, 1986). Spikes are unaffected by tetrodotoxin and blocked by L-type Ca channel blockers. The falling phase of the spike and the after-hyperpolarization are differentially affected by K channel blockers. Apamin (10^{-7}M) and 4-aminopyridine 4-AP (5×10^{-3}M) had no measurable effect on the rate of repolarization of the spikes, tetraethylammonium (TEA) (10^{-2}M) and quinidine (10^{-4}M) caused prolongation of the falling phase, and procaine (5×10^{-3}M) prolonged the falling phase by more than tenfold. At the above concentrations, procaine and apamin completely eliminated the after-hyperpolarization, 4-AP and TEA had little effect and quinidine reduced it (Fujii et al., 1990). All of the K-channel blockers tested can enhance the electrical and spontaneous mechanical activity in the guinea pig detrusor (Fujii et al., 1990), and K-channel opening drugs such as cromakalim blocked activity (Foster et al., 1989). These results strongly suggest that more than one type of K channel is present in guinea pig detrusor, and that K-channel modulation is a potential mechanism for affecting the behaviour of the bladder.

The spontaneous frequency of the spikes varies between about 6 and 30 spikes min^{-1}, and they often occur in bursts with quiescent intervals.

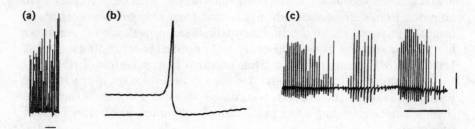

Figure 1 Spontaneous electrical and mechanical activity recorded from strips of guinea pig detrusor smooth muscle. (a) Mechanical activity: note variable sized contractions, and lack of fused tetanic activity; time bar 3 min. (b) Single spike showing after-hyperpolarization; time bar 0.1 s. (c) Spontaneous electrical activity: note nonuniform amplitude of the spikes; time bar 1 s, voltage bar 20 mV.

Mechanical activity recorded in separate strips usually consists of transient phasic contractions randomly variable in size, arising from and falling back to the baseline, and only occurring at a frequency of a few contraction per minute (Figure 1). Tetanic contractions do not occur in normal detrusor. Although we have not been able to correlate tension and electrical activity in the same strip the evidence strongly suggests that spikes recorded in a single cell do not correspond to the contractions in the whole strip. We postulate that the spikes do not occur synchronously in all the cells in a strip, and that the size of the contractions depends on the number of cells synchronously activated at any instant in time. A common occurrence with microelectrodes is the recording of small amplitude spikes which suggest that electrical activity does not propagate uniformly through the strip (Figure 1). Poor electrical continuity between detrusor cells is indicated by several other pieces of evidence. Extracellular impedance measurements carried out by Brading et al. (1989) show that the frequency-dependent impedance, which probably reflects the coupling pathways between cells, is considerably higher in guinea pig detrusor than in smooth muscles dissected from the gut. Double-sucrose gap recordings (Fujii, 1988) proved more difficult in guinea pig detrusor (and impossible in normal pig detrusor) than in other smooth muscles, and although activation of the nodal cells was possible, clear-cut action potentials were rarely recorded, again suggesting poor synchrony of the spikes in the nodes. N. Bramich (personal communication) recording with two microelectrodes positioned 30–40 μm apart in the axial direction has shown by direct injection of current into one cell and recording in the other that in the majority of cell pairs tested no electrical coupling existed, although activation of the intrinsic nerves initiated synchronous excitatory junction potentials (Figure 2).

Spontaneous activity combined with poor electrical coupling between the cells in the bladder wall is probably of considerable functional significance. *In situ*, the normal bladder is never a floppy bag, and during filling bladders take up the minimum surface area/volume ratio available to them anatomically because it is only in this condition that an intravesical pressure rise can occur

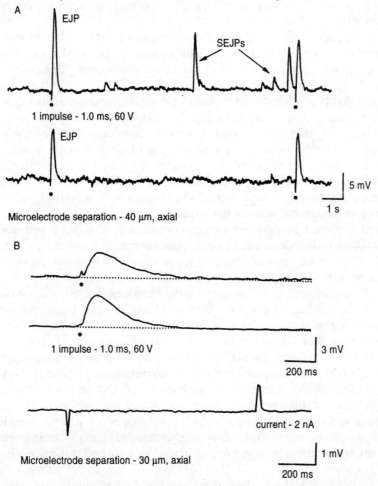

Figure 2 Microelectrode recordings obtained simultaneously from two cells of the same muscle strip in the presence of nifedipine to block action potentials. Intrinsic nerves were stimulated at the dots. A, Spontaneous excitatory junction potentials (SEJPs) occurring in the upper trace were not recorded in a cell 40 μm distant axially, although transmural nerve stimulation elicited simultaneous excitatory junction potentials (EJPs). B, Upper traces, simultaneous EJPs recorded in a pair of cells. Lower trace, voltage response from the upper cell in response to injection of current (2 nA for 1 s) in the lower cell. No evidence of electrical continuity was seen between these cells.

when the bladder wall contracts. Spontaneous electrical and mechanical activity of the individual cells will allow them to adjust their length to achieve this. This spontaneous adjustment of the bladder wall dimensions must, however, occur with the bladder wall remaining compliant, and without any increase in overall tone. This is achieved by poor electrical coupling which allows the cells to behave as individuals, or at most with limited interactions between them.

One frequently occurring clinical abnormality is that of bladder instability, a condition commonly seen in men with prostatic hypertrophy, and mimicked in animal models by partial bladder outlet obstruction (Speakman *et al.*, 1987). In unstable bladders the intravesical pressure rises spontaneously and uncontrollably, leading to urgency and often incontinence. Strips of detrusor smooth muscle from these bladders show spontaneous tetanic activity, and behave as if they have good electrical coupling. Double-sucrose gap recordings can be made from unstable pig bladder smooth muscle, again suggesting good coupling. We believe that the unstable contractions in the whole bladder arise because a focus of activity can spread and produce synchronous myogenic activation of the bladder wall, something that cannot happen in the normal bladder (Brading & Turner, 1994).

In the normal bladder emptying requires a synchronous and sustained contraction of the detrusor. In some animals which use urine for territorial marking, a mechanism is required to produce brief squirts of urine. The detrusor is activated through the parasympathetic nervous system, and is densely innervated by the post-synaptic neurones in this system. Detailed anatomical studies of the rat detrusor (Gabella, 1995) have shown that probably more than one close junction is made by a varicosity with each smooth muscle cell. Bramich has shown that spontaneous junction potentials can be recorded from the majority of cells in the guinea pig detrusor when muscle action potentials are eliminated with nifedipine (Figure 2). This dense innervation allows synchronous activation of the smooth muscle cells throughout the bladder wall. Since the early demonstration (Langely & Anderson, 1895) of atropine-resistant responses of animal bladders to parasympathetic nerve stimulation, numerous investigations have been made into the transmitters involved in this innervation (for references see Brading, 1987).

We have shown (Fujii, 1988) that transmural stimulation of detrusor strips elicits excitatory junction potentials that are noncholinergic, and presumably mediated by ATP since they were abolished by desensitization of the P_{2X} purinoceptors by α, β-methylene ATP, while atropine had no effect. Muscarinic agonists, when applied to strips, caused a slowly developing increase in the frequency of the spontaneous action potentials, with little change in the membrane potential. In other species muscarinic agonists also trigger significant depolarization. Detrusor smooth muscle myocytes from guinea pig, pig, rabbit and man (Inoue & Brading, 1990, 1991) develop fast inactivating inward currents on rapid application of ATP, suggesting that the receptors are probably directly coupled cationic ion channels, whereas muscarinic agonists cause predominantly activation of a delayed outward current, probably through Ca-activated K-channels (Figure 3).

It has been shown that muscarinic receptor activation in the guinea pig bladder leads to release of stored Ca (Mostwin, 1985) through synthesis of IP_3 (Iacovou et al., 1990). Functionally, these two mechanisms (excitatory junction potentials leading to rapid initiation of spikes and intracellular stored Ca release) could mediate the rapid contractions needed for fast expulsion of urine, and also the more sustained contraction needed for bladder emptying. It is interesting to note that atropine-resistant contractions are not seen in normal human bladder, although it clearly possesses receptors and channels activated by ATP. There is some evidence that in unstable human bladders some degree of atropine resistance is present.

We have studied the voltage-sensitive Ca channels in guinea pig detrusor in some detail (Nakayama & Brading, 1993a,b). These have the typical characteristics of L type Ca channels, and are responsible for the upstroke of the action potentials. The channels have been found to have some unusual properties. The normal activation by depolarization induces an open state of

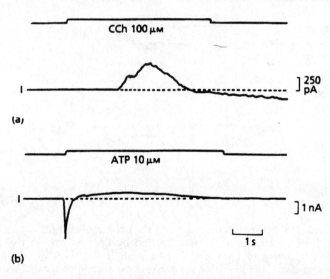

Figure 3 Current recordings of the response of isolated guinea pig detrusor smooth muscle cells to rapid application of 10 μM ATP and 100 μM carbachol. Whole-cell voltage-clamp, quasi-physiological conditions. The drugs were applied by a concentration jump protocol. Note instant, and rapidly inactivating inward current in response to ATP but delayed outward current slowly declining and converting to an inward current in the presence of carbachol.

the channels that undergoes Ca-dependent and voltage-dependent inactivation, and which deactivates rapidly on repolarization. This behaviour is commonly seen in L-type Ca channels, and is the dominant channel transition during the normal action potential. Prolonged depolarization however, leads to another transition into an open state with a longer dwell time, which undergoes no voltage-sensitive inactivation, and which deactivates slowly on repolarization (Figure 4.). In the normal action potentials, channel behaviour will limit Ca entry during the spike, but under conditions of more prolonged depolarization (such as will occur during agonist activation), there is a progressive transition of the channels into the long open state, which will allow significant amounts of Ca to enter the cell down its electrochemical gradient. This mechanism could be important for development of the sustained contractions that are needed for bladder emptying.

PROPERTIES OF THE URETHRA

Urethral smooth muscle is more difficult to obtain and we have confined our studies largely to the pig urethra. Studies on strips of smooth muscle

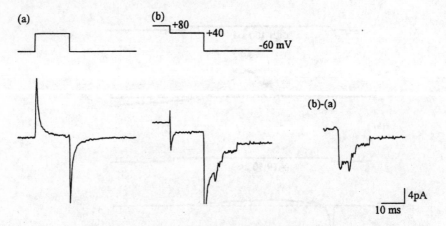

Figure 4 Cell-attached patch recording of Ca^{2+} channel currents in an isolated guinea pig detrusor myocyte. Current carried by Ba^{2+} (50 mM in the pipette). The cell was superfused with a Ca^{2+}-free high K solution. In (a) the patch membrane was depolarized with a simple test potential (+40 mV, 20 ms). In (b) the membrane was depolarized to +80 mV for 5 s before the test potential (only last 20 ms of conditioning step shown). (b)-(a). The capacitative surge in (a) was subtracted from (b) for the repolarizing step. Note the tail currents in (b)-(a) are hidden within the capacitative surge, whereas after the conditioning depolarization, slow switch-off of single channels can be seen during the large tail current.

dissected in the circular direction develop varying degrees of spontaneous tone, the highest amount being a few centimetres from the bladder neck. Smooth muscle strips dissected proximally and distally from here have progressively less spontaneous tone. The smooth muscle is multiply innervated, having cholinergic and adrenergic excitatory innervation and a dual inhibitory innervation, one using NO and the other an unknown transmitter (Bridgewater *et al.*, 1993). The adrenergic innervation is most highly developed close to the bladder neck in the proximal urethra, where the spontaneous tone is low, and declines in parallel with the rise in spontaneous tone more distally.

Extensive examination of the properties of smooth muscle cells isolated from the more proximal urethra, where the spontaneous tone is not well developed, is being carried out by N.T. Again, some interesting properties have beeen revealed. The isolated cells have a membrane potential of about

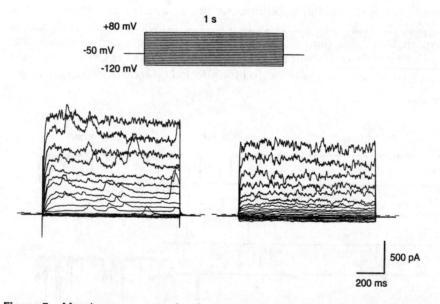

Figure 5   Membrane currents in pig urethra recorded in the whole-cell mode at a holding potential of $-50\,\text{mV}$. Quasi-physiological conditions, with extracellular Krebs' solution (Ca^{2+} 2.0 mM) and patch electrodes containing 140 mM K^+, 2 mM Mg^{2+}, 2 mM ATP, buffered to pH 7.4 with HEPES/Tris. The pipette solution in the left-hand panel contained 50 μM EGTA. In the right-hand panel the pipette contained 500 μM EGTA. Note that there is no inward current in these cells. Larger outward currents with superimposed spontaneous transient outward currents are seen in the cell on the left, in which the cellular Ca^{2+} is only weakly buffered.

−40 mV. If they are held at −50 mV under quasi-physiological conditions, and stepped to more positive potentials, a sustained outward current is seen, with little sign of any transient outward current or of any transient inward current (Figure 5). With little buffering of intracellular Ca^{2+}, spontaneous transient outward currents (STOCS) are superimposed randomly. Even when K channels are blocked with intracellular Cs, there is little evidence of significant voltage-dependent inward current in these cells. Prolonged recordings in current-clamp mode show no evidence of action potentials but, interestingly, show spontaneous transient hyperpolarizations. Single channel recordings, and the use of various recording conditions and K-channel blocking drugs has shown the cells to possess three types of K channel, a large and a small Ca-activated K channel both with Ca and voltage sensitivity, and another channel that is only seen with pipette solutions containing GDP or UDP but no ATP.

The Ca-activated K channels are remarkably sensitive to intracellular Ca (Figure 6), being fully activated at all potentials at free Ca levels of 5 × 10^{-8} M. Because the normal membrane potential under zero current conditions is considerably positive to the K equilibrium potential, it is unlikely that the free Ca exceeds this. The presence of the spontaneous hyperpolarizations (and STOCS seen under voltage clamp) suggests that intracellular Ca stores will to play a vital role in these cells. The membrane potential in current-clamp mode is little affected by application of Ca channel

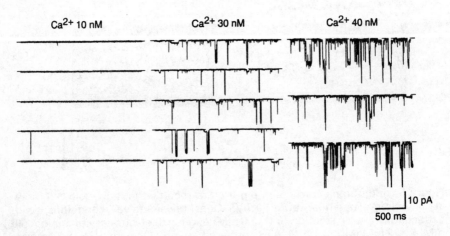

Figure 6 Effects of internal Ca^{2+} on large and small conductance K^+ channels in pig urethra. Currents were recorded from isolated membrane patches using the inside-out configuration. The pipette and bath solutions contained 140 mM K^+ and 5 mM EGTA, buffered to pH 7.4 with HEPES/Tris. Holding potential −60 mV. Note extreme sensitivity of both channels to internal Ca^{2+}.

blocking drugs, consistent with their being little involvement of L-type Ca channels. The low membrane potential could be explained by a relatively low resting K permeability, although TEA, 4-AP and elevation of K all cause significant depolarization of the cells (Figure 7), and the cell size and input resistant is virtually the same as in the detrusor smooth muscle cells.

On these mechanically quiescent cells, it would appear probable that agonist activation will produce contraction through release of intracellular Ca^{2+}, but in the absence of spike activity, since elevation of intracellular Ca^{2+}

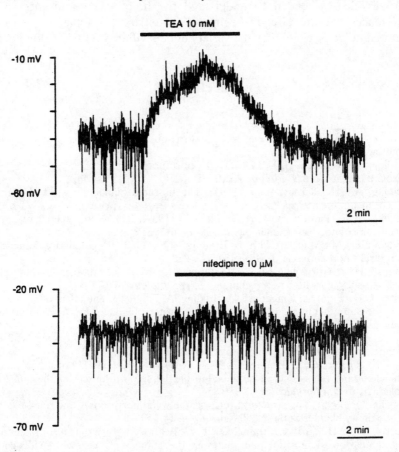

Figure 7 The effects of 10 mM tetraethyl ammonium (TEA) and 10 μM nifedipine on membrane potential of isolated smooth muscle myocytes from pig urethra. Current-clamp conditions using whole-cell recording. Patch electrode contained 140 mM K^+, 2 mM Mg^{2+}, 2 mM ATP, 50 μM EGTA buffered to pH 7.4 with HEPES/Tris. The extracellular solution was Krebs' solution with 2.0 mM Ca^{2+}. Note spontaneous hyperpolarizing potentials. Nifedipine had little effect, but TEA caused a marked depolarization and cessation of the spontaneous hyperpolarizations.

will hyperpolarize through the Ca sensitive K channels.

It will be of considerable interest to examine how the properties of the urethral smooth muscles change in the more distal parts of the urethra, as work on isolated strips has shown strips with high spontaneous tone, and the interesting property of relaxing to increases in extracellular K ions (Brading & Chen, 1990).

In conclusion, the electrophysiological properties of the different parts of the lower urinary tract do indeed show distinct properties. Although further work is clearly needed to understand the functional significance of the differences, we are already beginning to understand some of them, and continue to be fascinated by the variety of behaviours we have encountered.

REFERENCES

Brading, A.F. (1987). Physiology of bladder smooth muscle. In *The physiology of the Lower Urinary Tract* (Torrens, M.J. & Morrison, J.F.B. eds), pp. 161–191. Springer Verlag, New York.

Brading, A.F. & Chen, H.-I. (1990). High potassium solution induces relaxation in the isolated pig urethra. *J. Physiol.* **430**, 118P.

Brading, A.F. & Turner, W.H. (1994). The unstable bladder: towards a common mechanism. *Br. J. Urol.* **73**, 3–8.

Brading, A.F., Parekh, A.B. & Tomita, T. (1989). Tissue impedance of smooth muscles isolated from guinea pig. *J. Physiol.* **417**, 63P.

Bridgewater, M., MacNeil, H.F. & Brading, A.F. (1993). Regulation of tone in pig urethral smooth muscle. *J. Urol.* **150**, 223–228.

Clapp, L.H. & Gurney, A.M. (1991). Outward currents in rabbit pulmonary artery cells dissociated with a new technique. *Exper. Biology* **76**, 677–693.

Foster, C.D., Fujii, K., Kingdon, J. & Brading, A. F. (1989). The effect of cromakalim on the smooth muscle of the guinea pig urinary bladder. *Br. J. Pharmacol.* **97**, 281–291.

Fujii, K. (1988). Evidence for adenosine triphosphate as an excitatory transmitter in guinea pig rabbit and pig urinary bladder. *J. Physiol.* **404**, 39–52.

Fujii, K., Foster, C.D., Brading, A.F. & Parekh, A.B. (1990). Potassium channel blockers and the effects of cromakalim on the smooth muscle of the guinea pig bladder. *Br. J. Pharmacol.* **99**, 779–785.

Gabella, G. (1995). The structural relations between nerve fibres and muscle cells in the urinary bladder of the rat. *J. Neurocytol.* **24**, 159–187.

Iacovou, J.W., Hill, S.J. & Birmingham, T.A. (1990). Agonist-induced contraction and accumulation of inositiol phosphates in the guinea- pig detrusor evidence that muscarinic and purinergic receptors raise intracellular calcium by different mechanisms. *J. Urol.* **144**, 775–779.

Inoue, R. & Brading, A.F. (1990). The properties of the ATP-induced depolarization and current in single cells isolated from the gui nea-pig urinary bladder. *Br. J. Pharmacol.* **100**, 619–625.

Inoue, R. & Brading, A.F. (1991). Human pig and guinea pig bladder smooth muscle cells generate similar inward currents in response to purinoceptor activation. *Br. J. Pharmacol.* **103**, 1840–1841.

Langley, J.N. & Anderson, H.S. (1895). The innervation of the pelvic and adjoining viscera Part II. The Bladder. *J. Physiol.* **19**, 71–84.

Mostwin, J.L. (1985). Receptor operated intracellular stores in the smooth muscle of the guinea pig bladder. *J. Urol.* **133**, 900–905.

Mostwin, J.L. (1986). The action potential of guinea pig bladder smooth muscle. *J. Urol.* **135**, 1299–1303.

Nakayama, S. & Brading, A.F. (1993a). Evidence for mutiple open states of the Ca^{2+} channels in smooth muscle cells isolated from the guinea pig detrusor. *J. Physiol.* **471**, 87–105.

Nakayama, S. & Brading, A.F. (1993b). Inactivation of the voltage-dependent Ca^{2+} channel current in smooth muscle cells isolated from the guinea pig detrusor. *J. Physiol.* **471**, 107–127.

Speakman, M.J., Brading, A.F., Gilpin, C J., Dixon, J.S., Gilpin, S.A. & Gosling, J. (1987). Bladder outflow obstruction – a cause of denervation supersensitivity. *J. Urol.* **138**, 1461–1466.

Uvelius, B. & Gabella, G. (1980). Relation between cell length and force production in urinary bladder smooth muscle. *Acta Physiol Scand.* **110**, 357–365.

34

Electrical Rhythmicity in Gastrointestinal Muscles

KENTON M. SANDERS
SEAN M. WARD

Department of Physiology and Cell Biology,
University of Nevada School of Medicine,
Reno, Nevada, USA

INTRODUCTION

Electrical slow waves are generated in the stomach, small bowel and colon of most mammalian species, and in each region these events can elicit contractile responses. In some regions slow waves also serve as a stimulus for the generation of action potentials which elicit very strong contractions. Bozler's recordings from the stomach with extracellular electrodes demonstrated that slow waves are omnipresent, and changes in the amplitude and duration of these events correspond to the force of phasic contractions (Bozler, 1945). The concepts that arose from Bozler's work were supplemented by numerous studies of slow waves in the 1960s and 1970s that described the pharmacology and ionic dependencies of slow waves in various regions of the gastrointestinal tract (see reviews by Tomita, 1981; Szurszewski, 1987).

Tadao Tomita, who has contributed significantly toward our understanding of the mechanism(s) responsible for slow waves, utilized the double-sucrose gap technique to attempt to overcome some of the problems of voltage-clamping syncytial smooth muscle strips (Ohba *et al.*, 1975). Tomita concluded that there were two basic types of electrical slow waves: those of the stomach of guinea pig, and those of most other GI muscles (Tomita, 1981). Slow waves of guinea pig stomach consisted of a voltage-dependent and a voltage-independent component. To explain these observations, Tomita suggested that slow waves of the guinea pig stomach may result from a combination of an energy-dependent transport system (possibly Na^+/Ca^{2+} exchange) and ionic conductance changes (Ohba *et al.*, 1975). In reviewing

SMOOTH MUSCLE EXCITATION
ISBN 0-12-112360-X

the subject, however, Tomita (1981) also described other leading hypotheses to explain slow waves in other regions of the GI tract, such as: (1) the oscillating sodium pump hypothesis developed by Prosser and coworkers (Connor *et al.*, 1974) ; and (2) the ionic conductance hypothesis suggested by El-Sharkawy & Daniel (1975).

The patch-clamp technique has allowed characterization of ionic conductances present in enyzmatically dispersed smooth muscle cells, and studies of GI muscle cells have allowed refinements in the models proposed for GI rhythmicity. In some tissues it appears that conductance changes can explain many of the features of slow waves (Sanders, 1992), but in other cases, such as the guinea pig stomach, it is still unclear what ionic mechanisms are responsible for slow waves. Another important development in recent years is the realization that there may be a specialized class of pacemaker cells in GI muscles, referred to as interstitial cells of Cajal (ICCs), that initiate rhythmicity. This brief review will discuss studies of muscles of the small and large intestine and the role that ICCs may play in pacemaker activity.

CHARACTERISTICS AND MECHANISMS OF ELECTRICAL SLOW WAVES IN THE CANINE COLON

Electrical slow waves of the canine colon have been studied extensively (Smith *et al.*, Sanders, 1987; Huizinga *et al.*, 1991). These events can be divided into four components: (1) an upstroke depolarization that has a velocity of 0.1 to $1\,V\,s^{-1}$ and reaches a maximum depolarization level of about $-20\,mV$; (2) a partial repolarization following the peak of the upstroke that restores membrane potential to about -30 to $-50\,mV$; (3) a plateau phase in which membrane potential hovers between -30 and $-50\,mV$ for several seconds; and (4) a repolarization to the 'resting potential', which averages nearly $-80\,mV$ in the pacemaker region along the submucosal surface of the circular muscle layer of the canine colon (Smith *et al.*, 1987). Studies of the voltage-dependent conductances expressed in isolated myocytes have provided a hypothesis to explain each of these voltage transitions (see Figure 1).

The sharp upstroke depolarization appears to be due to an increase in Ca^{2+} conductance which activates at potentials positive to about $-60\,mV$ (Ward & Sanders, 1992a,b). Although it is difficult to block the upstroke with dihydropyridines (Huizinga *et al.*, 1991; Post & Hume, 1992; Ward & Sanders, 1992a,b), it appears that the inward current responsible for the upstroke is carried by 'L-type' Ca^{2+} channels (Rich *et al.*, 1993). The ineffectiveness of dihydropyridines is likely to be due to the voltage-

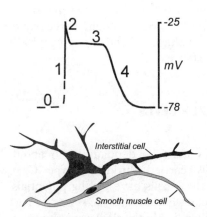

Phase 0 -- pacemaker current

*Activation of low threshold Ca²⁺ channels
in interstitial cells*

Phase 1 -- upstroke depolarization

Activation of voltage-dependent Ca²⁺ channels

Phase 2 -- partial repolarization

*Inactivation of voltage-dependent Ca²⁺ channels.
Activation of voltage-dependent K⁺ channels.*

Phase 3 -- plateau phase

*Sustained activation of voltage-dependent Ca²⁺
and K⁺ channels.
Inward and outward currents balance.*

Phase 4 -- repolarization

*Slow inactivation of voltage-dependent Ca²⁺ channels.
Activation of Ca²⁺-dependent K⁺ channels.
Deactivation of voltage-dependent Ca²⁺ and K⁺
channels.*

*Electrical slow waves originate in
interstitial cells and activate voltage-
dependent conductances in electrically
coupled smooth muscle cells.*

Figure 1 Electrical slow waves are composed of several phases (numbered on example slow wave). The initial depolarization (pacemaker activity) may be provided by interstitial cells of Cajal, which form an electrically coupled network and are coupled to smooth muscle cells. Depolarization activates voltage-dependent ionic conductances in smooth muscle cells which amplify and propagate the events. Ionic conductances expressed by smooth muscle cells can explain the waveform features denoted by 1–4. Proposed mechanisms are described for each phase.

dependence of the block of Ca^{2+} channels by these drugs (see Bean, 1984; Nelson & Worley, 1989). The upstroke depolarization slows and reaches a maximum depolarization at about $-20\,mV$. This peak appears to result from the development of inactivation of the Ca^{2+} current and activation of voltage-dependent K^+ currents (Thornbury *et al.*, 1992; Ward & Sanders, 1992a,b). This combination of events leads to reversal of the current to net outward current and initiates repolarization. Repolarization is incomplete at this point, however, because a potential is reached, typically between -35 and $-45\,mV$, at which remaining Ca^{2+} current, K^+ currents, and 'leak' currents balance, producing a quasi-stable 'plateau' potential (Thornbury *et al.*, 1992). Ca^{2+} enters cells continuously during the plateau phase as a result of the sustained inward current (Vogalis *et al.*, 1991), and this explains the association between the plateau potential and contractile force (Morgan & Szurszewski, 1980; Sanders & Smith, 1986; Ozaki *et al.*, 1991). Full repolarization eventually occurs when the balance between inward and outward currents is disrupted. This may result from continued inactivation of the inward current, perhaps as a result of Ca^{2+}-dependent inactivation as intracellular Ca^{2+} ($[Ca^{2+}]_i$) rises, and/or activation of Ca^{2+}-dependent K channels as $[Ca^{2+}]_i$ rises. Even a small imbalance between inward and outward current might precipitate repolarization and, as repolarization occurs, voltage-dependent Ca^{2+} and K^+ channels deactivate to restore resting conductance.

ROLE OF PACEMAKER CELLS

Most gastrointestinal smooth muscle cells must be depolarized to about $-50\,mV$ before inward current, typically carried through L-type Ca^{2+} channels, can be resolved. Since many of these cells have resting potentials 10–30 mV negative to this point, it is unclear what initiates slow waves. The initial depolarization, illustrated by the broken line in the slow wave shown in Figure 1, may result from electrical events in specialized, 'pacemaker' cells that form electrical connections with the smooth muscle syncytium.

Several investigators have suggested that electrical rhythmicity originates in a population of cells known as ICCs (Thuneberg, 1982; Thuneberg et al., 1983; Langton et al., 1989; Daniel & Berezin, 1992). These cells became possible candidates for the role of pacemakers when it was realized that ICCs populate specific sites within muscle layers found to be the local source of slow wave activity (Hara et al., 1986; Suzuki et al., 1986; Smith et al., 1987; Berezin et al., 1988). In many cases these cells form numerous gap junctions with each other and with neighbouring smooth muscle cells, thus creating a network of ICCs and forming an electrical conduit between the interstial cell network and the syncytium of smooth muscle cells. Morphological studies have been extremely important in establishing the structural basis for interactions between ICCs and smooth muscle cells (see review by Christensen, 1992), but morphology alone is not capable of testing the hypothesis that ICCs provide pacemaker input to the smooth muscle.

It has been rather difficult to test the hypothesis that ICCs are pacemakers because these small cells form rather diffuse networks with very fine processes. It is very difficult to locate and selectively record from ICCs in intact muscle strips with standard electrophysiological techniques. Even if it were possible to record directly from these cells, the fact that ICCs are electrically coupled to smooth muscle cells means that it would be difficult to be sure that the activity recorded from ICCs actually occurred in these cells (Barajas-Lopez et al., 1989). The question of the site at which electrical activity originates is further complicated by the need for multiple recording sites (Publicover & Sanders, 1984).

One approach to an understanding of the role of ICCs has been to use chemical agents to attempt to specifically lesion these cells while leaving smooth muscle syncytia functionally intact. Thuneberg and colleagues (1983) used methylene blue, chosen for its ability to be selectively taken up by ICCs, as a means to abolish interstial cell function. These authors found that exposure to methylene blue caused loss of slow waves in the mouse intestine, and this was associated with selective staining of ICCs. We have questioned the specificity of methylene blue because, along with the loss in slow-wave activity, this agent causes significant depolarization of membrane potential (Sanders *et al.*, 1989; Liu *et al.*, 1994), suggesting it has direct actions on the ionic mechanisms of smooth muscle cells which might contribute to the disruption in electrical rhythmicity.

One physical feature that helps to identify ICCs in some tissues is the large number of mitochondria found in these cells. We attempted to utilize this feature as a means to label and possibly damage ICCs of the canine colon by using a fluorescent dye, rhodamine 123, that is taken up by mitochondria (Ward *et al.*, 1990). Exposure to this agent resulted in uptake of the dye by ICCs and disruption or total loss of slow wave activity. ICCs appeared to be damaged by rhodamine 123, but labelling with this dye was not entirely specific. Therefore, as with most chemical agents, it is difficult to know whether pharmacological effects on smooth muscle cells or other cells contributed to the loss of rhythmicity.

For ICCs to be pacemaker cells, they must be excitable and capable of generating enough current to depolarize the electrically coupled smooth muscle syncytium to threshold. We have studied the excitability and ionic conductances of isolated ICCs to test whether these cells are capable of spontaneous rhythmicity. Patch-clamp studies of ICCs enzymatically dispersed from the pacemaker region along the submucosal surface of the circular muscle layer of the canine colon showed that: (1) ICCs are excitable cells; and (2) these cells are spontaneously rhythmic under conditions in which smooth muscle cells dissociated from the same region are quiescent (Langton *et al.*, 1989).

A comparison of voltage-dependent currents in ICCs and smooth muscle cells from the pacemaker region showed distinct differences (Lee & Sanders, 1993). Both cells generated Ca^{2+} currents upon depolarization, but ICCs expressed an inward current that activated near the resting potentials of the cells in the pacemaker region *in situ*, whereas the inward currents of smooth muscles were resolved positive to $-50\,mV$. The low threshold current in ICCs was almost entirely inactivated by holding cells at $-40\,mV$, and characterization of steady-state inactivation showed that the current inactivated at more negative potentials (half-inactivation $-45\,mV$) than the inward currents of smooth muscle cells (half-inactivation $-30\,mV$). Outward currents also inactivated at more negative potentials in ICCs and the non-Ca^{2+} dependent component was less sensitive to 4-aminopyridine than the delayed rectifier component of smooth muscle cells. The low threshold Ca^{2+}

current and negatively-inactivating K^+ current might participate in the generation of spontaneous electrical activity in these cells. Current spread via gap junctions (Berezin *et al.*, 1988) to neighbouring smooth muscle cells may depolarize these cells to a range in which voltage-dependent Ca^{2+} currents (L-type) can amplify and propagate the activity (Figure 1).

USING DEVELOPMENTALLY IMPAIRED ANIMALS TO STUDY THE INTERSTIAL CELL HYPOTHESIS

Although studies of isolated ICCs have provided insights into the mechanisms of electrical rhythmicity in GI muscles, in order to fully test the function of these cells in intact organs, a model is needed in which ICCs can be selectively manipulated. All known chemical agents appear to lack the necessary specificity (Sanders *et al.*, 1989), but it has recently become possible to affect the development of ICCs using immunochemical or genetic manipulations of the c-*kit* signalling pathway (Maeda *et al.*, 1992; Ward *et al.*, 1994; Burns *et al.*, 1995; Huizinga *et al.*, 1995; Torihashi *et al.*, 1995; Ward *et al.*, 1995).

Administration of antibodies to the proto-oncogene product, c-*kit*, to neonatal mice caused interference in c-*kit* signalling and impaired the development of normal phasic contractile activity in the intestine (Maeda *et al.*, 1992). These authors speculated that a lesion in the intestinal pacemaker system might be responsible for this effect. We investigated the identity of the cells that express c-*kit*-like immunoreactivity (c-*kit*-LI) in the mouse small intestine and colon (Ward *et al.*, 1994; Torihashi *et al.*, 1995). Cells in the small intestine were labelled with antibodies directed at the receptor portion of c-*kit* protein in the regions of the myenteric plexus and deep muscular plexus; cells in the colon were labelled in the subserosa, in the myenteric plexus region, within the circular and longitudinal muscle layers, and along the submucosal surface of the circular muscle. These locations match the distribution of ICCs. Cells expressing c-*kit*-LI formed an elaborate network, similar to the networks formed by cells stained with methylene blue, a standard marker for ICCs in the mouse gastrointestinal tract (Thuneberg, 1982; Thuneberg *et al.*, 1983). Immunocytochemistry confirmed that ICCs were labelled with antibodies to c-*kit* protein (Torihashi *et al.*, 1995). Repetitive injections of mice with antibodies to c-*kit* protein during the first week post partum caused a dramatic reduction in the number of ICCs. The loss of ICCs was accompanied by a loss in electrical rhythmicity, perhaps explaining the findings of Maeda and coworkers (1992), and supporting their hypothesis that c-*kit* signalling is critical for the proper development of the pacemaker apparatus in the mouse intestine. These results provide significant support for the notion that ICCs provide the pacemaker input for the generation of slow waves.

Another approach has been to study animals in which the c-*kit* signalling pathway is genetically impaired. For example, we studied the characteristiccs and distribution of ICCs and the electrical activity of small intestinal muscles from mice with mutations at the *White-spotting*/c-*kit* (*W*) locus (Ward *et al.*, 1994), which is allelic with c-*kit* (Chabot *et al.*, 1988). *W/W^v* mutants were viable and at days 3 to 30 post partum these animals had few ICCs in the myenteric plexus region of the small intestine compared with their wildtype (+/+) siblings. The few ICCs that were present were found close to neural elements between the myenteric ganglia and longitudinal muscle layer. Electrical slow waves, typically recorded from intestinal muscles of wildtype animals, were absent in *W/W^v* mutants, although irregular spike-like activity could be observed (Ward *et al.*, 1994; Huizinga *et al.*, 1995).

Studies have also been performed on animals with mutations at the *Steel* (*Sl*) locus, which codes for stem cell factor, the natural ligand for c-*kit* receptors (e.g. Williams *et al.*, 1990). Compound heterozygotes, such as *Sl/Sl^d*, survive to adulthood, but these animals have a severe lesion in the ICCs of the myenteric region of the small intestine (Ward *et al.*, 1995). An irregular network of ICCs associated with neural elements were found at about day 10 post partum, but none of these cells could be located in adult animals. Electrical recordings showed that slow waves are also absent in these animals, demonstrating that interference with c-*kit* signalling at multiple levels impairs the development of the intestinal pacemaker system.

SUMMARY AND CONCLUSIONS

Voltage-dependent currents in smooth muscle cells appear to explain the rhythmic electrical events referred to as slow waves. Initiation of slow waves in the smooth muscle syncytium may depend upon the generation of pacemaker activity in the ICCs. Support for this hypothesis comes from: (1) dissection experiments in which slow waves are blocked by removal of the pacemaker regions containing interstial cell networks; (2) chemical treatments in which agents, thought to have some selectivity for ICCs, cause damage to these cells and loss of electrical rhythmicity; (3) experiments on isolated ICCs showing that these cells are excitable and they express unique conductances that may facilitate spontaneous activity; and (4) developmental studies in which the formation or maturation of interstial cell networks is impaired by interference with the c-*kit* signalling pathway. Future studies may focus on more directed treatments to remove specific populations of ICCs and more efficient ways to isolate and culture interstitial cells of Cajal

ACKNOWLEDGEMENTS

This study was supported by a Program Project Grant from NIDDK, DK41315.

REFERENCES

Barajas-Lopez, C., Berezin, I., Daniel, E.E. & Huizinga, J.D. (1989). Pacemaker activity recorded in ICCs of the gastrointestinal tract. *Am. J. Physiol.* **257**, C830–C835.

Bean, B.P. (1984). Nitredipine block of cardiac calcium channels: High-affinity binding to the inactivated state. *Proc. Natl Acad. Sci. USA.* **81**, 6388–6392.

Berezin, I., Huizinga, J.D. & Daniel E.E. (1988). Interstitial cells of Cajal in the canine colon: a special communication network at the inner border of the circular muscle. *J. Comp. Neurol.* **273**, 42–51.

Bozler, E. (1945). The action potentials of the stomach. *Am. J. Physiol.* **144**, 693–700.

Burns, A.J., Torihashi, S., Harney, S.C., Sanders, K.M. & Ward, S.M. (1995). Regulation of the development of interstitial cells of Cajal in the gastrointestinal tract. *Gastroenterology* **108**, A719.

Chabot, B., Stephenson, D.A., Chapman, V.M., Besmer, P. & Bernstein, A. (1988). The proto-oncogene c-*kit* encoding a transmembrane tyrosine kinase receptor maps to the mouse *W* locus. *Nature* **335**, 88–89.

Christensen J (1992). A commentary on the morphological identification of ICCs in the gut. *J. Aut. Nervous Syst.* **37**, 75–88.

Connor, J.A., Prosser, C.L. & Weems, W.A. (1974). A study of pace-maker activity in intestinal smooth muscle. *J. Physiol.* **240**, 671–701.

Daniel, E.E. & Berezin, I. (1992). ICCs: are they major players in control of gastrointestinal motility ? *J. Gastroint. Motil.* **4**, 1–24.

El-Sharkawy T.Y. & Daniel, E.E. (1975). Ionic mechanisms of the intestinal electrical control activity. *Am. J. Physiol.* **229**, 1287–1298.

Hara, Y., Kubota, M. & Szurszewski, J.H. (1986). Electrophysiology of smooth muscle of the small intestine of some mammals. *J. Physiol.* **372**, 501–520.

Huizinga, J.D., Farraway, L. & den Hertog, A. (1991). Generation of slow-wave-type action potentials in canine colon smooth muscle involves a non-L-type Ca^{2+} conductance. *J. Physiol.* **442**, 15–29.

Huizinga, J.D., Thuneberg, L., Kluppel, M., Malysz, J., Mikkelsen, H.B. & Bernstein, A. (1995). W/kit gene required for intestinal pacemaker activity. *Nature* **373**, 347–349.

Langton, P., Ward, S.M., Carl, A., Norell, M.A. & Sanders, K.M. (1989). Spontaneous electrical activity of interstitial cells of Cajal isolated from canine proximal colon. *Pro. Natl Acad. Sci. USA* **86**, 7280–7284.

Lee, H.K. & Sanders K.M. (1993). Comparison of ionic currents from interstitial cells and smooth muscle cells of canine colon. *J. Physiol.* **460**, 135–152.

Liu, L.W.C., Thuneberg, L. & Huizinga, J.D. (1994). Selective lesioning of ICCs by methylene blue and light leads to loss of slow waves. *Am. J. Physiol.* **266**, G485–G496.

Maeda, H., Yamagata, A., Nishikawa, S., Yoshinaga, K., Kobayashi, S., Nishi, K., and Nishikawa S. (1992). Requirement of c-*kit* for development of intestinal pacemaker system. *Development* **116**, 369–375.

Morgan, K.G. & Szurszewski, J.H. (1980). Mechanism of phasic and tonic actions of pentagastrin on canine gastric smooth muscle. *J. Physiol.* **301**, 229–242.

Nelson, M.T. & Worley J.F. (1989). Dihydropyridine inhibition of single calcium channels and contractions in rabbit mesenteric artery depends on voltage. *J. Physiol.* **412**, 65–91.

Ohba, M., Sakamoto, Y. & Tomita, T. (1975). The slow wave in the circular muscle of the guinea pig stomach. *J. Physiol.* **253**, 505–516.

Ozaki, H., Blondfield, D.P., Stevens, R.J., Publicover, N.G., and Sanders, K.M. (1991). Simultaneous measurement of membrane potential, cytosolic calcium and muscle tension in smooth muscle tissue. *Am. J. Physiol.* **260**, C917–C925.

Post, J.M. & Hume, J.R. (1992). Ionic basis for spontaneous depolarizations in isolated smooth muscle cells of canine colon. *Am. J. Physiol.* **263**, C691–C699.

Publicover, N.G. & Sanders, K.M. (1984). A technique to locate the pacemaker in smooth muscles. *J.Appl. Physiol.* **57**, 1586–1590.

Rich, A., J.L. Kenyon, J.R. Hume, K. Overturf, B. Horowitz & K.M. Sanders. (1993). Dihydropyridine-sensitive calcium channels expressed in canine colonic smooth muscle cells. *Am. J. Physiol.* **264**, C745–C754.

Sanders, K.M. (1992). Ionic mechanisms of electrical rhythmicity in gastrointestinal smooth muscles. *Annu. Rev. Physiol.* **54**, 439–453.

Sanders, K. M. & Smith, T.K. (1986). Motoneurones of the submucous plexus regulate electrical activity of the circular muscle of the canine proximal colon. *J. Physiol.* **380**, 293–310.

Sanders, K.M., Burke, E.P. & Stevens, R.J. (1989). Effects of methylene blue on rhythmic activity and membrane potential in the canine proximal colon. *Am. J. Physiol.* **256**, G779–G784.

Smith, T.K., Reed, J.B. & Sanders, K.M. (1987). Origin and propagation of electrical slow waves in circular muscle of canine proximal colon. *Am. J. Physiol.* **252**, C215–C224.

Suzuki, N., Prosser, C.L. & Dahms, V. (1986). Boundary cells between longitudinal and circular layers: essential for electrical slow waves in cat intestine. *Am. J. Physiol.* **250**, G287–G294.

Szurszewski, J. (1987). Electrical basis for gastrointestinal motility. In *Physiology of the gastrointestinal tract* (Johnson, L.R. ed.), pp. 1435–1466. Raven Press, New York.

Thornbury, K.D., Ward, S.M. & Sanders, K.M. (1992). Participation of fast-activating, voltage-dependent potassium currents in electrical slow waves of colonic muscle. *Am. J. Physiol.* **263**, C226–C236.

Thuneberg, L. (1982). Interstitial cells of Cajal: intestinal pacemakers? *Adv. Anat. Embryol. Cell Biol.* **71**, 1-130.

Thuneberg, L., Johanson, V., Rumenssen, J.J., and Anderson, B.G. (1983). Interstitial cells of Cajal (ICC): selective uptake of methylene blue inhibits slow wave activity. In *Gastrointestinal Motility* (Roman, C. MTP ed.), pp. 495–502. Lancaster, UK.

Tomita, T. (1981). Electrical activity (spikes and slow waves). in gastrointestinal smooth muscle. In *Smooth Muscle: An Assessment of Current Knowledge* (Bulbring, E., Brading, A.F., Jones, A.W. & Tomita, T. eds), pp. 127–156. University of Texas Press, Austin.

Torihashi, S., Ward, S.M., Nishikawa, S-I., Nishi, K., Kobayashi, S. & Sanders, K.M. (1995). c-*kit*-dependent development of interstitial cells and electrical activity in the murine gastrointestinal tract. *Cell Tiss. Res.* **280**, 97–111.

Vogalis, F., Publicover, N.G., Hume, J.R. & Sanders, K.M. (1991). Relationship between calcium current and cytosolic calcium concentration in canine gastric smooth muscle cells. *Am. J. Physiol.* **260**, C1012–C1018.

Ward, S.M. & K.M. Sanders (1992a). Dependence of electrical slow waves of canine colonic smooth muscle on calcium current. *J. Physiol.* **455**, 307–319.

Ward, S.M. & K.M. Sanders. (1992b). Upstroke component of electrical slow waves in canine colonic smooth muscle due to nifedipine-resistant Ca^{2+} current. *J. Physiol.* **455**, 321–337.

Ward, S.M., Burke, E.P. & Sanders, K.M. (1990). Use of rhodamine 123 to label and lesion interstitial cells of Cajal in canine colonic circular muscle. *Anat. Embryol.* **182**, 215–224.

Ward, S.M., Burns, A.J., Torihashi, S. & Sanders, K.M. (1994). Mutation of the proto-oncogene c-*kit* blocks development of interstitial cells and electrical rhythmicity in murine intestine. *J. Physiol.* **480**, 91–97.

Ward, S.M., Burns, A.J., Torihashi, S., Harney, S.C. & Sanders, K.M. (1995). Impaired development of interstitial cells and intestinal electrical rhymicity in steel mutants. *Am. J. Physiol.* **269**, C1577–C1585.

Williams, D.E., Eisenman, J., Baird, A., Rauch, C., van Ness, K., March, C.F., Park, L.S., Martin, U. Mochizuki, D.Y., Boswell, H.S., Burgess, G.S., Cosman, D. & Lyman, S.D. (1990). Identification of a ligand for the c-*kit* proto-oncogene. *Cell* **63**, 167–174.

35

Interstitial Cells of Cajal as Pacemaker Cells of the Gut

JAN D. HUIZINGA
LOUIS W. C. LIU
JOHN MALYSZ
JONATHAN C. F. LEE
SUDIPTO DAS
LAURA FARRAWAY

*Department of Biomedical Sciences and
Intestinal Disease Research Programme,
McMaster University, Hamilton,
Ontario, Canada*

On routine radiological examination of the human small intestine one can see pacemaker cells at work. After a liquid barium meal is squirted across the pyloric sphincter, the liquid is quickly passed through the proximal part of the small intestine. This occurs through ring-like circular muscle contractions propagating over sections of the intestine. These propagating contractions occur in rapid succession when the intestine is filled with a barium liquid and at exactly the pacemaker (slow wave) frequency. The contents are efficiently moved to the jejunum. Interstitial cells, generating the slow waves, command this effective propagation.

In the 1960s it was clear to investigators such as Bortoff (1965) and Prosser (Kobayashi *et al.*, 1966) that slow waves were not recorded uniformly across a smooth muscle layer. Work on the small intestine of the cat suggested that slow waves were not recorded from isolated circular muscle, and it was concluded that longitudinal muscle was the site of origin of slow waves. Through similar experimentation it was concluded that in the cat colon it was the circular muscle that housed pacemaker activity (Christensen *et al.*, 1969). In the guinea pig stomach, Tomita concluded that both layers could generate the slow waves (Ohba *et al.*, 1975). Taking all these data together however, Tomita (1981) speculated 'It is thus possible that some particular cells located between the muscle layers act as pacemakers for the slow waves, and activate

SMOOTH MUSCLE EXCITATION
ISBN 0-12-112360-X

both the longitudinal and circular muscles'. An observation consistent with this hypothesis was that one could record slow waves of exceptional amplitude in the myenteric plexus region (Taylor *et al.*, 1975).

Tomita (1981) also concluded that: 'the slow waves are fundamentally of myogenic origin but at some regions of the preparations.... the slow waves may be markedly influenced by nervous activity'. It is interesting to note now that the interstitial cells of Cajal (ICCs) are by far the most heavily innervated cells of the gut. Tomita concluded that: 'If this kind of specialized pacemaker cell exists in all parts of the gastrointestinal tract, then it may be that when the longitudinal and circular muscle layers are separated from each other, these cells tend to attach to the longitudinal muscle in the cat small intestine and stomach, to the circular muscle in the cat colon and rabbit jejunum and to both the longitudinal and circular muscle in the guinea pig stomach and this determines the activity of the preparations' (Tomita, 1981).

Lars Thuneberg, working on his PhD thesis, noticed these accounts in the literature, in those moments when he was taking a break from the fascinating world of cells and cellular interactions related to the mouse small intestine he watched through his electron microscope. Then it occurred to him that the active sections of the intestine coincided with areas where he observed ICCs. He noted that electrophysiological data were consistent with active preparations always containing the myenteric plexus including ICCs. He also pointed out that the structural organization of ICCs, i.e. caveolae associated with SR, associated with mitochondria, formed a morphological basis for a metabolically driven 'ion pump' possibly involved in pacemaking (Thuneberg, 1982).

To prove his point Thuneberg used methylene blue. He knew that interstitial cells of the myenteric plexus of the small intestine of mice preferentially accumulated methylene blue and that exposure to strong light would make toxic products of methylene blue oxidation. He then saw that after the exposure of the ICCs stained with methylene blue, slow wave activity was abolished! (Thuneberg, 1989). We confirmed these observations later for the dog colon (Liu *et al.*, 1994) and found that this procedure very specifically destroys ICCs.

The first realization of highly localized pacemaker activity in the dog colon came from Nelson Durdle's paper in 1983 (Durdle *et al.*, 1983). El-Sharkawy was the external examiner of Nelson's Ph.D. work and when he returned to his laboratory where I worked, we were puzzled: clearly, slow wave activity disappeared when Nelson removed 'something' at the submucosal border of the circular muscle layer of the dog colon, but could 'submucosa' harbour slow wave activity? Then Lars Thuneberg started to talk about *ICCs* at international meetings.

It took a move to McMaster University and several years but then, together with Drs Berezin and Daniel, a fascinating network of ICCs was observed at the submucosal border of the dog colon circular muscle (Berezin et al, 1988). From several universities emerged evidence that ICC were critical in generating the typical slow wave activity of gastrointestinal smooth muscle (Daniel & Posey, 1984; Suzuki *et al.*, 1986; Christensen & Rick, 1987; Smith *et al.*, 1987; Faussone Pellegrini *et al.*, 1990; Taylor & Potter, 1990; Rumessen & Thuneberg, 1991; Christensen *et al.*, 1992). Slow waves of relatively large amplitude were generated in specific areas where ICCs were located, and thereafter the slow waves propagated into the muscle layers. The slow waves periodically depolarized the smooth muscle cells, evoking spiking activity on their plateaus, causing contraction. The intensity of the spiking activity was dependent on the level of excitation.

Tomita made another important speculation on slow waves which now has substantial evidence; however, it is still controversial. 'There seem to be active spots near the boundary between the longitudinal and circular muscle layers where the first component is generated by some rhythmic carrier-mediated transport system which functions electrogenically to depolarize the membrane and trigger the second component and which may also be involved in regulation the intracellular ions particularly the Ca concentration' (Tomita, 1981). Working in the guinea pig stomach, Tomita noticed that the 'first' component was not sensitive to voltage changes. In the dog colon, slow wave activity was subsequently seen not to be abolished by hyperpolarization up to $-120\,mV$ (Huizinga *et al.*, 1991a,b). Such experiments are done in the 'Abe-Tomita' bath. Extracellular current hyperpolarizes a section of tissue 2×2 mm. All cells are hyperpolarized, which is shown by recording the membrane potential at all corners. Furthermore, because the space constant in this preparation is approximately 7 mm, it is clear that all cells are sufficiently hyperpolarized. As the slow waves are also insensitive to L-type calcium channel blockers, a role of L-type calcium channels being activated at such negative voltages is excluded, although it should be noted that this hypothesis has been challenged. Another hypothesis is that L-type calcium channels are involved in initiation of the slow waves and that the failure of L-type calcium channel blockers to inhibit the activity is due to the voltage-dependent nature of the blocking action (Ward & Sanders, 1992a,b). Although voltage changes do not influence the upstroke potential of the slow waves (even though the plateau and superimposed spikes are very sensitive to hyperpolarization), temperature and intracellular metabolic components do (Huizinga *et al.*, 1991b). A hypothesis emerging from these and other (Liu *et al.*, 1993) studies is that inositol-trisphosphate induced Ca release from the ER activates the pacemaker channel, although this is still very speculative. We observed that influencing the rate of IP_3 synthesis strongly affects the slow wave frequency. Furthermore, we have observed that influencing ER calcium uptake markedly affects the slow wave frequency. This led to the hypothesis, entirely consistent with Tomita's hypothesis, that an intracellular metabolic clock activates the pacemaker system. Possibly, Ca periodically released from the ER activates the pacemaker channel. The exact nature of this channel has yet to be elucidated (Sanders 1992; Molleman *et al.*, 1994).

Recently it was shown that injection of antibody to the Kit receptor into newborn mice leads to changes in contraction patterns in the small intestine *in vitro* and an absence of Kit immunofluorescence in the myenteric plexus area (Maeda *et al.*, 1992). This led to the hypothesis that the Kit tyrosine-kinase receptor might be essential for intestinal pacemaker activity through its possible role as a signalling molecule required for the development of the ICCs. To determine whether mutations at the murine *W* locus, coding for the Kit receptor, might affect normal development of ICCs, we, in collaboration with Dr Thuneberg from the University of Copenhagen, first examined the morphology of the intestines of adult *W* mutant mice and their control littermates (Huizinga *et al.*, 1995). Control mice had a normal ICC network in the small intestine in the myenteric plexus region, visualized by selective accumulation of methylene blue and confirmed by electron microscopy. In contrast, this network of ICCs was absent in *W/W^v* mice. In the *W* mutant mice, only a few scattered methylene-blue-positive cells, now identified as genuine ICCs, were observed. Similar results were found in newborn mice (Ward *et al.*, 1994). In addition to this dramatic decrease in the number of ICCs, we observed the direct apposition of large stretches of the circular and longitudinal smooth muscle layers in *W/W^v* mice. The absence of the intermediary network of ICCs 'forced' the smooth muscle cells of both layers to communicate directly (Huizinga *et al.*, 1995).

In collaboration with Drs Bernstein and Klüppel from the University of Toronto and Dr Mikkelsen from the University of Copenhagen, Kit mRNA and protein expression were studied. In wild type and *W/+*, high levels of Kit expression, as measured by immunohistochemistry, were observed in a cell layer between the longitudinal and the circular muscle layers at the level of the Auerbach's plexus (Huizinga *et al.*, 1995). In contrast, no Kit immunoreactivity was seen in or between the muscle layers of *W* mutant mice. Whole-mount RNA *in situ* hybridization experiments on the ileum of wild type and *W/W^v* mice showed that the ileum of wild-type mice contained Kit mRNA-positive cells whose organization was identical to that of ICCs, as revealed by methylene blue staining. In contrast, no Kit positive cells were observed in the muscle layers of *W/W^v* mice. Because *Sl/Sl^d* mice, which lack Steel factor, (the growth hormone that is the ligand for the Kit receptor), showed similar abnormalities (J.D.H., H.B. Mikkelsen and L. Thuneberg, unpublished data), we propose that an interaction between Steel factor and the Kit receptor is essential for normal ICC development.

To determine whether lack of ICCs had effects on slow wave generation, we measured the electrical activities of the small intestinal muscle layers. Normal mice generated slow wave type action potentials with an amplitude of $22 \pm 6\,mV$, a frequency of 32 ± 1 cycles min^{-1} and a resting membrane potential of $-60 \pm 3\,mV$. In contrast, the ileum of W/W^v mice failed to display any slow wave type action potentials. The resting membrane potential was $-45 \pm 1\,mV$ ($n = 22$) and from it, at irregular frequency, fast spike-like action potentials arose. Their amplitude was $16 \pm 2\,mV$, and the frequency ranged from 4 to 20 cpm, and was irregular within all preparations. In particular, in the presence of an excitatory stimulus, a wide variety of patterns of electrical activities is present in W/W^v or Sl/Sl^d mice (Figure 1), whereas in their genetic controls only one pattern is found: slow waves at a constant frequency with superimposed spikes. The slow wave

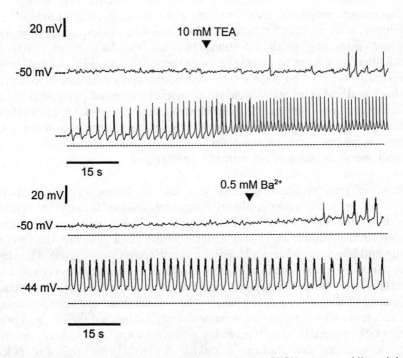

Figure 1 Activity in the small intestine of the Sl/Sl^d mouse. All activity is blocked by L-type calcium channel blockers. Two electrically quiescent preparations are shown that develop a variety of patterns of activity in response to blockade of K channels. Variable patterns of electrical activity result in variable contraction patterns.

component or pacemaker activity of gut smooth muscle is insensitive to L-type calcium channel blockers (Huizinga et al., 1991a). In the presence of the blockers nifedipine or D600, the slow wave component of the action potentials in wild-type mice remained unaltered, whereas the electrical activity of W/Wᵛ mice was completely abolished, proving the absence of the pacemaker component. These data demonstrate that W and Sl mutations lead to both the absence of the ICC network in the Auerbach's plexus region and pacemaker activity in the small intestine, demonstrating an essential role for ICCs in gut pacemaker activity.

It is of obvious interest to understand how the small intestine of W/Wᵛ mice generates propulsive contractile activity, without having intrinsic slow wave activity. Although the small intestine is shorter in W/Wᵛ mice, the defecation characteristics appear normal, giving no obvious clue as to motor abnormalities. The small intestine consists of rings of circularly oriented smooth muscle cells up to several millimetres wide (so-called lamellae) separated by connective tissue (the so-called septa). In normal mice, the slow waves are synchronized and ring-like contractions, involving several lamellae simultaneously, propagate anally, moving contents in an efficient manner. In W/Wᵛ mice, after we injected barium liquid into the stomach, the barium was delivered into the small intestine, but no ring-like circular muscle contractions were seen to propagate over the small intestine. Instead, large sections appeared to be contracting at random making intestinal contents flow back and fort. This activity did result in anally directed movement but at a speed many times slower than normal, consistent with other studies (Ha et al., 1983; Kamiya et al., 1985). It appears that in the mutant mice there is no intrinsic mechanism to have activity propagate from lamella to lamella, probably because there is no intrinsic gradient of slow waves (Liu et al., 1995).

These, in part preliminary, data give us the following picture: ICCs generate slow wave activity, thereby limiting spiking activity to periods coinciding with the plateaus of the slow waves. The slow waves propagate into the circular muscle layer and, at least within each lamellae, the spiking activity and hence the contractile activity is perfectly synchronized. The slow waves have therefore performed two functions: frequency regulation and synchronization. When the smooth muscle cells within a lamellae all contract in synchrony, a ring contraction occurs. In normal mice and man, this ring contraction is seen to propagate, predominantly in the anal direction. Again, the network of interstitial cells probably performs a crucial role here; this has been worked out for the cat (Conklin & Du, 1990) and dog colon (unpublished data). The electrical activity of the circular muscle layer propagates along the colon, not through the longitudinal muscle and not through septa, but through the network of interstitial cells joining the septa at the submucosal border.

The ideas of Tomita, as expressed in his 1981 review, have been substantiated and developed into a now widely accepted hypothesis that ICCs are the pacemaker cells of the gut, regulating contraction frequency, contraction synchronization and contraction propagation. There is evidence that the pacemaker clock is biochemical in nature. The pacemaker cells periodically initiate slow waves that then actively propagate into the circular muscle lamellae initiating spikes upon excitation to cause a ring-like contraction.

REFERENCES

Berezin, I., Huizinga, J.D. & Daniel E.E. (1988). Interstitial cells of Cajal in the canine colon: a special communication network at the inner border of the circular muscle. *J. Comp. Neurol.* **273**, 42–51.

Bortoff, A. (1965). Electrical transmission of slow waves from longitudinal to circular intestinal muscle. *Am. J. Physiol.* **209**, 1254–1260.

Christensen, J. & Rick, G.A. (1987). Intrinsic nerves in the mammalian colon: confirmation of a plexus at the circular muscle-submucosal interface. *J. Auton. Nerv. Syst.* **21**, 223–231.

Christensen, J., Caprilli, R. & Lund, G.F. (1969). Electric slow waves in circular muscle of cat colon. *Am. J. Physiol.* **217**, 771–776.

Christensen, J., Rick, G.A. & Lowe, L.S. (1992). Distributions of interstitial cells of Cajal in stomach and colon of cat, dog, ferret, opossum, rat, guinea pig and rabbit. *J. Auton. Nerv. Syst.* **37**, 47–56.

Conklin, J.L. & Du, C. (1990). Pathways of slow-wave propagation in proximal colon of cats. *Am. J. Physiol.* **258**, G89–G903.

Daniel, E.E. & Posey, D.V. (1984). Neuromuscular structures in opossum esophagus: role of interstitial cells of Cajal. *Am. J. Physiol.* **246**, G305–G315.

Durdle, N.G., Kingma, Y.J., Bowes, K.L. & Chambers, M.M. (1983). Origin of slow waves in the canine colon. *Gastroenterology* **84**, 375–382.

Faussone Pellegrini, M.S., Pantalone, D. & Cortesini, C. (1990). Smooth muscle cells, interstitial cells of Cajal and myenteric plexus interrelationships in the human colon. *Acta Anat. (Basel)* **139**, 31–44.

Ha, T.Y., Reed, N.D. & Crowle, P.K. (1983). Delayed expulsion of adult *Trichinella spiralis* by mast cell-deficient *W/W^v* mice. *Infec. Immun.* **41**, 445–447.

Huizinga, J.D., Farraway, L. & Den Hertog, A. (1991a). Generation of slow-wave-type action potentials in canine colon smooth muscle involves a non-L-type Ca^{2+} conductance. *J. Physiol. (London)* **442**, 15–29.

Huizinga,. JD., Farraway, L. & Den Hertog, A. (1991b). Effect of voltage and cyclic AMP on frequency of slow wave type action potentials in colonic smooth muscle. *J. Physiol. (London)* **442**, 31–45.

Huizinga, J.D., Thuneberg, L., Kluppel, M., Malysz J., Mikkelsen,. H.B & Bernstein, A. (1995). The *W-kit* gene is required for interstitial cells of Cajal and intestinal pacemaker activity. *Nature* **373**, 347–349.

Kamiya, M., Oku, Y., Itayama, H. & Ohbayashi, M. (1985). Prolonged expulsion of adult *Trichinella spiralis* and eosinophil infiltration in mast cell-deficient W/W^v mice. *J. Helminthol.* **59**, 233–239.

Kobayashi, M., Nagai, T. & Prosser, C.L. (1966). Electrical interaction between muscle layers of cat intesine. *Am. J. Physiol.* **211**, 1281–1291.

Liu, L.W.C., Thuneberg, L. & Huizinga, J.D. (1993). Regulation of colonic pacemaker frequency by intracellular calcium in sarcoplasmic reticulum. *J. Gastroint. Motil.* **5**, 201.

Liu, L.W.C., Thuneberg, L. & Huizinga, J.D. (1994). Selective lesioning of interstitial cells of Cajal by methylene blue and light leads to loss of slow waves. *Am. J. Physiol.* **266**, G485–G496.

Liu, L.W.C., Sperelakis, N. & Huizinga, J.D. (1995). Pacemaker Activity and intercellular communication in the gastrointestinal musculature. In *Pacemaker Activity and Intercellular Communication* (Huizinga, J.D. ed.), pp. 159–174. CRC Press, Ann Arbor.

Maeda, H., Yamagata, A., Nishikawa, S., Yoshinaga, K., Kobayashi, S. & Nishi, K. (1992). Requirement of c-kit for development of intestinal pacemaker system. *Development* **116**, 369–375.

Molleman,. A, Sims,. S, Lee, J.C.F. & Huizinga, J.D. (1994). Ion channels involved in gastrointestinal action potential generation. In *Pacemaker Activity and Intercellular Communication*, (Huizinga,. J.D. ed.), CRC Press. Baton Rouge.

Ohba, M., Sakamoto, Y. & Tomita, T. (1975). The slow wave in the circular muscle of the guinea pig stomach. *J. Physiol. (London)* **253**, 505–516.

Rumessen, J.J. & Thuneberg, L. (1991). Interstitial cells of Cajal in human small intestine. Ultrastructural identification and organization between the main smooth muscle layers. *Gastroenterology* **100**, 1417–1431.

Sanders, K.M. (1992). Ionic mechanisms of electrical rhythmicity in gastrointestinal smooth muscles. *Annu. Rev. Physiol.* **54**, 439–453.

Smith, T.K., Reed, J.B. & Sanders K.M. (1987). Origin and propagation of electrical slow waves in circular muscle of canine proximal colon. *Am. J. Physiol.* **252**, C215–C224.

Suzuki, N., Prosser, C.L. & Dahms, V. (1986). Boundary cells between longitudinal and circular layers: essential for electrical slow waves in cat intestine. *Am. J. Physiol.* **250**, G287–G294.

Taylor, C.W. & Potter, B.V. (1990). The size of inositol 1,4,5-trisphosphate-sensitive Ca2+ stores depends on inositol 1,4,5-trisphosphate concentration. *Biochem. J.* **266**, 189–194.

Taylor, G.S., Daniel, E.E. & Tomita, T. (1975). Origin and mechanism of intestinal slow waves. In Proceedings of the 5th international symposium on GI motility (Vantrappen, G. ed.), pp. 102–106, Typoff Press, Leuven.

Thuneberg, L. (1982). Interstitial cells of Cajal: intestinal pacemaker cells? *Adv. Anat. Embryol Cell Biol.* **71**, 1–130.

Thuneberg, L. (1989). Interstitial cells of Cajal. In *Handbook of Physiology, The Gastrointestinal System*, (Schultz, G.S., Wood, J.D. & Rauner, B.B. eds), pp. 349–386. American Physiological Society, Bethesda,U.S.A.

Tomita, T. (1981). Electrical activity (spikes and slow waves) in gastrointestinal smooth muscles. In *Smooth Muscle* (Bulbring, E. ed.), pp. 127–156. Arnold, London.

Ward, S.M. & Sanders, K.M. (1992a). Dependence of electrical slow waves of canine colonic smooth muscle on calcium gradient. *J. Physiol. (London)* **455**, 307–319.

Ward, S.M. & Sanders, K.M. (1992b). Upstroke component of electrical slow waves in canine colonic smooth muscle due to nifedipine-resistant calcium current. *J. Physiol. (London)* **455**, 321–337.

Ward, S.M., Burns, A.J., Torihashi, S. & Sanders, K.M. (1994). Mutation of the proto-oncogene c-kit blocks development of interstitial cells and electrical rhythmicity in murine intestine. *J. Physiol. (London)* **480**, 91–97.

36

Membrane Depolarization Caused by Sodium Removal in the Circular Muscle of Guinea Pig Gastric Antrum

TADAO TOMITA*
YI-WEI PANG**

*Department of Physiology,
School of Health Sciences,
Fujita Health University,
Toyoake, Aichi, Japan

**Department of Physiology,
School of Medicine,
Nagoya University,
Nagoya, Japan

INTRODUCTION

In several smooth muscles removal of external Na^+ produces contraction accompanied by membrane depolarization (0-Na depolarization). 0-Na depolarization has been reported in pregnant mouse (Osa, 1971) and rat myometrium (Savinneau et al., 1987). The circular muscle of the guinea pig gastric antrum is also one of the typical tissues which produce 0-Na depolarization (Ohba et al., 1976; 1977; Tomita & Sakamoto, 1977; Sakamoto & Tomita, 1982; Tomita et al., 1985). Contraction produced by Na^+ removal can be explained by Na^+-Ca^{2+} exchange mechanism, i.e. an increase in Ca^{2+} influx coupled with Na^+ outflux (Blaustein, 1977, 1984; Ashida & Blaustein, 1987; Rapoport, 1993). This hypothesis, however, cannot be applied during 0-Na depolarization, because in 0-Na Na^+-Ca^+ exchange presumably reverses in direction and there is an of an outward movement of positive charges as a result of coupling of $3Na^+$ efflux to $1Ca^{2+}$ influx in the exchange under these conditions.

In this article, we discuss possible mechanisms underlying 0-Na depolarization mainly based on our own data obtained from the guinea pig gastric muscle.

SMOOTH MUSCLE EXCITATION
ISBN 0-12-112360-X

GENERAL PROPERTIES OF DEPOLARIZATION PRODUCED BY Na$^+$ REMOVAL

In the circular muscle of guinea pig gastric antrum, the degree and rate of depolarization produced by Na$^+$ removal vary in different preparations, but fundamentally similar depolarizations were produced by different substitutes for Na$^+$, such as N-methyl-D-glucamine (NMDG), dimethyldiethanol ammonium (DDA), Tris-hydroxy aminomethane (THAM), choline, or sucrose (Ohba *et al.*, 1976, 1977; Sakamoto & Tomita, 1982). Therefore, 0-Na depolarization is considered to be due to the lack of Na$^+$, not to the effect of these substitutes.

Muscle strips taken from the antral region generated spontaneous electrical activity and slow waves. When exposed to Na$^+$-free solution prolongation of slow wave usually appeared first. In some preparations the membrane failed to repolarize within 1 min and stayed roughly at the plateau level of the slow wave (about -30 mV). In other preparations, depolarization slowly developed as incomplete repolarization of each slow wave, taking several minutes to reach a steady depolarization and this was accompanied by a gradual decrease in amplitude and an increase in frequency of slow wave. It is likely that 0-Na depolarization consists of two components, an early rapid depolarization and a late slow depolarization, but the size of the early component is particularly variable in different preparations.

In some preparations rhythmic electrical activity ceased during the depolarization but in many preparations some rhythmic activity continued in Na$^+$-free solution for more than 10 min. Differences in the effect of Na$^+$ removal have been considered to be related to the relative size of the first component of the slow wave which is responsible for the potential-independent part of the slow wave which occurs in a more negative potential range (Sakamoto & Tomita, 1982), but in recent experiments we failed to observe any clear relationship between the slow wave configuration and the rate or pattern of 0-Na depolarization.

On readmission of Na$^+$, the depolarization slowly recovered, taking more than 2 min. The pattern of recovery of slow wave varied in different preparations and depended on the exposure time to Na$^+$ solution. When the slow wave was abolished or strongly inhibited by Na$^+$ removal, it reappeared during repolarization after Na$^+$ readmission, and slowly recovered to the control size, the recovery taking a much longer time than repolarization of the membrane. Conversely, when relatively large rhythmic slow waves had remained during exposure to Na$^+$-free solution, reapplication of Na$^+$ reduced their amplitude transiently and this was followed by gradual recovery of their size. Readmission of Na$^+$ after a prolonged exposure to Na$^+$-free solution often produced complete suppression of rhythmic activity for a few minutes before slow recovery of slow waves. When there was a long suppression, slow waves often suddenly started to appear with a relatively large amplitude or even greater amplitude than the control. The rate of recovery was in the order: mechanical response, membrane potential, and slow wave amplitude.

0-Na depolarization is considered to result from a direct action on smooth muscle cells because it is not affected by various substances which inhibit nerve activity and transmitter action, such as tetrodotoxin, atropine, phenoxybenzamine, or which inhibit endogenous prostaglandin production, such as indomethacin.

0-Na depolarization is temperature-dependent. When the temperature was lowered to 20–23°C no depolarization was produced by Na+ removal (Tomita & Sakamoto, 1977). At this temperature, the frequency of slow wave was markedly reduced and the configuration of slow wave often became irregular. Na+ removal transiently increased their frequency, but the slow wave disintegrated into irregular fluctuations of membrane potential. This suggests that a proper metabolic support is important for slow wave generation and 0-Na depolarization and also that synchronization of electrical activity in a group of cells may underlie the generation of slow waves. Disintegration of slow wave into noisy potential fluctuations has also been observed in the presence of phosphodiesterase inhibitors (Tsugeno et al., 1995).

POSSIBILITY OF AN INCREASE IN Ca^{2+} CONDUCTANCE

Effects of Ca^{2+} removal

When the external Ca^{2+} was removed, the early rapid phase of 0-Na depolarization was much reduced but the later slow depolarization was not much affected. Similarly, removal of Ca^{2+} during 0-Na depolarization (the late phase) had only a weak repolarizing effect, although contraction was markedly inhibited. This suggests that Ca^{2+} conductance is increased during the early phase of 0-Na depolarization but that the contribution of Ca^{2+} conductance to the late phase is relatively small, although some Ca^{2+} influx is maintained and supports contraction (Sakamoto & Tomita, 1982).

Effects of organic Ca^{2+} channel blockers

Verapamil (1 μM) inhibited contraction produced by Na+ removal but it had a negligible effect on 0-Na depolarization (Tomita et al., 1985). Recently, similar effects were confirmed with nifedipine (1 μM) and nicardipine (1 μM). The early phase of 0-Na depolarization was also little affected. This differs from the effects of Ca^{2+} removal.

Effects of inorganic Ca^{2+} channel blockers

In the presence of 0.3 mM Mn^+, 0-Na depolarization could still be produced. When 0.5 mM Mn^{2+} was applied during 0-Na depolarization, no repolarization was observed, although it produced relaxation (Tomita & Sakamoto, 1977). When the concentration was increased to 2 mM, Mn^{2+} could produce very weak repolarization which was similar to Ca^{2+} removal (Sakamoto & Tomita, 1982).

Cd^{2+} (0.3 mM), Co^{2+} (2 mM), and Ni^{2+} (2 mM) had essentially similar effects to those of Mn^{2+}. These divalent cations produced a transient depolarization and an increase in slow wave frequency upon the first application, but upon a second application they produced only inhibitory effects and their prolonged or repeated application slowly blocked the slow waves. The inhibitory effects of these divalent cations on 0-Na depolarization, particularly on the late phase, was much weaker compared with the effects on slow waves. The tonic contraction produced by Na^+ removal was inhibited by Cd^{2+} and Co^{2+} but potentiated by Ni^{2+} at a concentration (2 mM) which was sufficient to abolish slow waves and their accompanying phasic contractions.

These results suggest that an increase in Ca^{2+} conductance (verapamil-insensitive) may be partly involved in the early phase of 0-Na depolarization, but that this contribution to the late phase seems very minor.

POSSIBILITY OF A DECREASE IN K^+ CONDUCTANCE

Effects of changes in external K^+ concentration

Membrane depolarization would be produced if the K^+ conductance is decreased by Na^+ removal. One would then expect that membrane potential becomes less sensitive to changes in external K^+ concentration ($[K^+]_i$). However, changes in membrane potential produced by changing $[K^+]_i$ from 3 to 12 mM were greater in the absence of Na^+. During a prolonged exposure to K^+-free solution, 0-Na depolarization was markedly inhibited and reversed to hyperpolarization (Tomita et al., 1985).

Intracellular Na^+ concentration ($[Na^+]_i$) is likely to be slowly increased in K^+-free solution, so that under this condition Na^+ removal may markedly increase intracellular Ca^{2+} concentration ($[Ca^{2+}]_i$). This may lead to hyperpolarization due to activation of Ca^{2+}-activated K^+ channels. This possibility, however, needs to be investigated. It might be also possible that the inhibitory action of K^+ removal is not simply due to a shift of the K^+ equilibrium potential but due to a lack of K^+ in the medium because K^+ is necessary for some ionic transport system switched on by 0-Na and that blocking this transport by K+ removal prevents 0-Na depolarization, as previously speculated for slow wave generation (Tomita, 1981).

Effects of cromakalim

Cromakalim is known to activate a type of K+ channel which is blocked by sulphonylureas, such as glibenclamide (Cook, 1988; Weston, 1989). When applied during 0-Na depolarization, cromakalim ($10\,\mu M$) repolarized the membrane and restored the amplitude of the rhythmic electrical activity (Katayama *et al.*, 1993). The amplitude of this activity was similar to, but the frequency was higher than, that of the slow wave in normal solution. This result suggests that a decrease in K+ conductance could underlie the depolarization and further that Na+ may not be the major ion carrying inward current for the generation of the slow wave (or slow wave-like potential).

Involvement of Na+-activated K+ channel

A K+ channel which is activated by intracellular Na+ (K^+_{Na} channel) has been found in some tissues (cardiac muscle: Kameyama *et al.*, 1984; neurone: Bader *et al.*, 1985; Dryer *et al.*, 1989). If activation of this type of K+ channel is involved in a repolarizing phase of the slow wave, 0-Na depolarization may be explained by a closure of K^+_{Na} channel by a decrease in intracellular Na+ concentration ($[Na^+]_i$) on Na+ removal. The K^+_{Na} channel in guinea pig cardiac muscle was shown to be inhibited by intracellular acidification (Veldkamp *et al.*, 1994). As Na+ removal is expected to cause intracellular acidification, this factor is likely to potentiate 0-Na depolarization. There is, however, no convincing evidence to support this idea. In cultured brain stem neurones from chick, this K^+_{Na} channel was blocked by 4-aminopyridine (4-AP, $4\,mM$), but not by tetraethylammonium (TEA, $2\,mM$). In the guinea pig gastric muscle, TEA produces a larger depolarization than 4-AP. Patch-clamp experiments are necessary to prove whether this K+ channel actually contributes to 0-Na depolarization.

H+-regulated K+ channel

Intracellular acidification would be expected on Na+ removal owing to impairment of a Na+-H+ exchange, as observed in some smooth muscles (e.g. guinea pig vena cava: Tomita *et al.*, 1993). This acidification may result in a decrease in the K+ conductance, leading to membrane depolarization. As already mentioned, the K^+_{Na} channel in cardiac muscle was inhibited by intracellular acidification (Veldkamp *et al.*, 1994). Inhibition of Ca^{2+}-activated K+ channels by intracellular acidification was also shown in rabbit tracheal muscle cells by patch-clamp experiments (Kume *et al.*, 1990). If intracellular acidification is responsible for 0-Na depolarization, an application of propionate (a weak acid) may produce a similar depolarization and 0-Na depolarization may be prevented by ammonium chloride (NH_4Cl, a weak base), because they are known to cause intracellular acidification and alkalinization, respectively. Although propionate (20 mM) depolarized the membrane and NH_4Cl (20 mM) inhibited 0-Na depolarization in the guinea pig gastric muscle, their effects were relatively small; accordingly, intracellular acidification does not appear to be a major factor causing membrane depolarization.

POSSIBILITY OF INVOLVEMENT OF Ca^{2+}-ACTIVATED Cl^- CONDUCTANCE

Effects of Cl^- removal

The presence of a Cl^- channel which is activated by intracellular Ca^{2+} (Cl^-_{Ca} channel) has been reported for some smooth muscles (Baron *et al.*, 1991; Droogmans *et al.*, 1991; Pacaud *et al.*, 1989, 1992; Lamb *et al.*, 1994). Na^+ removal may first increase intracellular Ca^{2+} concentration ($[Ca^{2+}]_i$) by Na^+-Ca^{2+} exchange and/or possibly by intracellular Ca^{2+} release and this may in turn activate Cl^-_{Ca} channels.

Because intracellular Cl^- concentration ($[Cl^-]_i$) is likely to be higher than that expected from a passive distribution (Aickin & Vermüe, 1983), activation of Cl^-_{Ca} channels may produce membrane depolarization, provided that this effect is stronger than that of activation of K^+_{Ca} channels. If Cl^- efflux through this channel were responsible for 0-Na depolarization one would expect gradual recovery of the membrane potential as $[Cl^-]_i$ is lowered in Cl^- deficient solution, but no such tendency was observed. Even after complete relaxation produced by Ca^{2+} removal or various Ca^{2+} channel blockers, when $[Ca^{2+}]_i$ would be expected to be significantly lowered, no marked repolarization was produced. Furthermore, sucrose substitution for NaCl did not produce larger depolarization compared with NMDG substitution where Cl^- concentration remains constant. Therefore, it is rather unlikely that activation of Cl^-_{Ca} channels plays a major role in 0-Na depolarization.

Effects of Cl^- channel blockers

Niflumic acid (Pacaud *et al.*, 1989; White & Aylwin, 1990; Hogg *et al.*, 1994; Janssen & Sims, 1994) and DIDS (Baron *et al.*, 1991; Lamb *et al.*, 1994) are considered to block Cl⁻ channels. Both slow waves and 0-Na depolarization were strongly inhibited by 200 μM niflumic acid. The recovery, particularly of slow waves, was poor and after wash-out of niflumic acid, only partial recovery of slow waves was observed on Na⁺ removal. The inhibitory action of DIDS was also stronger on slow waves than 0-Na depolarization but the recovery was better than with niflumic acid. At a concentration of 300 μM, DIDS completely abolished slow waves, but when Na⁺ was removed relatively large slow waves reappeared accompanied by much-reduced depolarization. The configuration of slow wave observed in Na⁺-free solution containing DIDS was not much different from that of slow waves in the normal solution. Thus, the effects of these Cl⁻ channel blockers suggest a contribution of Cl⁻ channels to 0-Na depolarization and also to slow wave generation, but this is not clearly supported by the results of Cl⁻ removal experiments.

Effects of caffeine

If Ca^{2+} release from sarcoplasmic reticulum (SR) is involved in the activation of Cl^{-}_{Ca} channels in Na⁺-free solution, caffeine may affect 0-Na depolarization because caffeine is known to release Ca^{2+} from SR in many types of smooth muscle. In the guinea pig gastric muscle, however, no clear evidence that caffeine releases Ca^{2+} has been obtained. In normal solution, the main effect of caffeine was to inhibit spontaneous activity at low concentrations (0.3-1 mM) and to increase Ca^{2+} influx through the plasma membrane at relatively high concentrations (3–10 mM), causing a sustained contraction accompanied by small depolarization (Chowdhury et al., 1995).

Caffeine had an inhibitory action on 0-Na depolarization. The inhibitory action of caffeine is considered to be mainly due to an increase in cyclic AMP through its inhibition of phosphodiesterase, because other inhibitors, such as isobutylmethyl- xanthine (IBMX, 10 μM) and theophylline (100 μM) also inhibited 0-Na depolarization. When these inhibitors were applied during the depolarization the membrane was repolarized, accompanied by the recovery of slow wave. Slow waves in normal solution were suppressed by these inhibitors (Tsugeno et al., 1995), but removal of Na⁺ during the suppression of slow waves restored nearly normal slow wave activity with little membrane depolarization. The configuration of slow wave and the pattern of activity in Na⁺-free solution containing the phosphodiesterase inhibitors was similar to the slow wave in normal solution and thus this differed from that observed in Na⁺-free solution containing cromakalim. In the latter the electrical activity had higher frequency and shorter duration.

POSSIBILITY OF INVOLVEMENT OF ELECTROGENIC CARRIER-MEDIATED TRANSPORT

Inhibition of Na^+–K^+ pump

If contribution of a Na^+–K^+ pump to membrane potential was large enough, one would expect depolarization by Na^+ removal because of inhibition of an electrogenic component of the membrane potential. Some depolarization produced by K^+ removal and also by ouabain suggested some contribution by this component, but this component was less than 10 mV and not large enough to explain 0-Na depolarization of about 20 mV. Furthermore, 0-Na depolarization could still be produced in the presence of 5–10 μM ouabain.

Na^+–Ca^{2+} exchange

The contraction produced by Na^+ removal can be explained by reversed Na^+–Ca^{2+} exchange (Blaustein, 1977; Ozaki & Urakawa, 1981; Ashida & Blaustein, 1987). In guinea-pig taenia caeci (Pritchard & Ashley, 1987) and vena cava (Tomita et al., 1993) this contraction was shown to be accompanied by an increase in $[Ca^{2+}]_i$. The increase in $[Ca^{2+}]_i$ can also be at least partly explained by reversed Na^+-Ca^{2+} exchange.

Under conditions in which Na^+, K^+, and Ca^{2+} channels and also the Na^+–K^+ pump were inhibited, the membrane currents which appeared to be carried by the Na^+–Ca^{2+} exchange mechanism can be recorded in single cells dispersed from rabbit portal vein and guinea-pig taenia caeci by the whole-cell voltage-clamp method (Tomita et al., 1993). When the external medium contained 130 mM Na^+ and no Ca^{2+} and the solution in a patch pipette (intracellular medium) contained 5 mM Na^+, an intracellular application of 0.2 μM Ca^{2+} through the pipette produced inward currents. Furthermore, when the ionic concentration gradient was reversed, i.e. when the external medium contained no Na^+ and the pipette contained 30 mM Na^+ and 0.2 μM Ca^{2+}, an external application of 1.2 mM Ca^{2+} produced outward current. Therefore, currents flowed in the direction of the Na^+ concentration gradient, which fits the hypothesis that $3Na^+$ ions are coupled to one Ca^{2+} ion in the process of Na^+–Ca^{2+} exchange. When the external Na^+ is removed, therefore, the outward currents carried by the Na^+–Ca^{2+} exchange are expected to produce hyperpolarization of the membrane, not the depolarization actually observed.

OTHER ELECTROGENIC IONIC TRANSPORT SYSTEMS

In order to produce depolarization, therefore, the original Na^+–Ca^{2+} exchange mechanism must be modified. For example, inward movement of

Ca^{2+} may be assumed to couple not only with outward movement of Na$^+$ but also with inward movement of K$^+$ (Tomita, 1981). This was proposed to explain 0-Na depolarization and slow wave generation, but was without much experimental basis. There may be several other possible electrogenic ionic transports to explain 0-Na depolarization or generation of slow wave, but our knowledge is still too limited to construct any reasonable model. Although the presence of external K$^+$ is necessary to produce 0-Na depolarization, it is not clear whether a negative shift of the K$^+$ equilibrium potential due to K$^+$ removal simply prevents the membrane from depolarizing or the absence of external K$^+$ stops an electrogenic ionic transport producing depolarization. If outward movement of Na$^+$ were driving an electrogenic transport in the plasma membrane to produce 0-Na depolarization, a slow recovery would be expected because intracellular Na$^+$ is depleted during exposure to Na$^+$-free solution, however, no such tendency was observed. The slow component of 0-Na depolarization developed gradually and also recovered slowly on Na$^+$ reapplication. This suggests that a decrease in [Na$^+$]$_i$ is responsible for depolarization rather than outward movement of Na$^+$.

SUMMARY

Based on the weak voltage-dependency and high temperature-dependency of slow wave frequency we have previously considered that some metabolic control is involved in the generation of slow waves and this leads to a hypothesis that an electrogenic ionic (Na$^+$–Ca^{2+}–K$^+$ coupled) transport might be responsible for the depolarizing phase of the slow wave (Tomita, 1981). However, the same idea does not appear to explain 0-Na depolarization. It is more likely that a slow decrease in [Na$^+$]$_i$ is responsible for the depolarization. We think that some ionic gating system is involved, but cannot propose a plausible ionic pathway. Inward currents may flow through some nonselective cationic channels which may be activated by intracellular Ca^{2+} or kept open by removal of a blocking action of intracellular Na$^+$. It is also possible that inward currents flow through Cl$^-$ channels activated by intracellular Ca^{2+} which are increased by reversed Na$^+$–Ca^{2+} exchange. Currently, neither of these possibilities is supported by firm experimental evidence but cannot be disproved. We hope that the mechanism underlying 0-Na depolarization will be clarified in the near future.

REFERENCES

Aickin, C.C. & Vermüe, N.A. (1983). Microelectrode measurement of intracellular chloride activity in smooth muscle cells of guinea pig ureter. *Pflügers Arch.* **397**, 25–28.

Ashida, T. & Blaustein, M.P. (1987). Regulation of cell calcium and contractility in mammalian arterial smooth muscle: the role of sodium-calcium exchange. *J. Physiol.* **392**, 617–635.

Bader, C.R., Bernheim, L. & Bertrand, D. (1985). Sodium-activated potassium current in cultured avian neurones. *Nature* **317**, 540–542.

Baron, A., Pacaud, P., Loirand, G., Mironneau, C. & Mironneau, J. (1991). Pharmacological block of Ca^{2+}-activated Cl^- current in rat vascular smooth muscle cells in short-term primary culture. *Pflügers Arch.* **419**, 553–558.

Blaustein, M.P. (1977). Sodium ions, calcium ions, blood pressure regulation, and hypertension: a reassessment and a hypothesis. *Am. J. Physiol.* **232**, C165–173.

Blaustein, M.P. (1984). Sodium transport and hypertension. Where are we going? *Hypertension* **6**, 445–453.

Chowdhury, J.U., Pang, Y.-W., Huang, S.-M., Tsugeno, M. & Tomita, T. (1995). Sustained contraction produced by caffeine after ryanodine treatment in the circular muscle of the guinea pig gastric antrum and rabbit portal vein. *Br. J. Pharmacol.* **114**, 1414–1418.

Cook, N.S. (1988). The pharmacology of potassium channels and their therapeutic potential. *Trends Pharmacol. Sci.* **9**, 21–28.

Droogmans, G., Callewaert, G., Declerck, I. & Casteels, R. (1991). ATP-induced Ca^{2+} release and Cl^- current in cultured smooth muscle cells from pig aorta. *J. Physiol.* **440**, 623–634.

Dryer, S.E., Fujii, J.T. & Martin, A.R. (1989). A Na^+-activated K^+ current in cultured brain stem neurones from chicks. *J. Physiol.* **410**, 283–296.

Hogg, R.C., Wang, Q. & Large, W.A. (1994). Action of niflumic acid on evoked and spontaneous calcium-activated chloride and potassium currents in smooth muscle cells from rabbit portal vein. *Br. J. Pharmacol.*, **112**, 977–984.

Janssen, L.J. & Sims, S.M. (1994). Spontaneous transient inward currents and rhythmicity in canine and guinea pig tracheal smooth muscle cells. *Pflügers Arch.* **427**, 473–480.

Kameyama, M., Kakei, M., Sato, R., Shibasaki, T., Matsuda, H. & Irisawa, H. (1984). Intracellular Na^+ activates a K^+ channel in mammalian cardiac cells. *Nature* **309**, 354–356.

Katayama, N., Huang, S.-M., Tomita, T. & Brading, A.F. (1993). Effects of cromakalim on the electrical slow wave in the circular muscle of guinea pig gastric antrum. *Br. J. Pharmacol.* **109**, 1097–1100.

Kume, H., Takagi, K., Satake, T., Tokuno, H. & Tomita, T. (1990). Effects of intracellular pH on calcium-activated potassium channels in rabbit tracheal smooth muscle. *J. Physiol.* **424**, 445–457.

Lamb, F.S., Volk, K.A. & Shibata, E.F. (1994). Calcium-activated chloride current in rabbit coronary artery myocytes. *Circ. Res.*, **75**, 742–750.

Ohba, M., Sakamoto, Y. & Tomita, T. (1976). Spontaneous rhythmic activity of the smooth muscle of the guinea pig stomach and effects of ionic environment. In *Smooth Muscle Pharmacology and Physiology* (Worcel, M. & Vassort, G. eds), pp. 301–316. INSERM, Paris.

Ohba, M., Sakamoto, Y. & Tomita, T. (1977). Effects of sodium, potassium and calcium ions on the slow wave in the circular muscle of the guinea pig stomach. *J. Physiol.*, **267**, 167–180.

Osa, T. (1971). Effect of removing the external sodium on the electrical and mechanical activities of the pregnant mouse myometrium. *Jpn. J. Physiol.*, **21**, 607–625.

Ozaki, H. & Urakawa, N. (1981). Involvement of a Na–Ca exchange mechanism in contraction induced by low-Na solution in isolated guinea pig aorta. *Pflügers Arch.* **390**, 107–112.

Pacaud, P., Loirand, G., Lavie, J.L., Mironneau, C. & Mironneau, J. (1989). Calcium-activated chloride current in rat vascular smooth muscle cells in short-term primary culture. *Pflügers Arch.* **413**, 629–636.

Pacaud, P., Loirand, G., Grégoire, G., Mironneau, C. & Mironneau, J. (1992). Calcium-dependence of the calcium-activated chloride current in smooth muscle cells of rat portal vein. *Pflügers Arch.* **421**, 125–130.

Pritchard, K. & Ashley, C.C. (1987). Evidence for Na^+/Ca^{2+} exchange in isolated smooth muscle cells: a fura-2 study. *Pflügers Arch.* **410**, 401–407.

Rapoport, R.M. (1993). Regulation of vascular smooth muscle contraction by extracellular Na^+. *Gen. Pharmacol.* **24**, 531–537.

Sakamoto, Y. & Tomita, T. (1982). Depolarization produced by sodium removal in the circular muscle of the guinea pig stomach. *J. Physiol.* **326**, 329–339.

Savinneau, J.P., Mironneau, J. & Mironneau, C. (1987). Influence of the sodium gradient on contractile activity in pregnant rat myometrium. *Gen. Physiol. Biophys.* **6**, 535–560.

Tomita, T. (1981). Electrical activity (spikes and slow waves) in gastrointestinal smooth muscles. In *Smooth Muscle: An Assessment of Current Knowledge* (Bülbring, E., Brading, A.F., Jones A.W., & Tomita, T. eds), pp. 127–156. Edward Arnold, London.

Tomita, T. & Sakamoto, Y. (1977). Electrical and mechanical activities in the guinea pig stomach muscle. In *Excitation-Contraction Coupling in Smooth Muscle* (Casteels, R., Godfraind, T. & Rüegg, J.C. eds), pp. 37–46. Elsevier/North-Holland Biomedical Press, Amsterdam.

Tomita, T., Tokuno, H. & Nakayama, S. (1985). Effects of Na-removal on the membrane potential in the circular muscle of the guinea pig stomach. In *Calcium Regulation in Smooth Muscles* (Mironneau, J. ed.), pp. 193–200. INSERM, Paris.

Tomita, T., Tokuno, H. & Matsumoto, T. (1993). Roles of sodium ions in mechanical and electrical activities in smooth muscles. In *Seventh Symposium on Salt*, Vol. II, pp. 365–370. Elsevier Science Publishers B.V., Amsterdam.

Tsugeno, M., Huang, S.-M., Pang, Y.-W., Chowdhury, J.U. & Tomita, T. (1995). Effects of phosphodiesterase inhibitors on spontaneous electrical activity (slow waves) in the guinea pig gastric muscle. *J. Physiol.* **485**, 493–502.

Veldkamp, M.W., Vereecke, J. & Carmeliet, E. (1994). Effects of intracellular sodium and hydrogen ion on the sodium activated potassium channel in isolated patches from guinea pig ventricular myocytes. *Cardiovas. Res.* **28**, 1036–1041.

Weston, A.H. (1989). Smooth muscle K^+ channel openers: their pharmacology and clinical potential. *Pflügers Arch.* **414** (Suppl. 1), S99–105.

White, M.M. & Aylwin, M. (1990). Niflumic and flufenamic acids are potent reversible blockers of Ca^{2+}-activated Cl^- channels in *Xenopus* oocytes. *Mol. Pharmacol.* **37**, 720–724.

37

Role of Magnesium Ions in Myometrial Motility

TAKURO OSA

Department of Physiology,
School of Medicine,
Yamaguchi University,
Ube, Japan

INTRODUCTION

Mg ions appear to play an important role during agonist–receptor interaction in the regulation of the ionic permeability of the plasma membrane and also in the transduction of many intracellular signals. Despite this, the role of Mg ions has not been much investigated compared with Ca ions. In this article the effects of changes in the external Mg concentration ($[Mg]_o$) on myometrial activity are described. The action of Mg is of clinical interest in relation to pregnancy and parturition, and particularly relevant to the treatment of premature labour and pre-eclampsia.

The concentration of Mg in body fluid has been measured by several investigators. Values of $1.2\,mmol\,l^{-1}$ plasma in rats and $1.8\,mmol\,l^{-1}$ plasma in dogs have been reported; it is very high in marine invertebrates ($56.9\,mmol$ $l^{-1}\,H_2O$ in sepia) (Prosser & Brown, 1965). Plasma Mg concentrations of $1.5\,mM$ in rat and $0.9\,mM$ in guinea pig are also documented (Marshall, 1974). About a half of the Mg is bound to plasma proteins. Less attention has been directed on the homeostasis of the plasma Mg concentration which is maintained in mammals perhaps mainly by the parathyroid hormone (Aikawa, 1981) and partly by mineralocorticoid hormones (Massry *et al.*, 1968). In human pregnancy the concentration of plasma Mg is reported to decrease from $1.87\,mE\,l^{-1}$ for non-pregnant to $1.39\,mE\,l^{-1}$ for women at term (De Jorge *et al.*, 1965).

Physiological saline solutions for mammals have been improved, starting from Locke solution (1901) in which the ionic constituents were more or less similar to those in frog solution made by Ringer (1883). Particular attention has been paid to Mg concentration and to buffering of pH in these solutions (Lockwood, 1961). As for myometrial tissues, the plasma constituents may differ depending on whether the animal is gravid, nongravid or spayed. Nevertheless, investigators generally use their favourite solution. The effects of applied drugs, hormones, and even divalent cations are, however, considered to vary during prolonged exposure to saline solution and also depend on the region of the uterus from which the muscle strips are obtained. These points are often overlooked in *in vitro* experiments.

INHIBITORY ACTION OF EXTRACELLULAR Mg

In most myometrial tissues *in vitro*, action potentials accompanied by phasic contractions are generated spontaneously or by electrical stimulation. Myometrial tissues are regarded as an example of highly excitable smooth muscle (Bülbring & Tomita, 1987). In mice and rats, the burst discharge of spike-type action potentials in longitudinal muscles, and action potentials with a plateau in circular muscles, underlie the phasic contractions. Ca ions are mostly responsible for the generation of both spike and plateau potentials. The strength and duration of contraction are closely related to the configuration of action potential and to the pattern of electrical activity.

When the longitudinal muscle of myometrium from ovariectomized rats was exposed to Mg-free Krebs solution, the muscle exhibited vigorous spontaneous contractions. The spontaneous and also the electrically evoked contractions were depressed by adding 0.6 mM Mg to the external medium. However, spontaneous activity was absent in Mg-free Krebs solution in longitudinal myometrium muscle taken from oestrogen-treated rats. Phasic contractions and also action potentials produced by electrical stimulation were only slightly depressed by 0.6 mM Mg (Osa & Maruta, 1986).

The plateau potential and contraction generated in the circular muscle of rat myometrium became progressively less depressed by 0.5 mM Mg as the duration of oestrogen-treatment of the rat was increased (Osa & Ogasawara, 1979). A similar observation has been reported for the contractions and electrical activity generated in pregnant human myometrial preparation *in vitro* (Kawarabayashi, 1994). In gravid rat myometrium, the electrically evoked contraction of circular muscles was less strongly depressed by 0.6 mM Mg during delivery than at mid-pregnancy (Osa & Ogasawara, 1983). In contrast, the membrane activity and contraction of longitudinal muscles became increasingly strongly depressed by 1.2 mM Mg from day 20 to day 22 of pregnancy (Osa *et al.*, 1983). Thus, Mg effects differ depending on hormonal influences and also between longitudinal and circular muscle layers. Nevertheless, the inhibitory effect of Mg on excitation may be the main physiological basis for its use for tocolytic therapy. Inhibition of excitation by divalent cations such as Ca and Mg is generally called a stabilizing action, but whether inhibition of the generation of spontaneous activity is playing a major role, or whether blocking of Ca channels is the dominant factor is still not clear. According to whole-cell voltage-clamp experiments on single cells freshly isolated from the longitudinal muscle of pregnant rat uterus, Ca current, particularly its transient component, was inhibited by about 40% by increasing Mg from 1 to 10 mM (Ohya & Sperelakis, 1990).

It is notable that in pregnant human myometrium an application of 4.8 mM Mg inhibited contractions induced by Na-depletion whereas it potentiated contractures induced by high K (Morishita et al., 1995). The inhibition of the former is probably due to suppression of Na–Ca exchange, as is known for other tissues, but the potentiation of K-contracture requires further investigation. Mg may exert intracellular actions on Ca stores and on the contractile machinery, where Mg may have not only an inhibitory but also a potentiating action depending on the experimental conditions.

ENHANCEMENT OF OXYTOCIN ACTION BY Mg

Oxytocin plays an important role in parturition (Fuchs, 1966). Oxytocin increased the frequency and duration of spike bursts generated in the longitudinal muscle of mouse and rat myometria in vitro (Kuriyama, 1961; Marshall, 1974) and prolonged the plateau potential in the circular muscle of rat myometrium (Chamley & Parkington, 1984). The accompanying phasic contractions were accordingly enhanced. It was recently reported that in polarized rat myometrium the strength and duration of phasic contractions induced by oxytocin were linearly related to the Ca transients, measured with fura-2, and that the relationship was not changed by the treatment with cyclopiazonic acid, an inhibitor of the Ca pump in the intracellular store sites (Kasai et al., 1994). Therefore, it may be reasonable to assume that the mechanical activity in rat myometrium produced by oxytocin depends mostly on the increase in membrane excitability. Oxytocin also potentiated Ca-induced contracture in rat myometrium depolarized by excess K and this is likely to be due to increased Ca-influx (Schild, 1969).

As early as 1939, Frazer reported that the stimulant action of oxytocin (and vasopressin) on the guinea pig uterus was enhanced when $[Mg]_o$ was increased. Historical works have been reviewed by Marshall (1974). In isolated uteri from ovariectomized rats, the concentration–response curve of oxytocin was studied in the presence of Mg ranging between 0 and 8 mM; a peak potentiating effect was found between 0.2 and 0.5 mM (Ishida &

Moritoki, 1966). It was later shown that the oxytocin receptor density in the plasma membrane was increased by the treatment of rats with oestrogen (Soloff et al., 1977), and that the potentiating effect was also observed with Mn (Bentley, 1965) and other polyvalent cations such as Cu, Ni, and Zn (Schild, 1969). The enhancement of oxytocin action on electrical activity by Mg and Mn was demonstrated in the longitudinal muscle of oestrogen-treated rats (Osa et al., 1981). A similar action of Mg was also shown in pregnant human myometrium in vitro (Kawarabayashi et al., 1990).

Schild (1969) proposed a ternary complex between receptor, metal and oxytocin as an initial step in the activation of a receptor-operated Ca channel, based on bioassay experiments. This idea has been further extended by measuring high-affinity sites for [^{3}H]oxytocin in particulate fractions from the myometrial tissues of rat, sow, ewe and human (Soloff et al., 1977; Kaneko et al., 1995). Using a radioiodinated oxytocin-receptor antagonist, it was shown that 3 mM Mg increased the affinity of oxytocin for the receptor in rat uterus by about 1500-fold (Antoni & Chadio, 1989). The potentiating action of Mg can easily be explained by the positive cooperativity found between oxytocin, Mg and receptor (Pliška & Albertin, 1991).

ROLE OF INTRACELLULAR Mg

More than 15 years have passed since the excellent review by Bolton (1979) on the action of transmitters and hormones including oxytocin. Since then, Ca-induced Ca release from sarcoplasmic reticulum has been demonstrated in smooth muscles and several intracellular signal pathways have also been clarified (Somlyo & Somlyo, 1994). These provided a new understanding of the initiation and regulation of contraction in which many enzymes are involved and their function under the influence of ions, particularly Ca and Mg. The emphasis has, however, been more towards modulation of myosin light chain kinase, the final step of contraction, and less towards regulation of ionic channels in the plasma membrane. Although the importance of Mg is implicated in many enzymatic processes, identification of sites and modes of action and also physiological significance of Mg involvement are not yet well understood.

The intracellular ionized Mg concentration ($[Mg]_i$) has been measured in various tissues by different methods (Romani & Scarpa, 1992); the values appear to be generally high in cardiac muscle (around 3 mM) and relatively lower in skeletal muscle (less than 1 mM), but the difference could be due mainly to the methods used rather than a real difference between the tissues. $[Mg]_i$ of cultured smooth muscle cells from rat aorta was estimated to be 680 μM and was easily increased by raising $[Mg]_o$ (Zhang et al., 1992). In the taenia of guinea pig caecum $[Mg]_i$ was estimated to be about $310\,\mu M$ by the NMR method, using the dissociation constant (K_d) of $41\,\mu M$ for Mg-ATP at $32°C$, and it was relatively resistant to alteration of $[Mg]_o$ (Nakayama & Tomita, 1990). The $[Mg]_i$ of rat myometrium was reported to be $200\,\mu M$, assuming the K_d for Mg-ATP to be $68\,\mu M$ at $4°C$ (Degani et al., 1984). In the longitudinal muscle of oestrogen-treated rat myometrium, $[Mg]_i$ was estimated to be $380\,\mu M$ utilizing mag-fura-2 fluorescence and this was increased only by $40\,\mu M$ on exposure to a solution containing $15\,mM$ Mg and $40\,mM$ K (Osa et al., 1994). Therefore, changes in the $[Mg]_i$ produced by changes in $[Mg]_o$ are suspected to be too small to influence intracellular enzymatic activity. Nevertheless, the inhibitory effects on mechanical and electrical activities of db-cAMP, forskolin and relaxin, the agents regarded as initiators of cAMP-dependent processes, were strongly enhanced by pretreatment with $15\,mM$ Mg.

The technical bottlenecks in the measurement of $[Mg]_i$ include the poor time resolution of the NMR method and difficulty in evaluating for the fluorescence method the real K_d for Mg·mag-fura-2 complex inside the cells. It can be expected that further information on changes in Mg concentration at various intracellular sites and also the relationship between $[Mg]_i$ and cellular functions will be accumulated in the near future.

EFFECTS OF Mn IN COMPARISON WITH Mg

Mn is a well-known inorganic Ca channel blocker. The action is much stronger than that of Mg. In the longitudinal muscle of rat uterus, an increase in $[Mg]_o$ to $10\,mM$ reduced spike frequency by inhibiting the slow potential without causing significant changes in the amplitude of the spike potential (Marshall, 1965), whereas only $0.5\,mM$ Mn inhibited both slow potential and spike potential (Osa et al., 1981).

It has been argued that in addition to the blocking action on Ca-influx, Mn has a potentiating action on the mechanical response by penetrating into the cells (Shibata, 1969; Ogasawara et al., 1980; Lategan & Brading, 1988). Mn appears to enter myometrium longitudinal cells more readily than Mg. The results shown in Figure 1 may be taken as evidence for Mn influx. Mn is known to bind to fura-2 and quenches its fluorescence (Hallam et al., 1988). The basal fluorescence of fura-2, loaded in the cells and recorded at $510\,nm$ emission with $360\,nm$ excitation wave length (F_{360}, isosbestic point), was quickly decreased by $0.6\,mM$ Mn applied in Mg-free Krebs solution (N. Todoroki and K. Mogami, unpublished data). The recovery was very poor after removal of Mn. The absolute value of the intracellular Mn concentration has not been estimated and the pathway of Mn influx has not

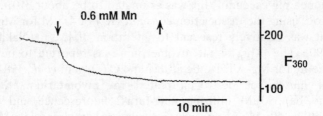

Figure 1 A decrease in fura-2 fluorescence signal by Mn in a longitudinal muscle strip taken from oestrogen-treated rat uterus. Fura-2 was excited at 360nm and measured at 510nm (36°C). 0.6 mM Mn was applied to Mg-free solution for 15 min as indicated.

been clarified. Mn may enter through voltage-gated Ca channels, as Mn is classified as a permeator as well as a blocker of the voltage-gated Ca channel in guinea pig ventricular cells (Lansman *et al.*, 1986).

When the longitudinal muscle of oestrogen-treated rat myometrium was treated with porcine relaxin together in the presence of 0.6 mM Mg, the mechanical and electrical activities became highly susceptible to the inhibitory action of Mg for more than 3 h after the removal of relaxin (Osa *et al.*, 1991). However, pretreatment with 0.6 mM Mn for 15–30 min attenuated the inhibitory effects of relaxin, and also of db-cAMP, whereas it enhanced the inhibitory effects of isoprenaline, forskolin and 8-bromo cGMP (Osa *et al.*, 1994). The mechanisms underlying these observations are difficult to understand at present; they are unlikely to be related to the channel blocking action of Mg and Mn. It is more probable that these cations modify some enzymatic activities resulting in alteration of membrane excitability and contraction.

SUMMARY

In myometrium, extracellular Mg depresses the slow potential responsible for generation of a burst of action potentials and this leads to a decrease in spike frequency or a block of spike activity in longitudinal muscle. The main action of Mg on circular muscle is to inhibit a plateau component of the action potential. These changes are considered to be mainly responsible for the mechanical depression. Because the plasma Mg concentration is likely to be maintained reasonably constant, however, modification of the electrical activity brought about by changes in $[Mg]_o$ cannot be a major regulatory factor modulating cellular function *in vivo*.

The potentiating action of Mg on oxytocin-induced contraction has attracted many investigators. Mg is likely to be involved in receptor activation by oxytocin. Modification of membrane properties (e.g., receptors, ionic channels, ionic transport systems) by ovarian steroid hormones may alter susceptibility of the membrane to divalent cations as well as to agonists such as oxytocin and catecholamines. Furthermore, similar considerations apply to enzymes involved in intracellular signal transduction. Other components, such as intercellular communication and contractile machinery are also possible sites which cannot be neglected. Similarity and dissimilarity of Mg and Mn actions are also interesting problems which should be investigated further to obtain more insight into the regulation of myometrial contractility.

REFERENCES

Aikawa, J.K. (1981). *Magnesium: Its Biologic Significance.* CRC Press, Boca Raton.

Antoni, F.A. & Chadio, S.E. (1989). Essential role of magnesium in oxytocin-receptor affinity and ligand specificity. *Biochem. J.* **257**, 611–614.

Bentley, P.J. (1965). The potentiating action of magnesium and manganese on the oxytocin effect of some oxytocin analogues. *J. Endocrinol.* **32**, 215–222.

Bolton, T.B. (1979). Mechanisms of actions of transmitters and other substances on smooth muscle. *Physiol. Rev.* **59**, 606–718.

Bülbring, E & Tomita, T. (1987). Catecholamine action on smooth muscle. *Pharmacol. Rev.* **39**, 49–96.

Chamley, W.A. & Parkington, H.C. (1984). Relaxin inhibits the plateau component of the action potential in the circular myometrium of the rat. *J. Physiol.* **353**, 51–65.

Degani, H., Shaer, A., Victor, T.A. & Kaye, A.M. (1984). Estrogen-induced changes in high-energy phosphate metabolism in rat uterus: ³¹P NMR studies. Biochemistry. **23**, 2572–2577.

De Jorge, F.B., Delascio, D., Cintra, A.B. & Antunes, M.L. (1965). Magnesium concentration in the blood serum of normal pregnant women. *Obstet. Gynecol.* **25**, 253–254.

Frazer, A.M. (1939). Effect of Mg on response of uterus to posterior pituitary hormones. *J. Pharmacol. Exp. Ther.* **66**, 85–94.

Fuchs, A.-R. (1966). The physiological role of oxytocin in the regulation of myometrial activity in the rabbit. Mem. Soc. *Endocrinol.* **14**, 229–248.

Hallam, T.J., Jacob, R. & Merritt, J.E. (1988). Evidence that agonists stimulate bivalent-cation influx into human endothelial cells. *Biochem. J.* **255**, 179–184.

Ishida, Y. & Moritoki, H. (1966). Potentiating actions of magnesium ion to oxytocin and vasopressin on the isolated rat uterus. *Folia Pharmacol. Jap.* **62**, 42.

Kaneko, Y., Kawarabayashi, T., Sugimori, H. & Tsukamoto, T. (1995). Changes in kinetic properties of oxytocin receptors in longitudinal muscle membranes of rat uterus during gestation. *J. Mol. Recog.* **8**, 179–183.

Kasai, Y., Iino, M., Tsutsumi, O., Taketani, Y. & Endo, M. (1994). Effects of cyclopiazonic acid on rhythmic contractions in uterine smooth muscle bundles of the rat. Br. *J. Pharmacol.* **112**, 1132–1136.

Kawarabayashi, T., Izumi, H., Ikeda, M., Ichihara, J., Sugimori, H. & Shirakawa, K.

(1990). Modification by magnesium of the excitatory effect of oxytocin in electrical and mechanical activities of pregnant human myometrium. *Obstet. Gynecol.* **76**, 183–188.

Kawarabayashi, T. (1994). Electrophysiology of the human myometrium. In *The Uterus* (Chard T. & Grudzinska G. eds), pp. 148–172. Cambridge University Press, Cambridge.

Kuriyama, H. (1961). The effect of progesterone and oxytocin on the mouse myometrium. *J. Physiol.* **159**, 26–39.

Lansman, J.B., Hess, P. & Tsien, R.W. (1986). Blockade of current through single calcium channels by Cd^{2+}, Mg^{2+}, and Ca^{2+}. *J. Gen. Physiol.* **88**, 321–347.

Lategan, T.W. & Brading, A.F. (1988). Contractile effects of manganese on taenia of guinea pig caecum. *Am. J. Physiol.* **254**, G489–494.

Locke, F.S. (1901). Die Wirkung der Metalle des Blutplasmas und verschiedener Zucker auf das isolierte Säugetierherz. *Zbl. Physiol.* **14**, 670–672.

Lockwood, A.P.M. (1961). 'Ringer' solutions and some notes on the physiological basis of their ionic composition. *Comp. Biochem. Physiol.* **2**, 241–289.

Marshall, J.M. (1965). Calcium and uterine smooth muscle membrane potentials. In *Muscle* (Paul, W.M., Daniel, E.E., Kay, C.M. & Monckton, G. eds), pp. 229–238. Pergamon Press, Oxford.

Marshall, J.M. (1974). Effects of neurohypophysial hormones on the myometrium. In *Handbook of Physiology, Endocrinology, IV, Part 1*, pp. 469–492. Am. Physiol. Soc., Washington, D.C.

Massry, S.G., Coburn, J.W., Chapman, L.W. & Kleenman, C.R. (1968). The effect of long term desoxy corticosterone acetate administration on the renal excretion of calcium and magnesium. *J. Lab. Clin. Med.* **71**, 212–219.

Morishita, F., Kawarabayashi, T., Sakamoto, Y. & Shirakawa, K. (1995). Role of the sodium-calcium exchange mechanism and the effect of magnesium on sodium-free and high-potassium contractures in pregnant human myometrium. *Am. J. Obstet. Gynecol.* **172**, 186–195.

Nakayama, S. & Tomita, T. (1990). Depletion of intracellular free Mg^{2+} in Mg^{2+}- and Ca^{2+}-free solution in the taenia isolated from guinea pig caecum. *J. Physiol.* **421**, 363–378.

Ogasawara, T., Kato, S. & Osa, T. (1980). Effects of estradiol-17β on the membrane response and K-contracture in the uterine longitudinal muscle of ovariectomized rats studied in combination with the Mn action. *Jpn. J. Physiol.* **30**, 271–285.

Ohya, Y. & Sperelakis, N. (1990). Tocolytic agents act on calcium channel current in single smooth muscle cells of pregnant rat uterus. *J. Pharmacol. Exp. Ther.* **253**, 580–585.

Osa, T. & Ogasawara, T. (1979). Influence of magnesium on the β-inhibition of catecholamines in the uterine circular muscle of estrogen-treated rats. *Jpn. J. Physiol.* **29**, 339–352.

Osa, T. & Ogasawara, T. (1983). Effects of magnesium on the membrane activity and contraction of the circular muscle of rat myometrium during late pregnancy. *Jpn. J. Physiol.* **33**, 485–495.

Osa, T. & Maruta, K. (1986). Comparative effects of Mg, Ca, Sr, and verapamil on the uterine longitudinal muscle of spayed and estrogen-treated rats. *Jpn. J. Physiol.* **36**, 871–889.

Osa, T., Ogasawara, T. & Kato, S. (1981). Modification by magnesium and manganese ions of the effects of oxytocin on the electrical and mechanical activity of the longitudinal muscle of estrogen-treated rat uterus. *Jpn. J. Physiol.* **31**, 317–329.

Osa, T., Ogasawara, T. & Kato, S. (1983). Effects of magnesium, oxytocin, and prostaglandin F_{2a} on the generation and propagation of excitation in the longitudinal muscle of rat myometrium during late pregnancy. *Jpn. J. Physiol.* **33**, 51–67.

Osa, T., Inoue, H. & Okabe, K. (1991). Effects of porcine relaxin on contraction, membrane response and cyclic AMP content in rat myometrium in comparison with the effects of isoprenaline and forskolin. *Br. J. Pharmacol.* **104**, 950–960.

Osa, T., Inoue, H., Todoroki, N. & Cui, D. (1994). Effects of Mg and Mn ions on the inhibitory action of cyclic nucleotides in the longitudinal myometrium of rat. *Jpn. J. Physiol.* **44**, 49–66.

Pliška, V. & Albertin, H.K. (1991). Effect of Mg²⁺ on the binding of oxytocin to sheep myometrial cells. *Biochem. J.* **227**, 97–101.

Prosser, C.L. & Brown, F.K. (1965). *Comparative Animal Physiology.* Saunders. Philadelphia.

Ringer, S. (1883). A third contribution regarding the influence of the inorganic constituents of the blood on the ventricular contraction. *J. Physiol.* **4**, 222–225.

Romani, A. & Scarpa, A. (1992). Regulation of cell magnesium. *Arch. Biochem. Biophys.* **298**, 1–12.

Schild, H.O. (1969). The effect of metals on the S-S polypeptide receptor in depolarized rat uterus. *Br. J. Pharmacol.* **36**, 329–349.

Shibata, S. (1969). Effects of Mn on ⁴⁵Ca content and potassium-induced contraction of the aortic strips. *Can. J. Physiol. Pharmacol.* **47**, 827–829.

Soloff, M.S., Schroeder, B.J., Chakraborty, T. & Pearlmutter, A.R. (1977). Characterization of oxytocin receptors in the uterus and mammary gland. *Fed. Proc.* **36**, 1861–1866.

Somlyo, A.P. & Somlyo, A.V. (1994). Signal transduction and regulation in smooth muscle. *Nature.* **372**, 231–236.

Zhang, A., Cheng, T.P.O., Altura, B.T. & Altura, B.M. (1992). Extracellular magnesium regulates intracellular free Mg²⁺ in vascular smooth muscle cells. *Pflügers Arch.* **421**, 391–393.

38

Membrane Channels in Smooth Muscle Cells of Arteries from Hypertensive Rats

YUSUKE OHYA
ISAO ABE
KOJI FUJII
MASATOSHI FUJISHIMA

Second Department of Internal Medicine,
Kyushu University,
Fukuoka, Japan

Membrane channels in smooth muscle cells of arteries are considered to play a crucial role in controlling vascular tone (Nelson 1990). Alterations to membrane channels in arteries may contribute to the development and maintenance of hypertension. The patch-clamp technique has been used to examine the membrane channels in various tissues (Hamill *et al.*, 1981). The patch-clamp technique allows us to examine the characteristics of membrane channels directly. In the present paper, our recent studies on alterations of membrane channels in arteries from spontaneously hypertensive rats (SHRs) and Dahl salt-sensitive rats using the patch-clamp technique are reviewed.

Ca^{2+} CHANNELS IN ARTERIES FROM SHR

Current density

The SHR develops hypertension as it maturates. In SHRs at about 10 weeks old or later the blood pressure is significantly elevated compared with its normotensive control, Wistar–Kyoto rats (WKYs). In adult SHRs after the development of hypertension, the resting vascular tone is elevated and its reactivity to various agonists is enhanced compared with WKYs. These alterations are considered to contribute to the maintenance of hypertension. It has been reported that administration of drugs such as angiotensin-converting enzyme inhibitors or blockers of the sympathetic nervous system

SMOOTH MUSCLE EXCITATION
ISBN 0-12-112360-X

(plus vasodilating drugs) to neonatal and young SHRs delayed or abolished the development of hypertension (Harrap *et al.*, 1990). This observation thus suggests that factors which act in the prehypertensive period play a crucial role in the development of hypertension in SHR. In voltage-clamp experiments, Rusch & Hermsmeyer (1988) reported that the L-type Ca^{2+} channel current in cultured azygos venous cells from neonatal SHR was increased compared with that of WKY. They suggested that the alteration of L-type Ca^{2+} channels may result from a strain-difference between SHRs and WKYs.

We therefore conducted experiments using freshly isolated single cells from a mesenteric resistance artery from young (4–6 weeks old; before the development of hypertension) and adult rats (16–20 weeks old; after the development of hypertension)(Ohya *et al.*, 1993). These cells were used because it was desired to investigate the alteration of Ca^{2+} channels in a resistance artery which is relevant to the control of the blood pressure and to investigate whether the alteration of Ca^{2+} channels observed in neonatal rats continues into the adult.

The cell size, input resistance, cell capacitance, and membrane specific capacitance were nearly the same between SHRs and WKYs both when young and when adult. The cell size was larger in adult rats than in young rats. Ca^{2+} channel currents were recorded with 50 mM Ba^{2+} as the charge carrier. The pipette solution contained a high Cs^+ solution with 3 mM ATP to record Ca^{2+} channel current. Under these conditions, most of the inward Ca^{2+} current was found to be of the L-type (Ohya & Sperelakis, 1989). The density (current amplitude normalized by cell capacitance) of Ca^{2+} current was significantly higher in cells from young SHRs than in cells from young WKYs. The difference in the current densities was evident after inhibiting the T-type Ca^{2+} channel current by depolarizing the membrane to $-40\,mV$ suggesting that the alteration of L-type Ca^{2+} channels mainly contributed to the difference in the current densities. Since the blood pressure level did not differ between young SHRs and young WKYs, the increased current densities were not considered to contribute to the maintenance of hypertension. The alteration of Ca^{2+} channels in young rats may be related to the development of hypertension; however, the role of the enhanced Ca^{2+} channel activity in the development of hypertension is presently unknown. One possible hypothesis is that the increased Ca^{2+} channel activity may be related to the vascular hypertrophy and the remodelling of the artery which occurs during the development of hypertension (Mulvany & Aalkaer, 1990).

Blood pressure of adult SHRs was significantly elevated compared with adult WKYs; however, the Ca^{2+} current densities, of adult SHRs and adult WKYs were nearly the same. Thus, changes in the Ca^{2+} current density cannot explain the increased vascular tone in adult SHRs. A recent study by

Wilde *et al.* (1994) showed that Ca^{2+} channel current in cerebral arterial cells from stroke prone SHRs (SHR-SPs) at adult age (> 17 weeks old) was increased compared with WKYs. The authors suggested that alteration of Ca^{2+} channels which persisted to adulthood may contribute to the maintenance of hypertension. Differences between our study and their study may be due to the use of different strains (SHR versus SHR-SP) or different arteries (mesenteric resistance artery vs. cerebral artery). Blood pressure of SHR-SPs increases to reach a higher level than that of SHRs until finally a stroke occurs. In contrast, the blood pressure of SHRs reaches a plateau level after about 30 weeks old. Therefore, the limitation in the enhancement of Ca^{2+} channel activity may protect SHRs from vascular damage.

Dihydropyridine sensitivity

Ca^{2+} channel antagonists are used clinically as a treatment for hypertension and angina pectoris. Ca^{2+} channel antagonists are very effective for decreasing the blood pressure. The degree of decrease in the blood pressure by Ca^{2+} channel antagonists is larger in hypertensives than in normotensives. This observation may imply that the sensitivity of Ca^{2+} channels to Ca^{2+} channel antagonist in arteries of hypertensives may thus be altered.

It has been reported that Bay K 8644, a dihydropyridine Ca^{2+} channel agonist, contracted the femoral artery from adult SHRs but did not contract the same artery from adult WKYs (Aoki & Asano, 1986). Studies using a Ca^{2+}-sensitive dye also revealed that Bay K 8644 caused a greater increase in intracellular Ca^{2+} ($[Ca^{2+}]_i$) in aortic smooth muscle cells from SHRs compared with WKYs (Sada *et al.*, 1990). Thus, alteration of the dihydropyridine sensitivity of Ca^{2+} channels in SHRs has been postulated. However, the dihydropyridine sensitivity of Ca^{2+} channels in arteries from SHRs has not yet been examined by the voltage clamp technique.

Ca^{2+} channel agonist

We compared the action of Bay K 8644 on Ca^{2+} channel currents in mesenteric arterial cells from adult SHRs and adult WKYs (18–26 weeks old). Conditions for the current recording were same as those in experiments for the current density. Application of Bay K 8644 increased the amplitude of Ca^{2+} channel current. The dose-dependent enhancement of the current amplitude was similar between SHRs and WKYs. Bay K 8644 also shifted the threshold potential of channel activation in a hyperpolarized direction. The degree of shift was similar between SHRs and WKYs. These results suggest that there was essentially no difference between the actions of Bay K 8644 on Ca^{2+} channels of SHRs and WKYs. The differences in the actions of Bay K

8644 observed on contraction and on $[Ca^{2+}]_i$ thus cannot be explained by alterations of Ca^{2+} channels.

Ca^{2+} channel antagonists

Action of Ca^{2+} channel antagonists on Ca^{2+} channel currents in mesenteric arterial cells from adult SHRs and adult WKYs were examined. Application of nicardipine, one of the dihydropyridine Ca^{2+} channel antagonists, concentration-dependently inhibited the Ca^{2+} channel current. A concentration–response relationship was obtained under the conditions where the current was evoked from a fully hyperpolarized holding potential (-90 mV) and with a low stimulation-frequency (0.033 Hz). Under these conditions, the concentration-response relationship is considered to reflect the sensitivity to nicardipine of Ca^{2+} channels in the resting state (Bean, 1984). There was no difference in the concentration–response curve between SHRs and WKYs, which suggested that the sensitivity to nicardipine of the resting channels was not different between SHRs and WKYs.

Nicardipine shifted the steady-state inactivation curves in a hyperpolarized direction. The shift of the steady-state inactivation curves was similar between SHRs and WKYs. The shift of the steady-state inactivation curve is considered to result from the difference in K_d value of the drug for the channels in the resting state and in the inactivated state (Bean, 1984). Therefore, the similar concentration–response curve and the similar shift in steady-state inactivation curve between SHRs and WKYs may suggest that the nicardipine-sensitivity of Ca^{2+} channels, both in the resting state and in the inactivated state was not altered in SHRs.

ALTERATION OF K^+ CHANNELS IN ARTERIES
FROM SHRs

It has been reported by other groups that Ca^{2+} dependent K^+ channel activity was enhanced in hypertensive rats (SHRs, coarctation of the aorta) (Rusch *et al.*, 1992; Rusch & Runnells, 1994). Antihypertensive treatment for several weeks decreased the blood pressure and normalized the alteration in Ca^{2+} dependent K^+ channels, which suggested that chronic hypertension may secondarily cause an alteration in Ca^{2+} dependent K^+ channels. The activation of K^+ channels hyperpolarizes the membrane and decreases $[Ca^{2+}]_i$. Therefore the increased activity of Ca^{2+} dependent K^+ channels is considered to work against the $[Ca^{2+}]_i$ -overload in arterial cells of hypertensive rats.

The ATP sensitive K^+ channel is known to be a target for K^+ channel openers. It has been reported using the open cranial window technique to observe the basilar artery, that the vasodilatation by K^+ channel opener, aprikalim decreased in stroke-prone SHR compared with WKY (Kitazono *et al.*, 1993). We examined the action of a K^+ channel opener, levcromakalim on the ATP-sensitive K^+ channel in mesenteric artery from adult SHRs and adult WKYs (18–26 weeks old). The bath contained a physiological salt solution. The pipette solution was a high K^+ solution containing 1 mM GDP. Application of levcromakalim evoked the current concentration-dependently. The evoked current was inhibited by glibenclamide, a specific blocker for ATP-sensitive K^+ channels. The current induced by levcromakalim was smaller in SHRs than in WKYs. It was apparent from the concentration–response curve, that the ED_{50} value was larger in SHRs than in WKYs. Our findings may thus explain the decreased vasodilator action of K^+ channel opener on arteries in hypertensive rats.

Ca^{2+} channels in arteries from Dahl salt-sensitive rats

Dahl salt-sensitive rats and Dahl salt-resistant rats are model rats for salt-sensitive hypertension (Iwai & Heine, 1986). In Dahl salt-sensitive rats, the hypertension develops after the salt loading, while with a low salt diet the blood pressure remains low. In contrast, hypertension does not develop by salt loading in Dahl salt-resistant rats.

We examined electrophysiological features of the mesenteric artery from Dahl salt-sensitive rats fed a high salt diet (8% NaCl) and a low salt diet (0.3%). Hypertension developed only in rats fed a high salt diet. The resting membrane potential in mesenteric artery of the rats fed a high salt diet was depolarized compared with the rats fed a low salt diet (Fujii *et al.*, 1992). In addition, spontaneous electrical activity was recorded in most of the arteries from rats fed a high salt diet, while such activity was not observed in arteries from rats fed a low salt diet. This spontaneous electrical activity was inhibited by Ca^{2+} channel antagonist, suggesting that activity of L-type Ca^{2+} channels was enhanced in the artery from Dahl salt-sensitive rats fed a high salt diet.

A voltage-clamp study was performed to record Ca^{2+} channel currents. The conditions used were same as those in the studies for Ca^{2+} channels of SHRs. The maximal Ca^{2+} current density (observed at a command potential of 20 or 30 mV) was not increased in rats fed a high salt diet. However, the threshold potential for channel activation was shifted in a negative direction and the current densities at negative command potentials (-40 to -20 mV) were larger in the rats fed a high salt diet. The difference in the current densities was evident after inhibiting the T-type Ca^{2+} channel current by depolarizing the membrane to -40 mV, suggesting that the L-type Ca^{2+} channels may be altered. Accordingly, the voltage-dependent activation curve was shifted significantly in a negative direction in the rats fed a high salt diet compared with the rats fed a low salt diet. Because the steady-state inactivation curve for the Ca^{2+} current was unchanged between the rats fed a high salt diet and those fed a low salt diet, window current (the non-inactivating component of the Ca^{2+} channels current) was increased by the salt-loading. In summary, the high salt diet made L-type Ca^{2+} channels more available near the resting membrane potential. At the depolarized membrane potentials which are observed with high salt diets, the enhanced Ca^{2+} channel activity may therefore contribute to the increased vascular tone of Dahl S rats fed these diets. Further study of which factors cause alterations of Ca^{2+} channels as a result of salt-loading are being carried out.

REFERENCES

Aoki, K. & Asano, M. (1986). Effects of Bay K 8644 and nifedipine on femoral arteries of spontaneously hypertensive rats. *Br. J. Pharmacol.* **88**, 221–230.

Bean, B.P. (1984). Nitrendipine block of cardiac calcium channels: high-affinity binding to the inactivated state. *Proc. Natl Acad. Sci. USA* **81**, 6388–6392.

Fujii, K., Ohmori, S., Tominaga, M., Abe, I., Takata, Y. & Fujishima, M. (1992). Hypertension impairs endothelium-dependent hyperpolarization, while it promotes spontaneous electrical activities in the isolated rat mesenteric artery (abst). *J. Hypertens.* **10**, S53.

Hamill, O.P., Marty, A., Nehr, E., Sackmann, B. & Sigworth, F.J. (1981). Improved patch-clamp techniques for high-resolution current recordings from cell and cell-membrane patches. *Pflügers Arch.* **391**, 85–100.

Harrap, S.B., Van der Merwe, W.M., Griffin, S.A., Macpherson, F. & Lever, A.F. (1990). Brief angiotensin converting enzyme inhibitor treatment in young spontaneously hypertensive rats reduces blood pressure long term. *Hypertension* **16**, 603–617

Iwai, J. & Heine, M. (1986). Dahl salt-sensitive rats and human essential hypertension. *J. Hypertens.* **4** (Suppl. 3), S29–S31.

Kitazono, T., Heistad, D.D. & Faraci, F.K. (1993). ATP-sensitive potassium channels in the basilar artery during chronic hypertension. *Hypertension* **32**, 677–681.

Mulvany, M.J. & Aalkaer, C. (1990). Structure and function of small arteries. *Physiol. Rev.* **70**, 921–961.

Nelson, M.T., Patlak, J.B., Worley, J.F. & Standen, N.B. (1990). Calcium channels, potassium channels, and voltage dependence of arterial smooth muscle tone. *Am. J. Physio.* l **258**, C3–C18.

Ohya, Y. & Sperelakis, N (1989). ATP regulation of the slow calcium channels in vascular smooth muscle cells of guinea pig mesenteric artery. *Circ. Res.* **64**, 145–154.

Ohya, Y., Abe, I., Fujii, K., Takata, Y. & Fujishima, M. (1993). Voltage-dependent Ca^{2+} channels in resistance arteries from spontaneous hypertensive rats. *Circ. Res.* **73**, 1090–1099.

Rusch, N.J. & Hermsmeyer, K. (1988) Calcium currents are altered in the vascular muscle cell membrane of spontaneously hypertensive rats. *Circ. Res.* **63**, 997–1002.

Rusch, N.J. & Runnells, A.M. (1994). Remission of high blood pressure reverses arterial potassium channel alterations. *Hypertension* **238** (part 2), 941–945.

Rusch, N.J., De Lucena, R.G., Wooldridge, T.A., England, S.K. & Cowley Jr, A.W.

(1992). A Ca^{2+}-dependent K^+current is enhanced in arterial membranes of hypertensive rats. *Hypertension* **19**, 301–307.

Sada, T., Koike, H., Ikeda, M., Sato, K., Ozaki, H. & Karaki, H. (1990). Cytosolic free calcium of aorta in hypertensive rats: Chronic inhibition of angiotensin converting enzyme. *Hypertension* **16**, 245–251.

Wilde, D.W., Furspan, P.B. & Szocik, J.F. (1994). Calcium current in smooth muscle cells from normotensive and genetically hypertensive rats. *Hypertension* **24**, 739–746.

39

Transmission of Excitation at Autonomic Neuroeffector Junctions

G. D. S. HIRST
H. M. COUSINS

*Department of Zoology,
University of Melbourne,
Parkville, Victoria,
Australia*

All autonomic effector organs receive an excitatory innervation which, when activated, causes an increase in the activity of that organ. As examples, sympathetic nerve stimulation causes most arteries, arterioles and veins to contract, parasympathetic nerve stimulation causes increased insulin secretion, stimulation of intrinsic cholinergic nerves causes contraction of intestinal smooth muscle, sympathetic nerve stimulation causes an increase in heart rate and an increase in the contractile response. Each of these responses invariably involves an increase in the free concentration of calcium ions, $[Ca^{2+}]_i$, inside the effector cells. However the way in which $[Ca^{2+}]_i$ is increased varies from tissue to tissue. At this stage it is clear that neurally released transmitters may trigger an increase $[Ca^{2+}]_i$ in smooth muscle by one of at least three different mechanisms:

1. In systemic arteries, arterioles and the vas deferens, sympathetic nerve stimulation releases a transmitter, probably adenosine triphosphate, ATP, (Sneddon & Burnstock, 1984; Sneddon & Westfall, 1984; Kügelgen & Starke, 1985) which interacts with sets of ligand gated channels. Activation of these channels causes a depolarization which leads to the opening of voltage dependent Ca^{2+} channels (Hirst & Edwards, 1989). Ca^{2+} enters from the extracellular fluid either in sufficient amount to trigger contraction or after augmentation by Ca^{2+} release from intracellular stores.
2. In intestinal muscle, intrinsic nerve stimulation causes the release of acetylcholine (ACh) which activates a muscarinic receptor and triggers a depolarization. Again the depolarization causes the opening of voltage

SMOOTH MUSCLE EXCITATION
ISBN 0-12-112360-X

dependent Ca^{2+} channels. However, when intestinal voltage dependent Ca^{2+} channels are blocked by organic Ca^{2+} antagonists it becomes apparent that the neurally released ACh itself causes a dramatic increase in $[Ca^{2+}]_i$ (Cousins *et al.*, 1993, 1995).

3. In pulmonary arteries, veins, iris dilator muscle and anococygeous muscle, sympathetic nerve stimulation causes the release of noradrenaline which activates a-adrenoceptors. The subsequent increase in $[Ca^{2+}]_i$ results from the activation of a pathway that is independent of membrane potential changes in the smooth muscle cells: rather it relies on Ca^{2+} release from intracellular stores (van Helden, 1991).

In each case nerve stimulation initiates a membrane potential change; this review will discuss the membrane potential changes associated with each of these three mechanisms in a range of tissues largely composed of smooth muscle.

NEUROEFFECTOR TRANSMISSION INVOLVING THE ACTIVATION OF LIGAND-GATED CHANNELS

In the vas deferens, systemic arteries and arterioles, sympathetic nerve stimulation triggers a characteristic excitatory junction potential or e.j.p. In each tissue, e.j.ps are resistant to α-adrenoceptor blockade (Holman & Surprenant, 1980; Burnstock & Holman, 1964; Angus *et al.*, 1988). When initiated by local field stimulation e.j.ps have short latencies, 10–20 ms, rising phases lasting some 50–100 ms and total durations of 0.3–1 s (Burnstock & Holman, 1961; Bell, 1969; Bennett, 1972; Hirst, 1977; Hirst & Neild, 1978; Cheung, 1982; Hill *et al.*, 1983; Itoh *et al.*, 1983; Kajiwara *et al.*, 1981; Hottenstein & Kreulen, 1987). E.j.ps themselves do not initiate contraction; usually, several e.j.ps must sum together to produce a large enough depolarization to activate smooth muscle voltage-dependent Ca^{2+} channels (Hirst, 1977; Hirst & Edwards, 1989; Blakely *et al.*, 1981). When these Ca^{2+} channels are blocked nerve stimulation continues to evoke e.j.ps but fails to initiate a contraction.

The time course of the excitatory junctional current, e.j.c., underlying an e.j.p. is much briefer than that of the e.j.p. The peak current occurs after 10 ms and the current has a total duration of about 200 ms with the decay of current being described by a single exponential having a time constant of some 25–50 ms. This has been shown in three different ways – by directly measuring the e.j.c. using a single-electrode voltage clamp technique (Finkel *et al.*, 1984); by determining the cable constants of the tissue and calculating the time course of the e.j.c. (Hirst & Neild, 1978; Holman & Suprenant, 1979; Bywater & Taylor, 1980; Cassell *et al.*, 1988); by measuring the time course of the e.j.c. using an extracellular electrode (Astrand *et al.*, 1988; Brock & Cunnane, 1988). The amplitudes of e.j.cs vary linearly with membrane potential and have a reversal potential of about 0 mV (Finkel *et al.*, 1984). The rapid rising phase and the short latency of the e.j.c. indicate that sympathetic transmitter at these junctions is activating sets of ligand-gated channels.

At junctions where the transmitter activates ligand-gated channels, spontaneously released quanta of transmitter produce detectable potential changes, termed spontaneous excitatory junction potentials or s.e.j.ps. As might be expected, s.e.j.ps are readily detected in systemic arteries, arterioles and vas deferens. This being the case, it is possible to describe the release of transmitter from single varicosities or groups of varicosities. There is now uniform acceptance that the probability of release at individual varicosities per nerve impulse is very low. The idea was first suggested by Burnstock & Holman (1961) who noted that during trains of stimuli only a few e.j.ps had rapid rising phases. They commented that if the rapid rising phases resulted from the local release of a packet of transmitter, then this occurred infrequently. These observations were confirmed by Blakeley & Cunnane (1979) who showed that the likelihood that a quantum of transmitter would be released near the recording electrode was extremely low. When the properties of s.e.j.ps and e.j.ps were compared in short isopotential segments of arteriole, it was found that the amplitudes of e.j.ps were either similar to, or a small multiple of, those of s.e.j.ps. As the preparations contained about 200 varicosities this observation suggested that the probability of release from an individual varicosity was low or that most varicosities did not release transmitter (Hirst & Neild, 1980). When Cunnane and his colleagues applied extracellular recording techniques to record the output of transmitter from a string of varicosities along with the arrival of the nerve impulse in the varicosities, they showed that a nerve impulse invariably invaded the nerve terminal but that a quantum of transmitter was rarely released (Cunnane & Stjärne, 1982; Brock & Cunnane, 1988; Astrand & Stjärne, 1989; Lavidis & Bennett, 1992; Brock & Cunnane, 1993). It was also shown that the interval between the arrival of a nerve impulse in a varicosity and the start of junctional current flow was some 2–3 ms (Brock & Cunnane, 1993), an observation again supporting the idea that groups of ligand-gated channels were being activated.

It seems likely that transmitter is released at the organised neuroeffector junctions found in tissues innervated by sympathetic post-ganglionic axons (Luff *et al.*, 1987; Luff & McLachlan 1988, 1989; Klemm *et al.*, 1992, 1993; Choate *et al.*, 1993; Hill *et al.*, 1993). Characteristically, sympathetic varicosities approach a muscle membrane and form a close apposition with an area of smooth muscle membrane. Vesicles concentrate towards the region of close apposition; although presynaptic specializations are occasionally detected, no post-junctional specializations are found (Klemm *et al.*, 1993). Furthermore, it appears unlikely that after release, transmitter spreads in appreciable concentration far from the point of release. If transmitter were to diffuse freely through the extracellular space, one might expect applied and neurally released transmitter to produce very similar responses. In the case of purinergic junctions this is clearly not the case. As indicated, nerve stimulation evokes an e.j.c. with a latency of some 2–3 ms. The resulting current has a rapid rising phase and does not trigger a contraction. In contrast, ATP applied by ionophoresis produces a response with a minimum latency of some 50 ms (Benham *et al.*, 1987). The channels activated by applied ATP have high Ca^{2+} selectivity (Benham, 1989). In some tissues such as the vas deferens, the responses to nerve stimulation are abolished by suramin whereas those produced by applied ATP are little affected. Moreover although the responses to nerve stimulation are abolished by blocking muscle voltage-dependent Ca^{2+} channels, those to applied ATP are only partly affected (Reilly & Hirst, 1996). The simplest explanations for each of these observations are either that ATP is not the transmitter, or if it is, that it activates pools of junctional receptors located under sympathetic varicosities which differ from extra-junctional receptors which are most readily activated by added ATP.

Thus, although vasa deferentia, arteries and arterioles are densely innervated, transmitter will only be released at a few regions following a nerve impulse. Moreover, neurally released transmitter appears to be confined to the junctional region and does spread to neighbouring cells. Because contraction of these tissues depends upon the opening of voltage-dependent Ca^{2+} channels, for non-innervated smooth muscle cells to contribute, junctional depolarizations must spread to the non-innervated cells. This is clearly the case; an e.j.p. is recorded from every cell following a nerve impulse, thus individual smooth muscle cells must be coupled to neighbouring cells so that they form an electrical syncytium. Electrical coupling has been demonstrated in every preparation examined. The analyses show that arteries and vasa deferentia behave as simple linear cables with electrical length constants in the range 0.3–2 mm (Bolton, 1974; Mekata, 1974; Casteels *et al.*, 1977; Bywater and Taylor, 1980; Holman & Surprenant, 1980; Kajiwara *et al.*, 1983; Cassell *et al.*, 1988). Electrical coupling between arteriolar cells has been demonstrated using two independent intracellular electrodes, one to pass current and the other to record potential changes (Hirst & Neild, 1978, 1980). When a current was passed through one electrode, a membrane potential change was detected at the second electrode.

Together, the observations suggest that at junctions where ligand gated channels are involved in transmission:

1. Transmitter is released at organized neuroeffector junctions where it activates pools of junctional receptors.
2. The probability that an individual varicosity will release a quantum of transmitter per nerve impulse is low.
3. Individual smooth muscle cells are electrically coupled to their neighbours so that depolarization can spread to cells which are not influenced by transmitter.
4. An increase in $[Ca^{2+}]_i$ following nerve stimulation results entirely from the entry of Ca^{2+} via muscle voltage dependent Ca^{2+} channels.

NEUROEFFECTOR TRANSMISSION INVOLVING THE ACTIVATION OF MUSCARINIC RECEPTORS IN INTESTINAL MUSCLE

Both smooth muscle layers of the mammalian intestine are innervated by cholinergic nerves whose cell bodies lie in the enteric nervous system. When stimulated these nerves initiate e.j.ps which are abolished by muscarinic receptor antagonists (Bennett, 1972; Bauer & Kuriyama, 1982; Bauer et al., 1991; Cousins et al., 1993). In control solutions, e.j.ps initiate action potentials, an associated increase in $[Ca^{2+}]_i$ which in turn triggers a contraction (Ito et al., 1988). However, in intestinal muscle the contractile responses to nerve stimulation are only partly reduced by blocking muscle voltage-dependent Ca^{2+} channels with organic Ca^{2+} antagonists (Zar & Goopta, 1983; Cousins et al., 1993, 1995). Thus a part of the increase in $[Ca^{2+}]_i$ involved in the generation of a contractile response arises from the opening of muscle voltage-dependent Ca^{2+} channels and part arises from an action of the transmitter itself.

As with 'ligand gated' junctions, single stimuli initiate detectable e.j.ps at muscarinic junctions in intestinal muscle; unlike 'ligand gated' junctions e.j.ps evoked at 'muscarinic junctions have latencies in excess of 100 ms (Bennett, 1966; Furness, 1969; Bauer et al., 1991; Bauer & Kuriyama, 1982; Cousins et al., 1993). In addition, s.e.j.ps which result from the release of single quanta of transmitter are not detected. In preparations of guinea pig ileal longitudinal muscle in which muscle Ca^{2+} channels have been blocked, single supramaximal stimuli initiate e.j.ps with maximum amplitudes of about 10 mV. At 25°C the depolarization starts after delay of some 200 to 500ms: the rising phase lasts some 300 to 600 ms and the e.j.p. has a total duration of some 1 to 2 s (Cousins et al., 1993). Both the latencies and time courses of e.j.ps are sensitive to temperature, with each approximately halving with a 10°C increase in bathing temperature (Cousins et al., 1993). When the time course of the e.j.c. underlying a muscarinic e.j.p. was calculated, using the measured electrical cable

constants of the muscle layer, it was found that the current had a long
latency and a duration approaching that of the e.j.p. Presumably, the long
latencies and slow time courses of muscarinic e.j.ps, each of which are
sensitive to small changes ($\sim10°C$) in temperature, reflect the kinetics of
activation and deactivation of a second messenger formed after muscarinic
receptor stimulation. Unlike the e.j.ps recorded from 'ligand gated'
junctions, even when smooth muscle Ca^{2+} channels are blocked, e.j.ps in
intestinal muscle are associated with brisk contractions (Cousins et al.,
1993). When the changes in $[Ca^{2+}]_i$ associated with an e.j.p. were measured
it was found that $[Ca^{2+}]_i$ increased with a time course very similar to that of
the underlying e.j.c. There are a number of explanations for these
observations. One is that the e.j.c. and increase in $[Ca^{2+}]_i$ are causally
related. This would imply that a second messenger causes the opening of a
set of Ca^{2+} selective channels. The resulting current would produce a
depolarization and a simultaneous increase in $[Ca^{2+}]_i$. The second is that
the messenger substance could activate a set of cation selective channels
and simultaneously cause the release of Ca^{2+} from an intracellular store.
Alternatively, the increase in $[Ca^{2+}]_i$ might cause the opening of sets of
nonselective cation channels.

Whichever the case may be it is clear, as with 'ligand gated' junctions, that
neurally released ACh produces a different response to that produced by
applied ACh. In the guinea-pig ileum, applied ACh causes a membrane
depolarization that results from the opening of nonselective cation channels
(Benham et al., 1985; Inoue et al., 1987; Inoue & Isenberg, 1990a,b; Vogalis
& Sanders, 1990). Channel opening is influenced by membrane potential and
$[Ca^{2+}]_i$ (Benham et al., 1985; Lim & Bolton, 1988; Inoue & Isenberg, 1990b)
and occurs after activation of a complex pathway (Komori & Bolton, 1990;
Inoue & Isenberg, 1990a,b; Pacaud & Bolton, 1991). In addition, applied
ACh releases Ca^{2+} from intracellular stores through the involvement of
inositol trisphosphate, IP_3, (Bolton & Lim, 1989; Komori & Bolton, 1990,
1991). Ca^{2+} release from the intracellular stores occurs in a pulsatile manner.
The 'quanta' of Ca^{2+} transiently increase $[Ca^{2+}]_i$ and activate several Ca^{2+}
activated K^+ channels. These in turn give rise to a series of transient
hyperpolarizations which are abolished by barium ions or charybdotoxin.
Thus, ionophoretically applied ACh produces depolarizations which are
interrupted by transient hyperpolarizations (Cousins et al., 1995). In marked
contrast, although e.j.ps were associated with an increase in $[Ca^{2+}]_i$ they
were never interrupted by transient hyperpolarizations (Cousins et al., 1993;
1995).

The latencies of ionophoretic potentials were longer than those of e.j.ps. In
a series of experiments an ACh pipette was placed within $5\,\mu m$ of the
recording electrode and within $2\,\mu m$ of the muscle surface. E.j.ps had
latencies of about 550 ms while the ionophoretic potentials had latencies of

about 650 ms. The differences were significantly different (Cousins *et al.*, 1995).

The most convincing evidence that neurally released ACh may activate a novel conductance change comes from the experiments in which ACh was allowed to escape from cholinerigic neuroeffector junctions by treating the preparations with the cholinesterase inhibitor eserine. When this was done, e.j.ps increased in amplitude and many were then interrupted by transient hyperpolarizations. Moreover, e.j.ps and the associated changes in muscle $[Ca^{2+}]_i$ recorded in control solutions, could be abolished by high concentrations of any of nicardipine, verapamil or diltiazem by a post-junctional action (see Cousins *et al.*, 1993). In the presence of these agents, eserine restored a 'slow' e.j.p. which was invariably associated with a smaller increase in muscle $[Ca^{2+}]_i$ than was associated with a comparably sized e.j.p. recorded in control solutions (Cousins *et al.*, 1995).

Again, the simplest explanation for the observations is that neurally released ACh activates a subset of junctional muscarinic receptors that differ from those more readily activated by applied ACh. Presumably, these receptors are located at the cholinergic neuroeffector junctions found in this tissue (Klemm, 1995).

As with tissues in which transmission relies on ligand-gated channels, intestinal muscle cells are linked together to form an electrical syncytium. This was first shown unequivocally by Tomita and his colleagues (Abe & Tomita, 1968). More recently the cable properties of the longitudinal muscle layer of the guinea-pig ileum were determined using two intracellular electrodes (Cousins *et al.*, 1993). These experiments showed that current flowed more readily along the muscle layer than in a circumferential direction. In the longitudinal muscle layer the innervation is largely confined to the inner surface, adjacent to the myenteric plexus (Klemm, 1995). The electrical connections between cells allow membrane depolarizations to spread to non-innervated cells and so activate voltage dependent Ca^{2+} channels present in their membranes. Perhaps in these tissues the connections may also serve to allow second messengers to pass to non-innervated cells so that they may also participate in the part of the contractile response that is not dependent on the entry of Ca^{2+} via muscle voltage-dependent Ca^{2+} channels.

Thus, at junctions where muscarinic receptors are involved in transmission:-

1. Transmitter is released at organized neuroeffector junctions where it activates pools of junctional receptors.
2. Since s.e.j.ps cannot be detected little is known about the probability of release of transmitter from an individual varicosity.
3. Individual smooth muscle cells are electrically coupled to their

neighbours so that depolarization can spread to cells which are not influenced directly by transmitter; the electrical connections may also allow the movement of Ca^{2+} or other second messengers between cells.

4. An increase in $[Ca^{2+}]_i$ following nerve stimulation results partly from the entry of Ca^{2+} via muscle voltage-dependent Ca^{2+} channels and partly from a receptor mediated pathway.

NEUROMUSCULAR TRANSMISSION AT JUNCTIONS WHICH INVOLVE THE ACTIVATION OF α-ADRENOCEPTORS

In pulmonary arteries, most veins and iris dilator cells, sympathetic nerve stimulation produces membrane depolarizations that last for several seconds (Suzuki, 1981, 1983; van Helden, 1988a; Hill et al., 1993). Unlike both 'ligand gated' and 'muscarinic' junctions, single supramaximal nerve stimuli fail to evoke detectable depolarizations. When triggered by a few stimuli, a small e.j.p. with an amplitude of some 2–3 mV is detected after a long latency of some 1–2 s. These small depolarizations are associated with muscle contraction indicating that the opening of muscle voltage-dependent Ca^{2+} channels are not involved in the increases in muscle $[Ca^{2+}]_i$ induced by sympathetic nerve stimulation. Repetitive nerve stimulation evokes larger more sustained e.j.ps. In each preparation large e.j.ps have complex shapes, frequently an initial transient component is followed by a sustained component. These responses to nerve stimulation are blocked by α-adrenoceptor antagonists (Suzuki, 1981, 1983; van Helden, 1988b, Hill et al., 1993). In mesenteric veins and dilator cells (van Helden, 1988a,b, 1991) an ongoing discharge of spontaneous transient depolarizations, s.t.ds, is detected. S.t.ds are not to be confused with s.e.j.ps, they do not result from the spontaneous release of quanta of transmitter from sympathetic nerve terminals since they persist in the presence of a-adrenoceptor antagonists (Hill et al., 1993). S.t.ds result from the pulsatile release of Ca^{2+} from intracellular stores (van Helden, 1991). Ca^{2+} then activates sets of Ca^{2+}-activated Cl^- channels to produce a series of transient depolarizations. S.t.ds increase in frequency shortly after a period of sympathetic nerve stimulation and sum to give the slow e.j.p. (van Helden, 1991; Hill et al., 1993). The pathway leading to an increased rate of release of Ca^{2+} from intracellular stores is very similar to that described for the release of intracellular Ca^{2+} in the intestine following the addition of ACh. At neuroeffector junctions where transmission involves the activation of α-adrenoceptors, noradrenaline is released and activates an adrenoceptor which in turn leads to the activation of phospholipase-C and the formation of IP_3. Ca^{2+} is then released in a pulsatile manner from intracellular stores (Berridge, 1987).

In tissues where α-adrenoceptors are activated by sympathetic nerve stimulation, sympathetic varicosities also form organized neuroeffector junctions (Hill et al., 1993; Klemm et al., 1993). Individual sympathetic varicosities form close appositions with accumulations of synaptic vesicles. In mesenteric veins, presynaptic specializations are frequently detected. However, since spontaneous junction potentials which reflect the release of individual quanta of transmitter are not detected, little is known about the probability of release of transmitter from individual varicosities. If the release pattern follows that described for 'ligand gated' junctions, again it seems likely that some form of electrical coupling must exist in smooth muscle tissues where neuroeffector transmission involves the activation of α-adrenoceptors, as e.j.ps are readily recorded from all cells following a few nerve impulses. The electrical properties of arterioles in the dilator muscle of the rat iris have recently been determined using two intracellular electrodes (D. Gould, C. Hill & G.D.S.H. unpublished observations). In these vessels where sympathetic transmission involves the activation of α-adrenoceptors, it was apparent that smooth muscle cells were coupled to their neighbouring cells to form a syncytium. Because it is clear that in these vessels that Ca^{2+} entry via muscle voltage-dependent Ca^{2+} channels is of little importance in the generation of tension, one must speculate that electrical connections between cells allow the passage of Ca^{2+} or another second messenger between cells. In this way cells not directly affected by neurally released transmitter will participate in the generation of tension.

To summarize, at junctions where α-adrenoceptors are activated:

1. Transmitter is released at organized neuroeffector junctions where it activates α-adrenoceptors.
2. Again, little is known about the probability of release of transmitter from an individual varicosity.
3. Individual smooth muscle cells are electrically coupled to their neighbours and the electrical connections may allow the movement of Ca^{2+} or other second messengers from cell to cell.
4. An increase in $[Ca^{2+}]_i$ following nerve stimulation results mainly from the activation of a receptor-mediated pathway which releases Ca^{2+} from intracellular stores.

SIMILARITIES AND DISSIMILARITIES BETWEEN PROCESSES OF TRANSMISSION AT 'LIGAND GATED', 'MUSCARINIC' AND 'α-ADRENOCEPTORS' MEDIATED NEUROMUSCULAR JUNCTIONS

Several features are common to each of the three junctions discussed. At each, histological studies indicate that autonomic varicosities form organized neuroeffector junctions. Varicosities lie within 100 nm of the effector cell and vesicles accumulate at these points of close apposition. At each type of junction the individual effector cells are coupled together to form an electrical syncytium which allows the movement of ions between cells and may also allow the movement of second messenger substances. In each tissue contraction results from an increase in $[Ca^{2+}]_i$ but the way in which this is achieved varies with junction type. At 'ligand gated' junctions the entry of Ca^{2+} from the extracellular fluid is critical. At 'muscarinic' junctions the increase in $[Ca^{2+}]_i$ results partly from Ca^{2+} entry from the extracellular space and partly from the activation of a poorly understood receptor-mediated pathway. At 'α-adrenoceptor' junctions the increase in $[Ca^{2+}]_i$ results from the release of Ca^{2+} from intracellular stores. The differences between the processes of transmission at the three junction types are most readily distinguished on the basis of the time course of the e.j.ps recorded from each junction. At 'ligand gated' junctions, an e.j.p. has a short latency, (2–5 ms), a rapid rising phase (about 100 ms), with the decay of potential being determined by the passive electrical properties of the effector tissue. At 'muscarinic' junctions an e.j.p. has a moderate latency (100–500 ms), a slow rising phase lasting in excess of 200 ms and the decay of potential largely reflects the rate of channel closure. At 'α-adrenoceptor' junctions, the e.j.p. has a very long latency (1–2 s), with prolonged rising and falling phases that reflect the activation of Ca^{2+} activated Cl^- channels. At both 'ligand gated' and 'muscarinic' junctions single stimuli initiate detectable e.j.ps whereas at 'α-adrenoceptor' junctions several stimuli are required before an e.j.p is detected. A further difference between the three junction types may be detected in their behaviour during repetitive nerve stimulation. At 'ligand gated' junctions, successive e.j.ps facilitate and sum to give a large depolarization. At 'muscarinic' junctions profound depression is noted, with full recovery noted only when successive stimuli are separated for periods in excess of 20 s. At 'α-adrenoceptor' junctions, e.j.ps show profound facilitation, with single impulses evoking barely detectable responses while brief trains of stimuli evoke substantial depolarizations.

REFERENCES

Abe, Y. & Tomita, T. (1968). Cable properties of smooth muscle. *J. Physiol.* **196**, 87–100.

Angus, J.A., Broughton, A. & Mulvany, M.J. (1988). Role of α-adrenoceptors in constrictor responses of rat, guinea-pig and rabbit small arteries to neural activation *J. Physiol.* **403**, 495–510.

Astrand, P. & Stjärne, L. (1989). On the secretory activity of single varicosities in the sympathetic nerves innervating rat tail artery. *J. Physiol.* **409**, 207–220.

Astrand, P., Brock, J.A. and Cunnane, T.C. (1988). Time course of transmitter action at the sympathetic neuroeffector junction in vascular and non-vascular smooth muscle. *J. Physiol.* **401**, 657-670.

Bauer, V. & Kuriyama, H. (1982) Evidence for non-cholinergic, non-adrenergic transmission in the guinea-pig ileum. *J. Physiol.* **330**, 95-110.

Bauer, V., Holzer, P. & Ito, Y. (1991). Role of extra- and intracellular calcium in the contractile action of agonists in the guinea-pig ileum. *Naunyn-Schmiedeberg's Arch. Pharmacol.* **343**, 58-64.

Bell, C. (1969). Transmission from vasoconstrictor and vasodilator nerves to single smooth muscle cells of the guinea-pig uterine artery. *J. Physiol.* **205**, 695-708.

Bennett, M.R. (1966). Transmission from intramural excitatory nerves to the smooth muscle cells of the guinea-pig taenia coli. *J. Physiol.* **185**, 132-147.

Bennett, M.R. (1972). Autonomic neuromuscular transmission. Monographs of the Physiological Society No. 30. Cambridge University Press.

Benham, C.D. (1989). ATP activated channels gate calcium entry in single smooth muscle cells from rabbit ear artery. *J. Physiol.* **419**, 689-701.

Benham, C.D., Bolton, T.B. & Lang, R.J. (1985). Acetylcholine activates an inward current in single mammalian smooth muscle cells. *Nature* **316**, 345-347.

Benham, C.D., Bolton, T.B., Byrne N.G. & Large, W.A. (1987). Action of externally applied adenosine triphosphate in single smooth muscle cells dispersed from rabbit ear artery. *J. Physiol.* **387**, 473-488.

Berridge, M.J. (1987). Inositol trisphosphate and diacylglycerol: two interacting second messengers. *Annu. Rev. Biochem.* **56**, 159-193.

Blakeley, A.G.H. & Cunnane T.C. (1979). The packeted release of transmitter from the sympathetic nerves of the guinea-pig vas deferens; an electrophysiological study. *J. Physiol.* **296**, 85-96.

Blakeley, A.G.H., Brown, D.A., Cunnane, T.C., French, A.M., McGrath, J.C. & Scott, N.C. (1981). Effects of nifedipine on electrical and mechanical responses of rat and guinea-pig vas deferens. *Nature* **294**, 759-761.

Bolton, T.B. (1974). Electrical properties and constants of longitudinal muscle from the avian anterior mesenteric artery. *Blood Vessels* **11**, 65-78

Bolton, T.B. & Lim, S.P. (1989). Properties of calcium stores and transient outward currents in single smooth muscle cells of rabbit intestine. *J. Physiol.* **409**, 385-401.

Brock, J.A. & Cunnane, T.C. (1988). Electrical activity at the sympathetic neuroeffector junction in the guinea-pig vas deferens *J. Physiol.* **399**, 607-632.

Brock, J.A. & Cunnane, T.C. (1993). Neurotransmitter release mechanisms at the sympathetic neuroeffector junction. *Exp. Physiol.* **78**, 591-614.

Burnstock, G. & Holman, M.E. (1961). The transmission of excitation from autonomic nerve to smooth muscle. *J. Physiol.* **155**, 115-133.

Burnstock, G. & Holman, M.E. (1964). An electrophysiological investigation of the actions of some autonomic blocking drugs on transmission in the guinea-pig vas deferens. *Br. J. Pharmacol.* **23**, 600-612.

Bywater, R.A.R. & Taylor, G.S. (1980). The passive membrane properties and excitatory junction potentials of the guinea-pig vas deferens *J. Physiol.* **300**, 303-316.

Cassell, J.F., McLachlan, E.M. & Sittiracha, T. (1988). The effect of temperature on neuromuscular transmission in the main caudal artery of the rat. *J. Physiol.* **397**, 31-49.

Casteels, R., Kitamura, K., Kuriyama, H. & Suzuki, H. (1977). The membrane properties of the smooth muscle cells of the rabbit main pulmonary artery. *J. Physiol.* **271**, 4-61.

Cheung, D.W. (1982). Two components in the cellular response of the rat tail artery to nerve stimulation. *J. Physiol.* **328**, 461–468.

Choate, J.K., Klemm M.F. & Hirst, G.D.S. (1993) Sympathetic and parasympathetic neuromuscular junctions in the guinea-pig sino-atrial node. *J. Auton. Nerv. Syst.* **44**, 1–16.

Cousins, H.M., Edwards, F.R., Hirst, G.D.S. & Wendt, I.R. (1993). Cholinergic neuromuscular transmission in the longitudinal muscle of the guinea-pig ileum. *J. Physiol.* **471**, 61-86.

Cousins, H.M., Edwards, F.R. & Hirst, G.D.S. (1995). Neuronally released and applied acetylcholine on the longitudinal muscle of guinea-pig ileum. *Neuroscience* **65**, 193–207.

Cunnane, T.C. & Stjarne, L. (1982). Secretion of transmitter from individual varicosities of guinea-pig and mouse vas deferens: all-or-none and extremely intermittent. *Neurosci.* **7**, 2565–2576.

Finkel, A.S., Hirst, G.D.S. & van Helden, D.F. (1984). Some properties of excitatory junction currents recorded from arterioles of the submucosa of guinea pig ileum. *J. Physiol.* **351**, 87–98.

Furness, J.B. (1969). An electrophysiological study of the innervation of the smooth muscle of the colon. *J. Physiol.* **205**, 549–562.

Hill, C.E., Hirst, G.D.S. & van Helden, D.F. (1983). Development of the sympathetic innervation of proximal and distal arteries of the rat mesentery. *J. Physiol.* **338**, 129–147.

Hill, C.E., Klemm, M., Edwards, F.R. & Hirst, G.D.S. (1993). Sympathetic transmission to the dilator muscle of the rat iris. *J. Auton. Nerv. Syst.* **45**, 107–123.

Hirst, G.D.S. (1977). Neuromuscular transmission in arterioles of guinea pig submucosa. *J. Physiol.* **273**, 263–275.

Hirst, G.D.S. & Neild, T.O. (1978). An analysis of excitatory junction potentials recorded from arterioles. *J. Physiol.* **280**, 87–104.

Hirst, G.D.S. & Neild, T.O. (1980). Some properties of spontaneous excitatory junction potentials recorded from arterioles of guinea pig. *J. Physiol.* **303**, 43–60.

Hirst, G.D.S. & Edwards, F. R. (1989). Sympathetic neuroeffector transmission in arteries and arterioles. *Physiol. Rev.* **69**, 546–604.

Holman, M.E. & Surprenant, A.M. (1979). Some properties of the excitatory junction potentials recorded from saphenous arteries of rabbits. *J. Physiol.* **287**, 337–351.

Holman, M.E. & Surprenant, A.M. (1980). An electrophysiological analysis of the effects of noradrenaline and receptor antagonists on neuromuscular transmission in mammalian muscular arteries. *B. J. Pharmacol.* **71**, 337–351.

Hottenstein, O.D. & Kreulen, D.L. (1987). Comparison of the frequency dependence of venous and arterial responses to sympathetic nerve stimulation in guinea-pigs. *J. Physiol.* **384**, 153–167.

Inoue, R. & Isenberg, G. (1990a). Effect of membrane potential on acetylcholine-induced inward current in guinea-pig ileum. *J. Physiol.* **424**, 57–71.

Inoue, R. & Isenberg, G. (1990b). Intracellular calcium ions modulate acetylcholine-induced inward current in guinea-pig ileum. *J. Physiol.* **424**, 73–92.

Inoue, R., Kitamura, K. & Kuriyama, H. (1987). Acetylcholine activates single sodium channels in smooth muscle cells. *Pflügers Arch.* **410**, 69–74.

Ito, Y., Kuriyama, H. & Parker, I. (1988). Calcium transients evoked by electrical stimulation of smooth muscle from guinea-pig ileum recorded by the use of Fura-2. *J. Physiol.* **407**, 117–134.

Itoh, T., Kitamura, K. & Kuriyama, H. (1983). Roles of extra-junctional receptors in the response of guinea-pig mesenteric and rat tail arteries to adrenergic nerves. *J. Physiol.* **345** 409–422.

Kajiwara, M., Kitamura, K. & Kuriyama, H. (1983). Neuromuscular transmission and smooth muscle membrane properties in the guinea-pig ear artery. *J. Physiol.* **315** 283–302.

Klemm, M.F. (1995). Neuromuscular junctions made by nerve fibres supplying the longitudinal muscle of the guinea-pig ileum. *J. Auton. Nerv. Syst.* **45**, 155–164.

Klemm M.F., Hirst, G.D.S. & Campbell, G.D. (1992). Structure of the autonomic neuromuscular junctions in the sinus venosus of the toad. *J. Auton. Nerv. Syst.* **39**, 139–150.

Klemm M.F., van Helden D.F. & Luff S.E. (1993). Ultrastructural analysis of sympathetic neuromuscular junctions on mesenteric veins of the guinea pig. *J. Comp. Neurol.* **334**, 159–167.

Komori, S. & Bolton, T.B. (1990) Role of G-proteins in muscarinic receptor inward and outward currents in rabbit jejunal smooth muscle. *J. Physiol.* **427**, 395–419.

Komori, S. & Bolton, T.B. (1991) Calcium release induced by inositol 1,4,5-trisphosphate in single rabbit intestinal smooth muscle cells. *J. Physiol.* **433**, 495–517.

Kügelgen, I.V. & Starke, K. (1985). Noradrenaline and adenosine triphosphate as co-transmitters of neurogenic vasoconstriction in rabbit mesenteric arteries. *J. Physiol.* **367**, 435–455.

Lavidis, N.A. & Bennett, M.R. (1992). Probabilistic secretion of quanta from visualized sympathetic nerve varicosities in mouse vas deferens. *J. Physiol.* **454**, 9–26.

Lim, S.P. & Bolton, T.B. (1988). A calcium-dependent rather than a G-protein mechanism is involved in the inward current evoked by muscarinic receptor stimulation in dialysed single smooth muscle cells of small intestine. *J. Pharmacol.* **95**, 325–327.

Luff, S.E. & McLachlan, E.M. (1988). The form of sympathetic postganglionic axons at clustered neuromuscular junctions near branch points of arterioles in the submucosa of the guinea pig ileum. *J Neurocytol.* **17**, 451–463.

Luff, S.E. & McLachlan, E.M. (1989). Frequency of neuromuscular junctions on arteries of different dimensions in the rabbit, guinea pig and rat. *Blood Vessels* **26**, 95–106.

Luff, S.E., McLachlan, E.M., and Hirst, G.D.S. (1987). An ultrastructural analysis of the sympathetic neuromuscular junctions of arterioles of the submucosa of the guinea pig ileum. *J. Comp. Neurobiol.* **257**, 578–594.

Mekata, F. (1974). Current spread in the smooth muscle of the rabbit aorta. *J. Physiol.* **242**, 143–155.

Pacaud, P. & Bolton, T.B. (1991). Relation between muscarinic receptor cationic currents and internal calcium in guinea-pig jejunal smooth muscle cells. *J. Physiol.* **441**, 477–499.

Reilly, M.J. & Hirst, G.D.S. (1996). Differences in the responses to purinergic nerve stimulation and applied ATP in the guinea pig vas deferens. *J. Auton. Nerv. Syst.* **57**, 93–100.

Sneddon, P. & Burnstock. G. (1984). ATP as a co-transmitter in rat tail artery. Europ. *J. Pharmacol.* **106**, 149–152.

Sneddon, P. & Westfall, D.P. (1984). Pharmacolgical evidence that adenosine triphosphate and noradrenaline are co-transmitters in the guinea-pig vas deferens. *J. Physiol.* **347**, 561–580.

Suzuki, H. (1981). Effects of endogenous and exogenous noradrenaline on the smooth muscle of guinea-pig mesenteric vein. *J. Physiol.* **321**, 495–512.

Suzuki, H. (1983). An electrophysiological study of excitatory neuromuscular transmission in the guinea-pig main pulmonary artery. *J. Physiol.* **336**, 47–59.

van Helden, D.F. (1988a). Electrophysiology of neuromuscular transmission in guinea-pig mesenteric veins. *J. Physiol.* **401**, 469–488.

van Helden, D.F. (1988b). An a-mediated chloride conductance in mesenteric veins of the guinea-pig. *J. Physiol.* **401**, 489–501.

van Helden, D.F. (1991). Spontaneous and noradrenaline induced transient depolarizations in the smooth muscle of guinea-pig mesenteric vein. *J. Physiol.* **437**, 543–562.

Vogalis, F. & Sanders, K.M. (1990) Cholinergic stimulation activates a non-selective cation current in canine pyloric circular muscle cells. *J. Physiol.* **429**, 223-236.

Zar, M.A. & Goopta, D. (1983). Effect of nifedipine on the contractile responses of human colonic muscle. *J. Clin. Pharmaacol.* **16**, 339–340.

40

Junction Potentials in the Intestines of Guinea Pigs and Mice

ROBERT A. R. BYWATER
DAVID J. K. LYSTER
MICHAEL J. WATSON
KENICHIRO FURUKAWA
GRAHAME S. TAYLOR

Neuropharmacology Group,
Department of Physiology,
Monash University,
Clayton, Victoria,
Australia

INTRODUCTION

The excitation of the smooth muscle cells is influenced by myogenic, neurogenic and hormonal mechanisms. The muscle layers of the gastrointestinal tract primarily aid in the digestion of foods through mixing movements and in addition propel the intestinal contents along the gut. In the intestine the muscle layers are primarily innervated by neurones whose cells bodies lie within the enteric nervous system. These intrinsic motorneurones thus play a vital role in contraction and relaxation of the muscle layers. Electrophysiological studies offer many advantages in investigating the characteristics of neurotransmission to the smooth muscle. It is possible to record the electrical changes in the smooth muscle cells following application of putative neurotransmitter substances to whole tissues or isolated cells and subsequently to study the mechanisms by which these substances affect the level of excitation of the cells. However, there is increasing evidence that applied substances may not mimic the effects of neurally released transmitter (Cousins *et al.*, 1995). A further complication is that neurotransmission probably occurs both indirectly, via the interstitial cells of Cajal, as well as directly from the neurone terminals to the smooth muscle cells. Thus, in order to properly understand the excitatory or inhibitory effects and the second messenger systems activated by neurally released substances, it is preferable to investigate these effects following release of the substances from nerve terminals. In this paper we discuss aspects of the neurotransmission to the circular muscle layer in the intestines of guinea pigs and mice.

Although neurotransmitters have actions on smooth muscle other than through altering their membrane potential, changes in the latter are important in determining the state of voltage-dependent calcium channels in their cell membranes and thus the contractile state of the smooth muscle. It is clear that there are several neurotransmitters that are released onto circular muscle cells by the enteric motor neurones. In this paper we emphasize the methods that may be used to distinguish between the junction potentials arising from different neurotransmitters substances acting via their respective receptors.

METHODS

All the experiments described below were carried out *in vitro*. Guinea pigs or mice were killed by cervical dislocation and exsanguination, and strips of small or large intestine (either full-thickness or devoid of the longitudinal muscle layer, myenteric plexus or mucosa) were pinned out in an organ bath and superfused with modified Krebs' solution at 30–36°C. The strips, 3–50 mm long, were cut either parallel to the circular muscle layer, or to the longitudinal muscle layer or as 'T'-shaped preparations (see Figure 1A). Nifedipine (1–2 µM) was included in the Krebs' solution in all experiments (unless otherwise indicated) to reduce tissue movement. Conventional KCl-filled glass microelectrodes were used to record the membrane potentials of cells in the circular muscle layer. Recordings were made onto FM tape (Tandberg, Instrument Series 115 or TEAC RO80) and later digitized using a personal computer. Figures were produced using Sigmaplot Version 5 (Jandel).

It was possible to test whether or not the microelectrode was in a circular muscle cell by producing electrotonic potentials using the partition stimulation technique described by Abe & Tomita, (1968). If tissue cut parallel to the circular muscle cells is placed between large external stimulating electrodes, application of current through these electrodes produces significant alterations in the membrane potential of cells in the circular muscle layer with minimal changes in the membrane potential of cells in the longitudinal muscle layer. We have used the partition stimulation method in 'T'-shaped preparations. In these preparations, we activated the enteric pathways projecting along the oral–aboral axis of the intestine using a

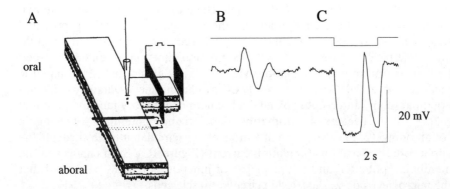

Figure 1 Confirmation that the microelectrode is in a circular muscle cell using the partition stimulation technique. A, Schematic diagram of a 'T' - shaped preparation consisting of a half-width strip of tissue cut parallel to the longitudinal muscle cells (the cross-part of the 'T'), with a peninsula of tissue (the vertical-part of the 'T'), cut parallel to the circular muscle cells, placed between the large external partition stimulation electrodes. The microelectrode was confirmed to be recording from a circular muscle cell if the membrane potential of the impaled cell was significantly changed when current was passed between the partition stimulation electrodes. Wire stimulating electrodes (here placed aboral to the recording microelectrode) were used to activate intramural nerve fibres. A second microelectrode (not shown) was placed near the recording microelectrode in the extracellular fluid and used to reduce the potential changes due to current leak into the recording compartment (see text). B, During recording from a preparation from the guinea pig ileum, a single transmural nerve stimulus, (10 V, 0.1 ms), via the wire electrodes (placed 4.5 mm aboral to the recording electrode), was used to activate intramural nerve fibres. This produced in the impaled cell (situated adjacent to the partition electrode), at the resting membrane potential, a biphasic junction potential consisting of a cholinergic e.j.p. interrupted by an i.j.p. C, When current was passed for 2 s between the partition stimulation electrodes (upper trace), the membrane potential of the cell was hyperpolarized by 25 mV (lower trace) indicating that the microelectrode was recording from a circular muscle cell. Activation of the intramural nerve fibres, same stimulus parameters as in B, now produced a large depolarizing junction potential.

pair of wire electrodes placed above and below the tissue at various distances from the recording microelectrode using stimulus durations up to 1 ms. At the same time it was possible to alter the membrane potential of the circular muscle cells using partition stimulation with low stimulus currents and with stimulus durations lasting up to tens of seconds. Although the partition technique reduces extracellular current spread from the partition stimulating electrodes into the recording chamber, we have in addition, used a second microelectrode, (not shown in Figure 1A) which we placed in the extracellular fluid to record the small changes in extracellular potential caused by residual current spread into the recording chamber; this potential was then subtracted from the potential recorded by the intracellular microelectrode. Figure 1B shows a compound junction potential recorded following transmural stimulation via the wire electrodes. The biphasic junction potential was composed of a cholinergic excitatory junction potential (e.j.p.) interrupted by a noncholinergic inhibitory junction potential (i.j.p.). This became a primarily depolarizing potential following a conditioning (25 mV) hyperpolarization of the circular muscle through the application of partition stimulation current (Figure 1C). Such changes in the membrane potential and in the shapes of junction potentials confirmed that the microelectrode was located in circular muscle cells.

RESULTS

Excitatory Junction Potentials

Cholinergic Excitatory Junction Potentials – Guinea Pigs

There are few reports in the literature using electrophysiological techniques that describe transmission which is likely to be cholinergic in origin in the circular muscle layer. The lack of detailed reports in this area may result from the fact that transmission produces significant movement despite the presence of Ca^{2+} channel antagonists such as nifedipine (R.A.R.B. & G. S.T. unpublished observations and Cousins *et al.*, 1993). The cholinergic e.j.p.s in the longitudinal muscle layer are associated with increases in intracellular Ca^{2+}, (Cousins *et al.*, 1995; see Hirst & Cousins in this volume). These authors speculated that the rise in Ca^{2+} may occur through the opening of postsynaptic ion channels by the neurotransmitter.

The cholinergic e.j.p.s in circular muscle cells are most easily recorded oral to the site of stimulation, especially if relatively low stimulus strengths are used. It is likely, that in these circumstances, that cholinergic motorneurones situated oral to the site of stimulation are synaptically activated by ascending (orally projecting) interneurones. There is often an i.j.p. evoked simultaneously, (as in Figure 1B), possibly owing to antidromic activation of descending interneurones which synapse onto inhibitory motorneurones or to direct antidromic activation of inhibitory motorneurones themselves. The neurotoxin apamin can be added to the Krebs' solution to antagonize the i.j.p. (see below).

The cholinergic e.j.p. is sensitive to the muscarinic antagonists hyoscine and atropine. The substance P analogue antagonist D-Arg[1], D-Pro[2],D-Trp[7,9], Leu[11]-substance P (RPWWL-SP) appears not to antagonize these e.j.p.s in the circular muscle layer of the guinea pig ileum, (Figure 2A–C).

In preparations free of myenteric plexus and in the presence of apamin (250 nM), we have recorded cholinergic e.j.p.s following single stimuli (e.g. see Figure 3A) when the recording microelectrode is less than 2 mm from the stimulating electrodes. The addition of hyoscine antagonized the cholinergic e.j.p. revealing a slower apamin-resistant i.j.p. (Figure 3B). The latter is likely to be due to the release of nitric oxide (see below). Thus, cholinergic e.j.p.s in the guinea pig ileum can be studied through activation of intramural nerves whilst antagonizing noncholinergic e.j.p.s with an antagonist such as RPWWL-SP, in combination with apamin to antagonize the fast i.j.p. and an inhibitor of nitric oxide synthase to prevent the synthesis and release of nitric oxide (see further below). In other experiments (Anna Windle, personal communication), a rise in intracellular Ca^{2+} was associated with the cholinergic e.j.p. in the circular muscle layer in the guinea pig ileum.

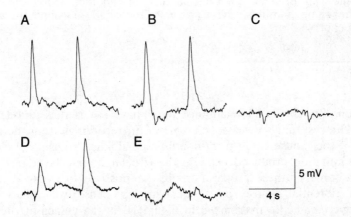

Figure 2 Effects of a substance P analogue on cholinergic and noncholinergic e.j.p.s in recordings from circular muscle cells in the guinea pig ileum. A, In the absence of atropine, two volleys, 4 s apart, of transmural nerve stimulation each produced a cholinergic e.j.p. B, In the presence of the substance P analogue antagonist (RPWWL-substance P, 6.7 μM), cholinergic e.j.p.s persist. C, Following the addition of atropine (1.4 μM), the e.j.p.s were abolished. D, In the presence of atropine (1.4 μM) and apamin (250 nM), two volleys of transmural nerve stimulation, 4 s apart, produced noncholinergic e.j.p.s. E, The noncholinergic e.j.p.s were abolished after the addition of RPWWL-substance P, (6.7 μM). The recordings in A,B and C were from one preparation, where each volley of transmural nerve stimulation was 3 pulses at 50 Hz, each 0.6 ms and 30 mA. The recordings in D and E were from another preparation where each volley of transmural nerve stimulation was 3 pulses at 50 Hz, each 0.6 ms and 35 mA.

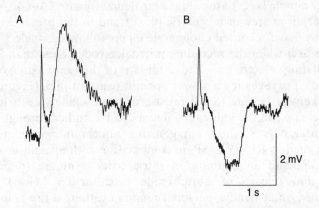

Figure 3 Junction potentials in the presence of apamin (250 nM) in a preparation of guinea pig ileum free of longitudinal muscle and myenteric plexus. A, A single transmural nerve stimulus (20 mA, 0.6 ms) using wire electrodes placed 250 μm aboral to the recording microelectrode produced a cholinergic e.j.p. B, In the same tissue, after the addition of hyoscine (1 μM), using the same stimulus, the e.j.p. was abolished revealing an apamin-resistant i.j.p.

Mice

The colon of the piebald lethal mouse (S^l/S^l) has been used as a model of the human Hirschsprung's disease (see below). In recordings from the circular muscle of the mouse colon from nondiseased siblings, transmural electrical nerve stimulation produced i.j.p.s in the circular muscle layer (see Figure $4A_1$). In some of these preparations it was possible to evoke a biphasic junction potential whose initial depolarizing phase was likely to be cholinergic (similar to that shown in Figure 1B in the guinea-pig ileum). It has not been possible to completely block the i.j.p. in the mouse colon with a combination of apamin and a nitric oxide synthase antagonist (see below). Thus, in order to investigate the time course of the cholinergic e.j.p. in the mouse colon we employed the partition stimulation technique to hyperpolarize the membrane potential to reduce the amplitude of the i.j.p. After conditioning hyperpolarization (e.g. of 43 mV; see Figure $4A_2$) a cholinergic e.j.p. was revealed. This may be shortened in its timecourse by the onset of a (reduced amplitude) i.j.p. Further hyperpolarization (e.g. to 61 mV more negative than the resting membrane potential, see Figure $4A_3$) produced a cholinergic e.j.p. whose recovery phase now is probably prolonged by a positive-going i.j.p. These experiments indicated the approximate time-course of cholinergic e.j.p.s in the mouse colon.

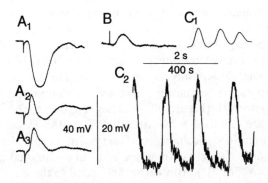

Figure 4 Cholinergic e.j.p.s in the circular muscle of mouse colon. A, In a circularly cut preparation, recordings of junction potentials from the same cell at different membrane potentials. A_1, At the resting potential, a single transmural nerve stimulus (20 mA) produced an i.j.p. A_2, Partition stimulation was used to hyperpolarize the cell by 43 mV; the same nerve stimulus now revealed an underlying cholinergic e.j.p. A_3, after further hyperpolarization (to 61mV negative of the resting potential, that is negative of E_K), the same nerve stimulus produced a cholinergic e.j.p. which was prolonged on its recovery phase by a 'reversed' (positive-going) i.j.p. NB: the downwards vertical displacements of the recordings A_2 and A_3 from that of A_1 represent the degree of conditioning hyperpolarization in traces A_2 and A_3. B, Recording from a circular muscle cell from the 'funnel' region of the colon (8 mm from the anus) in a preparation from a piebald-lethal mouse. A single transmural nerve stimulus (14 mA, 0.6 ms, and in the absence of nifedipine), produced a cholinergic e.j.p. whose time-course was not modified by a co-evoked i.j.p. C, Recordings from a circular muscle cell, in an unstimulated full-length strip of colon showing spontaneously occurring cyclical migrating myoelectric complexes; C_1, shows 2 Hz oscillations in membrane potential (which occur superimposed on the depolarizations seen in C_2), which are sensitive to hyoscine and atropine. Each oscillation has a timecourse similar to a cholinergic e.j.p. C_2, four myoelectric complexes are shown on a slower timebase. Vertical calibration is 40 mV in A and 20 mV in B and C. Horizontal calibration is 2 s in A, B and C_1 and 400s in C_2.

The colon of the homozygous piebald lethal diseased mouse is dilated proximately and constricted distally where there is a loss of innervation of the muscle by enteric neurones. We have noted that in the transition zone (the 'funnel' region where the colon narrows), there is an area which is devoid of i.j.p.s. In this area, transmural nerve stimulation produces cholinergic e.j.p.s which are therefore not interrupted by an i.j.p. (Figure 4B). These responses thus probably show the full duration of cholinergic junction potentials in the circular muscle layer of the mouse colon (at least in these diseased animals).

In full-length preparations of colon of the nondiseased siblings, membrane potential recordings in the circular layer show ongoing cycles of depolarization (lasting about 1 min) and hyperpolarization lasting about 2–6 min (Figure $4C_2$). These membrane potential cycles (myoelectric complexes), progress predominately aborally along the colon. During the depolarization phase of these migrating complexes, there are superimposed 2 Hz oscillations in membrane potential (Figure $4C_1$). They appear to be positive-going potentials and are abolished by atropine (Bywater *et al.*, 1989). These potentials are therefore probably cholinergic in origin. Each oscillation appears to resemble a single cholinergic e.j.p. in its time course (cp Figure $4C_1$ with Figure $4A_{2,3}$ or 4B). But carbachol added to the Krebs' solution did not produce the oscillations although it did depolarize the smooth muscle cells (Lyster *et al.*, 1995). These experiments suggest that in full-length segments of mouse colon, there are spontaneous periods of excitatory activity when cholinergic motorneurones fire either cyclically approximately every 500 ms, or that they fire asynchronously and the release of acetylcholine from cholinergic nerve terminals (perhaps onto localised post-junctional receptors) produces responses in the muscle that are not readily reproduced by the application of a muscarinic agonist. This is reminiscent of the suggestions made for the actions of acetylcholine on the longitudinal muscle layer in the guinea pig ileum (Cousins *et al.*, 1995). After muscarinic blockade, there is little evidence for other e.j.p.s in the mouse colon.

Non-cholinergic Excitatory Junction Potentials – Guinea Pigs

In the circular muscle layer of the guinea pig ileum, after the addition of atropine or hyoscine to the Krebs' solution, single transmural stimuli usually evoked i.j.p.s (Figure 5A). However increasing the number of stimuli in a volley evoked non-cholinergic e.j.p.s (see Figure 5B) after the second and subsequent volley. This is not because the i.j.p.s are severely depressed by increasing the number of stimuli in each volley, but because the e.j.p.s are greatly enhanced by such stimuli (see also Figure 6B). In the absence of nifedipine, the e.j.p.s readily depolarize the smooth muscle sufficiently to open voltage-dependent Ca^{2+} channels leading to muscle contraction. In the presence of nifedipine and atropine, muscle movement is not a feature despite large depolarizations. This suggests that the depolarization produced by the noncholinergic transmitter probably occurs through the opening of ion channels which have a low permeability for Ca^{2+} ions. The application of RPWWL-SP antagonizes these e.j.p.s (Figure 2E) as does prolonged (>15 min) application of substance P itself, the latter presumably through desensitization of the receptor or the postsynaptic messenger systems involved. These experiments suggest that the e.j.p.s are probably due primarily to tachykinin release. Enhancement of the e.j.p. amplitude with

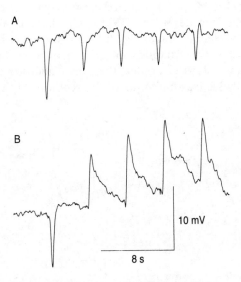

Figure 5 Effects of altering the stimulus parameters on the evoked junction potentials in a circular muscle cell from the guinea pig ileum in the presence of atropine (1.4 μM). A, Single transmural nerve stimulus (45 mA, 0.6 ms), repeated at 4-s intervals, produced i.j.p.s. B, Volleys (3 pulses, 50 Hz) of stimuli (35 mA, 0.6 ms), repeated at 4-s intervals, produced an i.j.p. following the first volley but noncholinergic e.j.p.s following the subsequent volleys.

increasing number of stimuli may be due to processes activated within the smooth muscle cells or to facilitation of release of tachykinin. In unpublished experiments we have noted that noncholinergic e.j.p.s similar to those in the ileum were not present in colonic muscle. Longer trains of stimuli, however, do produce depolarizations in the presence of hyoscine.

After the antagonism of cholinergic responses and the tachykinin responses described above, noncholinergic e.j.p.s with a slower time-course are seen following transmural nerve stimulation in the guinea pig ileum. These appear to be due to the release of nitric oxide as they are abolished by a nitric oxide synthase inhibitor. This response will be described below.

Inhibitory Junction Potentials

Guinea Pigs

As mentioned above, in the circular muscle layer of the guinea pig ileum, following the addition of atropine or hyoscine to the Krebs' solution, single transmural stimuli usually evoked i.j.p.s (Figure 5A or Figure 6A). The i.j.p.s result from an increase in conductance of the postsynaptic membrane to K^+ ions (Tomita, 1972; Bywater *et al.*, 1981). The i.j.p. is abolished by the addition of the K^+ channel blocking drug apamin (see Figure 6B). The mechanisms between postsynaptic receptor activation and K^+ channel opening are unknown. It is clear that there is a neurotransmitter(s) other than nitric oxide involved, as inhibition of the synthesis of the latter with N^G-

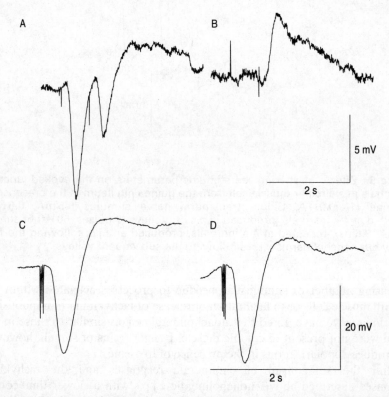

Figure 6 The effects of apamin and the nitric oxide synthase inhibitor NOLA on the (fast) noncholinergic apamin-sensitive i.j.p. in the circular muscle of the guinea pig ileum after muscarinic blockade. A, in the presence of atropine (1.4 µM) the first of two stimulus pulses (each 50 mA, 0.6 ms) produced an i.j.p., whereas the second pulse (given 700 ms later) produced a smaller amplitude i.j.p. followed by a period of depolarization. B, In the same cell after the addition of apamin (250 nM) the i.j.p.s were abolished but a noncholinergic e.j.p. was now evident following the second stimulus pulse. C and D are recordings from another preparation in the presence of hyoscine (1 µM). C, A volley of transmural nerve stimulation (3 pulses, 50 Hz, 0.6 ms, 10 mA) produced an i.j.p. followed by a period of depolarization. D, Following the addition of NOLA (100 µM) for 60 min the i.j.p. was increased in amplitude (same stimulus parameters as in D).

nitro-L-arginine (NOLA) does not abolish the i.j.p. (Figure 6D). It has been suggested that the neurotransmitter is ATP (Crist *et al.*, 1992). This suggestion needs confirmation.

In addition to the i.j.p. which is sensitive to apamin, there is an additional i.j.p. which is insensitive to this drug. In the guinea-pig ileum, the latter i.j.p. is slower in onset and is smaller in amplitude. It is best observed following blockade of the cholinergic e.j.p. by a muscarinic antagonist combined with blockade of the 'fast' i.j.p. with apamin (Figure 3B). It is readily obscured by the atropine-resistant e.j.p. if this has been enhanced using repeated volley stimulation. However, such a stimulus regimen may be used when the e.j.p.s resulting from tachykinin release have been antagonised as described above. The ions channel(s) involved in the hyperpolarization is unclear. It has been suggested that the hyperpolarization is caused by a reduction in membrane chloride conductance (Crist *et al.*, 1991) or perhaps by mixed conductance changes or activation of a membrane ion pump (Lyster *et al.*, 1992). The transmitter appears to be nitric oxide (Lyster *et al.*, 1992; He & Goyal, 1993). As nitric oxide is readily diffusible, the mechanisms of action of nitric oxide on smooth muscle cells may perhaps be more easily investigated by exogenous application rather than from stimulated release from nerves as discussed above for other neurotransmitters. Cyclic-GMP is clearly produced but additional pathways may be involved.

Following the 'slow' nitric oxide i.j.p. there is a 'slow' e.j.p. which is also sensitive to inhibition by NOLA, although the timecourse of the relative sensitivities of the e.j.p. and i.j.p. may vary. The e.j.p. appears to be associated with a membrane conductance increase, Lyster *et al.* (1992).

In the colon, both the apamin-sensitive and NOLA-sensitive i.j.p.s are evoked in the circular muscle layer by transmural nerve stimulation. The NOLA-sensitive i.j.p. is prominent in the colon, especially in the proximal colon (unpublished observations). In both the ileum and the colon a combination of apamin and NOLA effectively abolishes i.j.p.s.

Mice

The i.j.p. is readily evoked in the mouse colon following transmural nerve stimulation and is possibly due to an increase in membrane conductance to K^+ ions as the i.j.p. is reversed at potentials more negative than about $-90 \, mV$ (see Figure 4A). The i.j.p. is reduced in amplitude by approximately 50% by apamin but, in contrast to the guinea pig, the time-course of the remaining response is not obviously slower (Okasora *et al.*, 1986). Also in contrast to the guinea pig, in the presence of hyoscine and NOLA (the latter to inhibit nitric oxide synthesis), the addition of apamin does not abolish the i.j.p. in the mouse colon. This suggests that in addition to the apamin sensitive K^+ ion channel another ion channel or channels must be modulated by the non nitric oxide neurotransmitter(s) in the mouse colon.

As described above, in full-length segments of mouse colon cycling migrating myoelectric complexes could be recorded from the circular muscle layer. The membrane potential in the periods between the complexes is about −55 mV. In this period, the smooth muscle cells appear to be under the influence of ongoing inhibitory nerve activity as the membrane potential depolarizes between 10 and 20 mV if NOLA or tetrodotoxin is added to the Krebs' solution. This indicates that the 'resting' membrane potential of the circular muscle in the mouse colon may be around −35 to −40 mV, a level at which some voltage-dependent calcium channels may be conductive.

As part of our studies we have investigated whether the recordings from a given smooth muscle cell in the circular muscle of the mouse colon are representative of its neighbours. Figure 7 shows the recordings from two smooth muscle cells when the microelectrodes were separated by 0.5 mm in the circumferential direction. It is clear that ongoing inhibitory nerve activity (enhanced by the application of 100 μM 4-aminopyridine) is almost identical in the two cells. Our studies have indicated that ongoing junction potential activity is well correlated between two cells when the cells are separated by < 0.5 mm in the longitudinal direction and up to 1 mm in the circumferential direction. The latter estimate may be an underestimate owing to the small size in the circular direction of the experimental preparations.

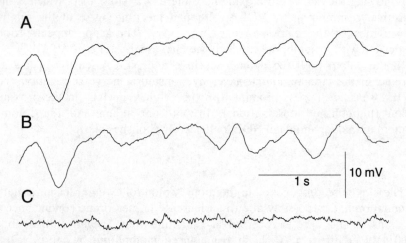

Figure 7 Simultaneous membrane potential recordings of spontaneous i.j.p.s from two circular muscle cells in the mouse colon separated by 500 μm in the circular direction. A, Recording from cell 1. B, Recording from cell 2. C, The difference between the recordings in A and B. This trace indicates that the spontaneous i.j.p.s recorded in these two cells were essentially identical. NB: the frequency of spontaneous i.j.p.s had been increased by the addition of 4-aminopyridine (100 μM).

SUMMARY

This paper describes the types and characteristics of the junction potentials which can be recorded using intracellular electrophysiological recording techniques in vitro from the circular muscle of the intestinal tracts of guinea pigs and mice.

ACKNOWLEDGEMENTS

Many of the experiments described above were supported by grants from the Australian N.H. & M.R.C

REFERENCES

Abe, Y. & Tomita, T. (1968). Cable properties of smooth muscle. *J. Physiol.* **196**, 87–100.

Bywater, R.A.R., Holman, M.E. & Taylor, G.S. (1981). Atropine-resistant depolarization in the guinea-pig small intestine. *J. Physiol.* **316**, 369–378.

Bywater, R.A.R., Small, R.C. & Taylor, G.S. (1989). Neurogenic slow depolarizations and rapid oscillations in the membrane potential of circular muscle of mouse colon. *J. Physiol.* **413**, 505–519.

Crist, J.R., He, X.D. & Goyal, R.K. (1991). Chloride-mediated junction potentials in circular muscle of the guinea pig ileum. *Am. J. Physiol.* **261**, G742–G750.

Crist J.R., He, X.D. & Goyal, R.K. (1992). Both ATP and the peptide VIP are inhibitory neurotransmitters in the guinea-pig ileum circular muscle. *J. Physiol.* **447**, 119–131.

Cousins, H.M., Edwards, F.R., Hirst, G.D.S. & Wendt, I.R. (1993). Cholinergic neuromuscular transmission in the longitudinal muscle of the guinea-pig ileum. *J. Physiol.* **471**, 61–86.

Cousins, H.M., Edwards, F.R. & Hirst, G.D.S. (1995). Neuronally released and applied acetylcholine on the longitudinal muscle of the guinea-pig ileum. *Neuroscience* **65**, 193–207.

He, X.D. & Goyal, R.K. (1993). Nitric oxide involvement in the peptide VIP-associated inhibitory junction potential in the guinea-pig ileum. *J. Physiol.* **461**, 485–9.

Lyster, D.J.K., Bywater, R.A.R., Taylor, G.S. & Watson, M.J. (1992). Effects of a nitric oxide synthase inhibitor on non-cholinergic junction potentials in the circular muscle of the guinea pig ileum. *J. Auton. Nerv. Syst.* **41**, 187–196.

Lyster, D.J.K., Bywater, R.A.R. & Taylor, G.S. (1995). Neurogenic control of myoelectric complexes in the mouse isolated colon. *Gastroenterology* **108**, 1371–1378.

Okasora, T., Bywater, R.A.R. & Taylor, G.S. (1986). Projections of enteric motor neurons in the mouse distal colon. *Gastroenterology* **90**, 1964–1971.

Tomita, T. (1972). Conductance change during the inhibitory potential in the guinea-pig taenia coli. *J. Physiol.* **225**, 693–703.

41

Endothelium-dependent Hyperpolarization in Cerebral and Peripheral Arteries

C. J. GARLAND
F. PLANE

*Department of Pharmacology,
University of Bristol,
Bristol, UK*

SUMMARY

1. Smooth muscle relaxation evoked by agonists such as acetylcholine (ACh) and bradykinin, and the calcium ionophore, A23187 is associated with hyperpolarization. The increase in membrane potential appears to reflect the release of a diffusible factor that is distinct from nitric oxide (NO), which has been termed endothelium-derived hyperpolarizing factor (EDHF). In some arteries under some conditions NO itself can also cause hyperpolarization.

2. In contrast to NO, which acts mainly through the generation of guanosine 3',5'-cyclic monophosphate (cGMP), EDHF leads to relaxation probably by hyperpolarization indirectly reducing the open probability of voltage-dependent calcium channels.

3. It is not clear how important hyperpolarization is for endothelium-dependent smooth muscle relaxation, compared with the increases in cGMP stimulated by NO. In large arteries, hyperpolarization may not normally be important for relaxation to ACh. However, changes in smooth muscle membrane potential appear to be more dominant in relaxation in small resistance vessels which rely more on voltage-dependent calcium influx for maintained contraction.

4. In our laboratory, simultaneous recording of tension and membrane potential in segments of large and small peripheral arteries (rabbit femoral artery and rat small mesenteric artery) and a cerebral blood

vessel (the rabbit basilar artery) suggest marked differences in the importance of hyperpolarization in endothelium-dependent relaxation between arteries.

5. In the femoral and basilar arteries, which are relatively large conducting vessels, ACh-evoked relaxation and hyperpolarization can be accounted for by the release of endothelium-derived NO. Furthermore, the change in membrane potential does not appear to make a major contribution to the relaxation evoked by ACh.

6. In contrast, in the rat mesenteric resistance artery, ACh-evoked hyperpolarization appears to be mediated by an EDHF distinct from NO, with both factors providing a major drive to relaxation.

INTRODUCTION

Endothelium-dependent relaxation of vascular smooth muscle is often associated with an increase in membrane potential (repolarization and/or hyperpolarization). This was first demonstrated with cholinomimetics (Bolton et al., 1984) but has subsequently been reported with a number of agonists such as bradykinin (Nagao & Vanhoutte, 1992) and substance P (Chen et al., 1991). The increase in potential appears to be independent of changes in cGMP (Taylor et al., 1988) and persists in the presence of either oxyhaemoglobin or methylene blue which block the actions of endothelium-derived NO (Chen, et al., 1988; Taylor & Weston, 1988; Brayden, 1990). These observations led to the suggestion that endothelium-dependent hyperpolarization reflected the release of an additional factor, distinct from NO. The factor, termed EDHF (Weston et al., 1988), is thought to cause relaxation by increasing the membrane potential of the muscle cells thereby reducing the open probability of voltage-operated calcium channels (Feletou & Vanhoutte, 1988; Taylor et al., 1988) and is the subject of a recent review (Garland et al., 1995).

In certain blood vessels, such as the guinea-pig uterine and coronary arteries (Tare et al., 1990; Parkington et al., 1993), NO itself can cause smooth muscle hyperpolarization. However, in many preparations, NO evoked relaxation appears not to be accompanied by changes in membrane potential (Garland et al., 1995).

The importance of smooth muscle hyperpolarization in mediating endothelium-dependent relaxation is unclear, whereas the role of NO-evoked increases in guanosine-3',5'-cyclic monophosphate (cGMP) has been demonstrated in many preparations (Moncada et al., 1991).

Two studies in rat aorta and pulmonary artery have indicated that hyperpolarization may play only a minor role, contributing to around only 20–30% of the response evoked by ACh in these vessels (Chen et al., 1988;

van de Voorde *et al.*, 1992). However, in these experiments, membrane potential and tension were recorded in separate experiments, making a direct comparison between the two components of the response somewhat difficult. In addition, hyperpolarization may play a more prominent role in the relaxation of small arterioles, in which the smooth muscle cells appear to be more dependent on extracellular Ca^{2+}-influx during contraction than muscle cells in larger arteries (Nilsson *et al.*, 1994).

We have investigated the relative contribution made to endothelium-dependent relaxation by NO and EDHF in both large and small peripheral vessels (the rabbit femoral artery and rat small mesenteric arteries) and in a cerebral blood vessel, the rabbit basilar artery.

METHODS

In the experiments described, small arterial segments were mounted in a Mulvany–Halpern myograph for simultaneous recording of tension and membrane potential as previously described (Garland, 1987). In these studies, the synthesis of NO was blocked with the NO synthase inhibitors nitromonomethyl arginine (L-NMMA), nitro-arginine (NO-ARG) or nitro-arginine methyl ester (L-NAME), all at a concentration of $100\,\mu M$. The actions of EDHF were inhibited with raised extracellular potassium ($25\,mM$).

RESULTS

Endothelium-dependent relaxation and hyperpolarization

Smooth muscle cells in the rabbit femoral, rabbit basilar and rat mesenteric arteries were electrically quiescent and had resting membrane potentials around $-60\,mV$. In all three vessels studied, the application of ACh (0.01-$10\,\mu M$) evoked sustained, endothelium-dependent hyperpolarization of the resting membrane potential and, in segments depolarized and preconstricted with noradrenaline or phenylephrine, ACh caused both relaxation and repolarization. All vessels had a similar sensitivity to ACh and the threshold concentration required to elicit hyperpolarization was consistently 10-fold higher than that which initiated relaxation.

However, there was considerable variation in the amplitude of the maximal hyperpolarization that accompanied ACh-evoked relaxation in segments from the different arteries, even though they were contracted and depolarized to a similar extent. In the rabbit femoral and basilar artery, the maximal hyperpolarization to ACh was around $9\,mV$; thus, the membrane potential of the smooth muscle cells was still significantly depolarized even when the increase in tone was completely reversed. In the rat mesenteric artery, the maximal change in membrane potential stimulated by ACh was around 20 mV and the depolarization stimulated by the contractile agonist was completely reversed and the tissue was fully relaxed (Figure 1).

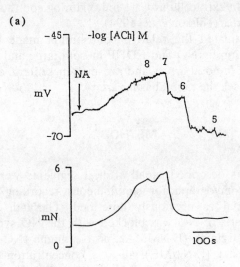

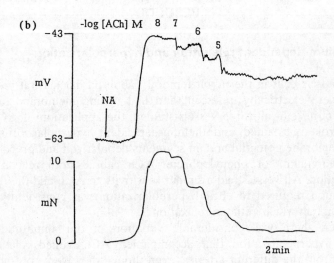

Figure 1 Effect of ACh on tone and membrane potential in isolated segments of (a) rat small mesenteric artery and (b) rabbit femoral artery.

The calcium ionophore A23187 $(0.01–100\,\mu M)$ elicited endothelium-dependent relaxation of preconstricted arterial segments from the rabbit femoral artery which was accompanied by pronounced repolarization. As with ACh, the concentration required to initiate repolarization was higher than for relaxation $(0.01\,\mu M$ and $0.03\,\mu M$, respectively). The maximal change in membrane potential was around $23\,mV$, which is considerably larger than the maximum response evoked by ACh in this vessel $(9\,mV)$.

Contribution of NO to endothelium-dependent hyperpolarization

Exogenous NO can evoke changes in smooth muscle membrane potential. This was initially shown in the guinea-pig uterine (Tare *et al.*, 1990) and coronary arteries (Parkington *et al.*, 1993). Thus, NO may contribute directly to the hyperpolarization which accompanies endothelium-dependent relaxation. In the three vessels studied, bolus doses of exogenous NO, applied close to the tissue, initiated transient, concentration-dependent relaxation of preconstricted artery segments. However, simultaneous measurement of smooth muscle membrane potential showed that the effects of NO on membrane potential varied.

In the rabbit basilar artery, exogenous NO, even at concentrations 10-fold higher than those required to elicit maximal relaxation $(150\,\mu M)$, did not alter smooth muscle membrane potential in either unstimulated or depolarized preparations. In contrast, in the rabbit femoral artery, at concentrations above $5\,\mu M$, smooth muscle NO-evoked relaxation was accompanied by a small, transient increases in membrane potential. The maximal hyperpolarization evoked by NO $(10\,\mu M)$ was around $8\,mV$, which was similar in size to the maximal hyperpolarization evoked by ACh.

In the rat mesenteric artery, in the absence of stimulation, NO induced an increase in the resting membrane potential which, as with the NO-evoked hyperpolarization in the rabbit femoral artery, was blocked by glibenclamide, an inhibitor of ATP-sensitive potassium channels. However, in contrast to the femoral artery, in precontracted tissues, NO-evoked relaxations were not accompanied by a change in membrane potential. This observation indicated that, in the rat mesenteric artery, NO-evoked changes in membrane potential were inhibited by prior depolarization whereas, in contrast, the amplitude of ACh-evoked hyperpolarization was increased in stimulated preparations.

The relative contribution of NO to endothelium-dependent hyper-polarization also varied between the different agonists and the different vessels studied. Inhibition of NO synthase with L-NAME, L-NMMA or NO-ARG $(100\,\mu M; 20\,mins)$, abolished the repolarization and relaxation to ACh in the isolated femoral artery and either abolished or markedly inhibited both components of the response in the basilar artery. These observations indicate that in these two relatively large arteries, the release of endothelium-derived NO may fully account for both components of the ACh-evoked response.

In contrast, both the relaxation and repolarization to A23187 in the femoral artery were unchanged by preincubation with L-NAME or L-NOARG for up to 1 h indicating that an alternative mechanism(s) mediates the responses to this agonist. Thus, NO-independent pathways are present in this artery and can mediate complete relaxation of induced tone, although this mechanism does not appear to be linked to the activation of muscarinic receptors.

In rat mesenteric resistance arteries, exposure to NO synthase inhibitors for up to 1 h caused a small rightward shift in the concentration–response curves for both ACh-evoked relaxation and repolarization. The amplitude of the maximal change in membrane potential was not altered and the maximal relaxation was depressed by only around 20%, indicating that, as in other small arteries, a large component of the endothelium-dependent relaxation is mediated by mechanisms independent of NO (Figure 2).

Furthermore, in the presence of NO synthase inhibitors the temporal relationship between ACh-evoked increases in membrane potential and relaxation was altered. Under control conditions, there was no difference in the time taken to initiate an increase in membrane potential and relaxation with ACh, or in the time taken to attain the maximal responses. Following the inhibition of NO synthase, both the onset of repolarization and the plateau phase of the maximal change in potential occurred about 4 s before the respective changes in relaxation. Therefore, it appears that when NO synthesis is blocked, an increase in membrane potential provides the major drive for relaxation to ACh.

In the same artery, endothelium-dependent relaxations evoked by bradykinin were completely resistant to blockade by NO synthase inhibitors, with no alteration in sensitivity to the relaxant and no change in the maximal response (Figure 4). Thus, whereas ACh-evoked relaxations are mediated in part by the release of endothelium-derived NO, bradykinin-evoked changes in smooth muscle tone appear to be completely independent of NO release in this artery. The contribution of repolarization to this response has not yet been examined.

Importance of membrane potential increases in endothelium-dependent relaxation

The importance of membrane potential changes to endothelium-dependent relaxation was examined using raised extracellular potassium (25 mM) to inhibit membrane potential change without reducing the production of, or responses to, endothelium-derived NO.

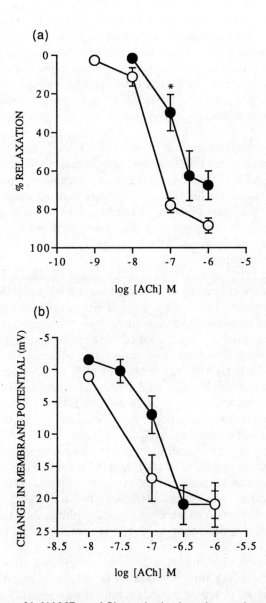

Figure 2 Effect of L-NAME on ACh-evoked relaxation and repolarization in rat mesenteric arteries. Mean concentration–response curves for ACh-evoked relaxation (a) and repolarization (b) in the presence (●) and absence (○) of L-NAME (100 μM). All points are mean ± SE mean, n=4. *P<0.05. From Waldron & Garland (1994) with permission of Stockton Press.

In the rabbit basilar and femoral arteries, raising the extracellular potassium chloride concentration to 25 mM abolished ACh-evoked repolarization but did not alter the relaxation. In fact, in the basilar artery, raising the extracellular potassium concentration to as much as 65 mM had no effect on ACh-evoked relaxations, with the maximal response still around 95% reversal of induced tone. Exposure to glibenclamide (10 μM) inhibited ACh-evoked repolarization in both the basilar and femoral arteries without reducing relaxation. Similarly, glibenclamide also inhibited the increases in membrane potential elicited by exogenous NO in the femoral and mesenteric arteries.

These observations indicate that in the rabbit femoral and basilar arteries, increase in membrane potential do not play a major role in ACh-evoked relaxation. As ACh-stimulated changes in membrane potential were abolished by NO synthase inhibitors, it appears that the release of NO can fully account for both components of the response to ACh in these large vessels. This proposal is supported by the finding that the hyperpolarization to NO and ACh are both mediated by the activation of glibenclamide-sensitive potassium channels.

In contrast, A23187-evoked changes in both tension and membrane potential in the femoral artery were both reduced by about 50% in raised extracellular potassium, but were unaltered by exposure to glibenclamide, indicating that the potassium channels underlying this response are different from those which mediate ACh-evoked hyperpolarization in this vessel. Exposure to L-NAME further attenuated the relaxation to A23187 in potassium-contracted arterial segments but did not further reduce the membrane repolarization. Thus, it appears that although repolarization does not make a major contribution to ACh-evoked relaxation in this vessel, a pathway mediating endothelium-dependent increases in membrane potential is present and can be activated by A23187.

In segments of the rat mesenteric artery, increasing the extracellular potassium concentration to 25 mM abolished ACh-evoked repolarization and reduced the maximal relaxation by around 50–60% (Figure 3). The remaining relaxation was then abolished by L-NAME. In addition, bradykinin-evoked relaxations were significantly inhibited by the presence of increased extracellular potassium with the maximal relaxation reduced by 75% (Figure 4).

Although glibenclamide inhibited smooth muscle cell hyperpolarization evoked by exogenous NO, this compound was without effect on ACh-evoked changes in membrane potential and tone, indicating a role for other types of potassium channel in this response. In the presence of L-NAME, tetraethylammonium (TEA) had no effect on ACh-evoked relaxation in rat mesenteric arteries, while individually charybdotoxin and apamin caused only a small shift in the concentration-response curves. However, when used

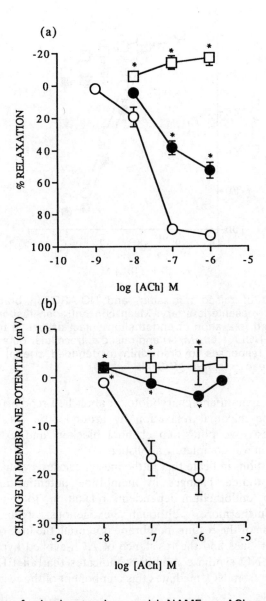

Figure 3 Effect of raised potassium and L-NAME on ACh-evoked relaxation and repolarization in rat mesenteric artery. Mean concentration–response curves for ACh-evoked relaxation (a) and repolarization (b) in the absence (() and presence of raised extracellular potassium (25 mM; •) and raised extracellular potassium together with L-NAME (100 μM; □). All points are mean ± SE mean, n=4. *P<0.05 compared with control. From Waldron & Garland (1994) with permission of Stockton Press.

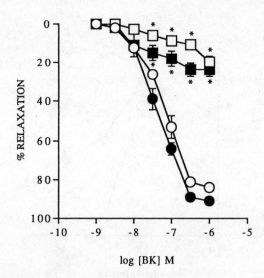

Figure 4 Effect of raised potassium and NO-ARG on bradykinin-evoked relaxation in rat mesenteric artery. Mean concentration–response curves for bradykinin-evoked relaxation of endothelium-intact tissues in the absence (○) and presence of NOLA (100 μM, (●) and raised extracellular potassium (25 mM, ■). (□) Denotes responses to bradykinin in denuded arterial segments. All points are the mean ± SE, n=4; *P<0.05.

in combination, apamin and charybdotoxin abolished repolarization to ACh and reduced the maximal relaxation by around 50%. In the combined presence of these two potassium channel blockers and L-NAME, ACh-evoked relaxation was completely abolished.

These observations indicate that in the mesenteric artery, in contrast to the larger vessels studied, changes in membrane potential make a major contribution to endothelium-dependent relaxation to both ACh and bradykinin. Furthermore, although exogenous NO can evoke hyperpolarization of the resting membrane potential, the lack of effect of NO on depolarized tissues and the resistance of ACh-evoked hyperpolarization to blockade by NO synthase inhibitors indicates that an EDHF, which is probably distinct from NO, mediates this component of the response.

CONCLUSIONS

Whereas NO may be the major factor mediating endothelium-dependent relaxations in large conducting arteries, in small resistance vessels NO-independent mechanisms such as membrane hyperpolarization may be at least as important in causing relaxation (Nagao *et al.*, 1992). Results from our laboratory support this proposal demonstrating that whereas in large peripheral and cerebral arteries ACh-evoked relaxation can be accounted for by the release of endothelium-derived NO, in a small-resistance artery both NO and EDHF contribute to reductions in tone. However, the finding that in the rabbit femoral artery A23187-evoked relaxations appear to be mediated by EDHF, with any contribution from NO only being revealed once hyperpolarization has been inhibited, demonstrates that EDHF can be released in this vessel, although not by ACh.

ACKNOWLEDGEMENTS

Work in the authors' laboratory is supported by the Wellcome Trust.

REFERENCES

Bolton, T.B., Lang, R.J. & Takewaki, T. (1984). Mechanisms of action of noradrenaline and carbachol on smooth muscle of guinea-pig anterior mesenteric artery. *J. Physiol.* **351**, 549–572.

Brayden, J.E. (1990). Membrane hyperpolarization is a mechanism of endothelium-dependent cerebral vasodilation. *Am. J. Physiol.* **259**, H668–H673.

Chen, G., Suzuki, H. & Weston, A.H. (1988). Acetylcholine releases endothelium-derived hyperpolarizing factor and EDRF from rat blood vessels. *Br. J. Pharmacol.* **95**, 1165–1174.

Chen, G., Yamamoto, Y., Miwa, K. & Suzuki, H. (1991). Hyperpolarization of arterial smooth muscle induced by endothelial humoral substances. *Am. J. Physiol.* **260**, H1888–H1892.

Feletou, M. & Vanhoutte, P.M. (1988). Endothelium-dependent hyperpolarization of canine coronary artery smooth muscle. *Br. J. Pharmacol.* **93**, 515–524.

Garland, C.J. (1987). The role of membrane depolarization in the contractile response of the rabbit basilar artery to 5-hydroxytryptamine. *J. Physiol.* **392**, 333–348.

Garland, C.J., Plane, F., Kemp, B.K. & Cocks, T.M. (1995). Endothelium-dependent hyperpolarization: a role in the control of vascular tone. *Trends Pharm. Sci.* **16**, 23–30.

Moncada, S., Palmer, R.M.J. & Higgs, E.A. (1991). Nitric oxide: physiology, pathophysiology and pharmacology. *Pharmacol. Rev.* **43**, 109–142.

Nagao, T. & Vanhoutte, P.M. (1992). Hyperpolarization as a mechanism for endothelium-dependent relaxations in the porcine coronary artery. *J. Physiol.* **445**, 355–367.

Nagao, T. Illiano, S. & Vanhoutte, P.M. (1992). Heterogeneous distribution of endothelium-dependent relaxations resistant to N^G-nitro-L-arginine in rats. *Am. J. Physiol.* **263**, H1090–H1094.

Nilsson, H., Jensen, P.E. & Mulvany, M.J. (1994). Minor role for direct adrenoceptor-mediated calcium entry in rat mesenteric small arteries. *J. Vasc. Res.* **31**, 314–321.

Parkington, H.C., Tare, M., Tonta, M.A. & Colman, H.A., (1993). Stretch revealed three components in the hyperpolarization of guinea-pig coronary artery in response to acetylcholine. *J. Physiol.* **465**, 459–476.

Tare, M., Parkington, H.C., Coleman, H.A., Neild, T.O. & Dusting, G.J. (1990). Hyperpolarization and relaxation of arterial smooth muscle caused by nitric oxide derived from the endothelium. *Nature* **346**, 69–71.

Taylor, S.G. & Weston, A.H. (1988). Endothelium-derived hyperpolarizing factor: a new endogenous inhibitor from the vascular endothelium. *Trends Pharm. Sci.* **9**, 272–274.

Taylor, S.G., Southerton, G.S., Weston, A.H. & Baker, J.R.J. (1988). Endothelium-dependent effects of acetylcholine in rat aorta: a comparison with sodium nitroprusside and cromakalim. *Br. J. Pharmacol.* **94**, 853–863.

Van de Voorde, J., Vanheel, B. & Leusen, I. (1992). Endothelium-dependent relaxation and hyperpolarization in aorta from control and renal hypertensive rats. *Circ. Res.* **70**, 1–8.

Waldron, G.J. & Garland, C.J. (1994). Contribution of both nitric oxide and a change in membrane potential to acetylcholine-induced relaxation in the rat small mesenteric artery. *Br. J. Pharmacol.* **112**, 831–836.

Weston, A.H., Taylor, S.G., Southerton, J.S., Bray, K.M., Newgreen, D.T. & Mcharg, A.D. (1988). Potassium channel-opening drugs in smooth muscle. In *Vascular Neuroeffector Mechanisms* (Bevan, J.A., Majewski, H., Maxwell, R.A. & Storey, D.F., eds), pp.193–200. IRL Press, Washington DC.

42

Vasodilatation Induced by Endothelium-derived Hyperpolarizing Factor

HIKARU SUZUKI
YOSHIMICHI YAMAMOTO
HIKARU HASHITANI

Department of Physiology,
Nagoya City University Medical School,
Nagoya, Japan

INTRODUCTION

Vasodilatation produced by many types of physiological stimuli is mediated by direct and indirect actions, and the latter involves endothelial products such as endothelium-derived relaxing factor (EDRF), hyperpolarizing factor (EDHF) and prostacyclin (Furchgott, 1983; Vanhoutte *et al.*, 1986; Rubanyi, 1991). EDRF is probably nitric oxide (NO) or a related nitro-containing substance metabolized from L-arginine through activation of NO-synthase (Moncada *et al.*, 1991). The production of cyclic GMP in smooth muscle cells accompanies the vasodilatation produced by EDRF; and nitro-containing substances such as sodium nitroprusside (SNP) or nitroglycerine have a similar action (Ignarro & Kadowitz, 1987). One of the important roles of endothelium-derived prostacyclin (PGI_2) in the physiology of blood circulation is to inhibit adhesion of blood cells or platelets to the vascular wall, and so avoid coagulation of the blood. However, this prostanoid also has stimulatory actions on adenylate cyclase in vascular smooth muscles, thus inducing vasodilatation by increased production of cyclic AMP (Moncada *et al.*, 1991).

Electrical responses of vascular smooth muscle in response to EDRF are estimated by using chemicals that inhibit the actions or the production of EDRF, but the results are equivocal. Inhibition of the actions of EDRF either inhibits the ACh-induced hyperpolarization (Tare *et al.*, 1990) or it does not change the membrane responses to ACh (Chen *et al.*, 1988, 1991; Chen & Suzuki, 1989). Inhibition of the production of EDRF by L-arginine analogues such as nitroarginine or nitro-L-arginine methylester either inhibits the ACh-induced hyperpolarization (Tare *et al.*, 1990; Parkington *et al.*, 1993), or produces no change in the membrane responses to ACh in vascular smooth muscle (Chen *et al.*, 1991; Suzuki *et al.*, 1993; Zhang *et al.*, 1994). Exogenously applied NO does not hyperpolarize the membrane (Beny & Brunet, 1988; Komori *et al.*, 1990; Garland *et al.*, 1995), and therefore it remains uncertain whether the inhibition by nitroarginine of the ACh-induced hyperpolarization is solely due to the reduced production of EDRF. PGI$_2$ hyperpolarizes the membrane of arterial smooth muscle, possibly by activating K$^+$-channels (Siegel *et al.*, 1990), and the ACh-induced hyperpolarization involves a component which can be inhibited by an inhibitor of cyclooxygenase, such as indomethacin (Parkington *et al.*, 1993). However, exogenously applied cyclic AMP produces a relaxation of muscles precontracted with either noradrenaline (NAd) or high-K solution (Itoh *et al.*, 1985), and therefore membrane potential-dependent and independent mechanisms may be involved in the vasodilatation produced by PGI$_2$.

The possible involvement of a hyperpolarizing factor from the endothelium has been suggested in several arteries (Bolton *et al.*, 1984; Komori and Suzuki, 1987; Kauser *et al.*, 1989), and the existence of a hyperpolarizing factor (EDHF) which is different from EDRF or PGI$_2$ is strongly suggested from the actions of inhibitors of these factors on the ACh-induced hyperpolarization in vascular smooth muscles, i.e., the dissociation of the electrical and mechanical responses produced by ACh appears in the presence of inhibitors of the actions of EDRF (Chen *et al.*, 1988; Huang *et al.*, 1988; Chen & Suzuki, 1989; Suzuki & Chen, 1990). However, the chemical nature of EDHF is uncertain, and the factor is not bioassayable (Kauser & Rubanyi, 1992). Recently, possible involvement of metabolites of arachidonic acid produced through epoxygenase pathways, such as epoxyeicosatrienoic acids (EETs), in the endothelium-dependent hyperpolarization is suggested from the inhibitory actions of the ACh-induced relaxation by an inhibitor of the enzyme cytochrome P450 (Hecker *et al.*, 1994). The physiological role of EDHF also remains obscure, and one of its actions on vascular smooth muscle may be the hyperpolarization-mediated inhibition of contraction.

PROPERTIES OF EDHF-INDUCED HYPERPOLARIZATION

The possible existence of endothelium-derived diffusible factors which hyperpolarize the membrane of vascular smooth muscle is suggested from two types of cascade experiment. In smooth muscle of the rat carotid artery, ACh hyperpolarized the membrane in an endothelium-denuded preparation when an intact segment of the artery was connected upstream of the recording vessel (Kauser et al., 1989). In experiments using the sandwich preparation (Chen et al., 1991), an endothelium-intact carotid artery was covered with an endothelium-denuded coronary arterial strip, so as to sandwich a single layer of carotid arterial endothelial cells between two smooth muscle layers. Membrane potentials recorded from the overlaying coronary smooth muscle cells by intracellular microelectrode revealed that application of ACh hyperpolarized the membrane of the endothelium-denuded coronary artery smooth muscles, possibly by a diffusible substance released from the endothelium. In the latter experiments, the observation that the ACh-induced hyperpolarization was not inhibited by nitroarginine or indomethacin indicated significant difference of EDHF from EDRF or PGI_2.

The hyperpolarization produced by EDHF is probably results from an increase in K^+ conductance of the smooth muscle membrane from the following evidence; (1) the amplitude of electrotonic potentials produced by extracellular stimulating electrodes is smaller during the endothelium-dependent hyperpolarization (Bolton et al., 1984; Komori & Suzuki, 1987); (2) the amplitude of the endothelium-dependent hyperpolarization is inversely related to the concentration of $[K^+]_o$ (Chen & Suzuki, 1989; Kauser et al., 1989); and (3) the accelerated efflux of incorporated ^{86}Rb from vascular smooth muscle tissues brought about by ACh is endothelium-dependent, and is not inhibited by oxyhaemoglobin, methylene blue or indomethacin (Chen et al., 1988); (4) inhibition by tetrabutylammonium (TBA), a non-selective K^+-channel blocker, of the ACh-induced hyperpolarization (Nagao & Vanhoutte, 1992) also indicates that the EDHF-induced hyperpolarization is indeed produced by activation of K^+-channels.

Many types of K^+-channels are reportedly distributed in the vascular smooth muscle membrane (Cook, 1988), and attempts made to determine the type of K^+-channel using several kinds of K^+-channel blockers have given equivocal results. Inhibition by glibenclamide of the ACh-induced hyperpolarization in the rabbit cerebral artery suggests a contribution of ATP-sensitive K^+-channels in the EDHF-induced hyperpolarization (Standen et al., 1989; Brayden, 1990). However, the inhibitory actions of glibenclamide on endothelium-dependent hyperpolarization are not found in other muscular arteries (Suzuki & Chen, 1990; Chen et al., 1991; Nagao & Vanhoutte, 1992; Garland et al., 1995).

In many cases, the ACh-induced hyperpolarization is transient, and contrasts with the sustained release of EDRF (Suzuki & Chen, 1990). The transient nature of the ACh-induced hyperpolarization is not due to the shortage of releasable EDHF in endothelial cells or reduced sensitivity of the smooth muscle membrane to EDHF (Chen & Suzuki, 1989). In the guinea-pig carotid artery, the hyperpolarizations produced by ACh are sustained while those by substance P are transient; the difference between these two agonists is considered to be related to the desensitization of endothelial receptors to the agonists (Zhang et al., 1994).

EDHF AND VASODILATATION

Possible involvement of membrane hyperpolarization in the endothelium-dependent relaxation is suggested from the effects of inhibitors of the actions of EDRF on the ACh-induced relaxation in muscles contracted with noradrenaline. In the aortic segment of the rat precontracted with NAd, ACh produced an endothelium-dependent relaxation, and the amplitude of the relaxation was reduced, but did not disappear, after inhibition of the actions of EDRF by oxyhaemoglobin or methylene blue (Chen et al., 1988; Chen & Suzuki, 1989). In muscles contracted with high-K^+ solutions, the endothelium-dependent relaxation can be blocked by inhibitors of the actions of EDRF (Suzuki & Chen, 1990). Thus, there is a possible contribution of hyperpolarization to the endothelium-dependent relaxation (Suzuki & Chen, 1990). These observations contrast with those observed in the rabbit aorta in which EDRF-inhibitors could block all but completely the ACh-induced relaxation (Furchgott & Zawadzki, 1980; Furchgott, 1983). Because the production of cyclic GMP is not increased by ACh in the presence of these inhibitors (Chen et al., 1988), the components of the relaxation insensitive to the EDRF-inhibitors are also considered to have a causal relation to the membrane hyperpolarization (Chen & Suzuki, 1989). The amplitude of the ACh-induced relaxation is small in muscles contracted with high-K^+ solution, possibly because when the endothelial membrane is depolarized (Laskey et al., 1989; Schilling, 1989) the potassium equilibrium potential and the membrane potential are close, so that increasing the potassium permeability of the membrane does not hyperpolarize it significantly: thus, there is no change in the number of open voltage-dependent Ca^{2+}-channels in the membrane and no change in Ca^{2+} influx into the cell (Schilling & Elliot, 1992). It is interesting that high-K^+ solution does not modify the resting and transient phases of the agonist-induced rise in endothelial $[Ca^{2+}]_i$ (Schilling & Elliot, 1992). Release of Ca^{2+} from endothelial store sites by agonists was accompanied by increased production of inositol trisphosphate, and therefore voltage-independent production of the second messenger in the endothelial cells contrasts with that of vascular smooth muscle in which the agonist-induced production of second messenger is voltage-sensitive (Itoh et al., 1992). Absence of membrane hyperpolarization of smooth muscle in high-K^+ solution may also be one of the factors reducing the amplitude of endothelium-dependent relaxation (Suzuki et al., 1989).

The components of the EDHF-induced relaxation involved in the endothelium-dependent relaxation could be estimated using inhibitors of the production of EDRF and PGI_2. In the guinea-pig carotid artery contracted with NAd, ACh produces a sustained relaxation, which is converted to a transient form with reduced amplitude after inhibiting production of EDRF by nitroarginine. The nitroarginine-resistant relaxation is not inhibited by indomethacin, and does not appear in muscles contracted with high-K^+ solution (Suzuki et al., 1993). Comparison between the nitroarginine-sensitive and insensitive components of the relaxation indicates that, in this artery, about 70–80% of the ACh-induced relaxation is produced by EDRF, and the remainder by EDHF (Suzuki et al., 1993). However, in the same artery, the relaxation produced by substance P (SP) is largely resistant to nitroarginine in muscles contracted with NAd, but is sensitive to this arginine analogue in muscles contracted with high-K^+ solution (Zhang et al., 1994). Therefore, SP releases both EDRF and EDHF in the guinea-pig carotid artery, and the latter is the main factor producing the endothelium-dependent relaxation.

In general, many types of agonists release both EDRF and EDHF, and the contribution of these factors to endothelium-dependent relaxation differs between vascular beds. ACh-induced relaxation or vasodilatation is more resistant to nitroarginine or related arginine analogues in peripheral vessels than in conducting arteries such as aorta or carotid artery (Garland et al., 1995); therefore EDHF is important for vasodilatation of small arteries.

Thus, it is clear that EDHF-induced hyperpolarization is one of the important factors in endothelium-dependent relaxation. However, the cellular mechanisms related to the hyperpolarization-induced vasodilatation remain obscure. The voltage-sensitive Ca^{2+}-channels in vascular smooth muscle are active at resting potential level. The membrane hyperpolarization has been calculated to reduce the amount of the Ca^{2+} influx from the extracellular fluids, and thus induce relaxation (Nelson et al., 1990). Generally, experiments have been carried out where tension has been raised by agonists such as NAd to facilitate observation of the endothelium-dependent relaxation. NAd contracts vascular smooth muscle by either pharmaco-mechanical or electro-mechanical coupling mechanisms (Kuriyama et al., 1982), and therefore the second messenger systems involved in the former mechanism may also be modulated by hyperpolarization, as in the case of the hyperpolarization produced by K^+-channel openers (Itoh et al., 1992). Further evidence for the inhibitory effects of membrane hyperpolarization on ion channels coupled to the NAd receptor is that the depolarizing actions of NAd are greatly reduced during hyperpolarization brought about by a K^+-channel opener (Itoh et al., 1994). Potential-dependency of the sensitivity of the contractile protein to Ca^{2+} has also been implicated in EDHF-induced vasodilatation, and hyperpolarization produced by K^+-channel openers is reported to reduce the Ca^{2+} sensitivity of vascular smooth muscle (Okada *et al.*, 1993).

The effects of EDHF on arterial $[Ca^{2+}]_i$ can be estimated using cultured arterial and endothelial cells (Fukuta *et al.*, 1994); stimulation of these cells with bradykinin elevates $[Ca^{2+}]_i$, which will cause contraction in the smooth muscles and elevated release of EDHF in the endothelial cells. Experiments using fura-2 reveal that in aortic smooth muscle cells, bradykinin elevates $[Ca^{2+}]_i$ with two components: an initial transient phase is followed by a sustained phase. The former component remains while the latter component disappears in the absence of $[Ca^{2+}]_o$. EDHF derived from the cultured endothelial cells by bradykinin reduces the fluorescence intensity of the sustained phase, i.e. EDHF can reduce $[Ca^{2+}]_i$ in vascular smooth muscles, possibly by reducing the influx of Ca^{2+}.

SUMMARY

Endothelial cells release a hyperpolarizing factor (EDHF) in response to many types of physiologically active substances, and this factor activates K^+-channels in vascular smooth muscles to hyperpolarize the membrane. Hyperpolarization of the membrane causes the vasodilatation, and thus EDHF is one of the factors involved in the endothelium-dependent relaxation.

REFERENCES

Beny, J.L. & Brunet, P.C. (1988). Neither nitric oxide nor nitroglycerine accounts for all the characteristics of endothelium-mediated vasodilation of pig coronary arteries. *Blood Vessels* **25**, 308–311.

Bolton, T.B., Lang, R.J. & Takewaki, T. (1984) Mechanism of action of noradrenaline and carbachol on smooth muscle of guinea-pig anterior mesenteric artery. *J. Physiol.* **351**, 549–572.

Brayden, J.E. (1990). Membrane hyperpolarization is a mechanism of endothelium-dependent cerebral vasodilation. *Am. J. Physiol.* **259**, H668–H675.

Chen, G. & Suzuki, H. (1989). Some electrical responses of the endothelium-dependent hyperpolarization in arterial smooth muscle cells of the rat. *J.Physiol.* 410, 91–106.

Chen, G., Suzuki, H. & Weston, A.H. (1988). Acetylcholine releases endothelium-derived hyperpolarizing factor and EDRF from rat blood vessels. *Br. J. Pharmacol.* **95**, 1165–1174.

Chen, G., Yamamoto, Y. Miwa, K. & Suzuki, H. (1991). Hyperpolarization of arterial smooth muscle induced by endothelial humoral substances. *Am. J. Physiol.* **260**, H1888–H1892.

Cook, N.S. (1988). The pharmacology of potassium channels and their therapeutic potential. *Trends Pharmacol. Sci.* **9**, 21–28.

Fukuta, H., Miwa, K., Yamamoto, Y. & Suzuki, H. (1994). Modulation of intracellular Ca ion concentrations in the guinea-pig aortic smooth muscles by hyperpolarizing factors derived from cultured bovine aortic endothelial cells. *Jpn. J. Physiol.* **44** (Suppl.), S138.

Furchgott, R.F. (1983). Role of endothelium in responses of vascular smooth muscle. *Circ Res.* **53**, 557–573.

Furchgott, R.F. & Zawadzki, J.V. (1980). The obligatory role of endothelial cells in the relaxation of arterial smooth muscle by acetylcholine. *Nature* **286**, 373–376.

Garland, C.J. & McPherson, G.A. (1992). Evidence that nitric oxide does not mediate the hyperpolarization and relaxation to acetylcholine in the rat small mesenteric artery. *Br. J. Pharmacol.* **105**, 429–435.

Garland, C.J., Plane, F., Kamp, B.K. & Cocks, T.M. (1995). Endothelium-dependent hyperpolarization: a role in the control of vascular tone. *Trends Pharmacol. Sci.* **16**, 23–30.

Huang, A.H., Busse, R. & Bassenge, E. (1988). Endothelium-dependent hyperpolarization of arterial smooth muscle is not mediated by EDRF. *Naunyn-Schmiedeberg's Arch. Pharmacol.* **338**, 438–442.

Hecker, M., Bara, A.T., Bauersachs, J. & Busse, R. (1994). Characterization of endothelium-derived hyperpolarizing factor as a cytochrome P450-derived arachidonic acid metabolite in mammals. *J. Physiol.* **481**, 407–414.

Ignarro, L.J. & Kadowitz, P.J. (1987) The pharmacological and physiological role of cyclic GMP in vascular smooth muscle relaxation. *Annu. Rev. Pharmacol. Toxicol.* **25**, 171–191.

Itoh, T., Kanmura, Y., Kuriyama, H. & Sasaguri, T. (1985). Nitroglycerine- and isoprenaline-induced vasodilation: assessment from the actions of cyclic nucleotides. *Br. J. Pharmacol.* **84**, 393–406.

Itoh, T., Seki, N., Suzuki, S., Ito, S., Kajikuri, J. & Kuriyama, H. (1992). Membrane hyperpolarization inhibits agonist-induced synthesis of inositol 1,4,5-trisphosphate in rabbit mesenteric artery. *J. Physiol.* **451**, 307–328.

Itoh, T., Ito, S., Shafiq, J. & Suzuki, H. (1994). Effects of a newly synthesized K$^+$-channel opener, Y-26763, on noradrenaline-induced Ca^{2+} mobilization in smooth muscle of the rabbit mesenteric artery. *Br. J. Pharmacol.* **111**, 165–172.

Kauser, K. & Rubanyi, G.M. (1992). Bradykinin-induced, nitro-L-arginine-insensitive endothelium-dependent relaxation of porcine coronary artery is not mediated by bioassayable substances. *J. Cardiovasc. Pharmacol.* **20** (Suppl. 12), S101–104.

Kauser, K., Stekiel, W.J., Rubanyi, G.M. & Harder, D.R. (1989). Mechanism of action of EDRF on pressurized arteries: effect on K$^+$ conductance. *Circ. Res.* **65**, 199–204.

Komori, K. & Suzuki, H. (1987). Electrical responses of smooth muscle cells during cholinergic vasodilation in the rabbit saphenous artery. *Circ. Res.* **61**, 586–593.

Komori, K., Lorenz, R.R. & Vanhoutte, P.M. (1990). Nitric oxide, ACh, and electrical and mechanical properties of canine arterial smooth muscle. *Am. J. Physiol.* **255**, H207–H212.

Kuriyama, H., Ito, Y., Suzuki, H., Kitamura, K. & Itoh, T. (1982). Factors modifying contraction-relaxation cycle in vascular smooth muscles. *Am. J.Physiol.* **243**, H641–H662.

Laskey, R.E., Adams, D.J., Johns, A., Rubanyi, G.M. & Van Breemen, C. (1989). Regulation of [Ca^{2+}]$_i$ in endothelial cells by membrane potential. In *Endothelium-Derived Relaxing Factors* (G.M. Rubanyi & P.M. Vanhoutte eds), pp.128–135. Karger, Basel.

Moncada, S., Palmer, R.M.J. & Higgs, E.A. (1991). Nitric oxide: physiology, pathophysiology and pharmacology. *Pharmacol. Rev.* **43**, 109–142.

Nagao, T. & Vanhoutte, P.M. (1992). Hyperpolarization as a mechanism for endothelium-derived relaxations in the porcine coronary artery. *J. Physiol.* **445**, 355–367.

Nelson, M.T., Patlak, J.B., Worley, J.F. & Standen, N.B. (1990). Calcium channels, potassium channels, and voltage dependence of arterial smooth muscle tone. *Am. J. Physiol.* **259**, C3–C18.

Okada, Y., Yanagisawa, T. & Taira, N. (1993). BRL 38227 (levcromakalim)-induced hyperpolarization reduces the sensitivity to Ca^{2+} of contractile elements in canine coronary artery. Naunyn-Schmiedeberg's *Arch. Pharmacol.* **347**, 438–444.

Parkington, H.C., Tare, M., Tonta, M.A. & Coleman, H.A. (1993) Stretch revealed three components in the hyperpolarization of guinea-pig coronary artery in response to acetylcholine. *J. Physiol.* **465**, 459–476.

Rubanyi, G.M. (1991). *'Cardiovascular Significance of Endothelium-Derived Vasoactive Factors'*. Futura Publishing, Mount Kisco, NY.

Schilling, W.P. (1989). Effect of membrane potential on cytosolic calcium of bovine aortic endothelial cells. *Am. J. Physiol.* **257**, H778–H784.

Schlling, W.P. & Elliott, S.J. (1992). Ca^{2+} signalling mechanisms of vascular endothelial cells and their role in oxidant-induced endothelial cell dysfunction. *Am. J. Physiol.* **262**, H1617–H1630.

Siegel, G., Wenzel, K., Schnalke, F., Mironneau, J., Schultz, G., Schroder, G., Schillinger, E., Grauhan, O. & Hetzer, R. (1990). Prostacyclin analogous as K^{+} channel openers. *Clin. Pharmacol.* **7**, 72–96.

Standen, N.B., Quayle, J.M., Davies, N.W., Brayden, J.E., Huang, Y. & Nelson, M.T. (1989). Hyperpolarizing vasodilators activate ATP-sensitive K^{+}-channels in arterial smooth muscle. *Science* **245**, 177–180.

Suzuki, H. & Chen, G. (1990). Endothelium-derived hyperpolarizing factor (EDHF): an endogenous potassium-channel activator. *News Physiol. Sci.* **5**, 212–215.

Suzuki, H., Chen, G. & Hashitani, H. (1989). Electrophysiological properties of acetylcholine-induced hyperpolarization in arterial smooth muscles. In *Endothelium-Derived Relaxing Factors* (Rubanyi, G.M. & Vanhoutte, P.M., eds), pp. 166–173. Karger, Basel.

Suzuki, H., Chen, G., Yamamoto, Y. & Miwa, K. (1993). Nitroarginine-sensitive and insensitive components of the endothelium-dependent relaxation in the guinea-pig carotid artery. *Jpn. J. Physiol.* **42**, 335–347.

Tare, M., Parkington, H.C., Coleman, H.A., Neild, T.O. & Dusting, G.J. (1990). Hyperpolarization and relaxation of arterial smooth muscle caused by nitric oxide derived from the endothelium. *Nature* **346**, 69–71.

Vanhoutte, P.M., Rubanyi, G.M., Miller, V.M. & Houston, D.S. (1986). Modulation of vascular smooth muscle contraction by the endothelium. *Annu. Rev. Pharmacol. Toxicol.* **48**, 307–320.

Zhang, G., Yamamoto, Y., Miwa, K. & Suzuki, H. (1994). Vasodilation induced by substance P in guinea-pig carotid arteries. *Am. J. Physiol.* **266**, H1132–H1137.

Index

Tables and figures in *italic* type.